Research and Practices in Child Maltreatment Prevention

Volume 1 of 2

Definitions of Abuse and Prevention

STM **Learning,** Inc.

Leading Publisher of Scientific, Technical, and Medical Educational Resources
Saint Louis
www.stmlearning.com

Our Mission

To become the world leader in publishing and information services on child abuse, maltreatment, diseases, and domestic violence. We seek to heighten awareness of these issues, and provide relevant information to professionals and consumers.

A portion of our profits is contributed to nonprofit organizations dedicated to the prevention of child abuse and the care of victims of abuse and other children and family charities.

Research and Practices in Child Maltreatment Prevention

Volume 1 of 2

Definitions of Abuse and Prevention

Randell Alexander, MD, PhD
Professor and Chief
Division of Child Protection and Forensic Pediatrics
Department of Pediatrics
Program Director
Pediatric Child Abuse Fellowship
University of Florida College of Medicine—Jacksonville
Director, Institute for Child Abuse Prevention
Wolfson Children's Hospital
Jacksonville, Florida

STM **Learning,** Inc.

Leading Publisher of Scientific, Technical, and Medical Educational Resources
Saint Louis
www.stmlearning.com

Publishers: Glenn E. Whaley and Marianne V. Whaley
Graphic Design Director: Glenn E. Whaley
Managing Editor: Paul K. Goode, III
Print/Production Coordinator: Jennifer M. Jones and G.W. Graphics
Cover Design: Jennifer M. Jones and G.W. Graphics
Acquisitions Editor: Glenn E. Whaley
Developmental Editors: Paul K. Goode, III
Copy Editors: Paul K. Goode, III and Lauren Plummer
Proofreaders: Paul K. Goode, III and Emily A. Ploch

Printed in the United States of America.

Publisher:
STM Learning, Inc.
Saint Louis, Missouri
Phone: (314) 434-2424
http://www.stmlearning.com orders@stmlearning.com

Library of Congress Cataloging-in-Publication Data

Names: Alexander, Randell, 1950- editor.
Title: Research and practices in child maltreatment prevention / [edited by] Randell Alexander.
Description: Florissant, MO : STM Learning, Inc., [2017] | Includes bibliographical references and indexes. Contents: volume 1. Definitions of abuse and prevention -- volume 2. Societal, organizational, and international approaches.
Identifiers: LCCN 2016055589 (print) | LCCN 2016056946 (ebook) | ISBN 9781878060396 (pbk. : v. 1 : alk. paper) | ISBN 9781878060839 (pbk. : v. 2 : alk. paper) | ISBN 9781936590469 (ebook : v. 1) | ISBN 9781936590384 (ebook : v. 2)
Subjects: | MESH: Child Abuse--prevention & control | Risk Factors
Classification: LCC RC569.5.C55 (print) | LCC RC569.5.C55 (ebook) | NLM WA 325 | DDC 362.76--dc23
LC record available at https://lccn.loc.gov/2016055589

Contributors

Randell Alexander, MD, PhD
Professor and Chief
Division of Child Protection and Forensic Pediatrics
Department of Pediatrics
Program Director
Pediatric Child Abuse Fellowship
University of Florida College of Medicine—Jacksonville
Director, Institute for Child Abuse Prevention
Wolfson Children's Hospital
Jacksonville, Florida

Sandra Alexander, MEd
Prevention Consultant
Division of Violence Prevention
Centers for Disease Control and Prevention
Atlanta, Georgia

Marla R. Brassard, PhD
Associate Professor of Psychology and Education
Teachers College
Columbia University
New York, New York

Melissa L. Brodowski, PhD, MSW, MPH
Child Welfare Program Specialist
Children's Bureau
Administration on Children, Youth and Families
Administration for Children and Families
US Department of Health and Human Services
Washington, DC

Alexandria R. Chambers, MPH
Research Assistant
Department of Health Policy and Management
University of Georgia College of Public Health
Athens, Georgia

Anne Cohn Donnelly, DPH, MPH
Senior Lecturer in Social Enterprise
Center for Nonprofit Management
Kellogg School of Management
Northwestern University
Evanston, Illinois

Phaedra Corso, PhD, MPA
Professor
Human Health
University of Georgia College of Public Health
Athens, Georgia

Jacqueline M. Counts, PhD, MSW
Associate Director
Programs and External Relations
University of Kansas
Lawrence, Kansas

Deborah Daro, PhD
Senior Research Fellow
Chapin Hall
University of Chicago
Chicago, Illinois

Diane DePanfilis, PhD, MSW
Professor
University of Maryland School of Social Work
Baltimore, Maryland

John Donovan, MPH
Health Education Specialist
Centers for Disease Control and Prevention
Atlanta, Georgia

Howard Dubowitz, MD, MS
Chief
Division of Child Protection
Department of Pediatrics
Co-Director
Center for Families
University of Maryland School of Medicine
Baltimore, Maryland

Jeffrey L. Edleson, PhD
Professor
School of Social Work
University of Minnesota
Saint Paul, Minnesota

Debra Esernio-Jenssen, MD
Medical Director
Child Protection Team
University of Florida at Gainesville
Gainesville, Florida

Corinne M. Graffunder, DrPH, MPH
Chief
Program Implementation and Dissemination Branch
Centers for Disease Control and Prevention
Atlanta, Georgia

Jordan Greenbaum, MD
Medical Director
Child Protection Center
Children's Healthcare of Atlanta
Atlanta, Georgia

Neil Guterman, PhD
Dean
University of Chicago School of Social Service Administration
Chicago, Illinois

Patricia Y. Hashima, PhD
Senior Public Health Service Fellow
Research, Synthesis, and Application Team
Program Implementation and Dissemination Branch
Division of Violence Prevention
Centers for Disease Control and Prevention
Atlanta, Georgia

Caroline J. Kistin, MD
Division of General Pediatrics
Boston University School of Medicine
Boston, Massachusetts

Joanne Klevens, MD, MPH, PhD
Epidemiologist
Sexual Violence and Child Maltreatment Team
Research and Evaluation Branch
Division of Violence Prevention
Centers for Disease Control and Prevention
Atlanta, Georgia

Rebecca T. Leeb, PhD
Epidemiologist
Etiology and Surveillance Branch
Division of Violence Prevention
Centers for Disease Control and Prevention
Atlanta, Georgia

Lisa R. Melmed, PhD
School Psychologist
Greenwich Public Schools
Greenwich, Connecticut

Jim Mercy, PhD
Director
Division of Violence Prevention
Centers for Disease Control and Prevention
Adjunct Associate Professor
Department of Sociology
Emory University
Adjunct Professor
Institute of Public Health
College of Health and Human Sciences
Georgia State University
Atlanta, Georgia

Marilyn Metzler, RN, MPH
Senior Analyst
Health Equity
Centers for Disease Control and Prevention
Atlanta, Georgia

Cindy Miller-Perrin, PhD
Professor of Psychology
Pepperdine University
Malibu, California

Rita Noonan, PhD
Associate Director for Program Development and Integration
National Center for Injury Prevention and Control
Centers for Disease Control and Prevention
Atlanta, Georgia

Beverly A. Parsons, PhD
Executive Director
InSites: A Support Network for Educational Change
Fort Collins, Colorado

Richard W. Puddy, PhD, MPH
Behavioral Scientist
Research Synthesis and Application Team
Program Implementation and Dissemination Branch
Division of Violence Prevention
National Center for Injury Prevention and Control
Centers for Disease Control and Prevention
Atlanta, Georgia

Janet Saul, PhD
Branch Chief
Prevention Development and Evaluation Branch
Division of Violence Prevention
National Center for Injury Prevention and Control
Centers for Disease Control and Prevention
Atlanta, Georgia

Robert Sege, MD, PhD
Division of General Pediatrics
Boston University School of Medicine
Boston, Massachusetts

Lynn Sheets, MD, FAAP
Medical Director and Professor
Child Advocacy and Protection
Children's Hospital of Wisconsin and Medical College of Wisconsin
Milwaukee, Wisconsin

Helen Singer, MPH
Research Analyst
Division of Violence Prevention
National Center for Injury Prevention and Control
Centers for Disease Control and Prevention
Atlanta, Georgia

Nathaniel H. Taylor, MPH
Research Analyst
University of Georgia College of Public Health
Athens, Georgia

Sally Thigpen, MPA
Public Health Analyst
Business Computer Applications
Centers for Disease Control and Prevention
Atlanta, Georgia

Richard M. Tolman, LMSW, PhD
Professor
University of Michigan School of Social Work
Ann Arbor, Michigan

Linda Anne Valle, PhD
Lead Behavioral Scientist
Division of Violence Prevention
Centers for Disease Control and Prevention
Atlanta, Georgia

Vanessa Vorhies Klodnick, LCSW, PhD
Lecturer
University of Chicago School of Social Service Administration
Senior Researcher
Thresholds Research & Evaluation
Chicago, Illinois

Tova B. Walsh, PhD
Assistant Professor
School of Social Work
University of Wisconsin—Madison
Madison, Wisconsin

Natalie J. Wilkins, PhD
Behavioral Scientist
Centers for Disease Control and Prevention
Atlanta, Georgia

Sandy K. Wurtele, PhD
Associate Dean for Community Partnerships & Programs
Professor of Psychology
University of Colorado
Colorado Springs, Colorado

Adam J. Zolotor, MD, MPH
Associate Professor
Department of Family Medicine and Department of Pediatrics
Associate Medical Director
North Carolina Child Medical Evaluation Program
University of North Carolina School of Medicine
Chapel Hill, North Carolina

Foreword

The essence of pediatrics is prevention, beginning with counseling during the prenatal period and continuing with well-baby visits and child care during the years of growth and development of each child. Since Jenner's inoculation of James Phipps in 1796 with the pus from cowpox blisters on the hands of Sarah Nelmes, a milkmaid who had contracted cowpox from a cow called Blossom, to the most recent vaccine for the prevention of the spread of human papilloma virus, immunizations have repeatedly proven the value of prevention. These vaccines have virtually eliminated a host of infectious diseases, such as smallpox, chickenpox, diphtheria, tetanus, whooping cough, polio, measles, mumps, rubella, most forms of bacterial meningitis, hepatitis A and B, influenza, and rotavirus. Other prevention programs, particularly those initiated by the Council on Injury, Violence and Poison Prevention of the American Academy of Pediatrics, have reduced the incidence of serious injuries and deaths in childhood by their prevention strategies. Educational programs and promotion of the use of condoms to prevent the spread of HIV has reduced the scourge of HIV/AIDS all over the world.

Now comes the first comprehensive book on the prevention of child maltreatment. A vaccine against this cause of morbidity and mortality in children and young adults is devoutly to be wished, but this would be too simple, since the etiologies for these harms to children are multiple and are not amenable to monovalent solutions. The reasons for child maltreatment are woven into the fabric of our society, our collective consciousness, our own medical and psychosocial histories, and belief systems that have deep roots in our earliest days as a species. Understanding the origins of this historical problem is challenging, but it is essential to prevention.

Prevention programs should meet certain criteria: measurability of results, ease of accessibility and understandability for clients, broad goals, sufficient control of variables, service provision for a reasonable period of time, adaptability to diverse populations, and provision of continuing education to providers. This book will help to guide the design and implementation of prevention programs dedicated to reducing the number of children affected by child abuse and neglect. It is a welcome new addition to the literature on violence against children.

Robert M. Reece, MD
Clinical Professor (Ret.)
Department of Pediatrics
Tufts University School of Medicine
Boston, Massachusetts

FOREWORD

Child maltreatment is a significant yet preventable problem. According to the Centers for Disease Control and Prevention, more than 1 in 10 children and youth experienced at least one form of child maltreatment in the past year, and more than 1400 children died from abuse and neglect in the United States in 2013. Globally, a quarter of adults are reported to have been physically abused as children, while 1 in 5 women and 1 in 13 men have been sexually abused as children. The statistics, however, only portray part of the picture of child maltreatment. Apart from the criminal justice, special education, and child welfare costs associated with child maltreatment, there are health care costs not only for the victims as abused children but also when they grow up as adults. There is now a substantive body of knowledge attesting to the long-lasting effects of child maltreatment on victims' health throughout the life span. For example, the Adverse Childhood Experiences (ACEs) Study has clearly demonstrated that children who are abused or neglected are at higher risk for health problems as adults, including alcoholism, smoking, drug use, depression, obesity, eating disorders, high-risk sexual behaviors, and chronic diseases, with cost to the health care system and society. And yet, child maltreatment is preventable and can be stopped before it occurs.

Which strategies and programs to prevent child maltreatment are effective? This is a question that may have been asked many times ever since child maltreatment was brought to the public's attention decades ago. *Research and Practices in Child Maltreatment Prevention* addresses the complexity of child maltreatment and its prevention by examining the complex interplay of individual, family, and environmental factors that may contribute to child maltreatment, thus reinforcing the importance of fostering safe, stable, and nurturing relationships and environments to preventing child abuse and neglect. Whether your interest is in primary, secondary, or tertiary prevention, and whether your focus is on individual interventions or changing societal norms, you will find what you need in this detailed and well-resourced title.

The authors and editor are to be commended for their expertise and excellent contributions to child maltreatment prevention. This book is a valuable resource for those who are committed to preventing child abuse and neglect.

Agnes Tiwari, PhD, RN, FAAN
Professor and Head
School of Nursing
Li Ka Shing Faculty of Medicine
University of Hong Kong

PREFACE

Child abuse in its various forms is miserable, degrading, often repetitive or chronic, emotionally adverse, and a human rights violation. Child abuse is expensive. It leaves scars on the individual and society. Evaluation, intervention, and treatment can never fully repair the damage of child abuse once it has occurred. Thus prevention is the ultimate solution.

When a child is born, many possibilities exist as to what his/her future may be. Genetics, the social environment, and external events may limit some possibilities. But child abuse further restricts life options, whether it is the acute trauma of abuse or the grinding harm of neglect. Prevention is not only about keeping options open, it should be about shaping the brain and body to create the best adult that a child can become.

This book approaches aspects of child abuse prevention in a variety of ways. Most of the prevention in these chapters is primary (before abuse occurs) or universal (strategies to reach out to an entire population). Prevention is not about program improvement—often erroneously cited as "prevention." It is important that at the end of the day, a child is safer because of some improvement, not that some agency program works better. Prevention should be less about "fixing" an environment and more about dynamically shaping the future. As events occur and the world evolves, prevention should be part of that change and be an agent for change. Ultimately, social norms and the policies that reflect them must change. Most people would revolt against the notion of young children working in mines, would put their children in seat belts, and ensure safe water sources for their children. Years ago, these concepts were not universally agreed or adhered to, but times have changed.

Through the wisdom of a diverse team of authors, it is hoped that a deeper understanding of current prevention efforts will be achieved. The range includes programs, non-programmatic efforts, governmental efforts at national and international levels, agencies and concepts, theory, and human change.

Prevention of child abuse has made some successes, but changing human behavior is hard. But in the words of Dr. Seuss, "unless someone like you cares a whole awful lot, nothing is going to get better. It's not." The children depend on you.

Randell Alexander, MD, PhD

Reviews

Research and Practices in Child Maltreatment Prevention *is an in-depth and conceptually rich 2-volume set that reviews the history, present, and potential future of child maltreatment prevention. Prevention should be a top priority for every professional, agency, and institution addressing child maltreatment. Without the unified vision and effort of everyone involved in mitigating the terrible toll of child maltreatment, we risk the perception, and perhaps even the reality, of becoming a child abuse industry, merely processing victims and perpetrators rather than effecting the revolutionary social movement to ensure a better future for children, families, and societies that I, and most of my colleagues, envision.*

With more than 80 contributors representing business, child advocacy, counseling, economics, education, government, law, medicine, psychology, public health, social science, and social work, these 2 volumes are the most current and comprehensive resource addressing child maltreatment prevention. Every private and public agency, educational department, hospital, library, and most professionals involved in the child maltreatment field should have ready access to this information, whether it be on their bookshelves or online. Thanks to Randy Alexander for leading this effort and to all the contributors for their dedication to a brighter tomorrow.

David L. Corwin, MD
Professor and Director of Forensic Services
Pediatrics Department
University of Utah School of Medicine
Board Chair
Academy on Violence and Abuse
Vice-President
American Professional Society on the Abuse of Children
Salt Lake City, Utah

Child abuse and neglect are preventable public health issues. Research and Practices in Child Maltreatment Prevention, Volume 1: Definitions of Abuse and Prevention *outlines the remarkable progress that has been made over the last several decades in understanding how to prevent child abuse and neglect. Leading researchers in the field provide information on the different types of abuse and neglect, prevention programs and their effectiveness, and other nonprogrammatic approaches to child abuse and neglect prevention.*

In particular, Chapter 14, "Nonprogrammatic approaches to Child Maltreatment Prevention" highlights a deliberate shift toward enhancing protective factors at all levels of the social ecology, including the community and societal levels, with a specific focus on changing norms, changing the narrative of the critical importance of early childhood, and assuring the conditions that support safety, security, and nurturance. This chapter reinforces the idea that a broad public health impact on child abuse and neglect prevention will likely require a comprehensive focus that includes attention to social norms, policy, and systems approaches, in addition to individual- and relationship-focused programs.

This text is an important resource for all child abuse and neglect prevention professionals. It will be an excellent resource for those new to prevention and for the seasoned professional who needs an update on the latest research across the different varieties of abuse and neglect.

Beverly L. Fortson, PhD
Behavioral Scientist
Division of Violence Prevention
Centers for Disease Control and Prevention

As the first major textbook dedicated exclusively to research on the prevention of child maltreatment, Research and Practices in Child Maltreatment Prevention, Volume 1 *provides a multidimensional, state-of-the-art perspective from leading experts in the field. This book is highly relevant to professionals from a broad array of disciplines who are committed to preventing various forms of child maltreatment. Chapters cover such critical areas as social determinants of child maltreatment, the role of the CDC in child maltreatment prevention, research designs in prevention, and expanding definitions of evidence in child maltreatment prevention. A particularly interesting chapter addresses nonprogrammatic approaches to child maltreatment prevention. It includes a comprehensive discussion of prevention interventions that go beyond the customary "one-to-one" approaches (eg, home visitation, parenting classes) and provides examples of creative macro-level prevention approaches.*

This book is highly recommended for all professionals who work with children and for policymakers concerned with child welfare. Readers will find this book an invaluable resource that expands visions and perspectives on child maltreatment prevention.

Susan J. Kelley, RN, PhD, FAAN
Associate Dean and Chief Academic Officer for Nursing
Byrdine F. Lewis School of Nursing and Health Professions
Professor
School of Nursing
Georgia State University
Atlanta, Georgia

Research and Practices in Child Maltreatment Prevention, Volume 1: Definitions of Abuse and Prevention *will fill a void in the library of any professional concerned with child welfare. The authors offer a dynamic perspective on the issue, taking into account changes in culture, public policy, the economy, technology, and other issues affecting children and families. So doing, they define the impact these changes can have on parenting, child safety, and service delivery systems. The multidisciplinary nature of child welfare professions is evident in the credentials of the contributing authors and the various conceptual frameworks utilized in defining and analyzing information about various types of maltreatment. Practitioners from any allied profession will find practical resources in this volume. From syntheses of critical research on preventing different types of child maltreatment to calls to action to researchers, practitioners, and policymakers, this volume has the potential to define the agenda and elevate education and practice in maltreatment prevention.*

Janet F. Rosenzweig, MS, PhD, MPA
Executive Director
American Professional Society on the Abuse of Children
Lecturer
University of Pennsylvania
Philadelphia, Pennsylvania

Contents in Brief

CONTENTS IN DETAIL

Research and Practices in

Child Maltreatment Prevention

Volume 1 of 2

Definitions of Abuse and Prevention

STM **Learning,** Inc.

Leading Publisher of Scientific, Technical, and Medical Educational Resources

Saint Louis

www.stmlearning.com

Section I

Introduction

Chapter 1

Etiology and Risk and Protective Factors in the Context of Primary Prevention

Rebecca T. Leeb, PhD

At the heart of child maltreatment prevention efforts lies the origins and causes of child abuse and neglect. Why does abuse and neglect of children by caregivers occur, and continue to occur, despite widespread recognition of the problem and its sequelae? What factors place children at risk? What factors protect children from harm? Child maltreatment is now widely recognized by experts as a public health problem and one that is amenable to public health prevention strategies; however, in order to design effective primary prevention programs and strategies, it is necessary to know as precisely as possible what causes the condition one intends to prevent and what factors influence the likelihood that the condition will occur and perpetuate. Answering questions about the etiology of child maltreatment is critical and provides fundamental information for designing effective prevention strategies and programs that can be widely implemented.

In this chapter a brief overview of a public health-based definition of child maltreatment and definitions of the various types of abuse and neglect is presented. Additionally, the magnitude of the problem and etiology of child maltreatment are discussed. Risk and protective factors for child maltreatment in general, including both factors that buffer against risk and those that protect children from harm independent of risk status, and the specific types of child abuse, ie, physical, sexual, and psychological abuse, and neglect, will be reviewed with respect to the ecological model. Finally, implications for primary prevention will be examined.

The Public Health Framework

Child maltreatment is a substantial problem in the United States with wide-ranging short- and long-term impacts on the health of children and adults. The public health model offers a framework to address public health problems in a coordinated manner.[1] Four distinct steps make up the public health approach and each step is designed to inform the next:

1. Public health surveillance and epidemiology are used to determine the magnitude and impact of the problem.
2. Etiologic research is conducted to identify risk and protective factors that can be modified with prevention programs and policies.
3. Prevention strategies are developed and tested empirically to determine the most effective and efficacious strategies.
4. Empirically supported prevention strategies are broadly disseminated.

All 4 steps of this model are action oriented and aimed at the primary prevention of public health issues. This chapter will focus on the first 2 steps of the model.

Definitions, Magnitude, and Etiology of Child Maltreatment

Before it is possible to identify those factors that may be key to protecting children from harm and developing prevention strategies for child maltreatment, we must agree on what we are trying to prevent. Defining and operationalizing child maltreatment has challenged professionals in the field since Kempe and colleagues first coined the term "battered child syndrome."[2] To date, the multiple sectors addressing this issue, including Child Protective Services (CPS), legal and medical communities, public health officials, researchers, practitioners, and advocates, often use their own definitions, thus limiting communication across disciplines and hampering efforts to identify, assess, track, treat, and prevent child abuse and neglect effectively. All too often, the definition of child maltreatment depends on the context in which it is being used.

To aid in the collection of public health–based data on child maltreatment, the Centers for Disease Control and Prevention embarked on a collaborative effort with professionals in child maltreatment research, prevention, and surveillance from settings including universities, state health departments, hospitals, contracted research firms, and other federal agencies to develop conceptual definitions of child maltreatment and guidelines for their use in public health settings. The definitions are intended to aid state and local health department staff in the collection of public health surveillance data on child maltreatment. Because the definitions were developed through a collaborative effort, they draw heavily upon definitions already in use in other sectors, complement existing definitions, and have been modified to fit the needs of public health professionals whose mission is to prevent child abuse and neglect before it occurs.[3]

Child Maltreatment Defined

The CDC defines child maltreatment as "Any act or series of acts of commission or omission by a parent or other caregiver that results in harm, potential for harm, or threat of harm to a child."[3] In addition to the overall definition, CDC also provides definitions for the individual types of abuse and neglect, ie, physical abuse, including abusive head trauma; sexual abuse; psychological abuse; and 2 forms of neglect: failure to provide and failure to supervise. (**Table 1-1** provides CDC definitions for each type of maltreatment.)

Although the CDC definitions of child abuse and neglect limit perpetrators to parents and caregivers, a parent or caregiver is broadly defined to be inclusive of anyone who is in a permanent or temporary custodial role at the time of the maltreatment incident and who is responsible for the care and control of the child and for the child's overall health and welfare. Perpetrators of child maltreatment are not limited to adults, but in order to differentiate child maltreatment from peer violence, perpetrators must be responsible for the child at the time of the incident. Thus peer bullying and peer-to-peer sexual harassment would not be included as forms of child maltreatment in this public health–based definition. Furthermore CDC definitions require that sexual abuse be perpetrated by a caregiver who is known to the child. Although rape of a child by a stranger is a violent act against a child, it is considered assault rather than abuse and is not included as a form of child maltreatment in the CDC definition of sexual abuse. These exclusions and caveats provide a definition that is broad enough to cast a wide net in determining the number of children who experience maltreatment within the population in order to provide a foundation from which to launch large-scale primary prevention efforts.

Table 1-1. CDC Definitions of Maltreatment Types*

Type of Abuse	Definition‡
Physical abuse	Physical abuse is defined as the intentional use of physical force against a child that results in, or has the potential to result in, physical injury. Physical abuse includes physical acts ranging from those which do not leave a physical mark on the child to physical acts which cause permanent disability, disfigurement, or death. Physical abuse can result from discipline or physical punishment. Physical abuse can include: — Hitting — Kicking — Punching — Beating — Stabbing — Biting — Pushing — Shoving — Throwing — Pulling — Dragging — Dropping — Shaking — Strangling/choking — Smothering — Burning — Scalding — Poisoning *Exceptions* Physical injuries to the anal or genital area or surrounding areas, eg, anal or genital bruising or tearing; internal injuries resulting from penetration by a penis, hand, finger, or other object that occur during attempted or completed sexual abuse; or other physical injuries that result from attempted or completed sexual abuse, eg, bruises due to restraint, hitting, and pushing, are considered sexual abuse and do not constitute physical abuse.
Abusive head trauma	Assault of infants and children (< 5 years of age) resulting in injury to the skull or intracranial contents from impact and/or violent shaking. *Exclusions* — Neglect — Gunshot wounds/ stab wounds/ penetrating trauma
Sexual abuse	Any completed or attempted (noncompleted) sexual act, sexual contact with, or exploitation, ie, noncontact sexual interaction, of a child by a caregiver.
Psychological abuse	Intentional caregiver behavior, ie, act of commission, that conveys to a child that he/she is worthless, flawed, unloved, unwanted, endangered, or valued only in meeting another's needs. Psychological abuse can be continual, ie, chronic and pervasive, or episodic, ie, triggered by a specific context or situation, eg, caregiver substance use/abuse. Psychologically abusive behaviors may include: — Blaming — Belittling — Degrading — Intimidating — Terrorizing — Isolating — Restraining — Confining — Corrupting — Exploiting — Spurning or otherwise behaving in a manner that is harmful, potentially harmful, or insensitive to the child's developmental needs or can potentially damage the child psychologically or emotionally.

(continued)

Table 1-1. CDC Definitions of Maltreatment Types* *(continued)*

Type of Abuse	Definition‡
Neglect	The failure to provide for a child's basic physical, emotional, or educational needs or to protect a child from harm or potential harm.
Failure to provide	Failure by a caregiver to meet a child's basic physical, emotional, medical/dental, or educational needs—or combination thereof.
Failure to supervise	Failure by the caregiver to ensure a child's safety within and outside the home given the child's emotional and developmental needs.

**Adapted from Leeb et al.*[3]
‡For complete definitions, see Leeb et al.[3]

Magnitude of Child Maltreatment

Despite the lack of consensus across the various disciplines that are engaged in the prevention of child maltreatment on definitional issues related to abuse and neglect, it is evident from available statistics that regardless of the definition used the problem of maltreatment is substantial. The Office of Child Abuse and Neglect at the federal Administration for Children and Families estimates that during 2008 an estimated 3.3 million referrals, involving the alleged maltreatment of approximately 6 million children, were referred to CPS agencies throughout the United States. Of these, approximately 63% (1.5 million children) were screened in for investigation or assessment. Of the cases investigated approximately 772 000 children were determined to be victims of abuse or neglect, based on reports to Child Protective Services. In 2008 the rate of victimization for American children was 10.3 per 1000 children in the population.[4]

Calculation of child victimization rates for maltreatment depends on how the definition of maltreatment is operationalized. As mentioned previously, the multiple sectors addressing this issue often use their own definitions, resulting in variations in the number of cases counted as "actual" cases of child maltreatment. Because of the National Child Abuse and Neglect Data System's (NCANDS) reliance on social services data, the statistics provided by the United States Department of Health and Human Services (HHS) reflect only those cases that come to the attention of, and are investigated by, social welfare authorities. The fact that one-third of all cases reported to CPS were not investigated raises the possibility that the prevalence of maltreatment exceeds the numbers reported.[5]

The National Incidence Study (NIS)[6] attempts to address the problem of relying solely on reports to social services to determine the magnitude of child maltreatment. Initially mandated by congress in 1974, the NIS periodically collects data from both CPS and community professionals who have contact with children and families, ie, "sentinels," such as police and sheriffs' departments; public schools; daycare centers; hospitals; mental health agencies; juvenile probation departments; public housing; shelters for runaways, homeless youth, and victims of domestic violence; and public health departments. Data are collected from a nationally representative sample of US counties and have been gathered on 4 occasions: 1979-1980, 1983, 1993, and 2005-2006.

The NIS uses 2 definitional standards: the Harm Standard and the Endangerment Standard. The Harm Standard has been in use since the First NIS and requires demonstrable harm or injury by a parent in order for an act of commission or omission to be classified as abuse or neglect. Thus, a case in which a child is brought to the emergency room with visible injuries characteristic of shaken baby syndrome and his father reports shaking the child to get him to stop crying would meet the Harm Standard. Beginning with the Second NIS, cases that met a less stringent standard, the Endangerment Standard, were also included in the estimate of the magnitude of child maltreatment. The Endangerment Standard counts all children who meet the Harm Standard as well as those children who have not yet been harmed by abuse or neglect but are deemed by a sentinel to be likely to experience harm from abuse or neglect. The Endangerment Standard also includes cases in which a CPS investigation substantiated or indicated their maltreatment even when there was no evidence of specific harm to the child. Thus a case in which a social services case worker removes a child from a home with a meth lab kept by her parents—addicts who sell other illicit substances—would meet the Endangerment Standard because, although the child has not been harmed in a demonstrable way, her living situation puts her in a position where she is very likely to experience harm at some point. Furthermore, the Endangerment Standard also allows for a broader array of perpetrators, eg, adult caregivers other than parents. Based on the NIS definitional standards, an estimated 1.25 million (1 in every 58 US children [Harm Standard]) to 3 million (1 in every 25 US children [Endangerment Standard]) were determined to have experienced abuse or neglect in 2005-2006. This is a significantly higher incidence of maltreatment than is found by reports to CPS alone; however, these numbers are still subject to differences in how the definition of maltreatment is operationalized, and data need to be collected at regular intervals in order to accurately assess changes in the incidence and prevalence.

The best method of gathering data on the incidence and prevalence of maltreatment is to ask children themselves. In studies where children are asked directly about their experiences of any type of maltreatment, the rate of child maltreatment in the general population is substantially higher (136 per 1000 children in the population,[7] or approximately 1 in 10 US children[8]).

Although the exact number of children impacted by abuse and neglect in the United States is unknown, the burden placed on children, families, and society is substantial and the estimated cost of maltreatment to society is staggering. In 2008 the direct economic costs of child maltreatment, eg, hospitalization, chronic physical health problems, mental health care, welfare, law enforcement, and court action, and the indirect, long-term economic costs of child maltreatment, eg, loss of educational attainment and work productivity and burden on insurers, were estimated at $104 billion annually, making the impact on societal health and the public economy significant.[9]

The Ecological Model: An Etiologic Model for Child Maltreatment

A variety of frameworks are available for understanding risk and protective models. Early models to explain the origins and causes of abuse and neglect focused on single risk factors, such as parental psychopathology, caregiver history of abuse and neglect, and child temperament, as possible primary causes of maltreatment; however, no single risk factor or set of risk factors has emerged from this research as constituting a necessary or sufficient cause of abuse and neglect. As a result, a variety of interactive etiologic models have been developed that consider the complex interplay of individual, family, and environmental factors that may contribute to child maltreatment.[5] The ecological model, which posits that individuals develop within a number of nested social contexts, provides a useful framework for examining risk and protective factors for child maltreatment. As conceptualized by Belsky[10] the ecological model has 4 primary levels: ontogenic, microsystem, exosystem, and macrosystem.

More recently the World Health Organization (WHO) expanded the application of the framework to additional types of violence beyond child maltreatment, including youth violence, intimate partner violence, sexual violence, and elder abuse, and described the levels using less burdensome language, ie, the individual, relationship, community, and societal levels.[11] The individual level (ontogenic) is primarily concerned with biological and personal factors that increase the likelihood of becoming a victim or perpetrator of violence, specifically issues of caregiver childhood experience of abuse and neglect, cognitive models of caregiver-child relationships, and biological aspects of the child and caregiver. The relationship level (microsystem) represents the immediate environment and context in which violence perpetration and victimization takes place as well as the proximal social relationship that may increase risk for violence. The community level (exosystem) includes more distal relationships in the formal and informal social structures that impact and influence victimization and perpetration, such as schools, workplaces, and neighborhoods. Finally, the societal level (macrosystem) examines greater factors that may create a climate in which violence is encouraged or inhibited. This level subsumes cultural values and beliefs that foster violence within families and communities.[11-12]

Each context within the model provides increasingly distal influences on individual development, beginning with the most proximal influence and characteristics of the individual and expanding outward to characteristics of the individual's family, community, and society/culture. In the ecological model, individuals actively shape their environments and are shaped by them. Each of the levels functions in a transactional manner with interactional influences existing across contextual boundaries. Proximal variables most often have a direct influence on potential for maltreatment, while more distal variables may have direct or indirect influence, working through more proximal variables, on the individual's likelihood of experiencing maltreatment. Furthermore, distal characteristics and contexts may have a delayed effect and their impact may not be evident until later in a child's development.

How each of these 4 levels of the model is operationalized for research is often based on the research question, available sample, and other factors related to the study at hand. For the purposes of this chapter the levels of the ecological model have been operationalized as follows:

1. Individual: individual/child, parent/caregiver
2. Relationship: parent/caregiver-child relationship, family
3. Community: neighborhood
4. Societal: society/culture

Factors discussed at each level will relate to both perpetration by the caregiver and victimization of the child. (See **Figure 1-1**.)

Risk Factors for Child Maltreatment and Implications for Prevention

Risk Factors for Child Maltreatment

Risk factors for child maltreatment have been identified within all levels of the ecological model. The Surgeon General's report on youth violence defined risk factors as those elements that increase the chances of a person acting violently or being the victim of a violent act.[13] More specifically, a risk factor is a characteristic, variable, hazard, event, or circumstance that if present for a given child makes it more likely that the child will experience abuse or neglect. It is important to note, however, that many risk factors are not static and factors that may increase risk for child maltreatment at one life stage may

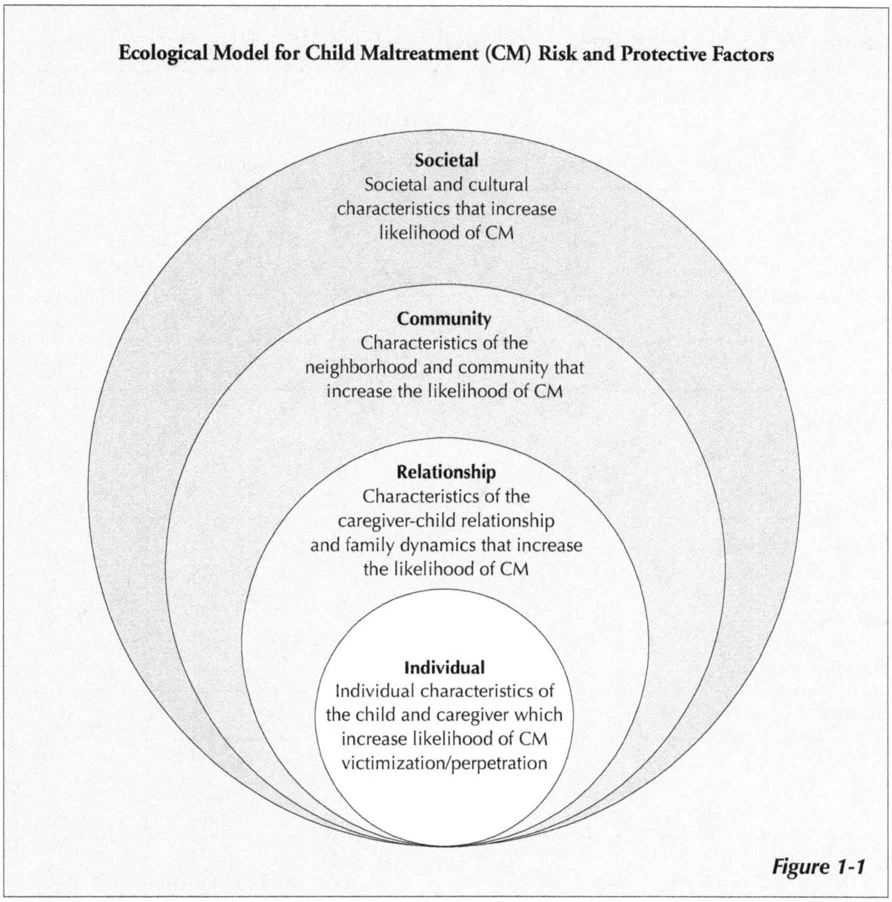

Figure 1-1. *Ecological model for child maltreatment risk and protective factors. Adapted from Krug EG, Dahlberg LL, Mercy JA, Zwi AB, Lozano L, eds.*[11]

or may not put the same individual at risk at a later stage in development.[5] Further, the presence of a risk factor, or multiple risk factors, in a child's life does not ensure that the child will experience abuse or neglect.

Tables 1-2 through **1-7** provide an overview of risk factors at each level of the model based on a review of recent literature. At each ecological level risk factors are grouped within general domains and the type of maltreatment for which risk has been identified is indicated.

The vast majority of the early research on risk factors for child maltreatment focused on the most proximal levels of the social ecology, ie, child characteristics, characteristics of the caregiver, and factors related to child-caregiver interaction.

Individual Level

Child Characteristics

Psychological and personality characteristics of the child have received substantial empirical attention. Child demographics, such as age, sex, and race have been studied extensively, and although most studies find these factors to be correlated with maltreatment in general, causal effects are unclear and have not been established. It is likely that demographic factors act as proxies for other indirect risk factors.[14-15] For example, Sedlak[15] found that risk status for maltreatment varied with children's age, but the relationship was modified by interactions with other risk factors, such as race/ethnicity and family structure. Similarly, minority race and ethnicity, eg, African-American or Latino/Hispanic, have been associated with higher risk of maltreatment in some studies,[15-19] but as noted above, demographic factors interact with risk factors at other levels of the ecological model.

Table 1-2. Risk Factors for Child Maltreatment (Ecological Level: Child)

Risk Factor	Type of Maltreatment					
	Any/Multiple	Fatal	Physical	Sexual	Psychological	Neglect
Demographic						
Age		X	X*	X	X	
Race	X					
Gender				X		
Emotional/Behavioral						
Temperament (irritability, crying)	X		X*			
Behavioral problems/ negative behavior			X			X
Externalizing behavior			X			X
Internalizing behavior			X			X
Psychiatric symptoms			X			
Psychological						
Disability	X		X	X		
Premature birth						X
Infant illness	X					
Low birth weight	X					X
Prenatal substance exposure						X
Less physical attractiveness						X
Prior Victimization						
Victimization/assault by non-family member	X			X		
History of maltreatment	X			X		
Witnessing physical/ sexual maltreatment/ assault of family member	X			X		

**Abusive head trauma only*

Table 1-3. Risk Factors for Child Maltreatment (Ecological Level: Caregiver)

Risk Factor	Type of Maltreatment					
	Any/Multiple	Fatal	Physical	Sexual	Psychological	Neglect
Demographic						
Biological parent		X		X		
Low educational attainment	X	X		X		X
Early childbearing/ young parental age	X	X	X			X
Race/ethnicity						
Gender/sex		X*‡	X‡			
Single parent	X					
Family structure	X	X	X			
Unrelated adults in home	X	X	X	X		X
Parenting/Behavioral						
Harsh discipline	X		X			X
Hostile caregiving			X		X	X
Poor caregiving skills	X	X				X
Low maternal motivation						X
Low parenting satisfaction						X
Low locus of control over child			X*			X
Low satisfactions/enjoyment with parenting				X		X
History of abuse/neglect of same or other child	X	X	X	X	X	X
History of neglect of child		X		X		X
Perceptions of Child						
Negative attributions about child behavior		X				X
Unrealistic expectations of child		X	X			X
Poor understanding of developmental norms		X	X			X
Inability to read child emotional cues			X			

(continued)

Table 1-3. Risk Factors for Child Maltreatment (Ecological Level: Caregiver) *(continued)*

Risk Factor	Type of Maltreatment					
	Any/Multiple	Fatal	Physical	Sexual	Psychological	Neglect
Emotional/Psychological						
Psychopathology/ mental illness	X	X	X			X
Depression	X	X	X			X
Maternal dysphoria (unhappiness [not depression], emotional distress, anxiety)		X				
Paternal dysphoria (unhappiness [not depression], emotional distress, anxiety)			X			
Low self-esteem		X				
Substance abuse	X	X	X‡			X
Impulsivity/ hyper-reactivity	X	X				X
Poor stress management						
Lack of empathy						
Poor marital adjustment	X					
Poor marital satisfaction	X					
Low interpersonal social support						X
Unplanned/unwanted pregnancy			X			X
Physiological/Cognitive Characteristics						
Learning disability						X
Cognitive processing deficits			X			
Physical disability		X				
Chronic health problems		X				

(continued)

Table 1-3. Risk Factors for Child Maltreatment (Ecological Level: Caregiver) *(continued)*

Risk Factor	Type of Maltreatment					
	Any/Multiple	Fatal	Physical	Sexual	Psychological	Neglect
Historical Characteristics						
History of/current criminal behavior		X	X	X‡		
Poor relationship with parents	X				X	
No/little prenatal education	X					
Prior Victimization						
History of any child maltreatment	X		X	X	X	X
History of physical abuse			X			
History of sexual abuse				X		
History of emotional abuse					X	
History of witnessing family violence	X		X			X

**Abusive head trauma only*
‡ Boys only

Table 1-4. Risk Factors for Child Maltreatment (Ecological Level: Caregiver-Child Interaction)

Risk Factor	Type of Maltreatment					
	Any/Multiple	Fatal	Physical	Sexual	Psychological	Neglect
Low Emotional Responsiveness to Child/Indifference Toward Child						
Few positive physical verbal/social interactions with child	X		X			
Verbal aggression toward child	X		X	X		X
Birth complications/ separation after birth due to complications			X		X	X

(continued)

Table 1-4. Risk Factors for Child Maltreatment (Ecological Level: Caregiver-Child Interaction) *(continued)*

Risk Factor	Type of Maltreatment					
	Any/Multiple	Fatal	Physical	Sexual	Psychological	Neglect
Low Emotional Responsiveness to Child/Indifference Toward Child						
Low parental support for child	X					
Low affection toward child			X	X		X
Frequent TV watching by child			X	X		X
Child behavior perceived negatively						X

Table 1-5. Risk Factors for Child Maltreatment (Ecological Level: Family)

Risk Factor	Type of Maltreatment					
	Any/Multiple	Fatal	Physical	Sexual	Psychological	Neglect
Demographic						
Low SES/income	X	X	X	X	X	X
Unstable employment/ unemployment	X	X	X	X‡		X
Single parent	X		X	X		X
Single parent cohabiting with non-marital partner			X*	X		X
Unrelated adults in home	X			X		X
Large family size	X	X	X	X		X
Young father			X			X
Emotional/ Psychological						
Caregiver substance abuse	X	X	X	X	X	X
Poor family adaptability		X				
Poor family cohesion		X				

(continued)

Table 1-5. Risk Factors for Child Maltreatment (Ecological Level: Family) *(continued)*

Risk Factor	Type of Maltreatment					
	Any/Multiple	Fatal	Physical	Sexual	Psychological	Neglect
Emotional/Psychological *(cont)*						
Lack of expressiveness in family			X			
Lack of caregiver support for one another			X			X
Poor marital relationship			X		X	X
Lack of external support for family				X		
Stressors						
General stress	X		X			X
Parenting stress	X		X			X
Daily life stress	X		X			X
Multiple major life stressors			X	X		X
Residential mobility	X					
Perceived material hardship						X
Recent changes/instability in household structure	X			X		X
History of/Current Violence						
Current IPV	X		X	X	X	
History of IPV						
Caregiver history of child in current home	X					
Caregiver history of abuse of child in former home	X					
Family conflict	X		X	X	X	
Caregiver childhood history of CM or witnessing family violence			X			X
Current/past family contact with social services/child welfare	X	X	X	X		X
Physical Environment						
Dangerous physical home environment	X					

**Abusive head trauma only*
‡Boys only

Table 1-6. Risk Factors for Child Maltreatment (Ecological Level: Neighborhood)

Risk Factor	Type of Maltreatment					
	Any/Multiple	Fatal	Physical	Sexual	Psychological	Neglect
Demographic						
Poverty or low neighborhood/community SES				X		
Low female labor force participation	X					
High male unemployment	X					
High general unemployment	X					
Low school retention rate						X
High density single parent families						X
Racial/ethnic composition	X					
Ratio of children to adults in community	X					
Low property values	X					
Neighborhood Structure						
Residential instability						X
Vacant housing	X					
Overcrowding	X					X
Per capita density of alcohol outlets	X		X			X
Social impoverishment			X			X
Resource-poor	X					
Psychosocial						
Low cohesion	X					
Low collective efficacy	X					
Violence						
Community violence	X		X	X		X
High crime rate	X		X	X		X

Table 1-7. Risk Factors for Child Maltreatment (Ecological Level: Society/Culture)

Risk Factor	Type of Maltreatment					
	Any/Multiple	Fatal	Physical	Sexual	Psychological	Neglect
Social Norms						
Racism	X		X			
Social norms supporting violence	X		X			
Social norms supporting physical punishment of children	X		X			
Poverty						X

Physiological, emotional, and behavioral characteristics of the child have also been a focus of research on risk for maltreatment. Physiological child characteristics, such as premature birth status, low birth weight, prolonged infant illness, and prenatal substance exposure, have all been identified as risk factors for subsequent abuse[14,16,20-21] and may be useful markers for targeting primary prevention programs.

Difficult child temperament has been found to be associated with increased risk of maltreatment in general,[22] but child temperament is most often reported by the caregiver and may reflect the caregiver's perception of the child's temperament as difficult rather than a characteristic inherent to the child.[23] With the exception of crying and substantial fussiness by an infant or young child, difficult child temperament does not appear to have a significant relationship with risk for abuse or neglect when specific types of maltreatment are examined individually. Crying is the only temperament-specific variable that has consistently been identified as a trigger for shaking and abusive head trauma (AHT) and has been the focus of several large-scale programs designed to prevent Shaken Baby Syndrome before it occurs.[24-25]

Similar to difficult child temperament, child behavior problems, including internalizing and externalizing behaviors, have been identified as risk factors for child maltreatment. A vast array of internalizing behaviors, eg, depression and self-harm, and externalizing behaviors, eg, acting-out behaviors such as defiance, delinquency, and fighting, have been studied alone and in combination. In general, child behavior problems, including internalizing and externalizing behaviors, are associated with risk for maltreatment. In their meta-analytic review of the literature on risk for physical abuse and neglect, Stith et al[26] found externalizing behaviors to be moderately associated with risk for physical abuse and neglect and internalizing behaviors weakly, but significantly, associated with risk for physical abuse and neglect. It is important to note that many studies do not examine problem child behaviors prospectively, so it is often difficult to untangle the effects of maltreatment on child behavior versus the effect of child behavior on risk for maltreatment.

Psychiatric symptoms and child disabilities have also been identified as risk factors for abuse, although there is some disagreement about the strength of these associations and the type of maltreatment for which these characteristics may be risk factors. For example Stith et al[26] found no association between child disabilities and physical abuse nor between child disabilities and neglect; however, in their review of the literature on neglect, Scannapieco and Connell-Carrick[21] found evidence for an association between physical/mental disabilities and risk for neglect, and in a prospective longitudinal analysis of risk factors for child maltreatment, Brown et al[22] found that children with a physical handicap were approximately 12 times more likely to experience sexual abuse than their nonhandicapped peers.

Caregiver Characteristics

The vast majority of the research on risk factors for child maltreatment has focused on characteristics of the caregiver or perpetrator, and most of this research has focused on mothers or female caregivers. Far less research has focused on fathers and father figures.[27-28] As is the case for children, a variety of demographic factors, including age, sex, educational attainment, and single-parenthood, have been linked to risk for perpetration of child maltreatment. Results for parental age as a risk factor for maltreatment perpetration have been conflicting. Dubowitz[27] and Stith et al[26] found no direct relationship between young parental age and physical abuse or neglect. On the other hand, in a number of early studies of fatal maltreatment, young parents, particularly biological mothers and fathers, were more likely to perpetrate fatal maltreatment.[29] In contrast, Chance et al[30] found no relationship between parent age and fatal maltreatment. As suggested in the literature it is possible that parental age is a proxy for other risk factors, such as parental stress, depression, educational attainment, and employment.[14,26-27]

By far the strongest caregiver risk factors for perpetration of child maltreatment are negative parenting behaviors, maternal depression, caregiver substance abuse, and a childhood history of victimization. With the exception of childhood history of victimization all of these factors are modifiable and amenable to primary prevention. Negative parenting behaviors, such as harsh discipline practices, unrealistic expectations of child behavior and development, negative attributions about child behavior, and previous abuse of another child, have been strongly linked to the perpetration of child maltreatment in general and to all types of abuse and neglect. Similarly caregiver depression and substance abuse have been strongly linked to all forms of abuse and neglect. Children of caregivers who abuse alcohol and drugs were found to be almost 5 times more likely to experience physical abuse, greater than 6 times more likely to experience sexual abuse, and approximately 4 times more likely to experience neglect than children whose caregivers were not substance abusers.[27] Substance abusing caregivers are also more likely to have an infant injured or die as a result of accidental suffocation or abusive head trauma.[33-34]

There has been substantial attention paid to the intergenerational transmission of abuse, ie, the risk for caregivers who experienced victimization in childhood to subsequently abuse or neglect their own children. Research has shown that being victimized or witnessing family violence in childhood is a strong risk factor for subsequent perpetration of child maltreatment; however, not all parents who experience childhood maltreatment repeat the cycle of violence.[31,36] In fact, it is a small minority of parents with a history of abuse who go on to abuse or neglect their children.[12] It is important to look at the attributes of these parents in order to inform prevention efforts.

Relationship Level

Caregiver-Child Relationship Characteristics

Areas in the caregiver-child relationship that are often identified as risk factors include lack of parental support, affection, emotional responsiveness, and playfulness with the child; less positive verbal and nonverbal behavior with the child, including caregiver verbal aggression in response to child behavior[14,18,26,32,38]; and hyper-responsivity to aversive child behavior.[14,17,26,38] Other characteristics that have, in the past, been identified as possible risk factors at the caregiver-child interaction level, such as birth complications and separation of the caregiver and child immediately after birth, have not received support in recent literature reviews and empirical analyses. It may be that these characteristics interact with other risk factors and appear to impact risk for maltreatment if other more direct influences are not accounted. Similarly the combination of many child and caregiver characteristics described earlier can result in poor caregiver-child relationships. For example a fussy, crying infant with a caregiver prone to hyper-responsivity to aversive child behavior and ignorant of appropriate developmental norms and behaviors could result in abusive behavior, such as shaking.

Family Characteristics

After individual characteristics of the child and caregiver, characteristics and dynamics of the family have received considerable attention regarding what puts children at risk for maltreatment. As said by Cicchetti and Toth, "child maltreatment exemplifies a pathogenic relational environment that poses substantial risk for undermining biological and psychological development across a broad spectrum of domains of functioning."[5(p414)] Families provide the primary context in which children grow and develop, and therefore, families can have a substantial impact on risk. A family environment characterized by "toxic" stressors can have a profound effect on risk for maltreatment.[39] Stressors such as extreme poverty, severe maternal depression, caregiver substance abuse, and family violence strongly influence the likelihood that a child will experience direct or indirect abuse or neglect as well as the likelihood that the impact of abuse will be long-lasting. This is supported by recent research indicating that early child maltreatment can alter brain architecture in such a way that lower thresholds for stress responses are established, which consequently impairs health and increases risk for stress-related diseases, eg, obesity, heart disease, and certain types of cancer, and cognitive impairment across the lifespan.[39-40] As is the case for child and caregiver characteristics, numerous demographic characteristics related to the family have been identified as risk factors for maltreatment. Family socioeconomic status (SES) and economic hardship have consistently been shown to have a strong influence on violence in general and child maltreatment specifically.[28] In analyses using data from the Second National Incidence Study, Sedlak[15] found that children from low income families had greater than 20 times the risk of experiencing physical abuse, sexual abuse, or neglect; 13 times greater risk of experiencing psychological abuse; and 16 times the risk of experiencing multiple forms of maltreatment than children from higher income families. There is debate in the field about whether SES has a direct or indirect effect on maltreatment and whether it is actual or perceived economic hardship that increases risk for child maltreatment. SES is influenced by caregiver characteristics such as early childbirth/young caregiver age, education, and employment status as well as by other family demographic risk factors such as single parenthood, large family size, and the presence of unrelated adults living in the home. In studies where these factors have been statistically controlled, the potency of the effect of poverty has been attenuated.[32] Furthermore in an empirical investigation of economic and parenting characteristics that may influence risk of child neglect, Slack et al[32] found that perceived economic hardship, as reported by the primary caregiver, rather than actual material hardship, ie, difficulty paying rent, eviction, or experiencing any utility shutoffs, was a robust predictor of future social service reports of neglect. In fact, perceived economic hardship was the only poverty indicator in the study that remained significant in the final model once demographics and other correlates of neglect were accounted for.

Family stressors above and beyond finances have also been identified as significant risk factors for child maltreatment. The cumulative effects of daily stressors on caregivers increase small frustrations and have been shown to have small to moderate effects on physical abuse and neglect, particularly when caregiver coping and problem solving skills are limited.[26,38] Similarly major life stressors, such as chronic health problems, loss of employment, and household moves, increase likelihood of child maltreatment.[5,17,18]

A history of violence and/or current violence within the home have also been identified as strong and consistent risk factors for child maltreatment. Violence within the home, specifically violence between caregivers, has been identified as a risk factor for all types of maltreatment.[5,14,17-19,26,31] In her meta-analysis of risk factors for physical abuse and neglect, Stith and colleagues[26] found that the risk factors with the strongest effect size for physical abuse were high family conflict and low family cohesion. Similarly in an empirical investigation of the intergenerational transmission of violence, Dixon and her colleagues[31] found that living with a violent partner was a strong predictor of the perpetration of maltreatment in families regardless of whether the caregiver had a history of maltreatment. There are several ways that intimate partner violence can interact with child maltreatment risk[41]:

1. The perpetrator may target both spouse and child.
2. The child may become incidentally caught up in the violent episode by witnessing the event, choosing to intervene, or by accident.
3. The victimized caregiver may be unable to provide for the needs of the child due to the foremost need for self-protection.

These interactions are not well understood and additional research is needed to highlight ways in which to prevent additional violence within the context of family violence.

Other psychosocial family characteristics, such as poor family cohesion, lack of expressiveness, and low emotional and social support for family members, have also been identified as risk factors for various types of maltreatment.[14,17,19,38] For example, in their review of risk factors for neglect, Schumacher et al[38] report that although neglectful mothers' ratings of family cohesion did not differ from nonmaltreating mothers' ratings, neglected children perceived their families as significantly less cohesive than nonneglected children.

Community Level

Neighborhood Characteristics

Research focused on the outer levels of social ecology has lagged behind investigation of risk factors more proximal to children. Only in the last 2 decades have factors related to the neighborhood, cultural, and societal contexts begun to be examined to determine their effects on risk for, and rates of, maltreatment. In general researchers have found that child maltreatment cases tend to be concentrated in disadvantaged areas[42-43] but the processes that link neighborhood disadvantage to maltreatment are still uncertain.[42] Three aspects of neighborhoods have dominated the research literature: poverty and its correlates, eg, employment, school retention, and property values; neighborhood structure, eg, residential instability, vacant housing, social impoverishment, cohesion, and collective efficacy; and violence.

Poverty and its correlates appear as a risk factor for all forms of child maltreatment at almost every level of the ecological model. Collective neighborhood poverty, or a collective lack of resources within a neighborhood, puts additional stress on families, parents, and children. There is evidence that indicators of poverty, such as concentrated areas of unemployment, low school retention, low property values, concentrated areas of vacant property, and neighborhood overcrowding, are linked to higher rates of maltreatment reports and poor parenting practices[18-19,38,42]; however, it is uncertain whether neighborhood poverty has a direct or indirect relationship with maltreatment. To further complicate matters, research in this area is confounded by selection, or endogeneity, bias, ie, the possibility that parents and families may be constrained to live in disadvantaged areas not by choice but because they lack the resources to live elsewhere. As such, it is difficult to disentangle the effects of neighborhood context from parental characteristics as causal factors for child maltreatment.[42] When parental characteristics are included in analyses of the effect of poverty on maltreatment, as in Slack et al[32], it has been found that neighborhood poverty is indirectly related to neglect through maternal warmth and the physical quality of the home environment. There is also evidence that neighborhood poverty may impact types of maltreatment differently.[32,43] For example, Drake and Pandy[43] found that neglect was more strongly associated with neighborhood poverty than either physical or sexual abuse.

Similar to poverty, research on the relationship between neighborhood structure and maltreatment has been complicated by issues of residential bias[38,42] and the question of direct vs. indirect effects of neighborhood characteristics on maltreatment. Nevertheless, numerous studies have found a relationship between maltreatment and various neighborhood structural characteristics, such as residential instability, social impoverishment, cohesion, and collective efficacy. Coulton et al[44-45] found that poor social organization in communities had an indirect effect on child maltreatment by lowering the ability of the community to respond to and provide collective support for residents, thereby increasing family isolation and negative effects of other individual and family risk factors for child maltreatment.

Finally, there is a small but important literature on the effects of neighborhood violence on risk for maltreatment.[12,14,42] This effect is likely to be confounded by neighborhood poverty and selection bias because families of lower SES are more likely to live in communities with high levels of neighborhood violence, giving rise to speculation that continuous exposure to these conditions may predispose parents in these neighborhoods to view violence as an acceptable response or behavior.[14] In support of this speculation, it has been found that risk for physical abuse is greater for children living in high-violence neighborhoods than for children from lower violence neighborhoods.[46] However, not all families living in high-violence neighborhoods endorse or engage in intrafamilial violence; therefore, it is important to look at mediating and moderating variables in this relationship.

Societal Level

Societal and Cultural Characteristics

At the farthest reaches of the ecological model lie characteristics of society and culture that may impact risk for child maltreatment. While interest in this level of social ecology is growing, little empirical research has been conducted regarding specific aspects of society and culture, and much of the work in this area is theoretical. Other areas of interest at this level of social ecology include laws governing the care and treatment of children and policies related to maternal and paternal leave, health, education, and child welfare.

When examining the societal and cultural characteristics that increase risk for child maltreatment perpetration and victimization, researchers must consider and examine the embeddedness of the individual, family, and neighborhood within the larger fabric of culture and society. Two areas have received attention at this level of the model: social norms that support violence and physical punishment and racism.

Relative to other developed nations, the United States maintains a culture that accepts, if not approves of, violence. For example, corporal punishment is widely practiced and condoned by parents and other caregivers in the United States.[47-48] It has been posited that in cultures where violence is considered an acceptable response or behavior, an environment that fosters maltreatment is supported. Even in nations outside the United States the societal acceptance of corporal punishment has raised concerns. In a recent study in Spain examining the relationship between the reported necessity of corporal punishment in child rearing and the perceived frequency of child physical abuse in society, the authors found that parents who reported using corporal punishment as a necessary parenting strategy also reported perceiving lower rates of physical abuse in the general population.[49] The acceptance of cultural values that support violence has led many child maltreatment researchers and professionals to conclude that a change in societal attitudes toward and an acceptance of aggression as a means of controlling child behavior is essential to reducing the incidence of physical abuse.[48]

Like social norms supporting physical punishment of children, racism is another social norm that has been identified as a risk factor for child maltreatment. Racism's effect on child maltreatment is indirect. Societal belief systems about races and ethnic groups as well as disparities in goods and services accessible to these groups places undue stress on families and limits educational and economic opportunities as well as the distribution of resources, in turn, increasing the possibility of families and caregivers experiencing other, more proximal risk factors for child maltreatment, such as limited and unstable employment, increase in daily stressors, and caregiver mental health issues.[21]

Risk Factors and Implications for Prevention

Much of the application of our knowledge about risk factors to prevention efforts has centered on interventions to prevent revictimization of children and reduce harm from maltreatment once it has occurred. These efforts have focused primarily on social welfare, eg, out-of-home placement and other CPS-based programs, and the justice system, eg, prosecution of child maltreatment perpetrators, and have had some success in preventing further harm to many children.

Other prevention efforts have targeted specific families and children that are at high risk for maltreatment with the goal of early intervention preventing maltreatment before it occurs. These prevention efforts, for example Triple P[50-51] and Healthy Start home visitation,[52] include a wide range of activities and may incorporate primary prevention strategies such as community-wide media campaigns designed to facilitate caregiver access to parenting information, physicians and community agencies providing information directly to specific groups of parents, and direct skills training and counseling. Prevention programs such as Nurse Family Partnership Home Visitation programs[53-54] and Triple P,[50-51] have demonstrated success in reducing incidence of abuse, but prevention success has been mixed in other programs. First, many programs have not been designed to prevent child abuse and neglect specifically, but rather have been designed to reduce problem behaviors in children and families or to enhance the quality of the parent-child relationship. Consequently, demonstrated impact on maltreatment has been mixed. Second, the vast majority of programs have not been adequately evaluated for cost effectiveness. Finally, while a few prevention programs such as Nurse Family Partnership and Triple P have been widely disseminated, many of the available programs cannot easily be taken to scale, if they can be taken at all, thus limiting their application at the population level.

The public health framework emphasizes primary prevention at the population-level, ie, preventing adverse occurrences in the population before they happen. Preventing child maltreatment before it occurs requires understanding not only which factors put children at risk but also understanding which of these factors can be changed before they occur through prevention efforts. There is little sense in expending time, effort, and resources to change risk factors that cannot be changed or that go beyond the scope of the entity responsible for changing them. The focus of the public health model, therefore, is on identifying modifiable risk factors and working with these modifiable factors to develop prevention strategies targeting risk factors that are highly prevalent in a population.

As noted above, the vast majority of research on risk factors has focused on characteristics of the child, the caregiver, and the child-caregiver relationship. Many of the risk factors identified at these levels of social ecology are demographic, for example child sex as a risk factor for sexual abuse, child age as a risk factor for neglect and abusive head trauma; however, many demographic characteristics are not modifiable. Nevertheless, identifying demographic characteristics related to risk is an important aspect of both surveillance and designing effective public health prevention programs. There is some evidence that while many demographic characteristics may not have a direct effect on maltreatment in general, specific child demographic characteristics may have a direct bearing on individual types of abuse or neglect and can be useful for identifying populations that may be targeted by perpetrators. For example, girls are at significantly greater risk for sexual abuse than boys[55] but data on sexual abuse are confounded by reporting bias and the inclusion of noncaregiving perpetrators in rate estimates. With regard to age, infants and very young children (less than 5 years) are at the greatest risk for abusive head trauma and fatal maltreatment.[21,30] Young boys, those under the age of 13 or prior to puberty, are at greater risk for sexual abuse than older boys[16,55] and girls' risk for sexual abuse evidences a bimodal distribution with peak risk periods in early childhood and again in early adolescence.[55] Based on results from the Second National Incidence Study (NIS-2),[56] older children are at greater risk for experiencing psychological maltreatment than younger children. Although demographic factors such as child age and sex are not modifiable risk factors, as is usually the focus for public health, they do serve as important markers for prevention programs and resources targeted toward reducing perpetration in these areas.

As is the case with demographic factors, the intergenerational transmission of abuse, caregiver-child interaction characteristics, and poverty are all candidates for primary prevention efforts and a substantial body of literature exists in this area. Not all parents who experience childhood maltreatment repeat the cycle of violence.[31,36] Likewise, most risk factors at the caregiver-child interaction level of the ecological model are characterized by poor parenting skills[26,31] that can be identified early in the parent-child relationship and improved through effective parenting programs; therefore, the caregiver-child relationship realm of the ecological model presents many identified areas amenable to public health prevention efforts. Finally, despite lack of consensus regarding the direct or indirect effects of SES at various levels of the social ecology, it may still be an important and useful marker for targeted, large-scale prevention programs.

Klevens and Whitaker[57] provide an excellent review of primary prevention programs focused on modifiable risk factors aimed at reducing physical abuse and neglect. As noted by the authors, few of the prevention programs discussed in the literature have been rigorously evaluated and only a select few have demonstrated empirical evidence of reducing the incidence of child maltreatment or attenuating risk factors. This observation has been supported by other recent reviews of and commentaries on primary prevention programs.[58-62] There are still large gaps in primary prevention efforts at most levels of the ecological model. Klevens and Whitaker identify a need for additional attention to interventions that target prevalent risk factors such as poverty, racial and ethnic disparity, partner violence, teenage pregnancy, and social norms that tolerate violence toward children.

Protective Factors for Child Maltreatment and Implications for Prevention

Protective Factors

Offsetting risk factors in children's lives are those factors that buffer or protect a child from victimization. As defined by HHS[13] protective factors are aspects of the individual or environment that buffer or moderate the effect of risk. There is substantial debate in the literature about how to operationalize the relationship of risk to protective factors. Protective factors have generally been operationalized in the literature in 2 ways. First, protective factors have been defined as being at the opposing end of the risk factor continuum, in other words, the opposite of a risk factor. For example, while a difficult child temperament has been shown to be a risk factor for physical abuse and abusive head trauma[14,23,63] it is presumed that an easy-going child temperament will protect a child from abuse given the same social context. Likewise, Stith and colleagues[26] found that child social competence, as opposed to a lack of social competence in a child, was a significant protective factor for both physical abuse and neglect. Second, protective factors have been operationalized as the absence of a risk factor: for example, children whose parents do not have a childhood history of abuse or neglect will be protected from the intergenerational transmission of maltreatment. (See Stouthamer-Loeber et al[64] for full discussion of the relationship between risk and protective factors.)

Although both of these conditions may be true of protective factors, it is important to consider protective factors as unique conditions that, in and of themselves, create an environment in which children are shielded from harm. In addition, these factors and conditions work in a transactional manner with risk factors to buffer negative impacts. In ideal conditions, the combination of risk and protective factors in a child's life will create an environment in which the child thrives and excels. At the very least, it is hoped that the combination of risk and protective factors will create an environment in which harm to the child is minimized.

Given the confusion surrounding the precise definition of protective factors, it is not surprising that much less research has been devoted to identifying factors that protect children from maltreatment. There is a large literature on resiliency—factors that buffer the impact of maltreatment on developmental outcomes—but little information on characteristics, variables, events, or circumstances that prevent maltreatment from occurring in the first place.

The goal of primary prevention is, ideally, to prevent maltreatment before it occurs; however, when this is not possible, a second goal of primary prevention is to minimize risk for children and foster an environment in which children are able to maximize their potential to live happy and healthy lives. Thus, it is child well-being promotion rather than child maltreatment prevention that we seek.[58] **Table 1-8** lists protective factors found in a review of the recent literature, the level of the ecological model in which they reside, and the type of maltreatment buffered. These studies are discussed below within a new framework for developing positive environments for children as a means to preventing child maltreatment. As can be seen in **Table 1-8**, very few unique protective factors have been identified in the empirical literature. Substantial research is still needed to identify key factors that mediate or moderate risk in children's lives.

Table 1-8. Protective Factors for Child Maltreatment

Ecological Level	Protective Factor	Type of Maltreatment					
		Any/Multiple	Fatal	Physical	Sexual	Psychological	Neglect
Child	Child social competence	X		X			X
Caregiver	Stable, positive romantic relationship	X					
	Caregiver warmth						X
Family	Financial stability	X					
	Stable family structure	X					
	Family cohesion	X		X			
	Secure home environment	X					
Neighborhood	Social cohesion	X					
	Community pride	X					
	Perception of neighborhood as safe	X					

Safe, Stable, and Nurturing Relationships (SSNRs)

The Centers for Disease Control and Prevention has developed a framework for examining protective factors for child maltreatment and translating these factors into strategies and programs for the primary prevention of child maltreatment and promotion of child health and well-being. Safe, stable, and nurturing relationships (SSNRs) between children and their caregivers have been identified as a strategic framework for the primary prevention of child maltreatment.[65] SSNRs between children and their caregivers are the antithesis of abuse, neglect, and other adverse exposures that occur during childhood, and which compromise health over the lifespan. Young children experience their world through their relationships with parents and other caregivers in their environment.[66] These relationships are fundamental to the healthy development of the brain and consequently the development of physical, emotional, social, behavioral, and intellectual capacities.[66-67] From a public health perspective the promotion of SSNRs is, therefore, strategic in that, if done successfully, it can help foster a shift in the focus of professionals and researchers in child maltreatment and public health from viewing child maltreatment as a disease in and of itself to seeing child maltreatment as one symptom of a larger familial, communal, or societal disease[58] and will have synergistic effects on a broad range of health problems, as well as contribute to the development of skills that will enhance the acquisition of healthy habits and lifestyles.

SSNRs and Implications for Prevention

The 3 dimensions of SSNRs, safety, stability, and nurturance, each represent important aspects of the social and physical environments that may protect children, promote their optimal development, and be key points for prevention.[68] Protective factors identified in the literature fit into each of the 3 SSNR dimensions at various levels of the ecological model.

Safety

Safety refers to the extent to which a child is free from physical and/or emotional harm. Empirical studies have shown that children who grow up in home environments that are safe from physical danger and neighborhoods that are perceived by residents as a safe place for child and family development are less likely to experience maltreatment.[14,21,31,42] Further, caregivers can ensure the safety of children by (1) regulating their emotional response to their children, (2) protecting children under their care from others that may harm them, (3) disciplining their children in ways that do not cause harm and promote self-regulation, (4) monitoring their child's behavior and development, and (5) ensuring the child's environment is hazard free.[66,69] The nature of these vital functions for parents and other caregivers change as a child grows older but remain important through adolescence. Substantially more work in the area of safety is needed to identify those factors that have the greatest impact in creating relationships and environments that protect children.

Stability

Stability refers to the degree of predictability and consistency in a child's environment and is critical to providing the child with a sense of coherence, ie, seeing the world as predictable and manageable.[70-71] Stability includes consistency in the caregivers with whom the child has regular interactions as well as predictability in the nature of interactions with caregivers, other people in the child's environment, and the environment itself. Family structures and routines that provide stability buffer the impact of stressful experiences on children.[72]

Protective aspects of stability have been identified at the caregiver, family, and neighborhood levels of the ecological model. At the caregiver level, work by Dixon et al demonstrates that a mother with a childhood history of abuse or neglect is more likely to break the intergenerational cycle of abuse if she has a stable, positive romantic relationship and mental health status that is positive and stable.[31] Likewise at the family level of the model, financial stability, stable family structure, and a secure physical home environment have all been shown to protect children from experiencing maltreatment.[16,21,26,28,30-32,63] Finally, at the neighborhood level, social cohesion has been identified as a strong protective element for the prevention of child maltreatment.[42,44] Socially cohesive neighborhoods have strong stability in structural factors, such as employment, residential stability (vs. turnover), and social integration, all of which have been found to be significantly associated with lower levels of maltreatment as reported by caregivers and reports to social service agencies.[44]

Nurturance

Nurture refers to the extent to which a parent or caregiver is available and able to sensitively respond to and meet the needs of their child.[66] These include physical needs, eg, food, shelter, hygiene, and medical care; developmental needs, ie, experiences necessary for development; and emotional needs, eg, affection, empathy, acceptance, and affirmation. Early nurturing relationships contribute to the growth of a broad range of skills, competencies, and personality characteristics that children use throughout their lives, including their interest in and capacity to learn, sense of self-worth, social skills, and an understanding of important building blocks of human relationships, such as emotions, commitment, and morality.[73-74]

As is the case with safety and stability, dimensions of nurturance display protective properties at multiple levels of the social ecology. Caregiver characteristics of warmth and empathy have consistently been shown to protect children from multiple types of maltreatment. In an analysis of poverty and parenting characteristics, Slack found that parental warmth was inversely related to reports of neglect to Child Protective Services.[32] Characteristics of nurturance within the family, such as family cohesion and intrafamilial support, also show evidence of providing a protective buffer for children.[31,63] Similarly, a nurturing neighborhood environment in which there is a sense of social connectedness and bonding, where neighbors know and rely on one another and take pride in their community can protect children from maltreatment in the face of other risk factors.[14,21,42,63,75]

Next Steps for Risk, Protection, and Prevention

Substantially more theoretical and empirical work is needed to determine focal points for prevention based on risk and protective factors. Previous research suggests that prevention efforts in early childhood, particularly those that foster safe, stable, and nurturing relationships and environments, are promising and have great potential to improve children's health over a lifetime. It is clear that no one risk or protective factor nor one single programmatic approach will be the panacea for child maltreatment. While most available prevention programs lack strong empirical evidence for effective impact on child maltreatment, a few strategies have strong evidence for efficacy and have been rigorously evaluated: home visitation by a nurse or social worker, in-hospital parent education (most programs focus on normal infant crying and soothing techniques), and parent support/training programs.[58,60,68,76] The future of primary prevention of child abuse and neglect will employ what is known about effective programs, the concept of promoting child well-being through safe, stable and nurturing relationships and evaluating which mix of programs, at what developmental stage and dosage, and for what duration will achieve the greatest impact.[58] Furthermore incorporation of these programs into communities must be evaluated as to where they are most needed, and additional research is needed regarding how to take successful programs to meaningful scale in order to make a substantial difference.

References

1. Hammond WR. Public health and child maltreatment prevention: the role of the Centers for Disease Control and Prevention. *Child Maltreat.* 2003;8(2):81-83.

2. Kempe HC, Silverman FN, Steele BF, Droegemueller W, Silver HK. The battered-child syndrome. *JAMA.* 1962;181(1):17-24.

3. Leeb RT, Paulozzi L, Melanson C, Simon T, Arias I. *Child Maltreatment Surveillance: Uniform Definitions for Public Health and Recommended Data Elements.* Version 1.0. Atlanta, GA: Centers for Disease Control and Prevention, National Center for Injury Prevention and Control; 2008.

4. US Department of Health and Human Services, Administration for Children and Families, Children's Bureau. Child maltreatment 2008. Administration for Children and Families Web site. http://www.acf.hhs.gov/programs/cb/research-data-technology/statistics-research/child-maltreatment. Accessed February 14, 2013.

5. Cicchetti D, Toth SL. Child maltreatment. *Annu Rev of Clin Psychol.* 2005;1:409-438.

6. Sedlak AJ, Mettenburg J, Basena M, et al. *Fourth National Incidence Study of Child Abuse and Neglect (NIS–4): Report to Congress. Executive summary.* Washington, DC: US Department of Health and Human Services, Administration for Children and

Families; 2010. US Department of Health and Human Services, Administration for Children and Families Web site. http://www.acf.hhs.gov/programs/opre/resource/fourth-national-incidence-study-of-child-abuse-and-neglect-nis-4-report-to-0. Accessed March 23, 2015.

7. Finkelhor D, Ormrod R, Turner H, Hamby SL. The victimization of children and youth: a comprehensive national survey. *Child Maltreat.* 2005;10(1):5-25.

8. Finkelhor D, Turner H, Ormrod R, Hamby SL. Violence, abuse, and crime exposure in a national sample of children and youth. *Pediatrics.* 2009;124(5):1411-1423.

9. Pew Charitable Trusts. *Time For Reform: Investing in Prevention: Keeping Children Safe at Home.* Philadelphia, PA: Pew Charitable Trusts; 2007.

10. Belsky J. Child maltreatment: an ecological integration. *Am Psychol.* 1980;35(4):320-335.

11. Krug EG, Dahlberg LL, Mercy JA, Zwi AB, Lozano L, eds. *World Report on Violence and Health.* Geneva, Switzerland: WHO; 2002.

12. Cicchetti D, Lynch M. Toward an ecological/transactional model of community violence and child maltreatment: consequences for children's development. *Psychiatry.* 1993;56(1):96-118.

13. Office of the Surgeon General (US), National Center for Injury Prevention and Control (US), National Institute of Mental Health (US), Center for Mental Health Services (US). *Youth Violence: A Report of the Surgeon General.* Rockville, MD: Office of the Surgeon General (US); 2001.

14. Portwood SG. Physical abuse in childhood. In: Gulotta T, Blau GM, eds. *Family Influences on Childhood Behavior and Development: Evidence-based Prevention and Treatment Approaches.* New York: Routledge; 2008:267-292.

15. Sedlak AJ. Risk factors for the occurrence of child abuse and neglect. *J Agg Maltreat Trauma.* 1997;1(1):147-185.

16. Holmes WC, Slap GB. Sexual abuse of boys. *JAMA.* 1998;280(21):1855-1862.

17. Black DA, Heyman RE, Smith Slep AM. Risk factors for child physical abuse. *Aggress Violent Behav.* 2001;6(2-3):121-188.

18. Black DA, Smith Slep AM, Heyman RE. Risk factors for child psychological abuse. *Aggress Violent Behav.* 2001;6(2-3):189-201.

19. Black DA, Heyman RE, Smith Slep AM. Risk factors for child sexual abuse. *Aggress Violent Behav.* 2001;6(2-3):203-229.

20. Brodowski ML, Nolan CM, Gaudiosi JA, et al. Nonfatal maltreatment of infants—United States, October 2005–September 2006. *MMWR Morb Mortal Wkly Rep.* 2008;57(13):336-339.

21. Scannapieco M, Connell-Carrick K. Focus on the first years: an eco-developmental assessment of child neglect for children 0 to 3 years of age. *Child Youth Services Rev.* 2002;24(8):601-621.

22. Brown J, Cohen P, Johnson JG, Salzinger S. A longitudinal analysis of risk factors for child maltreatment: findings of a 17-year prospective study of officially recorded and self-reported child abuse and neglect. *Child Abuse Negl.* 1998;22(11):1065-1078.

23. Davies WH, Garwood MM. Who are the perpetrators and why do they do it? In: Lazoritz S, Palusci VJ, eds. *The Shaken Baby Syndrome: A Multidisciplinary Approach*. London: Hawthorn; 2001:41-54.

24. Dias MS, Smith K, deGuehery K, Mazur P, Li V, Shaffer ML. Preventing abusive head trauma among infants and young children: a hospital-based, parent education program. *Pediatrics*. 2005;115(4):e470-e477.

25. Barr RG, Barr M, Fujiwara T, Conway J, Nicole C, Brant R. Do educational materials change knowledge and behaviour about crying and shaken baby syndrome?: a randomized control trial. *CMAJ*. 2009;180(7):727-733.

26. Stith SM, Liu T, Davies LC, et al. Risk factors in child maltreatment: a meta-analytic review of the literature. *Aggress Violent Behav.* 2009;14(1):13-29.

27. Dubowitz, H. The families of neglected children. In: Lamb ME, ed. *Parenting and Child Development in "Nontraditional" Families*. Mahwah, NJ: Erlbaum; 1999:327-345.

28. Guterman NB, Lee Y. The role of fathers in risk for physical child abuse and neglect: possible pathways and unanswered questions. *Child Maltreat.* 2005;10(2):136-149.

29. Brewster AL, Nelson JP, Hymel KP, et al. Victim, perpetrator, family, and incident characteristics of 32 infant maltreatment deaths in the United States Air Force. *Child Abuse Negl.* 1998;22(2):91-101.

30. Chance T, Scannapieco M. Ecological correlates of child maltreatment: similarities and differences between child fatality and nonfatality cases. *Child Adolesc Social Work J.* 2002;19(2):139-161.

31. Dixon L, Browne K, Hamilton-Giachritsis C. Patterns of risk and protective factors in the intergenerational cycle of maltreatment. *J Fam Violence.* 2009;24(2):111-122.

32. Slack KS, Holl JL, McDaniel M, Yoo J, Bolger K. Understanding the risks of child neglect: an exploration of poverty and parenting characteristics. *Child Maltreat.* 2009;9(4):395-408.

33. Klevens J, Leeb RT. Child maltreatment fatalities in children under 5: findings from the National Violent Death Reporting System. *Child Abuse Negl.* 2010;34(4):262-266.

34. Millard, DD. Toxicology testing in neonates. *Clin Perinatol.* 1996;23(3):491-507.

35. Milner JS, Chilamkurti C. Physical child abuse perpetrator characteristics: a review of the literature. *J Interpers Viol.* 1991;6(3):345-366.

36. Widom CS. Does violence beget violence?: a critical examination of the literature. *Psychol Bull.* 1989;106(1)3-28.

37. Wilson LM, Reid AJ, Midmer DK, Biringer A, Carroll JC, Stewart DE. Antenatal psychosocial risk factors associated with adverse postpartum family outcomes. *CMAJ*. 1996;154(6):785-799.

38. Schumacher JA, Smith Slep AM, Heyman RE. Risk factors for neglect. *Aggress Violent Behav.* 2001;6(2-3):231-254.

39. Shonkoff JP, Boyce WT, McEwen BS. Neuroscience, molecular biology, and the childhood roots of health disparities: building a new framework for health promotion and disease prevention. *JAMA*. 2009;301(21):2252-2259.

40. National Scientific Council on the Developing Child. *Excessive Stress Disrupts the Architecture of the Developing Brain: Working Paper 3.* Cambridge, MA: Center on the Developing Child at Harvard University; 2005. Center on the Developing Child at Harvard University Web site. http://developingchild.harvard.edu/index.php/resources/reports_and_working_papers/working_papers/wp3/. Accessed March 24, 2015.

41. Edelson, JL. Studying the co-occurrence of child maltreatment and woman battering in families. In: Grahm-Berman SA, Edelson JL, eds. *Domestic Violence in the Lives of Children: The Future of Research, Intervention, and Social Policy.* Washington, DC: American Psychological Association; 2001:91-110.

42. Coulton CJ, Crampton DS, Irwin M, Spilsbury JC, Korbin JE. How neighborhoods influence child maltreatment: a review of the literature and alternative pathways. *Child Abuse Negl.* 2007;31(11-12):1117-1142.

43. Drake B, Pandey S. Understanding the relationship between neighborhood poverty and specific types of child maltreatment. *Child Abuse Neg.* 1996;20(11):1003-1018.

44. Coulton CJ, Korbin JE, Su M, Chow J. Community level factors and child maltreatment rates. *Child Devel.* 1995;66(5)1262-1276.

45. Coulton C, Korbin J, Su M. Neighborhoods and child maltreatment: a multi-level study. *Child Abuse Negl.* 1999;23(11):1019-1040.

46. Lynch M, Cicchetti D. An ecological-transactional analysis of children and contexts: the longitudinal interplay among child maltreatment, community violence, and children's symptomatology. *Dev Psychopathol.* 1998;10(2):235-257.

47. Christoffel KK. Violent death and injury in US children and adolescents. *Am J Dis Child.* 1990;144(6):697-706.

48. Straus MA. Corporal punishment and primary prevention of physical abuse. *Child Abuse Negl.* 2000;24(9):1109-1114.

49. Gracia E, Herrero J. Beliefs in the necessity of corporal punishment of children and public perceptions of child physical abuse as a social problem. *Child Abuse Negl.* 2008;32(11):1058-1062.

50. Prinz RJ, Sanders MR, Shapiro CJ, Whitaker DJ, Lutzker JR. Population-based prevention of child maltreatment: the US Triple P System Population Trial. *Prev Sci.* 2009;10(1):1-12.

51. Sanders MR, Markie-Dadds C, Turner KMT. *Theoretical, Scientific, and Theoretical Foundations of the Triple P-Positive Parenting Program: A Population Approach to the Promotion of Parenting Competence.* Parenting Research and Practice Monograph. Brisbane, Qld. Australia: The Parenting and Family Support Centre; 2003:1-24.

52. Duggan AK, McFarlane EC, Windham AM, et al. Evaluation of Hawaii's Healthy Start program. *Future Child.* 1999;9(1):66-90.

53. Olds DL, Eckenrode J, Henderson CR Jr, et al. Long-term effects of home visitation on maternal life course and child abuse and neglect. *JAMA.* 1997;278(8):637-643.

54. Olds D, Henderson CR Jr, Chamberlin R, et al. Preventing child abuse and neglect: a randomized trial of nurse home visitation. *Pediatrics.* 1986;78(1):65-78.

55. Snyder HN. *Sexual Assault of Young Children as Reported to Law Enforcement: Victim, Incident, and Offender Characteristics.* NCJ 182990. US Department of Justice, Bureau of Justice Statistics; 2000.

56. Sedlak AJ. *National Incidence and Prevlaence of Child Abuse and Neglect: 1988 (Revised Report).* Rockville, MD: Westat Inc; 1991.

57. Klevens J, Whitaker DJ. Primary prevention of child physical abuse and neglect: gaps and promising directions. *Child Maltreat.* 2007;12(4):364-377.

58. Greeley CS. The future of child maltreatment prevention. *Pediatrics.* 2009;123(3):904-905.

59. Krugman SD, Lane WG, Walsh CM. Update on child abuse prevention. *Curr Opin Pediatr.* 2007;19(6):711-718.

60. Reynolds AJ, Mathieson LC, Topitzes JW. Do early childhood interventions prevent child maltreatment? *Child Maltreat.* 2009;14(2):182-206.

61. Wekerle C. The dollars and senselessness in failing to prioritize childhood maltreatment prevention. *Child Abuse Negl.* 2011;35(3):159-161.

62. Wurtele SK. Preventing sexual abuse of children in the twenty-first century: preparing for challenges and opportunities. *J Child Sex Abus.* 2009;18(1):1-18.

63. Zielinski DS, Bradshaw CP. Ecological influences on the sequelae of child maltreatment: a review of the literature. *Child Maltreat.* 11(1):49-62.

64. Stouthamer-Loeber M, Loeber R, Wei E, Farrington DP, Wikströrm PO. Risk and promotive effects in the explanation of persistent serious delinquency in boys. *J Consult Clin Psychol.* 2002;70(1):111-123.

65. Centers for Disease Control and Prevention. Preventing child maltreatment through the promotion of safe, stable, and nurturing relationships between children and caregivers. Centers for Disease Control and Prevention Web site. http://www.cdc.gov/violenceprevention/pdf/CM_Strategic_Direction--Long-a.pdf. Accessed March 24, 2015.

66. National Scientific Council on the Developing Child. *Young Children Develop in an Environment of Relationships: Working Paper No. 1.* Cambridge, MA: Center on the Developing Child at Harvard University; 2004. Center on the Developing Child at Harvard University Web site. http://developingchild.harvard.edu/index.php/resources/reports_and_working_papers/working_papers/wp1/. Accessed March 24, 2015.

67. Committee on Integrating the Science of Early Childhood Development, Youth and Families Board on Children. Shonkoff JP, Phillips DA, eds. *From Neurons to Neighborhoods: The Science of Early Childhood Development.* Washington, DC: National Academies Press; 2000.

68. Mercy JA, Saul J. Creating a healthier future through early interventions for children. *JAMA.* 2009;301(1):2262-2264.

69. Barnard KE, Solchany JE. Mothering. In: Bornstien MH, ed. *Being and Becoming a Parent.* Mahwah, NJ: Erlbaum; 2002:3-25. *Handbook of Parenting;* vol 3.

70. Ainsworth MD. Patterns of infant-mother attachments: antecedents and effects on development. *Bull N Y Acad Med.* 1985;61(9):792-812.

71. Bowlby J. Developmental psychiatry comes of age. *Am J Psychiatry.* 1988;145(1):1-10.

72. Antonovsky A. How the sense of coherence develops over the lifespan. In: Antonovsky A, ed. *Unraveling the Mystery Of Health: How People Manage Stress and Stay Well.* San Francisco, CA: Jossey-Bass; 1987:89-127.

73. Seeman TE, Singer B, Horwitz R, McEwen BS. The price of adaptation–allostatic load and its health consequences: McArthur studies of successful aging. *Arch Intern Med.* 1997;157(19):2259-2268.

74. Waters E, Kondo-Ikemura K, Posada G, Richters JE. Learning to love: mechanisms and milestones. In: Gunnar M, Sroufe L, eds. *Self Processes and Development.* Hillsdale, NJ: Erlbaum; 1991:217-255. Minnesota Symposia on Child Psychology; vol 23.

75. Crouch JL, Milner JS, Thomsen C. Childhood physical abuse, early social support, and risk for maltreatment: current social support as a mediator of risk for child physical abuse. *Child Abuse Negl.* 2001;25(1):93-107.

76. Mikton C, Butchart A. Child maltreatment prevention: a systematic review of reviews. *Bull World Health Organ.* 2009;87(5):353-361.

The findings and conclusions in this chapter are those of the authors and do not necessarily represent the official position of the Centers for Disease Control and Prevention.

Chapter 2

A Conceptual Framework for Exploring the Social Determinants of Child Maltreatment

Marilyn Metzler, RN, MPH
Joanne Klevens, MD, MPH, PhD
Jim Mercy, PhD
Janet Saul, PhD

Introduction

Given the overall vulnerability of children, the number of children affected by child maltreatment, and the potential impact on life-long health and well-being, the prevention of child maltreatment is an important public health goal.[1] To be successful in this effort, there is a need to understand not only overall risk for maltreatment but also how risk for maltreatment is distributed—why are some children at greater risk than others? For example, children in households with low incomes experience maltreatment at more than 5 times the average rate, including being more than 3 times as likely to experience physical, sexual, or emotional maltreatment and nearly 7 times as likely to be neglected.[2] Can these findings be explained by parental/caregiver education level or limited parenting skills? Perhaps in some cases, but the fact that children living in families with low incomes are much more likely to experience maltreatment also raises important questions about how the conditions in which some parents and caregivers are raising children may contribute to greater risk for harm. It is known that education, housing, and other social conditions increase risk and that these do not act in isolation. Understanding how these conditions are distributed, including how they cluster and interact, is critical if the goal of preventing child maltreatment is to be achieved.

The relationship between the social context and health has been the subject of a rapidly growing body of evidence over the past 2 decades. This inquiry has shed light on how social conditions impact health and how health is differentially distributed between groups according to their location on social hierarchies. Generally referred to as the social determinants of health, this research has led to increased understanding of the need to address social and economic conditions if many public health goals, including the prevention of child maltreatment, are to be attained.

This chapter provides a framework for understanding the relationship between social determinants and risk for child maltreatment, with an emphasis on the differential access to conditions needed for health that may increase risk in families that experience social and economic disadvantages. Public health actions to address these risks are discussed, with examples from communities provided to illustrate the potential to improve conditions for health and safety for all children and their families.

Social Determinants of Health Inequities

A critical mass of evidence demonstrates persistent gradient relationships between social and economic conditions and virtually all health outcomes, even after controlling for individual behavior and access to health care. These relationships have been observed within and across countries. In the United States, a meta-analysis of the relationship between social conditions and adult all-cause mortality estimated that, in 2000, approximately 245 000 deaths were attributable to low education, 176 000 to racial segregation, 162 000 to low social support, 133 000 to individual-level poverty, 119 000 to income inequality, and 39 000 to area-level poverty.[3] An examination of trends in black-white standardized mortality ratios using 2002 data estimated that 83 570 excess deaths among African Americans could be prevented each year if the black-white mortality gap could be eliminated.[4] (See Braveman et al[5] for an overview of US findings.)

Exposure to unhealthy conditions is particularly harmful in-utero and during early childhood, and the impact can extend throughout the life-course, increasing risks for premature morbidity and mortality.[6,7] In a study of adults reporting exposure to childhood adversities, including child maltreatment and exposure to violence in the home, analyses capitalizing on the National Death Index revealed that participants reporting high exposure died, on average, nearly 20 years earlier than those reporting no exposure.[8] Hypotheses explaining the relations between social and economic conditions and health include limited access to material resources needed for health, eg, affordable, healthy food and safe neighborhoods; stress caused by lack of access to these resources; stress caused by social exclusion and other forms of discrimination, eg, racism; and interactions among these. (For more in-depth discussions of social determinants of health see Braveman et al,[9] Adler & Stewart.[10])

A Framework for Action

To provide a comprehensive understanding of how social determinants may impact health, the World Health Organization's Commission on Social Determinants of Health (CSDH), a global collaboration of policymakers, researchers, and civil society members, proposed the following framework to synthesize relevant evidence, theories, and pathways in order to support the development of effective actions.[11]

The CSDH framework draws on many models that preceded it, including the social-ecological model (SEM). Like the CSDH, the SEM situates health outcomes within a series of nested relationships and acknowledges the complex interplay between the inner and outer spheres; however, the CSDH framework provides greater specificity to inform more in-depth explorations of the mechanisms and pathways through which broader influences contribute to differential exposure, vulnerability, and inequitable outcomes. In this framework, outcomes are examined by comparing the health of more and less socially advantaged populations. The CSDH framework seeks to explain how the differential impact of structural policies and processes influence socioeconomic position based on race, ethnicity, gender, and other social categories and how this positioning creates vulnerability through limited access to living and working conditions needed for health. This distinction between structural and intermediate determinants is critical for developing plausible hypotheses leading to effective actions. For example, interventions addressing intermediate determinants may improve the situations of those currently living in vulnerable conditions, but addressing the structural determinants that give rise to these conditions in the first place is necessary to assure sustainable opportunities for health and safety. As such, expectations for outcomes must be reasonably based on the level of the intervention. Finally, and importantly, the CSDH framework accounts for human agency in the generation of structures, policies, and processes that create and distribute life chances and opportunities for health. The distinction between the determinants, eg, macro-level policies, and the processes that give rise to their distribution, eg, social and political power, is critical for development of effective actions to redress inequities.[12]

Critiques of the framework include the absence of overarching determinants, eg, racism, sexism, and classism, that not only inform how particular policies may be differentially implemented based on race, gender, and/or income, but also the fact that discrimination may be imbedded in actual policies or social and political processes.[13,14]

The following is a brief overview of the major elements of the CSDH framework:

Structural Determinants: Socioeconomic Political Context

Includes the broad array of structural, cultural, and functional aspects of how societies are organized—governance structures; macroeconomic policies; social policies, eg, labor market and housing; public policies, including education, health, and social protection; and cultural and societal values about children and the role of women. These aspects cannot be measured at the individual level. Policies at this level would seek to maximize health and life opportunities through the fair distribution of a society's resources to all its members.

Structural Determinants: Socioeconomic Position

Describes how structural policies and processes interact to effectively assign socioeconomic position based on social characteristics, eg, race/ethnicity or gender, through more or less access to essential resources, including education, occupation, and income. Policies at this level would seek to minimize the systematic assignment of socioeconomic position based on social characteristics as well as limit the inequitable burden of macro policies on members of society based on hierarchies.

Intermediary Determinants

Includes material circumstances, psychosocial, behavioral, and biological characteristics. Broadly encompassing living and working conditions, the availability of food, etcetera, this element also includes the health system, which has an independent and interacting effect on health. Policies at this level would seek to limit the effects of excess vulnerability and exposure to existing conditions that disproportionately impact groups disadvantaged by social status or socioeconomic position.

Cross-cutting Determinants, Including Social Capital and Social Cohesion

This element acknowledges the role of people in the shaping of policies and processes that effectively determine how societies are organized. The CSDH emphasized the need to include groups historically and currently excluded from decision-making processes that impact their health and life opportunities and placed special emphasis on empowerment theory and models where collective action is informed by a human rights and social justice approach.

Framing the Social Determinants of Child Maltreatment

The CSDH framework is a useful tool for exploring contextual conditions empirically associated with child maltreatment and the potential mechanisms through which these conditions, and their differential distribution, might contribute to increased risk for some children. It is important to note that many of the conditions described throughout this chapter are related both to children at risk of maltreatment as well as the perpetrators, reflecting an accumulation of risk across his/her life-course.

Intermediary Determinants: Living and Working Conditions

The choices parents make in caring for their children are shaped by the choices they have, including access to adequate income, stable jobs, secure housing, high quality affordable child care, high quality schools, and safe neighborhoods. Limited access to these resources can place undue stress on parents and contribute to increased rates of child maltreatment.

Living in Poverty or With a Low Family Income

Low income has long been associated with child maltreatment, and most consistently with child neglect.[15] Living in poverty and low-income conditions might contribute to child maltreatment through multiple mechanisms, with one or more mechanisms impacting families at any given point in time. Insufficient income may determine limited or differential access to resources or supports that could directly prevent child maltreatment, eg, access to quality child care might prevent supervisory neglect, or buffer the impact of other risk factors, such as opportunities for recreation or family vacations. Additionally, low income might limit access to other important resources for childrearing, such as family planning resources, mental health or substance abuse treatment, reliable transportation or resources to adequately heat or cool the home. Insufficient income may also limit access to safe and stable housing, sufficient and nutritious foods, and family-friendly work schedules. Lower-income working families often spend more than half of their income on housing, leaving less money to purchase important items such as health care and health insurance.

Insufficient income may also contribute to child maltreatment by acting as a psychological stressor. Descriptions of people who are near poor show how parents struggle to balance work and family and end up with little time to positively interact with and monitor their children,[16] both of which increase risk for neglect. Inadequate financial resources may generate stress for multiple reasons, including a mismatch between aspirations and opportunities, as a contributor to perceptions of being looked down on or devalued, or because of decreased control over life and work. Rising inequality may lead to longer working hours and increased debt because of status competition, ie, the pressure to "keep up with the Joneses."[17] Families living in poverty or with low incomes have fewer assets to serve as a buffer during periods of unexpected financial hardship (**Box 2-1**).

Adult poverty is often preceded by childhood poverty, which can lead to child maltreatment in another way. A parent who was exposed to poverty in early childhood, especially when compounded by other adverse conditions such as maltreatment and other forms of family violence, may have suffered "toxic stress."[18] Toxic stress during sensitive periods of early growth can impact brain structure and function, recalibrating the threshold for activating the stress response system. These stress-related changes can affect attention, decision-making abilities, impulse control, and emotional regulation that contribute to greater future susceptibility for emotional instability, anxiety and depressive disorders, learning disabilities, substance abuse, and aggression.[19]

Work

Access to a stable job that pays a living wage and allows employees some degree of control is important for securing family income, reducing stress, and providing adults the opportunity to participate in an important societal role. Families who are "near poor" have been characterized by working parents (sometimes in 2 and even 3 jobs), long commutes, and being uninsured or underinsured.[16] Constantly changing shifts increases risk for neglect, selection of inappropriate care givers, and can impact the ability to monitor and supervise children, making them more difficult to care for.[20]

Box 2-1. Raising Children Facing Multiple Hardships

Imagine a single mother working 50-60 hours a week as a nurse to support her 2 children. Imagine that she is in a car accident and unable to work for a year because of severe damage to her knee. With her loss of income she is unable to pay for the delivery of heating oil for her mobile home. She sleeps with her children in one room with 2 electric heaters, but the pipes freeze and then break, causing water damage to the carpet and floor. This family is under significant stress—they are now unable to shower or wash clothes, the kids struggle to keep up with school, and putting food on the table is a daily challenge. Eventually the children go stay with family and friends while their home is being repaired and heat restored. The family is now deep in debt and the mother is considering moving herself and her children into her parents' home, which is small and already crowded. Other family members resent the burden this places on the aging parents, and the children are upset because the move across town means they will have to change schools. This mother is clearly trying to do her best for her family, but even one unexpected hardship can destabilize families with few assets and increase the challenges of providing safe, stable, and nurturing care for children. Structural determinants contribute to parental stress in families such as this one by requiring a 60-hour work week to support a family while not making enough to build wealth to cover emergency expenses.

Unemployment is also a risk factor for child neglect,[21] parental physical aggression toward a child,[22] and physical abuse, especially by male perpetrators.[23] Chronic unemployment would likely contribute to child maltreatment in many of the same ways as low income, eg, increased stress and greater material hardship. Sudden job loss can also create additional risks for perpetrating child maltreatment. For example, in the case of male perpetrators of physical abuse, unemployed fathers or surrogates may be tasked with child care, increasing their contact with children. Because the role as provider is so strongly linked to masculinity, unemployed men may reassert their status through power and coercion.[23]

Neighborhood

In addition to a family's income level, one of the most consistent contextual factors associated with child maltreatment is living in neighborhoods of concentrated disadvantage.[24,25] These include neighborhoods characterized by high poverty rates, high unemployment rates, and low property values. Neighborhoods of concentrated disadvantage have fewer resources and services, leading to more stressors and less support for parents—both being risk factors for child maltreatment.

Residential instability is higher in neighborhoods of concentrated disadvantage and has been consistently associated with child maltreatment.[26-28] Whether a direct result of low income or its correlate, residential instability makes it difficult for families to develop and maintain a local support network. Weakness or lack of social support is a consistent risk factor for child maltreatment.[15,22] High turnover in a community may also contribute to lack of solidarity and trust in one's neighbors, a characteristic commonly referred to as social capital and associated with child neglect.[29]

In sum, multiple social and economic conditions contribute to increased risk for child maltreatment. The stress and challenges associated with being a parent intensify in neighborhoods of concentrated disadvantage with many other adults struggling financially and coping with alcohol and drug abuse, family members convicted of crimes, exposure to violence, under-resourced schools, limited job prospects, etc. Parents in these neighborhoods face substantial challenges to supervising and protecting their children.

Parental and caregiver access to time and resources are needed to reduce these risks and to provide safe, stable, nurturing environments for children. Given the strong relationship between living and working conditions and risk for child maltreatment, it seems reasonable to ask, how is access to these conditions achieved and why are some families less likely than others to have the opportunity to raise their children in healthy environments?

Socioeconomic Position

To comprehend how families access opportunities for healthy living and working conditions, which the previous section showed are associated with child maltreatment, it is important to understand how socioeconomic position is patterned in the United States. This includes understanding the underlying distribution of education, occupation, and income that effectively determines where groups land on social hierarchies that strongly correlate with race/ethnicity, class, gender, and other social characteristics and that are associated with multiple health inequities, including child maltreatment. For example:

Education: People who live below the poverty line are twice as likely to not complete high school than are those who live above the poverty line; black non-Latino, American Indian/ Alaska Native, and Latino students are at much greater risk of noncompletion than are white, non-Latino, and Asian/Pacific Islander students.[30] Similar patterns based on family income and race/ethnicity are seen with college enrollment[31] and college completion.[32]

Occupation: Workers in minority racial or ethnic groups are overrepresented in the service sector and low-paying jobs. The working poor, ie, workers who have been employed for at least 27 weeks and live below the federal poverty level, are disproportionately comprised of racial minorities, with blacks or Latinos twice as likely to be among the working poor than are whites or Asian Americans.[33] Lack of work is differentially distributed by education and race/ethnicity. Adults without a high school diploma are nearly 3 times as likely to be unemployed as college graduates; Latinos and African Americans are far more likely to be unemployed as are Asians and whites.[34]

Income level and wealth: In the section on living and working conditions we suggested different ways of how living with a low income might increase the risk for child maltreatment. In this section we describe how some families might end up at the low end of the income hierarchy.

Education level can improve employment opportunities, but it is not equally protective. At all levels of educational attainment, African Americans and Latinos earn less than whites; African Americans and Latinos with Master's degrees have lifetime earnings lower than whites with Bachelor's degrees.[35] Women make less than men at every level of educational attainment, even when they work as much as men. Overall, women who work full-time, full-year earn 19 percent less than men; at similar education levels, and in similar occupational categories, eg, service, managerial, executive, and professional positions, women earn 24% to 27% less than men.[36] The gender wage disparity is greatest for women of color: in 2010, the most recent year for which data are available, the wages of black women and Latino women were 64% and 55% respectively, compared to those of white men.[37] In 2013, the official poverty rate was 14.5% overall, with blacks and Latinos being 2.5-3 times more likely to be poor than whites or Asian Americans; children are more likely to live in poverty than are people aged 18 to 64.[38] However, living in poverty is not an equal experience for all children in poverty because some children are more poor than others: 36% of black children in poverty live in households with incomes *less than half* of the federal poverty line compared to white (30%) and Latino (30%) children.[39] The median wealth of white households is 20 times that of black households and 18 times that of Latino households.[40]

Persistent patterns based on race/ethnicity, class, and gender are seen across opportunities for education, work, and income—essential resources needed for healthy living—but identifying the distributions is not enough. Understanding *how* socioeconomic hierarchies are created is critical if effective actions to improve these distributions are to be developed. The CSDH framework encourages stepping back at this point to examine how structural policies and processes interact to effectively determine these patterns.

Structural Determinants: Socioeconomic and Political Contexts

Reducing inequitable risks for child maltreatment requires understanding the structural drivers of educational, occupational, and income levels in order to develop effective responses. A full exploration of all potential contributors to the distributions is beyond the scope of this chapter, but even a cursory look at a few structural domains in the CSDH framework—education, employment, economic, housing, and justice policies—sheds critical light on systematic and interacting policies and processes that may explain why some children and their families are less likely to have the resources needed for health and how this may create differential risk for maltreatment.

Education Policies

In the United States all children are guaranteed the right to an education through high school, but this is not an equal-opportunity experience. Black and Latino students, who are at greatest risk of school noncompletion, are more likely to attend racially segregated, high-poverty schools.[41] In 2005, school districts with the highest concentration of poor students received, on average, $938 less per pupil in state and local money than low-poverty school districts, a gap that was essentially unchanged, given inflation, from 1999.[42] High-poverty schools tend to have a less stable and less qualified teaching staff; a 2004 United States Department of Education report showed that in schools where 75% or more of the students were low income, there were 3 times as many uncertified or out-of-field teachers in both English and science.[41] Higher per-student spending is linked to higher achievement through the provision of better physical conditions, more qualified teachers, smaller classroom sizes, and more consistency and order in school learning environments.[43]

For students who do complete high school and seek postsecondary education, the rising cost of college makes this aspiration available to fewer and fewer. From 1982 to 2007 college tuition and fees increased 439% while median family income rose 147% during the same period.[31] Student borrowing has more than doubled in the last decade, and, on average, students from lower-income families get smaller grants from the colleges they attend than students from more affluent families.[31] College has become disproportionately unaffordable for low- and middle-income families; for the 2007-2008 school year, net college costs for families in the lowest income quintile represented 55% of median family income, compared to 9% for families in the highest income quintile.[31] And the situation is likely to get worse: at least 28 states cut funding for public colleges and universities and/or substantially increased college tuitions to balance their 2009 fiscal year budgets.[32]

In sum, funding decisions have led to fewer educational opportunities for minorities and those who are poor. Level of education may contribute to child maltreatment through several avenues. It may, for example, reduce access to knowledge that would enhance parental practices that contribute to optimal child development. In addition, lack of education is associated with lower income and could indirectly contribute to familial stress in making ends meet and thereby increase chances of physical abuse or neglect.

Labor Market

There are many reasons for work-related variations, including racist employment practices. For example, in a study of résumés submitted through online job boards, researchers found that, after controlling for education and experience, people with "white" names, eg, Carrie or Kirsten, got about 1 callback per 10 résumés, compared with people with "black" names, eg, Aisha or Tamika, who got 1 callback per 15 résumés.[44] Another study found that employers in the United States are more likely to hire a white person with a felony conviction than an African American with no felony convictions, even when both applicants have otherwise comparable credentials.[45] For African Americans even an advanced degree is not protective against employment-related racial bias. In an in-depth analysis of grant data from the United States National Institutes of Health (NIH), black PhD scientists were less likely to receive NIH funding for a research idea than a white scientist from a similar institution with the same research record.[46]

Unfair labor market practices can contribute to lower family income through reduced ability to secure employment as well as increased risk for unemployment. Both low income and unemployment are associated with increased risk for child maltreatment.

Economic

Managing financial resources, no matter the level of income or wealth, is a critical activity for individuals and families. Access to banking services at a federally insured institution provides people with the opportunity to conduct basic financial transactions, save for emergencies and long-term security needs, and access credit on affordable terms; however, many people in low-to-moderate income households do not have access to mainstream financial products, such as bank accounts and low-cost loans, reducing opportunities to build credit histories and achieve financial security such as building wealth or investing in assets. A 2009 study by the Federal Deposit Insurance Corporation (FDIC) found that 1 in 4 US households are currently unbanked, ie, no one in the household currently had a checking or savings account, or under-banked, ie, have had a checking or savings account but also rely on alternative financial services; low-income and minority households were disproportionately represented in the findings.[47] Most of these households used alternative financial services (AFS) instead, including pawn shops, payday loans, and rent-to-own agreements. AFS services are not cheap; for example, a payday loan of $325 with a term of 2 weeks and an average interest rate of 16% costs the typical customer $52, translating into an Annual Percentage Rate (APR) of 400%.[48] But AFS are more geographically accessible in predominantly low-income and minority neighborhoods, while traditional banks are more accessible in predominantly white neighborhoods.[49] In a national survey of banks' efforts to serve unbanked and under-banked individuals and families, banks stated that the primary reason they are less likely to provide services to these populations was concern about lack of profitability.[50]

Studies show low-income families may be further limited in their ability to build savings because means-tested income transfer programs, such as Temporary Assistance for Needy Families, Supplemental Nutrition Assistance Program, and Supplemental Security Income, discourage the accumulation of financial assets by requiring households to spend down or keep their financial assets below asset limits in order to be eligible for transfer benefits.[51,52]

Housing

The 2008 subprime mortgage and foreclosure crisis has impacted Americans across the socioeconomic spectrum, but those at the lower ends of social hierarchies experienced the greatest impacts of all. It is now well-documented that subprime mortgages were disproportionately marketed in communities of color; African Americans and Latinos were nearly twice as likely to have lost their homes to foreclosures compared to whites.[53]

An analysis of 2006 Home Mortgage Disclosure Act (HMDA) data for 100 metropolitan areas across the country documented striking racial disparities: in more than 70% of the communities, African American and Latino consumers were more likely to receive high-risk, high-cost loans than were white consumers *within their same income groups*. Similar patterns were observed between Latinos and Whites in 40 of the communities.[54] A companion study of 2007 HMDA data revealed similar mortgage lending inequities by gender, race, and class: in 84% of metropolitan areas examined, middle- to upper-income African American women were at least twice as likely to receive high-cost loans than were their white female counterparts, and in nearly 62% of metro areas, Latina women were at least twice as likely to receive high-cost loans as white females.[55]

High-cost loans translate into higher payments to lenders and reduced buying power, making home ownership in low-income neighborhoods of concentrated disadvantage the only option for many families and contributing to residential segregation by race/ethnicity in many US communities. Given the magnitude of wealth lost due to mortgage lending disparities and increased rates of foreclosure, excessive economic burden has been experienced by entire communities where families of color live and raise their children.

Housing insecurity is not limited to those with mortgages. The United States Department of Housing and Urban Development has established a 30 percent of net monthly income standard for housing affordability.[56] Yet low-income families who rent often pay far more than this to keep a roof over their heads; more than 5.6 million of the nation's lowest-income households are paying more than 50% of their income for rent.[57] Being behind on rent or mortgage correlates strongly with negative health outcomes for both mothers and children,[57] including increased risk for child maltreatment, possibly due to stress from not being able to pay the rent; eviction; doubling up, ie, multiple families living in one household[58]; or becoming homeless.[59] Families who are behind on rent or mortgage must make trade-offs among household expenses, including whether to pay rent instead of paying for utilities, food, medical care or other life necessities. In some housing assistance programs, having utilities shut off is automatic grounds for eviction.[57]

In sum, discriminatory mortgage lending practices or disproportionate housing costs relative to income can lead to housing insecurity. As noted in the section on living conditions, housing insecurity is independently associated with out-of-home placement of children and may also lead to increased risk of child maltreatment through increased psychological stress on families.

Justice

Communities of color are disproportionately affected through the massive increases in incarceration rates that have occurred in the United States over the past 3 decades. For example, although African Americans and whites have comparable rates of illicit drug use, African Americans are sentenced to prison for drug offenses at a rate of 34 times that of whites, African Americans comprise only 14% of regular users but make up 37% of those arrested for drug offenses, and drug possession as a first-time offense is more likely to result in incarceration for African Americans and Latinos than whites.[60] Time served in federal prison for drug offenses committed by African Americans is almost as long (58.7 months) as time served for violent offenses committed by whites (61.7 months).[60] If current trends continue 1 of every 3 African American males and 1 of every 6 Latino males born today can expect to go to prison in his lifetime, compared to 1 in 17 white males. The overall figures for women are lower, but the patterns are similar.[61]

The American Bar Association Standards for Criminal Justice defines a collateral sanction as "any legal penalty, disability, or disadvantage...that is imposed on a person automatically upon that person's conviction for a felony, misdemeanor or other offense, even if it is not included in the sentence"[62(p1)] and has identified hundreds of collateral sanctions, including limited access to employment, denial of public benefits, and loss of voting rights.[60] Felony disenfranchisement laws, which restrict the right to vote following criminal conviction, were first implemented in 1865 but are still on the books in some form in nearly all states. They range from no withdrawal of franchisement (2 states) to permanent disenfranchisement, unless clemency or specific government approval is received (10 states).[63] More than 5 million US citizens are not allowed to vote because of a felony conviction; 13% of all African American men have lost the right to vote, a rate that is 7 times the national average.[59]

Differential incarceration rates and resulting sanctions reduce opportunities to create stable, 2-parent families[64] and limit opportunities for successful reentry to community life following imprisonment. Both conditions may impact family income.

Complex, Interacting Obstacles Cannot be Solved by Families on Their Own

As seen earlier in this chapter, the literature shows associations between intermediary determinants, ie, living and working conditions, and risk for child maltreatment. The CSDH framework is useful for exploring how structural determinants may increase risk for child maltreatment through their effect on the intermediary determinants. For example, fewer educational opportunities may lead to lower family income, a known risk factor for child maltreatment. Unfair labor market practices can also contribute to lower family income through reduced ability to secure employment as well as increased risk for unemployment, which is independently associated with increased risk for child maltreatment. Housing insecurity resulting from discriminatory mortgage lending practices or disproportionate housing costs relative to income can increase psychological stress on families, which is also a known risk factor for child maltreatment.[58,59]

Using the CSDH framework, some paths to increased risk for maltreatment, such as low family income, are more readily apparent and clear cut. Other paths can be explored from a theoretical perspective, for example, the relationship between differential incarceration rates and lower income or the additive effect of concentrated neighborhood disadvantage where an entire community may have fewer economic opportunities or limited access to important resources, such as secure financial institutions. Complex, interacting policies and processes systematically and repeatedly create barriers for some groups over others in the ability to access life opportunities and essential resources needed for health. Understanding how these policies and processes effectively determine socioeconomic position and how they cluster based on, for example, race/ethnicity, is of critical importance in the quest to address child maltreatment.

The excessive stress experienced by families and communities dealing with several or all of these compounding obstacles no doubt places children at greater risk for maltreatment. Clearly, these societal obstacles cannot be solved by families on their own. Addressing these structural determinants may seem beyond the scope of public health; however, if the mission to eliminate health inequities, including in child maltreatment, is to be accomplished, the boundaries of research and practice roles must be expanded to address societal barriers inhibiting opportunities for health.

Public Health Role Addressing the Social Determinants of Child Maltreatment

Historically, public health has made a difference in the quality of life for Americans through the application of its fundamental problem-solving capacity.[65] Public health actions such as water quality control, immunization programs, and food inspection have prevented many deaths and illnesses. These successes exemplify what is possible as a result of organized efforts based on scientific and technical knowledge, combined with concern for the well-being of all members of society. Addressing social determinants of child maltreatment will require building upon and expanding the traditional problem-solving methods that public health has used to address other pressing public health problems. There are at least 4 key areas where public health can make substantive contributions to reducing child maltreatment by addressing the social determinants of health. One is to use the information we have to develop and implement evidence-informed strategies, including policies and programs, which could improve social and economic conditions for children and their families. The second is to develop partnerships with key sectors and organizations in order to develop and implement the most relevant strategies. The third is to monitor social determinants, and their differential distribution, that are important contributors to child maltreatment to see if our efforts are having any effects. The fourth is to undertake epidemiologic and social science research, including identifying and evaluating the full range of social and economic policies that could improve living conditions and life chances for children and families, in order to better understand the relationship between structural determinants and child maltreatment, the interactions between multiple determinants, and the pathways by which they contribute to child maltreatment. Each of these roles is linked to the others. Here each of these public health roles is considered in more depth.

Policies and Programs

The previous section on structural determinants discussed how policies can create the unequal distribution of income, wealth, employment, and safe and stable housing, but understanding the role of the social environment in shaping policy is also critical. For example, it is necessary to understand how specific interests and influences may hinder or enhance the adoption of a policy, what the existing organizational and community capacity is to implement a specific policy, how that capacity can be enhanced, and how broader political or social processes affect the dissemination and implementation of a policy.[66]

As noted by the CSDH, policy choices are guided by values, which may be implicit or explicit.[11] Current values-based framings for addressing the social determinants of health include a social justice approach, human rights, and human development, among others. In considering how to create equitable conditions for health, the CSDH considered the following approaches:

— Policies that focus solely on those who are most disadvantaged, eg, antipoverty programs. One problem with this approach is the lack of an explicit value on eliminating poverty vs. only ameliorating some of its impact. Also, these policies often exclude those who are near poor.

— Policies that seek to close the health gaps between high/low socioeconomic groups although this approach can obscure what is happening to those in the middle, eg, those who are near poor.

— Policies that address health across the gradient—a population health approach. The problem with this approach is that it may not close high/low gaps and, in some cases, may even increase gaps.

After exploring the options, the CSDH ultimately decided that a series of strategies across all 3 approaches is required to achieve health equity. The CSDH developed a useful model that provides a typology of entry points for addressing social determinants of health. This model can be used to map out policy actions relevant for addressing child maltreatment by addressing the social determinants of health. This model identifies 5 major options for addressing social determinants. The first domain of policy options are those that attempt to alter patterns of social stratification by reducing inequalities in power, prestige, income, and wealth that are linked to different socioeconomic positions. The second domain includes policy options that attempt to decrease exposures to health-damaging factors suffered by people in disadvantaged positions. The third domain involves policies that lessen the impact of health-damaging conditions that people living with disadvantages face. The fourth domain comprises those policies designed to intervene via the health system to mitigate the unequal consequences of ill-health and further socioeconomic degradation among disadvantaged people once they become ill; and the final domain includes those policies addressing macro-social conditions, such as social cohesion or social capital.[11] These 5 domains embrace policies that address both structural and intermediary determinants of health. Another dimension along which these policies can be distinguished is whether they are universal or targeted in nature. In universal policies, the entire population of a nation or region is the beneficiary, whereas in targeted or selective policies, eligibility for the benefits of the policy is limited to those groups deemed to be deserving of the particular benefit. Research suggests that both approaches are needed to reduce inequities in risk for violence at the neighborhood level.[67]

Partnering

A now massive literature, viewed through various lenses, including disease and injury, risk factors, populations, and geography, among others, has documented the pervasive and persistent nature of health inequities. Like other major public health challenges, these inequities are rooted in the distant past but impact the lives of current and future generations, playing out in the public eye and impacting a vast array of stakeholders. Solutions lie beyond the control of any single authority; tackling these inequities and achieving true health equity will only come through leadership—societal, organizational, and individual—that embraces the powerful integration of science, practice, and policy to create lasting change.[68]

Increasingly, public health agencies and other organizations are bringing attention to the need to not only document but to address health inequities. For example, Healthy People 2020 includes "achieve health equity, eliminate disparities" among its 4 over-arching goals and has a new focus area on social determinants of health[69]; the National Association of County and City Health Officials' now 12-year-old Health Equity and Social Justice unit leads multiple health equity initiatives for its constituents[70]; and many local and state health departments now have health equity units. Many of these efforts include the development of multi-sectoral partnerships, some of which have led to the adoption of an equity focus by other agencies or organizations. For example, in King County, Washington, a cross-sector partnership, including leadership from the Seattle-King County health department, was convened to bring the science of early childhood development to King County neighborhoods to promote optimal conditions for health for all children.[71] The work of the partnership revealed an array of policy and structural barriers, including disparities in access to education and employment, that inhibited achieving the desired goals and that ultimately led to the adoption of legislation by King County that established definitions and implementation steps related to the fair and just principle to be addressed through the 2010-2014 county-wide strategic plan.[72] This legislation requires regular assessment and reporting of practices and policies to improve fairness in county governmental agencies and specifically requires strategies to include participation in the implementation of the legislation by populations that experience the greatest inequities.

In its 2008 report the CSDH provided multiple recommendations related to the inclusion of marginalized groups in efforts to address the root causes of health inequities. Specifically, the Commission recommended that "National government acknowledges, legitimizes, and supports marginalized groups, in particular Indigenous Peoples, in policy, legislation, and programmes that empower people to represent their needs, claims, and rights."[73(p.159)]

The inclusion of marginalized groups is consistent with a social justice approach to improving conditions for health so that those who experience the greatest inequities can participate in societal decision-making processes that effectively determine their life chances and access to opportunities for health. Evidence suggests inclusion, especially in regards to political participation, is fundamentally linked to health, as evidenced, for example, by the positive association between voter participation and self-rated health.[74] A systematic review of political systems and health inequities suggested that political incorporation of subordinated racial/ethnic, indigenous, and gender groups reduced health gaps,[75] including in the United States in the 2 decades following the 1960s "War on Poverty" and the enactment of civil rights legislation.[76]

Public health has long worked in and with communities to improve health, most often through collaborative efforts focused on implementing programs aimed at reducing risks or increasing protective behaviors; however, growing evidence strongly suggests the need to expand the relationships with communities as more than recipients of programs but also as equitable and capable partners in the goal to improve social and economic conditions that underlie health inequities.

Monitoring

The importance of monitoring the social determinants of child maltreatment lies in the need to know and to be able to document whether efforts to address social and economic conditions are actually contributing to improve conditions and to reduce child maltreatment. Establishing or enhancing surveillance systems with social indicators in this arena builds a foundation for all of the other efforts by grounding them in timely and useful information that can be efficiently communicated to policymakers and the public. Developing viable monitoring strategies, for example, will enable federal, state, and local governments and communities to be more accountable for the impact of programs and policies intended to address the relationship between social determinants and child maltreatment. Both the public and private sectors increasingly set and monitor goals for the many programs and policies that are administered across these sectors. This emphasis on accountability requires timely, reliable, and useful data be collected systematically and on an ongoing basis.

There are several conditions and processes that would be especially valuable to monitor and address given understanding of the science linking social determinants to child maltreatment. For example, as noted throughout this chapter, there is a strong association between family income and risk for child maltreatment; therefore, monitoring social policies, eg, minimum income wage laws, and social processes, eg, the impact, including the differential impact, of recessions, on family income are important public health assessment activities that could provide critical information to guide the development of interventions. One valuable approach is to incorporate these indicators into child maltreatment surveillance systems for the ongoing and systematic collection, analysis, and interpretation of data on child maltreatment. While useful surveillance systems for child maltreatment are currently limited, options exist for enhancing other systems that collect data on the conditions in which children live. For example, recent measures of food insecurity and housing insecurity developed as an optional module for the Centers for Disease Control and Prevention's Behavioral Risk Factor Surveillance System[77] could, if routinely used by all states and territories, provide annual national, state, and county estimates of financial stresses reported by respondents with children.

Another approach to achieve better monitoring may be to incorporate or encourage the use of indicators that are used by many states and communities to track progress on issues they wish to change. The American Community Survey (ACS), a project of the United States Census Bureau, is a nationwide annual survey of 3 million respondents designed to provide communities with information about how they are changing.[78] The ACS collects data on age, race, income, employment, education, housing characteristics, and other measures and provides annual single- or multi-year estimates, depending on the size of a community, that could be used independently to assess and monitor local conditions for health or potentially in concert with data from other systems to more closely assess relationships between these conditions and health outcomes, including child maltreatment.

Public health could also partner with and learn from the hundreds of US communities that use publically available and/or locally collected data to assess and monitor community conditions across an array of domains to inform local decision-making processes. For example, since 1977, the Jacksonville Community Council, Inc. (JCCI), a nonpartisan civic organization, has developed annual reports on education, employment, housing, etc. Community members participate in surveys, research, and dialogue about findings to improve community conditions.[79] In addition to multi-domain reports, JCCI identifies a special topic each year to be explored more fully; past topics have included *Positive Development of Jacksonville's Children, Reducing Murder: A Community Response*, and *Beyond the Talk: Improving Race Relations*.[80]

Research

While the scientific literature suggests that many aspects of the social environment are associated with the risk of child maltreatment victimization and perpetration, there remains much that is not known that could potentially guide and refine future actions. Research in this area has focused largely on demonstrating simple associations between the social characteristics of a geographic area and child maltreatment, primarily using cross-sectional study designs and aggregate population data. Research is needed that helps to elucidate the causal pathways or mechanisms that help to explain these associations.[81] Prospective studies examining child maltreatment that incorporate key measures of the social environment would contribute greatly to this end. An emphasis should be placed on including structural determinants in research as the current literature primarily focuses on intermediate determinants. Theoretical models, such as those presented in this paper, that clearly conceptualize social conditions and their relationships to child maltreatment are important to guide the research into these mechanisms. Understanding these mechanisms will be extremely useful in the development of programs and policies to prevent child maltreatment through intervening upon the social environment. Research efforts should make use of multilevel or hierarchical modeling techniques to disentangle the influence that individual characteristics have on child maltreatment from those that are attributable to the social conditions and environments in which individuals live and interact.

Multifaceted community programs addressing child maltreatment that include at least one component addressing the social environment are rarely evaluated in a satisfactory way.[82] Given the expectation that ultimately the most effective approach to preventing child maltreatment will combine programs and policies targeting the social environment, it is important to understand and be able to disentangle the effects of these potentially complementary approaches in multi-faceted programs. Methodologies are also needed to evaluate policies for their potential impact on health. One such approach is the Health Impact Assessment (HIA), a tool that can be used by scientists, communities, and government and private sector policymakers to factor health and related costs into decision-making to improve health and enhance public well-being.[83] HIAs can support a "health in all policies" approach by examining federal educational, agricultural, transportation, and other policies and their impact on health.[84] For example, the Community Reinvestment Act, passed by Congress in 1977, was designed to reduce discriminatory credit practices against low-income neighborhoods, including encouraging commercial banks and savings associations to help meet the needs of borrowers in all segments of their communities; however, as seen earlier in this chapter, discriminatory lending practices plus reduced access to mainstream financial institutions still limit the opportunities of many families to access secure housing and safe neighborhoods, contributing to increased and differential risk for child maltreatment.

Another approach to advancing the knowledge base on preventing child maltreatment through a social determinants lens is to take advantage of "natural experiments" that are occurring in communities. The systems that influence living conditions are not stagnant. In fact, system and policy changes are fairly common. These changes provide an often untapped source for evaluating the effects on both intermediate determinants and the outcome of child maltreatment. In the area of youth violence, these types of evaluations have already been conducted to inform the prevention field. For example, Johnson[85] exploited quasi-random variation in the timing and scope of court-ordered school desegregation plans during the 1960s, 1970s, and 1980s to examine the long-term impacts on adult attainments among participants in the Panel Study of Income Dynamics. This study estimated that school desegregation led to reductions in class size and increases in per-pupil spending, and the accompanied increases in school quality resulted in significant improvements in educational attainment and adult earnings, reduced probability of incarceration, and improved adult health status for blacks with no effects, either positive or negative, on whites across each of these outcomes.

Unraveling the Complex Interplay of Social and Economic Determinants and Risks for Child Maltreatment

As described throughout this chapter risks for child maltreatment reflect poor living conditions for children *and* for their families. On a strict definition of child maltreatment the parent or caregiver is an abuser. While all who are entrusted with the care of children are ultimately responsible for their actions, when looked at from a social justice perspective, parents/caregivers at risk for maltreatment are frequently, and often systematically, also denied conditions and resources for health and a flourishing life. All children need and deserve safe, stable, and nurturing relationships as well as food, shelter, and healthy social interactions provided by parents and caregivers who also have these essential resources for themselves. The ultimate goal of eliminating child maltreatment, then, has to be framed as creating equitable conditions for health for all children and their parents and caregivers.

Raising children can be challenging in the best of circumstances; however, parents raising children in conditions described throughout this chapter face such excessive stress that it is amazing many do as well as they do. Children raised in these conditions are not only at increased risk for maltreatment but also have fewer opportunities to create better lives for the children they themselves may one day raise. Children living in these conditions, even if they are not being maltreated, are less likely to thrive and to reach their full human potential.

All parents and families may benefit from supportive interventions, such as parenting programs, at different points in time. These interventions are more likely to be effective if parents are not also worried about paying the rent, finding a job, or putting food on the table. Given complex, interacting systems of disadvantage, accessing these essential resources is simply beyond the ability of many families to manage on their own. The social determinants research has increased understanding of the relationship between childhood health and health across the life course. The evidence base for the protection of child health is solid. Public health practitioners must engage in relevant efforts to successfully achieve our mission, described by the Institute of Medicine as "the fulfillment of society's interest in assuring the conditions in which people can be healthy,"[65(p40)] including creating communities and a nation that foster the safety and well-being of all children and their families.

It is often said that children are our future. The truth of this statement has never been more apparent: the health and well-being of children today is a "down payment" on the health and well-being of the adults they will become, as well as that of their children. There is no better way to assure the health of future generations than to improve conditions for today's children.

References

1. Hammond WR. Public health and child maltreatment prevention: the role of the Centers for Disease Control and Prevention. *Child Maltreat.* 2003;8(2):81-83.

2. Sedlak AJ, Mettenburg J, Basena M, et al. *Fourth National Incidence Study of Child Abuse and Neglect (NIS–4): Report to Congress, Executive summary.* Washington, DC: US Department of Health and Human Services, Administration for Children and Families; 2010. US Department of Health and Human Services, Administration for Children and Families Web site. http://www.acf.hhs.gov/programs/opre/resource/fourth-national-incidence-study-of-child-abuse-and-neglect-nis-4-report-to-0. Accessed March 27, 2015.

3. Galea S, Tracy M, Hoggatt KJ, DiMaggio C, Karpati A. Estimated deaths attributable to social factors in the United States. *Am J Public Health.* 2011;101(8):1456-1465.

4. Satcher D, Fryer GE Jr, McCann J, Troutman A, Woolf SH, Rust G. What if we were equal?: a comparison of the black-white mortality gap in 1960 and 2000. *Health Aff (Millwood).* 2005;24(2):459-464.

5. Braveman PA, Cubbin C, Egerter S, Williams DR, Pamuk E. Socioeconomic disparities in health in the United States: what the patterns tell us. *Am J Public Health.* 2010;100(suppl 1):S186-S196.

6. Schonkoff JP, Boyce WT, McEwan BS. Neuroscience, molecular biology, and the childhood roots of health disparities: building a new framework for health promotion and disease prevention. *JAMA.* 2009;301(21):2252-2259.

7. Edwards V, Anda R, Dube S, Dong M, Chapman D, Felitti V. The wide-ranging health consequences of adverse childhood experiences. In: Kendall-Tackett K, Giacomoni S, eds. *Victimization of Children and Youth: Patterns of Abuse, Response Strategies.* Kingston, NJ: Civic Research Institute; 2005:8-1–8-12.

8. Brown DW, Anda RF, Tiemeier H, et al. Adverse childhood experiences and the risk of premature mortality. *Am J Prev Med.* 2009;37(5):389-396.

9. Braveman PA, Egerter S, Williams DR. The social determinants of health: coming of age. *Annu Rev Public Health.* 2011;32(3):381-398.

10. Adler N, Stewart J, eds. The biology of disadvantage: socioeconomic status and health. *Ann N Y Acad Sci.* 2010;1186:1-275.

11. Solar O, Irwin A. *A Conceptual Framework for Action on the Social Determinants of Health. Social Determinants of Health Discussion Paper 2 (Policy and Practice).* Geneva, Switzerland: World Health Organization; 2010. World Health Organization Web site. http://whqlibdoc.who.int/publications/2010/9789241500852_eng.pdf. Published 2010. Accessed March 27, 2015.

12. Graham H. Social determinants and their unequal distribution: clarifying policy understandings. *Milbank Q.* 2004;82(1):101-124.

13. Birn AE. Making it politic(al): closing the gap in a generation: health equity through action on the social determinants of health. *Social Medicine.* 2009;4(3):166-182.

14. Krieger N. Ladders, pyramids and champagne: the iconography of health inequities. *J Epidemiol Community Health.* 2008;62(12):1098-1104.

15. Schumacher JA, Smith Slep AM, Heyman RE. Risk factors for neglect. *Aggress Violent Behav.* 2001;6(2-3):231-254.

16. Newman KS, Chen VT. *The Missing Class: Portraits of the Near Poor in America.* Boston, MA: Beacon Press; 2007.

17. Frank R. *Falling Behind: How Rising Inequality Harms the Middle Class.* Berkeley, CA: California University Press; 2007.

18. National Scientific Council on the Developing Child. *Excessive Stress Disrupts the Architecture of the Developing Brain: Working Paper 3.* Cambridge, MA: Center on the Developing Child, Harvard University; 2005. Center on the Developing Child, Harvard University Web site. http://developingchild.harvard.edu/index.php/resources/reports_and_working_papers/working_papers/wp3/. Accessed February 13, 2013.

19. National Scientific Council on the Developing Child, National Forum on Early Childhood Policy and Programs. *The Foundations of Lifelong Health Are Built in Early Childhood.* Cambridge, MA: Center on the Developing Child, Harvard University; 2010. Center on the Developing Child, Harvard University Web site. http://developingchild.harvard.edu/resources/reports_and_working_papers/foundations-of-lifelong-health/. Accessed March 27, 2015.

20. Repetti R, Wang S. Parent employment and chaos in the family. In: Evans GW, Wachs TD, eds. *Chaos and Its Influence on Children's Development: An Ecological Perspective.* Washington, DC: American Psychological Association; 2001:191-208.

21. Connell-Carrick K. A critical review of the empirical literature: identifying correlates of child neglect. *Child Adolesc Social Work J.* 2003;20(5):389-425.

22. Black DA, Heyman RE, Smith-Slep AM. Risk factors for child physical abuse. *Aggress Violent Behav.* 2001;6(2-3):121-188.

23. Jones L. Unemployment and child abuse. *Families in Society.* 1990;71(10):579-588.

24. Coulton CJ, Crampton DS, Irwin M, Spilsbury JC, Korbin JE. How neighborhoods influence child maltreatment: a review of the literature and alternative pathways. *Child Abuse Negl.* 2007;31(11-12):1117-1142.

25. Freisthler B, Merritt DH, La Scala EA. Understanding the ecology of child maltreatment: a review of the literature and directions for future research. *Child Maltreat.* 2006;11(3):263-280.

26. Coulton C, Korbin JE, Su M, Chow J. Community level factors and child maltreatment rates. *Child Dev.* 1995;66(5):1262-1276.

27. Deccio G, Horner WC, Wilson D. High risk neighborhoods and high risk families: replication research related to the human ecology of child maltreatment. *J Soc Serv Res.* 1994;18(3-4):123-137.

28. Ernst JS. Community-level factors and child maltreatment in a suburban county. *Soc Work Res.* 2001;25(3):133-142.

29. Zolotar AJ, Runyan DK. Social capital, family violence, and neglect. *Pediatrics.* 2006;117(6):e1124-e1131.

30. Centers for Disease Control and Prevention. CDC health disparities and inequalities report — United States, 2013. *MMWR.* 2013;62(suppl 3):1-187. Centers for Disease and Prevention Web site. http://www.cdc.gov/mmwr/pdf/other/su6203. Accessed September 9, 2014.

31. National Center for Public Policy and Higher Education. *Measuring Up 2008: The National Report Card on Higher Education.* San Jose, CA: National Center for Public Policy and Higher Education; 2008. National Center for Public Policy and Higher Education Web site. http://measuringup2008.highereducation.org/print/NCPPHEMUNationalRpt.pdf. Accessed March 27, 2015.

32. Egerter S, Braveman P, Sadegh-Nobari T, Grossman-Kahn R, Dekker M. Education matters for health. Issue brief series: exploring the social determinants of health. Robert Wood Johnson Foundation Web site. http://www.rwjf.org/content/dam/web-assets/2011/05/education-matters-for-health. Published April 2011. Accessed February 14, 2013.

33. An J, Braveman P, Dekker M, Egerter S, Grossman-Kahn R. Work, workplaces and health. Robert Wood Johnson Foundation Web site. http://www.rwjf.org/en/library/research/2011/05/work-and-health-.html. Published May 1, 2011. Accessed March 27, 2015.

34. US Department of Labor, Bureau of Labor Statistics. *The Employment Situation—August 2014.* Washington, DC: US Department of Labor, Bureau of Labor Statistics; 2014. US Department of Labor Bureau of Labor Statistics Web site. http://www.bls.gov/news.release/archives/empsit_09052014.pdf. Accessed March 27, 2015.

35. Carnevale AP, Rose SJ, Cheah B. *The College Payoff: Education, Occupations, Lifetime Earnings.* Washington, DC: Georgetown University Center on Education and the Workforce; 2011. US Department of Education Web site. https://www2.ed.gov/policy/highered/reg/hearulemaking/2011/collegepayoff.pdf. Accessed March 27, 2914.

36. US Department of Labor, Bureau of Labor Statistics. *BLS Reports 1045: Highlights of Women's Earnings in 2012.* Washington, DC: US Department of Labor, Bureau of Labor Statistics; 2013. US Department of Labor, Bureau of Labor Statistics Web site. http://www.bls.gov/cps/cpswom2012.pdf. Published October 2013. Accessed September 28, 2014.

37. Ahmad F, Iverson S. *The State of Women of Color in the United States: Too Many Barriers Remain for This Growing and Increasingly Important Population.* Washington, DC: Center for American Progress; 2013. Center for American Progress Web site. http://cdn.americanprogress.org/wpcontent/uploads/2013/10/StateOfWomenColor-1.pdf. Accessed March 27, 2015.

38. DeNavas-Walt C, Proctor BD. *Income and Poverty in the United States: 2013.* Washington, DC: US Government Printing Office; 2014. http://www.census.gov/content/dam/Census/library/publications/2014/demo/p60-249.pdf. Accessed March 27, 2015.

39. Seith D, Kalof C. *Who are America's Poor Children?: Examining Health Disparities by Race and Ethnicity.* New York, NY: National Center for Children in Poverty; 2011. National Center for Children in Poverty Web site. http://nccp.org/publications/pdf/text_1032.pdf. Accessed March 27, 2015.

40. Kochhar R, Fry R, Taylor P. *Wealth Gaps Rise to Record Highs Between Whites, Blacks and Hispanics.* Washington, DC: Pew Research Center Social & Demographic Trends; 2011. Pew Research Center Social and Demographic Trends Web site. http://pewsocialtrends.org/files/2011/07/SDT-Wealth-Report_7-26-11_FINAL.pdf. Accessed March 27, 2015.

41. Orfield G, Lee C. *Why Segregation Matters: Poverty and Educational Inequality.* Cambridge, MA: Harvard University Civil Rights Project; 2005. Education Resources Information Center Web site. http://www.eric.ed.gov/PDFS/ED489186.pdf. Accessed March 27, 2015.

42. Arroyo CG. The funding gap. The Education Trust Web site. http://www.nvasb.org/Publications/Research_Data/the_funding_gap.pdf. Accessed February 14, 2013.

43. Condron DJ, Roscigno VJ. Disparities within: unequal spending and achievement in an urban school district. *Sociol Educ.* 2003;76(1):18-36.

44. Bertrand M, Mullainathan S. *Are Emily and Greg More Employable Than Lakisha and Jamal?: a Field Experiment on Labor Market Discrimination.* Cambridge, MA: National Bureau of Economic Research; 2003. NBER Working Paper No. 9873. National Bureau of Economic Research Web site. http://www.nber.org/papers/w9873. Accessed March 27, 2015.

45. Pager D. The mark of a criminal record. *Am J Sociol.* 2003;108(5):937-975.

46. Ginther DK, Schaffer WT, Schnell J, et al. Race, ethnicity, and NIH research awards. *Science.* 2011;333(6045):1015-1019.

47. Federal Deposit Insurance Corporation. 2009 FDIC national survey of unbanked and underbanked households. Federal Deposit Insurance Corporation Web site. http://www.fdic.gov/householdsurvey/2009/index.html. Published December 2009. Updated September 7, 2012. Accessed February 14, 2013.

48. Parrish L, King U; Center for Responsible Lending. *Phantom Demand: Short-term Due Date Generates Need for Repeat Payday Loans, Accounting for 76% of Total Volume.* Durham, NC: Center for Responsible Lending; 2009. Center for Responsible Lending Web site. http://www.responsiblelending.org/payday-lending/research-analysis/phantom-demand-final.pdf. Accessed March 27, 2015.

49. Cover J, Fuhrman Spring A, Garshick Kleit R. Minorities on the margins?: the spatial organization of fringe services. *J Urban Aff.* 2011;33(3):317-344.

50. Bachelder E, Alexander EK, Yu L, et al. *Banks' Efforts to Serve the Unbanked and Underbanked, for the Federal Deposit Insurance Corporation. Final Report, December 2008.* Boston, MA: Dove Consulting; 2008. Federal Deposit Insurance Corporation Web site. http://www.fdic.gov/unbankedsurveys/2008survey/unbankedstudy/FDICBankSurvey_Report.pdf. Accessed February 14, 2013.

51. Powers ET. Does means-testing welfare discourage saving? Evidence from a change in AFDC policy in the United States. *J Pub Econ.* 1998;68(1):33–53.

52. Gruber J, Yelowitz A. *Public Health Insurance and Private Savings.* Cambridge, MA: National Bureau of Economic Research; 1997. National Bureau of Economic Research Web site. http://www.nber.org/papers/w6041.pdf. Accessed March 27, 2015.

53. Gruenstein Bocian D, Li W, Ernst KS. *Foreclosures by Race and Ethnicity: the Demographics of a Crisis.* Durham, NC: Center for Responsible Lending; 2010. Center for Responsible Lending Web site. http://www.responsiblelending.org/mortgage-lending/research-analysis/foreclosures-by-race-and-ethnicity.pdf. Accessed March 27, 2015.

54. National Community Reinvestment Coalition. *Income Is No Shield Against Racial Differences in Lending II: a Comparison of High-cost Lending in America's Metropolitan and Rural Areas.* Washington, DC: National Community Reinvestment Coalition; 2008. Housing Preservation Project Web site. http://www.hppinc.org/_uls/resources/Racial_Gap_Report.pdf. Accessed March 27, 2015.

55. National Council of Negro Women. *Income Is No Shield, Part III: Assessing the Double Burden: Examining Racial and Gender Disparities in Mortgage Lending.* Washington, DC: National Council of Negro Women; 2009. National Council of Negro Women Web site. http://www.ncnw.org/images/double_burden.pdf. Accessed March 27, 2015.

56. Schwartz M, Wilson E. Who can afford to live in a home?: a look at data from the 2006 American Community Survey. US Census Bureau Web site. http://www.census.gov/hhes/www/housing/special-topics/files/who-can-afford.pdf. Accessed February 14, 2013.

57. Children's Health Watch. Behind closed doors: The hidden health impacts of being behind on rent. Children's Health Watch Web site. http://www.childrenshealthwatch.org/upload/resource/behindcloseddoors_report_jan11.pdf. Published January 2011. Accessed February 14, 2013.

58. Yang M. The effect of material hardship on child protective service involvement. *Child Abuse & Neglect.* In press, available online 5 June 2014 at http://www.sciencedirect.com/science/article/pii/S0145213414001859. Accessed 10/10/14.

59. Cowal K, Shinn M, Weitzman B, Stojanovic D, Labay L. Mother–child separations among homeless and housed families receiving public assistance in New York City. *Am J Comm Psych.* 2002; 30(5):711-730.

60. King RS, Mauer M. *Distorted Priorities: Drug Offenders in State Prisons.* Washington, DC: Sentencing Project; 2002. Sentencing Project Web site. http://www.sentencingproject.org/doc/File/Drug%20Policy/dp_distortedpriorities.pdf. Accessed March 31, 2015.

61. Mauer M, King RS. *Uneven Justice: State Rates of Incarceration by Race and Ethnicity.* Washington, DC: Sentencing Project; 2007. Sentencing Project Web site. http://www.sentencingproject.org/doc/publications/rd_stateratesofincbyraceandethnicity.pdf. Accessed March 31, 2015.

62. American Bar Association. *ABA Standards for Criminal Justice: Collateral Sanctions and Discretionary Disqualification of Convicted Persons.* 3rd ed. Washington, DC: American bar Association; 2004. American Bar Association Web site. http://www.americanbar.org/content/dam/aba/publishing/criminal_justice_section_newsletter/crimjust_standards_collateralsanctionwithcommentary.authcheckdam.pdf. Accessed March 31, 2015.

63. Wood E. *Restoring the Right to Vote.* 2nd ed. New York, NY: Brennan Center for Justice; 2009. Brennan Center for Justice Web site. http://brennan.3cdn.net/5c8532e8134b233182_z5m6ibv1n.pdf. Accessed February 14, 2013.

64. Arditti JA. Families and incarceration: an ecological approach. *Families in Society: The Journal of Contemporary Social Services.* 2005;86(2):251-260.

65. Committee for the Study of the Future of Public Health; Division of Health Care Services. *The Future of Public Health.* Washington D.C: National Academies Press; 1988.

66. Sogolow ED, Sleet DA, Saul JS. Dissemination, implementation, and widespread use of injury prevention interventions. In: Doll LS, Bonzo SE, Mercy JA, Sleet DA, eds. *Handbook of Injury and Violence Prevention.* New York, NY: Springer; 2007:493-510.

67. Cerdá M, Tracy M, Ahern J, Galea S. Addressing population health and health inequalities: The role of fundamental causes. *Am J Pub Health.* 2014;104(S4):S609-619.

68. Koh HK, Nowinski JM. Health equity and public health leadership. *Am J Public* Health. 2010;100(suppl 1):S9-11.

69. Healthy People 2020. Social determinants of health. http://www.healthypeople.gov/2020/topicsobjectives2020/overview.aspx?topicid=39. Updated September 6, 2012. Accessed February 14, 2013.

70. Healthy equity and social justice. National Association of County and City Health Officials Web site. http://www.naccho.org/topics/justice/. Accessed February 14, 2013.

71. Horsley K, Ciske SJ. From neurons to King County neighborhoods: partnering to promote policies based on the science of early childhood development. *Am J Public Health.* 2005;95(4):562-567.

72. Oleru N, Gedeon M, Valenzuela M. Institutionalizing health equity and social justice in King County, Washington. In: Hofrichter R, Bhatia R, eds. *Tackling Health Inequities through Public Health Practice: Theory to Action.* New York, NY: Oxford University Press; 2010:404-416.

73. Commission on Social Determinants of Health. *Closing the Gap in a Generation: Health Equity Through Action on the Social Determinants of Health.* Geneva, Switzerland: World Health Organization; 2008. World Health Organization Web site. http://whqlibdoc.who.int/publications/2008/9789241563703_eng.pdf. Accessed March 30, 2015.

74. Blakely TA, Kennedy BP, Kawachi I. Socioeconomic inequality in voting participation and self-rated health. *Am J Public Health.* 2001;91(1):99-104.

75. Beckfield J, Krieger N. Epi + demos + cracy: linking political systems and priorities to the magnitude of health inequities—evidence, gaps, and a research agenda. *Epidemiol Rev.* 2009;31(1):152-177.

76. Krieger N, Rehkopf DH, Chen JT, Waterman PD, Marcelli E, Kennedy M. The rise and fall of US inequities in premature mortality: 1966-2002. *PLoS Med.* 2008;5(2):e46.

77. Centers for Disease Control and Prevention. *Behavioral Risk Factors Surveillance System Questionnaire.* Atlanta, GA: Centers for Disease Control and Prevention; 2009. Centers for Disease Control and Prevention Web site. http://www.cdc.gov/brfss/questionnaires/pdf-ques/2009brfss.pdf. Published December 30, 2008. Accessed March 30, 2015.

78. US Department of Commerce, US Census Bureau. The American community survey. http://www.census.gov/acs/www/. Updated February 1, 2013. Accessed March 30, 2015.

79. Jacksonville Community Council Inc. Home page. http://www.jcci.org/. Accessed March 30, 2015.

80. JCCI annual reports. Jacksonville Community Council Inc Web page. http://www.jcci.org/library. Accessed March 19, 2013.

81. Yen IH, Syme SL. The social environment and health: a discussion of the epidemiologic literature. *Annu Rev Public Health.* 1999;20:287-308.

82. Mercy JA, Mack KA, Steenkamp M. Changing the social environment to prevent injuries. In: Doll LS, Bonzo SE, Mercy JA, Sleet DA, eds. *Handbook of Injury and Violence Prevention.* New York, NY: Springer; 2007:277-294.

83. Committee on Health Impact Assessment; National Research Council. Improving health in the United States: the role of health impact assessment. The National Academies Press Web site. http://www.nap.edu/catalog.php?record_id=13229. Published 2011. Accessed March 30, 2015.

84. Collins J, Koplan JP. Health impact assessment: a step toward health in all policies. *JAMA.* 2009;302(3):315-317.

85. Johnson RC. *Long-run Impacts of School Desegregation & School Quality on Adult Attainments.* Cambridge, MA: National Bureau of Economic Research; 2011. National Bureau of Economic Research Web site. http://www.nber.org/papers/w16664. Accessed March 30, 2015. NBER Working Paper No. 16664.

The findings and conclusions in this chapter are those of the authors and do not necessarily represent the official position of the Centers for Disease Control and Prevention.

Chapter 3

Emerging Opportunities in Prevention: Lessons From the Past

Deborah Daro, PhD
Anne Cohn Donnelly, DPH, MPH

Overview

In 1976, when asked to comment on the utility of child abuse prevention efforts, Edward Zigler labeled such efforts as doomed to failure. "Social change," he wrote, "is produced not by the stroke of a pen but by intensive and persistent efforts to change the human ecology in which the social target is embedded."[1] Despite his dire warnings, child maltreatment has progressed from a relatively obscure medical condition identified by forward thinking physicians and social workers to a widely recognized public health challenge.

At the forefront of this transformation was an engaged network of state and federal policymakers, service professionals, researchers, and a robust network of child welfare advocates. By the 1980s, combating child abuse had become a central theme among philanthropic and community service efforts being promoted by the National Basketball Association, Master Card, the Ad Council, corporations such as Freddy Mac and Target, and a number of social fraternities and sororities. Several nonprofit national organizations including the National Committee to Prevent Child Abuse and the Kempe Center for the Prevention and Treatment of Child Abuse and Neglect focused exclusively on maltreatment, coordinating child abuse intervention and prevention efforts across the country, and disseminating promising practices.

During this same period, the National Center on Child Abuse and Neglect (NCCAN) focused on implementing the Child Abuse Prevention and Treatment Act (Public Law 93-274) and on building more collaborative efforts across federal and state agencies and providing substantial investment in research and demonstration projects.[2] Almost every state established a Children's Trust and Prevention Fund that raised revenues to support a diverse array of emerging prevention strategies and provided a strong voice within state governments for the prevention message.[3] Collectively, these and similar efforts created a climate that fostered new ideas, generated greater public and private resources, ignited public interest, and inspired a generation of young professionals who focused on child maltreatment.

Today, the child abuse field stands at a critical juncture, at which its viability as a unique field of practice faces notable challenges. In many respects, current efforts to address child abuse are more diffuse and discipline-specific. A greater distance exists between those focusing on clinical and judicial interventions for victims and perpetrators and those promoting abuse prevention. While not a new situation, the problem has been exacerbated by the partnerships and fields of practice to which both sides are now drawn.

Those engaged in providing therapeutic services to victims and offenders are increasingly less likely to align with family support agencies. They seek clinical partnerships and shared learning with those implementing trauma-focused therapies that address a wide array of violent acts and social dilemmas that negatively impact children.[4] On the prevention side, robust alliances are being formed with early care and education professionals. Indeed, the framing of the child abuse prevention message has moved away from an explicit mention of maltreatment in favor of a more positive, strength-based messages that emphasize child development, positive parent-child interaction, and protective factors.[5-7] Most recently, the Centers for Disease Control (CDC) adopted the promotion of safe, stable, and nurturing relationships between children and caregivers as its primary strategy for preventing child maltreatment.[8]

One interpretation of these changes is that they represent the logical next step in the evolution of child abuse as a social dilemma. Decades of research on the maltreatment issue has resulted in a keener understanding of its complexity and its co-occurrence with other forms of violence and trauma.[9] Prevention developments in other domains, such as school readiness, violence prevention, and health promotion, have underscored the importance of altering social context as well as strengthening individual behaviors.[10] In addition to providing targeted services to remediate specific individual difficulties, efforts to prevent child abuse, youth violence, and school failure also incorporate strategies to increase overall service availability; to better align the efforts of health, education, and social service agencies; and to address normative standards that threaten a child's well-being. Creating synergy across these diverse efforts may be achieved by not focusing on a single problem but rather by focusing on a consolation of issues that impact a larger proportion of children and families.

On the other hand, it is possible that the absence of a coherent, well-focused child abuse and neglect field will leave some families unserved and some children unprotected. Families unable to effectively access and engage in broadly targeted prevention services but considered inappropriate for mandated child welfare interventions are at-risk of being lost in a sustained bifurcation between prevention and treatment. Indeed, the diversity of risk presented by families referred to the child welfare system for investigation contributed to the development of differential response systems that work to balance the need to support families facing challenges with the responsibility to protect children from harm.[11] Efficiently responding to all at-risk families requires a solid continuum of strategies that can support families at a level commensurate with their needs. Developing and sustaining this robust and diversified set of supports may best be served by invigorating interest in child abuse and neglect as a unique social dilemma that successfully integrates treatment, prevention, and protective factor frameworks. The purpose of this chapter is to reflect on the evolution of child maltreatment as a focus of public policy and identify how the strengths and limitations of past practice might illuminate future policy. After briefly reviewing this historical context, the chapter discusses the relative merits and shortcomings of allowing child abuse and neglect to become embedded in a range of dilemmas facing the nation's children. Regardless of how the issue is defined going forward, this chapter suggests 4 strategic directions that will be important in building a more integrated and holistic approach to protecting children and promoting optimal child development.

Historical Framework

Over the past 50 years, efforts to prevent child maltreatment have moved through various stages: public and professional recognition of the problem, experimentation with a wide range of programs addressing one or more factors believed to increase a child's risk for maltreatment or mitigate its consequences, and the development of systemic and contextual reforms to better integrate and sustain these diverse interventions.[12] At each evolutionary stage, those developing, implementing, and funding child abuse interventions have been driven, in part, by what they were learning from current practice and research. As a result, public policies responding to this problem have evolved from simply capturing the extent of the problem to understanding its underlying causes to determining how best to treat and ultimately prevent its occurrence.[13]

Definition and Awareness

Modern public and political attention to the issue of child maltreatment is often pegged to Henry Kempe's 1962 article in the *Journal of the American Medical Association* on the "battered child syndrome."[14] Although several medical articles had appeared as early as the 1940s describing subdural hematomas and long bone fractures suggestive of maltreatment,[15,16] Kempe's work differed from these earlier efforts in 2 key respects: (1) his choice of research methods and (2) his decision to link his findings to a specific public policy.[17] In contrast to those who had focused on developing detailed clinical case studies to explain maltreatment patterns, Kempe and his colleagues examined hospital emergency room X-rays for 1 year in 70 hospitals around the country and surveyed 77 district attorneys. These efforts painted a vivid and disturbing picture of children suffering physical and emotional trauma as a result of overburdened parents or caregivers using extreme forms of corporal punishment or depressed single mothers failing to provide for their child's basic emotional and physical needs.

Armed with these descriptions, Kempe persuaded federal and state policymakers to support the adoption of a formal child abuse reporting system that professionals and others concerned with a child's well-being could use to insure a child's safety and to obtain services for her parents. Between 1963 and 1967, all states and the District of Columbia passed child abuse reporting laws, a trend viewed by some as one of the most rapid diffusions of a legislative innovation in the twentieth century.[18] Federal reporting guidelines were established in 1974 with the authorization of the Child Abuse Prevention and Treatment Act (CAPTA). Although many factors played into the passage of this legislation, Kempe's data and the burgeoning body of clinical case studies and survey research provided policymakers with evidence of the problem and, more importantly, a way to deal with it.[2,17]

Over time, it became clear that the child abuse problem was more common and nuanced than initially imagined. Single-factor theories that located the cause of maltreatment solely within an individual's lack of knowledge, skill, or emotional competence proved insufficient in understanding the problem or generating reasonable public policy. Increasingly, the field embraced complex, ecological frameworks that called for a comprehensive approach offering myriad interventions targeting individuals as well as social conditions around them.[19-22]

This theoretical shift had implications on how treatment programs were developed and generated a strong interest in expanding investments in a diverse array of prevention strategies. Treatment services provided to families identified as being at risk or actively engaged in abusive or neglectful behaviors ranged from individual, family, and group counseling to various types of self-help groups and case management services.[23] Although such interventions netted changes in parental practices and access to ongoing support, over one-third of the participants in these programs continued to mistreat their children while enrolled.[24] As foster care caseloads grew and available resources for clinical services diminished, a prevention response that merely identified a child after they had been victimized proved unsatisfactory. Increasingly, both prevention and treatment professionals turned their attention to developing, implementing, and evaluating a continuum of services that addressed causal factors found at all levels of the ecological framework.[25]

Building a Service Continuum

The 1980s represented a period of significant expansion in public awareness of child maltreatment, research on its underlying causes and consequences, and the development and dissemination of both clinical interventions and prevention strategies. As more became known, unique subpopulations were singled out for specific programmatic options and legislative attention.[17] Explicitly differentiating types of maltreatment offered greater conceptual clarity as to which behaviors or risk factors might constitute a reportable act of maltreatment and provided greater specificity on how to develop more effective interventions.

Clinical interventions targeting child abuse victims and perpetrators became increasingly specialized. The skyrocketing number of sexual abuse cases reported during this period contributed to the rapid expansion of interventions that focused exclusively on families, victims, or perpetrators engaged in this form of maltreatment. The primary emphasis of these models was on altering behaviors and developing more positive ways to cope with external stress. In addition, specialized case management and family support programs as well as self-help groups emerged that addressed a narrow set of targeted behaviors or conditions. For example, some strategies exclusively addressed the socioeconomic issues and parental limitations commonly cited as the major contributors to chronic neglect and physical abuse. Other interventions played heavier emphasis on the psychological, family dynamics, and behavioral issues surfacing in cases of interfamilial sexual abuse. Families involved in specific forms of maltreatment were increasingly enrolled in interventions with more homogeneous caseload than had been true in the earliest years of addressing the problem.[17]

On the prevention front, this differentiated approach resulted in 2 distinct programmatic paths: (1) interventions targeting reductions in physical abuse and neglect, including emotional neglect and attachment disorders, and (2) interventions targeting reductions in child sexual abuse.[17] Prevention strategies targeting the first group emanated from research that suggested physical abuse and neglect generally reflected a parent's lack of knowledge, resources, and emotional capacity. The prevention strategies targeting families experiencing these difficulties included, among others, services to new parents, general parenting education classes, parent support groups, family resource centers, and crisis intervention services, such as hotlines and crisis nurseries.[26] In contrast, the target population for sexual abuse prevention became potential victims, not potential perpetrators. Strategies within this framework included a number of education-based efforts provided on a universal basis to children on the distinction between good, bad, and questionable touching and the concept of body ownership or the rights of children to control who touches their bodies and where they are touched.[27] These educational programs also encouraged children and youth who had been victimized to report these incidences and seek services.

Many more interventions were proposed and implemented than rejected during this period. On balance, programs were replicated based on their theoretical and emotional appeal rather than on any significant evidence of effectiveness. Program evaluations, while plentiful, often lacked strong comparison groups and suffered from poorly specified theories and outcomes that lacked reliable and valid assessment methods. Although exceptions to this pattern existed, families were generally directed to a specific model not because it was perceived as the best fit for their specific problems but rather because it was available in their community.

As with the initial generation of services, overall impacts were disappointing. Reabuse rates for offenders who had been provided intensive clinical interventions remained high.[28] Developmental outcomes for abused children were often not significantly improved, even when they were offered intensive therapeutic support.[29] Although general parent education and support programs improved parental capacity among their participants, the utility of such efforts were generally limited to parents able to access and utilize these options. Prevention efforts developed during this period were far less successful in attracting and retaining families who did not know they needed assistance or, if they recognized their shortcomings, did not know how to access help.[30] A prevention imagery that merely suggested a diverse array of service options without also offering explicit strategies on how to integrate these efforts across disciplines and intent proved disappointing and, in many instances, ineffective.

The Developmental Paradigm

In response to the disappointment with the child abuse service continuum, prevention planners explicitly shifted their imagery from the horizontal, in which prevention investments were equally distributed to programs serving children of all ages, to the vertical, which focused investments on the youngest children.[31] Within this new paradigm, emphasis was placed on establishing a strong foundation of support for every parent and child, initiating services when a child is born or a woman becomes pregnant. Although this conceptual shift suited the new prevention context, the approach was less salient among those tasked with responding to current cases. In the case of those addressing the needs of victims, resources continued to be needed across a diverse set of interventions which targeted a broad range of offenders and children of all ages. In addition to focusing on a specific developmental period, many prevention advocates galvanized around a single program strategy, expanding the availability of home visiting services to newborns and their parents. Drawing on the experiences of Western democracies with a long history of operating universal home visiting systems and emerging evidence of the strategy's utility in the United States, the US Advisory Board on Child Abuse and Neglect concluded that "no other single intervention has the promise of home visitation."[32] The seminal work of David Olds and his colleagues showing initial and long-term benefits from regular nurse visiting during pregnancy and a child's first 2 years of life provided the most robust evidence for this intervention.[33] Equally important, however, were the growing number of national home visiting programs being developed and successfully implemented by public agencies and community-based service organizations. Although initially less rigorous in their evaluation methodologies, programs such as Parents as Teachers, Healthy Families America, and the Parent-Child Home Program demonstrated respectable gains in parent-child attachment, access to preventive medical care, parental capacity and functioning, and early identification of developmental delays.[31]

To guide this phase, stronger linkages were established with the child development community to better understand how research in this domain (both basic and applied) might best inform child abuse prevention efforts. In addition, higher priority was placed on holding program planners accountable for outcomes, a standard shared with those developing treatment innovations. The importance of evidence-based practice across the child abuse field was reflected in more rigorous program evaluations, including an increase in the number of randomized controlled trials, more rigorous quasi-experimental designs, and an expanded use of quality assurance and monitoring systems to track performance.[13]

After implementing home visiting programs for over a decade, the prevention field is again critically examining its progress. In some cases, reviewers conclude that when well implemented, the strategy does produce significant and meaningful reduction in child abuse risk and improves child and family functioning.[34-37] Others are more sobering in their conclusions, emphasizing the lack of consistent rigor in how programs are evaluated and the unevenness in their documented impacts.[38,39]

Most reviewers, however, agree that all families are not equally well-served by the pool of intensive, long-term home visiting programs that have received the most focused attention in these reviews. A recent federally funded review of these evaluations identified several areas and populations in which impacts were far from consistent in part because of poor implementation.[40] Retention in these long-term interventions can be difficult—identifying, training, and retaining competent service providers is challenging, particularly when the number of program sites rapidly increase. And although these home visiting programs can be substantial in both dosage and duration, even intensive interventions cannot fully address the needs of the most challenged populations (eg, those struggling with serious mental illness, domestic violence, and substance abuse as well as those rearing children in violent and chaotic neighborhoods).

Faced once again with the inevitable limitations of any one program strategy, increased emphasis is being placed on approaches that seek change at a community or systemic level.[10] The objective of this paradigm is to create safe and nurturing environments for all children and communities in which parents are supported through both formal services and normative values that foster mutual reciprocity. The approach also embraces infrastructure reforms that support the replication and sustainability of high-quality, evidence-based direct services. Communities where residents share a belief in collective responsibility to protect children and advocate for expanding high-quality, evidence-based services and instrumental supports for parents is viewed as fertile ground for achieving population-level changes in maltreatment rates.[10]

Implications for Moving Forward

Protecting children from abuse and neglect is a complex task that requires a focused and well-integrated response. It remains unclear if this coordinated response will galvanize around a unique emphasis on child abuse and neglect or focus on a constellation of more generalized outcomes, such as reducing trauma, strengthening families, achieving optimal child development, or reducing the achievement gap. Sustaining a unique emphasis on child abuse would focus public attention on a public health dilemma that harms a significant number of children each year, highlight specific strategies to reduce the parental and societal conditions that enable abusive and neglectful behavior to develop and continue, and may afford children greater protection from physical assaults, sexual abuse, and chronic neglect. On the other hand, placing the issue within the context of broader social concerns potentially expands the resources available for addressing the problem, builds on progress being made in other domains, and advances the cause of child welfare beyond a narrow emphasis on the absence of physical abuse, sexual abuse, or parental neglect. It expands public responsibility for child well-being beyond simply avoiding the worst outcomes for children to achieving optimal child development.

Regardless of where the child maltreatment issue finds a policy and practice home going forward, maximizing the impacts of any investments in child safety and well-being will require an increased set of actors and new relationships. And whether one's focus is improving treatment efforts or expanding prevention opportunities, change is needed in 4 key domains: (1) how we influence and shape normative parenting practices, (2) how we expand and better integrate professional partners, (3) how we strengthen nonprofit service organizations, and (4) how we build a more appropriate research paradigm.

Building a More Supportive Context for Parents

A significant proportion of the parent population is self-motivated to seek out and utilized diverse opportunities to help them care for their children. These "consumer parents" read parenting magazines and books, enroll in parenting classes and attend parent support groups, and talk with family members and friends on how to address specific parenting challenges.[30] Over the years, these parents have made good use of the growing body of parenting information found in most communities. Unfortunately, other equally compelling and pervasive messages about parenting, supporting parents, and what child abuse prevention entails currently exists which inhibit the ability to implement more effective prevention efforts. These include a common perception that parenting is a personal issue, that "how I parent is my business, not yours" and that little is to be gained by trying to "learn" how to be a better parent.

In addition to facilitating a parent's willingness to seek out information and support, it is equally important to establish collective acceptance that certain behaviors are unacceptable and, indeed, harmful to a child's healthy development. An example of this type of explicit education around what parents should not do is reflected in efforts to prevent shaken baby syndrome (SBS). Repeated evaluations of these efforts have demonstrated the ability to reduce the frequency of this negative behavior and a corresponding decline in the types of abusive head injuries associated with violent shaking.[41-43]

A key element in these campaigns is encouraging parents to identify others in their social network that can be used to provide relief from the frustration of caring for a fussy baby. The messages are, "You are not alone." and "It is okay to rely on others for support in your effort to be a good parent. Asking for help is not a sign of weakness or failure." To the extent such messages focus on issues that might trigger abusive or neglectful behaviors (eg, persistent crying) rather than on the maltreatment itself, these efforts provide a more inclusive platform for normative change. The greater the proportion of parents who identify with a given situation, the more open parents might be to offers of assistance and to seek out assistance in times of stress.

Expanding Professional Partners, Perspectives, and Priorities

Engaging the public in addressing the maltreatment problem is important. Equally important, however, is creating among the full range of professionals who are or who should be concerned with maltreatment a common understanding of the problem and an awareness of how their specific discipline can contribute to reducing maltreatment incidence and minimizing its impacts. Child abuse is a multifaceted problem and, as such, benefits from a multifaceted, interdisciplinary perspective and response.

Although multidisciplinary teams have been flagged as an effective component of the response system to individual cases of child abuse for many years,[44] this approach has not been replicated at the systems level. Each professional discipline and each individual public agency generally defines standards of best practice and relevant policies within their respective operational silo. Too little time and energy is devoted to understanding the perspectives of other disciplines and to establishing enduring collaborations. As long as professionals remain somewhat insular from each other and not open to rigorous discussion about the limitations of their respective disciplines and professional and organizational perspectives, collaborative partnerships that focus on child maltreatment will be superficial and unable to create needed structural change.

Similarly, a viable multidisciplinary approach will require a more equitable balance between investments in response and investments in prevention. To the extent fiscal incentives favor treatment programs and reimburse agencies in a more generous and consistent manner for addressing the needs of confirmed cases, as they currently do, prevention programming will remain a residual or secondary activity. At the moment, the public's response to child abuse is dominated by questions of what happened and who made it happen and less on questions of why it might have happened and what can be done to prevent its reoccurrence. Priority is placed on ensuring an appropriate legal response in which parental rights and due process are protected. A policy and practice shift which placed equal emphasis on meeting the needs of children before any injury occurs could improve the overall effectiveness of our efforts. Establishing and sustaining such a shift will require substantial investments in new, more inclusive prevention efforts. Universal assessments of all new parents would reflect a collective interest in the well-being of all children and in supporting parents in meeting their basic care obligations.[45] The message of collective responsibility and social interest could be reinforced throughout a child's development by a corresponding investment in early education programs, primary health and preventive care, community-based family support centers, and school-based parent education efforts. This is not a recommendation to abandon or replace legal and remediation concerns with preventive ones but rather to strike a more appropriate balance.

Recognizing, Engaging, and Strengthening Our Nonprofit Partners

Both the public and private sectors have critical roles to play in preventing child abuse. While the public sector has primary responsibility and greater resources for responding to the problem and often for taking preventive programs to scale, the nonprofit world plays a significant role in providing the child abuse field with leadership, innovation, research, and knowledge. The nonprofit sector, including a variety of health-based organizations, is also home to a diverse workforce of paid professionals and volunteers, the majority of whom deliver direct services to families and often focus on specific geographic areas or neighborhoods. The nonprofit sector, by virtue of the relatively small size and nimble nature of most individual organizations, is in an ideal position to initiate as well as respond to a changing environment.

Much of the nonprofit sector's funding is fragile and many of the organizations are not as well managed.[46] However, the sector does shoulder primary responsibility for delivering the majority of preventive services funded through child welfare and public health agencies. Agency administrators, as well as the general public, often underestimate the role of nonprofits within the current delivery system and frequently fail to provide the institutional supports needed to insure consistent quality. The public sector has fostered a competitive funding environment among nonprofits, an environment which rewards serving the most families for lowest cost often at the expense of sustaining quality and achieving outcomes.[47]

To maximize the contribution of the nonprofit sector in preventing maltreatment, improvements are needed on 2 fronts. First, new strategies are needed to strengthen the relationship between nonprofits and large public agencies. Nonprofits have a legitimate, important role at the policy table. While nonprofits make up close to 10% of overall GNP, they occupy a much larger space in the social service sector.[48] In most respects, the work of nonprofits equals the importance of that of their public agency counterparts even if dwarfed by size. If public and private agencies in any given community worked together in a truly coordinated and effective manner, they would undoubtedly find that the community has a far broader pool of resources to provide families the support necessary to avoid abuse and neglect. An initial starting point for building this more coordinated network of public-private offerings is creating a common mission and purpose among all stakeholders concerned with children and families—not just social service and health-related agencies, but also early childhood and other community support organizations.[49] Building these new alignments begins with the robust use of strategic planning approaches that focus on a shared number of programmatic and policy objectives.

Second, greater attention is needed to strengthening the internal organization and management of community-based agencies. While public agencies may be burdened with too much bureaucracy and thus lack the ability to innovative and change with their environment, nonprofits are characterized by a perceived lack of consistency and sustainability. Most nonprofits would benefit from greater attention to the same principles that govern effective businesses. Regardless of size, these organizations need to establish a clear purpose or mission, define a strategic plan that articulates a limited set of goals with clear steps toward those goals, develop a strong governance structure, maintain a sustainable and diverse financial base, and identify clear metrics for measuring effectiveness.[50] With a strengthened infrastructure, nonprofit organizations can enhance their strategic position at the policy table and generate the types of innovations not easily achieved by large public institutions.

Altering the Research Paradigm

Defining the evidentiary base necessary for estimating the potential impact of a given intervention is complex. In general, 2 lines of inquiry guide the development of program evaluations: (1) Does the program make a measurable difference with participants (efficacy)? (2) Does a given strategy represent the best course of action within a given context (effectiveness)? Randomized clinical trials are often viewed as the best and most reliable method for determining if the changes observed in program participants over time are due primarily to the intervention rather than to other factors. Understanding how best to implement programs often requires additional information not captured in clinical trials. As noted by the American Evaluation Association in a February 2009 memo to Office of Management and Budget (OMB) Director Peter Orszag:

> There are no simple answers to questions about how well programs work, and there is no single analytic approach or method that can decipher the complexities that are inherent within the program environment and assess the ultimate value of public programs.[51]

The success of any promising prevention strategy hinges, in part, on how potential participants view early intervention services, on what service and provider characteristics will attract parents into these programs, and on the relation between these efforts and other elements within a community's existing service continuum. Although randomized clinical trials are excellent for assessing impacts, they offer little guidance in terms of how to integrate such efforts into existing health care and educational systems, the vehicles through which a comprehensive national effort to prevent child abuse and neglect needs to be based.

The knowledge and assurances needed to build this type of integrated system for at-risk children and their parents will be found in the evidence being generated by diverse analytic and research methods that focus on implementation and program fidelity as well as participant outcomes.[52] Identifying the appropriate investments in prevention will require efforts from both the research and policy communities aimed at recognizing the importance of linking learning and practice. It is not enough for scholars and program evaluators, on the one hand, to learn how maltreatment develops and what interventions are effective and for practitioners and, on the other, to implement innovative interventions in their work with families. Instead, initiatives must be implemented and assessed in a manner that maximizes both the ability of researchers to determine the effort's efficacy and the ability of program managers and policymakers to draw on these data to shape their practice and policy decisions.

Conclusion

The *National Incidence Study on Child Abuse and Neglect (NIS-4)* reported a 19-percent reduction in the overall rate of child maltreatment since the 1993 NIS.[53] This study highlights important and potentially meaningful drops in the rate of violence toward children. The trend suggests that comprehensive prevention strategies, high-quality clinical interventions, and holding those who harm children accountable for their actions have the capacity to keep children safe.

However, the findings also underscore the limitations of prevention efforts. Although rates of child maltreatment have dropped since 1993, they remain substantially higher than those documented in the first NIS report in 1980 and the second in 1986. No significant changes were documented in the rate of child neglect, the more chronic and pervasive form of child maltreatment and the form most often documented among children in the child welfare system.[54]

Further reductions in all forms of maltreatment will require a commitment to sustain a culture of continuous quality improvement on the part of practitioners, program managers, and researchers. Those engaged in working with families involved in child abuse and neglect may need to define new ways to frame and implement their work, initiate new relationships with a broader range of public and private partners, and utilize research methods that measure implementation as well as impacts. Specifically, the field would do well to address a number of key questions:

— Is there a commitment to creating a sustained and aggressive effort to motivate the public to support more extensive investment in addressing child maltreatment and to accept personal responsibility for insuring child protection?

— Is it possible to address social values that hinder prevention efforts, such as the prevailing belief that parenting is solely a personal issue and any intervention, voluntary or not, is unwelcome, and thereby create opportunities for parents to reach out for help?

— Can collaboration and partnerships become the hallmark of the child abuse field, allowing communities to take advantage of the expertise and wisdom of all disciplines and all participating organizations, thereby maximizing the use of all available fiscal and human resources?

— Can public institutions take full advantage of what the nonprofit sector has to offer the field and create opportunities for full and equal participation in decisions regarding the structure of key service delivery systems?

— Can the research community fully embrace and equally value diverse ways of measuring the implementation and impacts of prevention programs and policies?

A central determinate in how these questions are addressed will be the degree to which child maltreatment prevention and treatment professionals and advocates position themselves in relationship to each other as well as to those focusing on other social dilemmas. Over its history, child maltreatment has been an issue recognized as having multiple underlying causes and diverse manifestations. As such, the field has many stakeholders, including direct service providers and advocates, public institutions and community-based agencies, philanthropists and public funding streams, academic researchers and local program evaluators, civic leaders, and business executives. Opportunities for program and policy innovations might be found in federal legislation, state health care programs, child welfare or educational reform efforts, or demonstration projects promoted by local community volunteers or foundations. Failure to embrace this diversity and potential opportunities in shaping future prevention efforts may well stymie progress in the protection and well-being of children.

References

1. Zigler E. Controlling child abuse in America: an effort doomed to failure. *Proceedings of the First National Conference on Child Abuse and Neglect, January 4-7, 1976.* Washington, DC: US Department of Health, Education and Welfare; 1976:29-35.
2. Myers JEB. *Child Protection in America: Past, Present, and Future.* New York, NY: Oxford University Press; 2006.
3. Scott J, Birch T. *Summary of Children's Trust Funds: Working Paper No. 20.* Chicago, IL: National Committee to Prevent Child Abuse; 1986.
4. Briere J. *Child Abuse Trauma: Theory and Treatment of the Lasting Effects.* Newbury Park, CA: Sage Publications, Inc; 1992.
5. Committee on the Prevention of Mental Disorders and Substance Abuse Among Children, Youth and Youth Adults. *Preventing Mental, Emotional, and Behavioral Disorders Among Young People.* Washington, DC: The National Academies Press; 2009.
6. Kirkpatrick K. *Reframing Child Abuse and Neglect for Increased Understanding and Engagement: Defining the Need for Strategic Reform.* Chicago, IL: Prevent Child Abuse America; 2004.
7. Patel V, Goodman S. Researching protective and promotive factors in mental health. *Int J Epidemiol.* 2007;36(4):703-707.
8. Centers for Disease Control and Prevention. Preventing child maltreatment through the promotion of safe, stable, and nurturing relationships between children and caregivers. Centers for Disease Control and Prevention Web site. http://www.cdc.gov/ViolencePrevention/pdf/CM_Strategic_Direction--Long-a.pdf. Accessed September 14, 2016.
9. Daro D, Edleson JL, Pinderhughes H. Finding common ground in the study of child abuse, youth violence and adult domestic violence. *J Interpers Violence.* 2004;19(3):282-298.
10. Daro D, Dodge K. Creating community responsibility for child protection: possibilities and challenges. *Future Child.* 2009;19(2):67-94.
11. Waldfogel J. Prevention and the child protection system. *Future Child.* 2009;19(2):195-210.
12. Daro D, Cohn-Donnelly A. Charting the waves of prevention: two steps forward, one step back. *Child Abuse Negl.* 2002;(26):731-742.
13. Daro D. The history of science and child abuse prevention – a reciprocal relationship. In: Dodge K, Coleman D, eds. *Community-Based Prevention of Child Maltreatment.* New York, NY: Guilford Press; 2009:9-25.
14. Kempe CH, Silverman F, Steele B, Droegemueller W, Silver H. The battered child syndrome. *JAMA.* 1962;181(17):17-24.

15. Caffey J. Multiple fractures in the long bones of infants suffering from chronic subdural hematoma. *AM J Roentgenol Radium Ther.* 1946;56(2):163-173.

16. Silverman FN. The roentgen manifestations of unrecognized skeletal trauma in infants. *Am J Roentgenol Radium Ther Nucl Med.* 1953;69(3):413-427.

17. Daro D. *Confronting child abuse.* New York, NY: Free Press; 1988.

18. Nelson B. *Making An Issue of Child Abuse: Political Agenda Setting for Social Problems.* Chicago, IL: University of Chicago Press; 1984.

19. Belsky J. Child maltreatment: an ecological integration. *Am Psychol.* 1980;35(4):320-335.

20. Bronfenbrenner U. *The Ecology of Human Development: Experiments by Nature and Design.* Cambridge, MA: Harvard University Press; 1979.

21. Cicchetti D, Rizley R. Developmental perspectives on the etiology, intergenerational transmission, and sequelae of child maltreatment. *New Dir Child Dev.* 1981;(11):31-55.

22. Garbarino J. The human ecology of child maltreatment: a conceptual model for research. *J Marriage Fam.* 1977;(39):721-735.

23. Cohn AH. Effective treatment of child abuse and neglect. *Social Work.* 1979;24(6):513-519.

24. Daro D, Cohn A. Is treatment too late: what ten years of evaluative research tells us. *Child Abuse Negl.* 1987;11(3):433-442.

25. Helfer R. A review of the literature on the prevention of child abuse and neglect. *Child Abuse Negl.* 1982;6(3):251-261.

26. Cohn A. *An Approach to Preventing Child Abuse.* Chicago, IL: National Committee to Prevent Child Abuse; 1983.

27. Wurtele S, Miller-Perrin C. *Preventing Child Sexual Abuse: Sharing the Responsibility.* Lincoln, NB: University of Nebraska Press; 1992.

28. Joners PH, Alexander H. Treating the abusive family within the family care system. In: Helfer R, Kempe R, eds. *The Battered Child: Fourth Edition.* Chicago, IL: University of Chicago Press; 1987:339-359.

29. Kempe R. A developmental approach to the treatment of the abused child. In: Helfer R, Kempe R, eds. *The Battered Child.* 4th ed. Chicago, IL: University of Chicago Press; 1987:360-381.

30. Daro D. Child maltreatment research: implications for program design. In: Cicchetti D, Toth S, eds. *Child Abuse, Child Development, and Social Policy.* Norwood, NJ: Ablex Publishing Corporation; 1993:331-367.

31. Daro D. Child abuse prevention: new directions and challenges. In: Hansen DJ, ed. *Motivation and Child Maltreatment.* Lincoln, NB: University of Nebraska Press; 2000:161-219. *Nebraska Symposium on Motivation*; vol 46.

32. US Department of Health and Human Services, US Advisory Board on Child Abuse and Neglect. *Creating Caring Communities: Blueprint for an Effective Federal Policy for Child Abuse and Neglect.* Washington, DC: US Government Printing Office; 1991.

33. Olds D, Sadler L, Kitzman H. Programs for parents of infants and toddlers: recent evidence from randomized trials. *J Child Psychol Psychiatry.* 2007;48(3-4):355-391.

34. American Academy of Pediatrics, Council on Child and Adolescent Health. The role of home-visitation programs in improving health outcomes for children and families. *Pediatrics.* 1998;10(3):486-489.

35. Geeraert L, Van den Noorgate W, Grietens H, Onghena P. The effects of early prevention programs for families with young children at risk for physical child abuse and neglect: a meta-analysis. *Child Maltreatment.* 2004;9(3):277-291.

36. Guterman N. *Stopping Child Maltreatment Before It Starts: Emerging Horizons in Early Home Visitation Services.* Thousand Oaks, CA: Sage Publications, Inc; 2001.

37. Hahn RA, Bilukha OO, Crosby A, et al. First reports evaluating the effectiveness of strategies for preventing violence: early childhood home visitation. *MMWR Recomm Rep.* 2003;52(RR14):1-9.

38. Chaffin M. Is it time to rethink Healthy Start/Healthy Families? *Child Abuse Negl.* 2004;28(6):589-595.

39. Gomby D. *Home Visitation in 2005: Outcomes for Children and Parents.* Washington, DC: Committee for Economic Development; 2005.

40. Paulsell D, Avellar S, Sama Martin E, Del Grosso P. *Home Visiting Evidence of Effectiveness Review: Executive Summary.* Washington, DC: Office of Planning, Research and Evaluation; Administration for Children and Families; US Department of Health and Human Services; 2010.

41. Barr RG, Barr M, Fujiwara T, Conway J, Catherine N, Brant R. Do educational materials change knowledge and behavior about crying and shaken baby syndrome? *CMAJ.* 2009;180(7):727-733.

42. Dias MS, Smith K, DeGuehery K, Mazur P, Li V, Shaffer ML. Preventing abusive head trauma among infants and young children: a hospital-based parent education program. *Pediatrics.* 2005;115(4):e470-e477.

43. Showers J. Preventing shaken baby syndrome. *J Aggress Maltreat Trauma.* 2001;5(1):349-365.

44. Krugman R. The assessment process of a child protection team. In: Helfer R, Kempe R, eds. *The Battered Child.* 4th ed. Chicago, IL: University of Chicago Press; 1987:127-136.

45. Daro D. Home visitation. In Zigler E, Gilliam W, Barnett WS, eds. *The Pre-K Debates: Current Controversies and Issues.* Baltimore, MD: Brookes Publishing; 2011:169-172.

46. Bradley B, Jansen P, Silverman L. The nonprofits sector's $100 billion opportunity. *Harv Bus Rev.* 2003;81(5):94-108.

47. Frumkin P, Kim MT. Strategic positioning and the financing of nonprofit organizations: is efficiency rewarded in the contributions marketplace? *Public Administration Review.* 2001;61(3):226-275.

48. Sherlok M, Gravelle J. *An Overview of the Nonprofit and Charitable Sector.* Washington, DC: Congressional Research Service; 2009.

49. Kania J, Kramer M. Collective impact. *Stanford Social Innovation Review.* 2001;(winter):36-41.

50. Senge P, Kleiner A, Roberts C, Ross R, Smith B. *The Fifth Discipline Fieldbook: Strategies and Tools for Building a Learning Organization.* New York: Bantam Doubleday Dell Publishing Group; 1994.

51. American Evaluation Association, Evaluation Policy Task Force. *An Evaluation Roadmap for a More Effective Government*. Fairhaven, MA: American Evaluation Association, Evaluation Policy Task Force; 2009.

52. Schorr L, Farrow F. Expanding the evidence universe: doing better by knowing more. Paper presented at: Harold Richman Public Policy Forum; July 28, 2011; Washington, DC.

53. Sedlak AJ, Mettenburg J, Basena M, et al. *Fourth National Incidence Study of Child Abuse and Neglect (NIS–4): Report to Congress, Executive Summary*. Washington, DC: US Department of Health and Human Services, Administration for Children and Families; 2010.

54. Daro D. *Child Abuse Prevention: A Job Half Done*. Chicago, IL: Chapin Hall, University of Chicago; 2010.

Chapter 4

Promoting the Health and Well-being of Children: The Role of the Centers for Disease Control and Prevention in Preventing Child Maltreatment

Patricia Y. Hashima, Phd
Natalie J. Wilkins, PhD
James A. Mercy, PhD
Corinne M. Graffunder, DrPH, MPH

Introduction

Child maltreatment is a serious public health problem. The millions of children who experience maltreatment early in life encounter increased risks for illness, injury, and death, demonstrating a clear connection between child maltreatment and public health. Yet, society often still views the problem of child maltreatment solely as a child welfare service or criminal justice problem, in part because the consequences that child maltreatment has on health and development are still not well recognized. Public health can play an important and unique role in addressing the issue of child maltreatment because it places prevention at the forefront of its efforts, has the potential to create broad population-level impact at a comparatively low cost, makes science integral to identifying and developing effective policies and programs, and integrates the efforts of diverse organizations, communities, and scientific disciplines.[1] This approach to child maltreatment prevention complements other approaches such as those of the child welfare and criminal justice systems. This chapter discusses a public health approach to the prevention of child maltreatment. The chapter begins by discussing the magnitude of the problem and its health and social consequences. It then outlines the role of public health generally, and the Centers for Disease Control and Prevention (CDC) more specifically, in addressing child maltreatment through a public health approach.

Brief Overview of the Problem of Child Maltreatment

The Prevalence of Child Maltreatment

While more than 2 decades have passed since the US Advisory Board on Child Abuse and Neglect declared child maltreatment a national emergency, the magnitude of child maltreatment in the United States continues to be substantial. Data from state and local child protective service agencies (CPS) reveal that in 2008 more than 3.7 million children received CPS investigations.[2] Among approximately 772 000 children substantiated to have been maltreated (10 per 1000 children in the population), 71% suffered neglect, 16% were physically abused, 9% were sexually abused, and 7% were emotionally abused. The rate of substantiated child maltreatment is highest among children under 1 year of age at the rate of 22 per 1000 children, and approximately 80% of perpetrators among this age group were parents. Furthermore, based on data recorded by CPS and other agencies (eg, a coroner's office), an estimated 1740 children died of abuse or neglect in 2008.[2] Since many cases of child maltreatment go undetected and unreported, these numbers and rates are underestimates of the true magnitude of child maltreatment in the United States today.[3]

Indeed, the National Survey of Children's Exposure to Violence (NatSCEV), the most comprehensive nationwide survey of the incidence and prevalence of children's exposure to violence to date, paints an even more sobering picture. The survey, sponsored by the Office of Juvenile Justice and Delinquency Prevention (OJJDP) and supported by the Centers for Disease Control and Prevention (CDC), found that about 1 out of 10 children surveyed in 2008 were maltreated due to physical or emotional abuse, were neglected or abducted during the past year, and 1 out of 5 children is maltreated during their lifetime. Only a small fraction of these incidents come to the attention of authorities.[4]

The Impact of Child Maltreatment on Health

Child maltreatment is disruptive to the healthy development of a child and a pathway to poor health through a variety of immediate and long-term problematic outcomes. In the short term, children who are maltreated often suffer from injuries resulting directly from abuse and neglect. These injuries may result in permanent physical disabilities and even death. Another proximal consequence of child maltreatment is its potential impact on children's developing brains. During the first 6 years of life, there are major spurts of growth and refinement in the network of nerve cells in the brain, which enable the emergence of new physical and mental capacities.[5] Although biologically rooted, all these changes are facilitated by the social context, which is dominated by a child's relationship with parents and other caregivers. The child's social experiences during certain critical periods of development and integration of connective neural networks play an important role in shaping the development of the brain.[6] A number of studies have found differences in the size and structure of the brains of children who have been maltreated when compared to the brains of their peers who have not been abused or neglected.[7] A growing body of research now suggests that child maltreatment exposes children to "toxic stress" which can inhibit optimal brain development and lead to developmental delays, cognitive impairments, risky behaviors, and poor health outcomes.[8] This research shows that by exposing a child to enormous physical and emotional stress, child maltreatment can alter healthy brain development and, thereby, influence health-related behaviors and outcomes over the life course.[9]

Child maltreatment is linked to factors that increase the risk for long-term health problems. Research shows that children who are abused or exposed to other adversities are more likely to smoke,[10,11] be physically inactive and/or obese,[12-14] and engage in risky sexual behavior.[15-18]

Perhaps as a result of engagement in risky behaviors, children who experience abuse and neglect are also more likely to exhibit poor physical health outcomes than peers who have not been maltreated. Child maltreatment has been associated with poor adult health status, including ischemic heart disease,[12] chronic obstructed pulmonary disease (COPD),[19] diabetes,[20] chronic pain,[21] autoimmune diseases,[22] sexually transmitted diseases,[23] liver disease,[24,25] cancer,[13,26,27] and an increased risk of premature death.[28]

Child maltreatment has been linked to a variety of poor psychosocial health outcomes as well.[29-32] For example, research shows that adolescents who have been maltreated as children are more likely to have problems in school, including conduct disorders,[31] poor reading skills, and low academic achievement.[30,32] Studies also show that adults who were abused and/or neglected as children are more likely to be diagnosed with depression and/or anxiety,[29,33,34] struggle with drug and/or alcohol abuse,[34,35] and engage in self-directed violence, including suicide.[34,36,37] Still other studies show that abuse and neglect in childhood is linked to youth violence,[38] teen dating violence,[39] and intimate partner violence perpetration and victimization in adulthood.[40,41]

The consequences of child maltreatment affect not only individuals but have significant short- and long-term impacts on communities and society as well. Child maltreatment and its associated physical, behavioral, and mental health outcomes create significant costs to communities and societies through low educational attainment,[32] loss of productivity,[42] and medical care.[43]

The Role of Public Health in the Prevention of Child Maltreatment

Child maltreatment is a major, but preventable, public health issue. With its emphasis on population health and prevention strategies to improve the health and well-being of populations, public health is uniquely suited to make important contributions to reducing child maltreatment and its consequences. The unique features of public health's role in child maltreatment prevention can be captured within 4 general themes.[1,44] First, public health places an emphasis on the primary prevention of child maltreatment, meaning that it focuses on efforts to prevent child maltreatment from occurring in the first place. Much of the emphasis in our societal response to child maltreatment has been on identifying and addressing child maltreatment cases after they occur through the child welfare and criminal justice systems. A public health approach, therefore, provides an important complement by focusing on preventing or reducing cases of child maltreatment before they occur.

Second, the public health approach brings a strong commitment to developing a rigorous science base for strategies to prevent child maltreatment. In order to effectively prevent child maltreatment, it is first important to understand it. Monitoring and tracking the magnitude, nature, and trends of child maltreatment using public health surveillance and researching risk and protective factors for child abuse and neglect are both public health methods used to increase knowledge around the nature of child maltreatment as a health problem. Public health also provides methods for understanding how to prevent child maltreatment, including the rigorous evaluation of interventions, analyses of the costs of child maltreatment and the benefits of prevention strategies, and research on factors related to the successful dissemination, implementation, and utilization of effective child maltreatment prevention strategies.

Third, public health brings a cross-cutting perspective to problem-solving that seeks to integrate the efforts of diverse disciplines, organizations, and communities to prevent child maltreatment. Public health embraces a multi-disciplinary approach which is particularly useful for problems like child maltreatment which are caused by multiple factors. Sectors and disciplines that play potentially important roles in child maltreatment prevention include health, media, psychology, business, criminal justice, behavioral science, epidemiology, social science, advocacy, and education. The traditional response to child maltreatment has been fragmented across these sectors and disciplines. It is imperative that public health work to combine these diverse perspectives and resources to promote the well-being of children to successfully prevent child maltreatment.

Fourth, public health takes a population approach to addressing child maltreatment. Public health emphasizes population health, not solely the health of individuals. The long-term goal of public health is to reduce rates of child maltreatment in populations by impacting factors and conditions that place people at risk or protect them in families, communities, and society as a whole.

The Role of the Centers for Disease Control and Prevention in the Prevention of Child Maltreatment

The Centers for Disease Control and Prevention (CDC) is one of the 13 major operating components of the US Department of Health and Human Services, the principal agency responsible for providing essential human services and protecting the health and safety of all Americans. Founded in 1946, CDC is at the forefront of public health efforts to prevent and control infectious and chronic diseases, injuries, environmental health threats, workplace hazards, and disabilities; and to promote terrorism preparedness.

Although recognized worldwide as a leader in public health, the role that CDC has played in violence prevention for nearly 3 decades is often overlooked.[45] As a direct result of a National Research Council and Institute of Medicine report recommending the establishment of a federal center for injury control, the Division of Injury Epidemiology and Control was established in 1986.[45] Six years later, as the public health approach to violence shifted its focus to prevention, CDC established the National Center for Injury Prevention and Control (NCIPC) as the lead federal organization to prevent premature death and disability caused by injuries.[45] Due to its immediate and long-term health threats, one of the current priorities of NCIPC, through its Division of Violence Prevention (DVP), is the prevention of child maltreatment. The mission of DVP's child maltreatment prevention program is to prevent child maltreatment and its consequences through surveillance, research and development, capacity building, communication, and leadership.

Understanding Violence and the Effect of Potential Prevention Strategies at the CDC

Human development and behavior are best understood in context and Bronfenbrenner argued that:

> The understanding of human development demands going beyond the direct observation of behavior on the part of one or two persons in the same place; it requires examination of multiperson systems of interaction not limited to a single setting and must take into account aspects of the environment beyond the immediate situation containing the subject.[46]

Bronfenbrenner[46] proposed that there are 4 major dimensions of environment that surround an individual: the microsystem, or immediate setting containing the particular individual, eg, home or school; the mesosystem, or connections between microsystems, eg, interactions among family, school, and peer group; the exosystem, or extension of the mesosystem which indirectly influences the microsystem, eg, neighborhood; and the macrosystem, or the larger socio-cultural context.[46] His model of the ecology of human development, offers a framework for understanding the broader environment in which human behavior occurs.

CDC uses a similar social-ecological model[47] to conceptualize the causes and prevention of violence. CDC's model also has 4 levels (individual, relationship, community, and societal) of interactive, mutually nested spheres of influence, and it offers a framework for understanding the environment in which violence occurs. The first level is the individual level. It encompasses biological and personal history factors, eg, age, education, income, history of abuse, that may increase the likelihood of becoming a victim or perpetrator of violence. The second level is the relationship level. It includes close interpersonal relationships, eg, family, partners, peers, that may increase the likelihood of becoming a victim or perpetrator of violence, eg, the presence of marital conflict or other forms of conflict within a family. The third level is the community level. It examines the settings and social institutions, eg, neighborhoods, schools, workplaces, which may have an important influence on the risk of experiencing violence as a victim or perpetrator, eg, low level of social capital. The final level focuses on broad societal factors, eg, social and cultural norms, public policies, that help create a climate in which violence is encouraged or inhibited.

Ecologically based models[46,47] are useful for organizing risk and protective factors of violence and the prevention strategies that can be used to address them. It also helps recognize how the experiences and attributes of individuals which contribute specifically to child maltreatment and its prevention are nested within and influenced by increasingly broader social contexts.[48-52] As depicted in **Figure 4-1**, the social environment encompasses those ecological contexts that surround the individual, ie, the relationship, community, and societal levels. Each ecological level can have an impact on other levels within it.[53,54] For example, changing societal norms about the appropriate modes of child discipline may influence the nature of key relationships and interactions between individuals such as the extent to which bystanders intervene in public settings to prevent a caregiver from disciplining a child in a physically abusive manner.

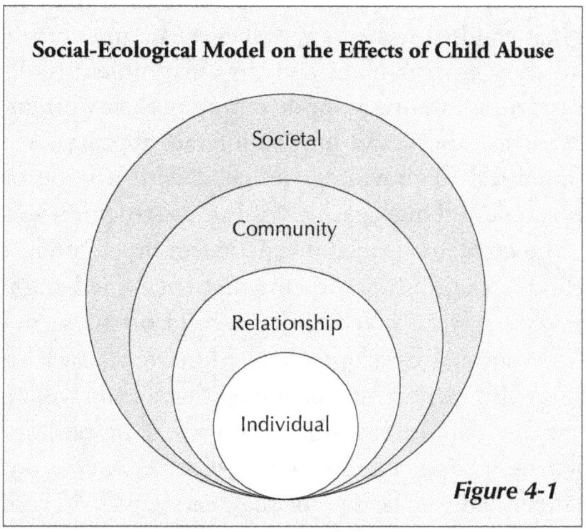

Figure 4-1. *The Social-Ecological Model. Reprinted from Centers for Disease Control and Prevention.*[55]

Essentials for Childhood: CDC's Strategic Approach to the Prevention of Child Maltreatment

"Essentials for Childhood" represents CDC's strategic direction for child maltreatment: to promote safe, stable, and nurturing relationships (SSNRs) for children.[44] SSNRs are the antithesis of maltreatment. The premise of this approach is that to the extent that we can be successful in promoting SSNRs, we will also be successful in reducing child maltreatment and its health consequences. The power of SSNRs lies in the fact that young children experience their world through their relationships with parents and caregivers.[56] These relationships are fundamental to the healthy development of the brain and, consequently, the development of physical, emotional, social, behavioral, and intellectual capacities.[56,57] From a public health perspective, the promotion of SSNRs is therefore strategic in that, if done successfully, it can have synergistic effects on a broad range of health problems as well as contribute to the development of skills that will enhance the acquisition of healthy habits and lifestyles.[58]

The 3 dimensions of SSNRs, safety, stability, and nurturing, each represent important aspects of the social and physical environments that protect children and promote their optimal development. Each can be thought of as the positive ends of continuums that extend from safe to neglectful. An example is with violent relationships/environments ranging from stable to unpredictable, chaotic relationships/environments ranging from nurturing to hostile, and cold or rejecting relationships/environments. These dimensions overlap, but each represents important and distinct aspects of a child's relationships and environments that are crucial to his or her healthy development. What follows is a more detailed description of each of these dimensions.[58]

Safety

Safety refers to the extent to which a child is free from fear and secure from physical or psychological harm within their social and physical environment. Childhood exposure to physical, sexual, or psychological violence is a direct threat to a child's safety. Neglect, or acts of omission, affect safety as well. For example, failure to properly secure a child in a car seat or ensure that poisons are stored securely in the home are clear threats to a child's safety. Caregivers ensure the safety of children by regulating their emotional response to their children, protecting children under their care from others that may harm them, disciplining their children in ways that do not cause harm and promote self-regulation, monitoring their child's behavior and development, and ensuring the child's environment is hazard free.[57,59] The nature of these vital functions for parents and caregivers change as a child matures but remain important through adolescence. The security of a child's broader social environment, which includes the magnitude of crime in their neighborhood and the presence of social supports within their community, are also important aspects of this dimension.

Stability

Stability refers to the degree of predictability and consistency in a child's environment. It encompasses consistency for those that children relate to as well as the nature of their interactions with caregivers, others in their environment, and the environment itself. A child's interaction with their environment is important for determining their working model of how the world performs, what to expect, and how to interact appropriately with those around them. Stability is critical to providing the child with a sense of coherence, ie, seeing the world as predictable and manageable.[60,61] Family structures and routines that provide stability buffer the impact of stressful experiences on children.[62] Disruptions in the stability of a child's relationships or environment, whether by divorce, death, or frequently changing caregivers, may deprive a child of the secure and nurturing attachments needed for optimal development.[63] Moreover, a lack of stable relationships or environments may also increase the likelihood that a child will be exposed to relationships and environments that are stressful and unsafe.[64] Instabilities in the lives of parents, as reflected by family conflict and violence, divorce, separation, or single parenthood, are also well-established risk factors for maltreatment.[64,65] These disruptions in family dynamics may contribute to caregiver stresses such as isolation or lack of social support, which also increase risk for maltreatment perpetration.[64,66]

Nurturing

Nurturing refers to the extent in which a parent or caregiver is available and able to sensitively respond to and meet the needs of their child.[56] These needs include physical, eg, food, shelter, hygiene, medical care; developmental, or experiences necessary for development, eg, access to education and appropriate social interaction; and emotional, eg, affection, empathy, acceptance, affirmation. Nurturing relationships reduce a child's fear in novel situations, allowing them to explore their world with confidence. Early nurturing relationships contribute to the growth of a broad range of skills, competencies, and personality characteristics that children use throughout their lives, including their interest in and capacity for learning, self-worth, social skills, and an understanding of the important building blocks of human relationships such as emotions, commitment, and morality.[67,68] For example, the negative consequences linked to lack of nurturing due to parental hostility or mental illness, eg, maternal depression, have been well documented in developmental research and studies of brain functioning.[69-71] Lack of nurturing in a caregiver-child relationship is a distinct feature of child maltreatment in that it can be expressed as both neglect and hostility towards a child.

There is substantial evidence that promoting SSNRs can be effective in reducing child maltreatment.[72-78] The most basic approach to facilitating positive relationships involves teaching parents safe and nurturing child-rearing and management skills. There is strong evidence that parent training programs or behavioral family interventions delivered in clinical settings and focused on influencing children's behavior through positive reinforcement are effective at influencing the child-rearing practices of families.[76,78] Some evidence also suggests that these types of programs can reduce child maltreatment. For example, a hospital-based program that disseminated information to new parents before discharge, which discussed the detrimental effects of violently shaking an infant, was found to have a substantial impact on reducing rates of abusive head trauma to infants.[79] Parent-child interaction therapy (PCIT), an intervention that teaches parents safety and nurturing skills, has also been effective in reducing physical child abuse in families who have been referred to child protective services or who are at risk of maltreatment for other reasons.[80]

SSNRs can also be facilitated by providing social support (such as receipt of emotional support or instrumental help during an emergency) to parents and families. The availability, adequacy, and use of social support by families has long been established as important correlates of child maltreatment.[72,74,75] Economic deprivation combined with a lack of social support places children at a higher risk for maltreatment.[72-74] Social support can help to buffer the effects of chronic and situational stress.[74,75] Support with baby-sitting or childcare appears to be particularly helpful in reducing parental behaviors that are harmful or neglectful to children.[74] Moreover, emerging evidence indicates that social support is one of the most important environmental factors in promoting resiliency against depression among maltreated children even in the presence of a genotype associated with greater vulnerability for psychiatric disorders.[81]

Parenting information and training and social support are often included within multi-component child development programs. Comprehensive child-parent centers, for example, that provide a stable, enriched learning environment and that actively promote parental involvement and parent-child interaction have been associated with lower levels of substantiated child maltreatment in participating families.[77] Nurse-Family Partnership (NFP) provides home visitation to low-income, first-time mothers from pregnancy through their child's infancy. NFP is perhaps the most rigorously evaluated example of a program that promotes SSNRs through efforts to systematically engage mothers and other family members in improving prenatal health-related behaviors, eg, smoking, alcohol use, health access; providing more responsible and competent care of infants and toddlers; and improving economic self-sufficiency. Several randomized controlled trials (RCTs) have found that this program effectively reduces abuse and injury, improves cognitive and socio-emotional outcomes in children, and demonstrates a very favorable cost-benefit ratio.[82-84] Triple P, another example of a comprehensive program that promotes SSNRs, provides a system of population-level parenting and family support that includes professional training on parent skills-based intervention to gatekeepers, eg, pediatricians, child welfare case workers, combined with media and communication strategies to normalize parenting interventions. It has been found to reduce substantiated child maltreatment cases, out-of-home placements, and child hospitalizations and emergency department visits for injuries.[82,85] A meta-analysis of Triple P programs globally found consistent evidence that this program is also linked to positive changes in parental skills, child problem behavior, and parental well-being.[86]

Child maltreatment and SSNRs emerge from and are sustained within the social contexts that help create and support them. Consequently, programs and policies designed to reduce social and economic disadvantage may also help in promoting SSNRs by alleviating individuals' stress and exposure to adversity. Various studies have found that social determinants such as neighborhood economic distress and disadvantage; housing stress, eg, density of vacant housing or residential instability; low social capital; low family income; and low parental education are associated with child maltreatment.[64,87-90] Intervention strategies that operate at a community or societal level might reach broader segments of the population and be influential in widespread promotion of SSNRs and reductions in child maltreatment. The contributions of programs or program components that focus on social and economic disadvantage, however, have not been well studied.

Current CDC Efforts in the Prevention of Child Maltreatment: The National Center for Injury Prevention and Control

Recognizing the need for a coordinated effort to prevent injuries in the United States, the National Research Council and the Institute of Medicine (IOM) in 1985 identified CDC as the federal agency best suited to lead injury research. Currently, CDC's National Center for Injury Prevention and Control (the Injury Center) functions as the focal point for the public health approach to preventing and treating injuries. In 1987, the Injury Center began funding Injury Control Research Centers (ICRCs) throughout the United States to study ways to prevent injuries and disabilities, including the prevention of child maltreatment. For example, the University of North Carolina Injury Prevention Research Center has supported LONGSCAN, a consortium of linked research studies designed to address critical issues in child maltreatment.[91] Recently the LONGSCAN data were used to document that maltreatment (of any type) before age 12 places children at a much greater risk of early initiation of sexual intercourse.[92]

There are a wide variety of programs and services aimed at supporting children and families. However, many of these programs and services are crisis-oriented and often do not focus on preventing problems before they happen. Within CDC's Injury Center is the Division of Violence Prevention (DVP) which brings a public health approach to the problem of child maltreatment[93] that complements that of child welfare services and law enforcement. Its approach has 4 steps: (1) defining and assessing the problem of child maltreatment, (2) identifying risk and protective factors associated with child maltreatment, (3) developing and evaluating child maltreatment prevention programs, and (4) supporting effective program implementation in the field and providing states and communities with information to guide child maltreatment prevention efforts. Each step is intended to provide knowledge and information to inform the next step.

Surveillance and Epidemiology

DVP undertakes work to define the problem of child maltreatment by establishing its magnitude and distribution and identifying its risk and protective factors. For example, in partnership with the US Department of Justice and several other partners including the Association of State and Territorial Health Officials, International Association of Chiefs of Police, National Association of Medical Examiners, and the Joyce Foundation, CDC funded the development of the National Violent Death Reporting System (NVDRS). This system integrates data from medical examiners, law enforcement, health departments, and child protective services to provide the public with information on the scope and nature of violence-related deaths and to help guide public health prevention efforts.[94] The NVDRS data elements are drawn in part from the 1999 National Violent Injury Statistics System (NVISS), a pilot for the system which was funded by 6 private foundations; this data system provides potentially valuable information on child maltreatment fatalities. Additionally, DVP is developing a coding system that will enable national and state level monitoring of the problem of abusive head injuries to children. DVP also conducts research on the factors that protect children from maltreatment. For example, DVP is funding a study to gather national-level data on SSNR behaviors by caregivers and assesses their value in protecting against, buffering, and/or compensating for high levels of violence exposure in childhood.

Development and Evaluation of Strategies to Prevent Child Maltreatment

DVP also develops and evaluates the effectiveness of child maltreatment prevention programs. For example, DVP funded the evaluation of the Triple P, or Positive Parenting Program, a parent-training program implemented in 9 counties in South Carolina, with 9 matched counties as wait-list comparison counties. Compared to the matched counties, the Triple P counties had a lower increase in substantiated abuse cases, lower rates of child out-of-home placements, and lower rates of hospitalizations and emergency room visits for child injuries.[85] DVP has also funded 2 studies to establish the effectiveness and cost-effectiveness of delivering abusive head trauma (AHT) prevention information to parents and other caregivers in hospitals at the time of delivery and in public health clinics or pediatricians' offices at the first postnatal visit(s). DVP also houses a team of economists to estimate the financial burden of child maltreatment to society and the economic benefits and costs of prevention policies and programs. For example, DVP is developing a concrete framework for estimating the long-term costs of child maltreatment. The division is exploring whether sufficient information exists in the current literature to make long-term cost estimates for (1) the effects of child maltreatment on future perpetration of violence, such as youth violence and intimate partner violence; (2) the inter-generational effects of child maltreatment, such as the increased probability that victims of child maltreatment may maltreat their own children; (3) the effects of child maltreatment on long-term physical and mental health; and (4) the effects of child maltreatment on educational attainment and future productivity. Another project in this area involves linking a sample from the National Survey on Child and Adolescent Well-Being (NSCAW) data with individual Medicaid claims to develop an analytic approach for estimating the annual medical costs of children that are attributable to child maltreatment.

Implementation and Dissemination of Child Maltreatment Prevention Programs

DVP helps state and local partners plan, implement, and evaluate child maltreatment prevention programs, and conducts research on the effective dissemination, implementation, and utilization of prevention strategies. It also provides states and communities with information and resources to guide and enhance their child maltreatment prevention efforts. For example, DVP is partnering with the CDC Foundation and the Doris Duke Charitable Foundation to investigate the core components of a state public health strategy for the promotion of SSNRs in the lives of children. This initiative includes an environmental scan of child maltreatment prevention efforts in the public health agencies of all 50 states, the District of Columbia, and United States territories. Findings from this scan, along with a select number of in-depth case studies, are providing information on emerging models and core/common components of promising state-level public health approaches to child maltreatment prevention. This information is also being used to develop concrete recommendations for state public health agencies to help enhance their work to promote SSNRs in their states, as well as a number of tools and resources to support these efforts. These recommendations and tools will then be disseminated to state and local public health agencies through national public health networks, child maltreatment prevention organizations, and other channels. Additionally, DVP is studying how to better translate the science behind child maltreatment prevention so that it is actionable and useful for practice in the field. Currently, DVP is exploring ways for the findings from the Adverse Childhood Experience studies[95,96] to shape changes in policy, practice, and community involvement to promote SSNRs at the community and societal level. The division is also involved in the development, implementation, and promotion of the Essentials for Childhood: Safe, Stable, Nurturing Relationships for Children.

Conclusion

The efforts of the child welfare system mainly focus on receiving and responding to reports of child maltreatment. In addition to child welfare, law enforcement and the courts have a statutory mandate to assume a major role to protect children from harm. However, protection of children should take "a more comprehensive holistic response."[97] Whereas child welfare and the justice system are focused on responding and alleviating the consequences of child maltreatment, public health can complement their services by focusing its efforts upstream to prevent child maltreatment.

Public health at the federal, state, and local level can provide leadership in child maltreatment prevention in a number of ways that are at the core of essential public health services, including surveillance of child and family health and well-being, eg, vital statistics, hospital and emergency department records, school-based health assessments; establishing policies and regulations, eg, mandates on abusive head trauma; and direct service provision, eg, well-baby visits, Women, Infants, and Children (WIC), immunization, mental health and substance abuse treatment. Health departments can also help educate the public about the issues of child maltreatment and use existing structures, such as the Early Childhood Comprehensive Systems (ECCS) to convene child maltreatment stakeholders for action. Furthermore, public health can frame the issue of child maltreatment as everyone's problem because public health moves it into the realm of a shared concern at the general population level – everyone is responsible for addressing the complex problem of child maltreatment and no one system or discipline has the capacity to address this issue on its own.

Furthermore, public health's role in the prevention of child maltreatment includes the development of a strong national prevention system to prevent child maltreatment by supporting programs and services that enhance family resiliency and foster the development of healthy children. Public health prevention infrastructure exists in every state and territory within the United States, with an average of about 2000 state employees in the workforce and state and federal funding of approximately $2.89 billion combined per state.[98] State public health systems also offer programs and services that promote healthy early child development, and promote the physical, emotional, and social well-being of children. Whereas the child welfare system serves an important role in intervening in situations where child maltreatment is already suspected, public health agencies commonly come in contact with children age 6 years and under, when parent receptivity for support is likely to be the highest, through prevention programs such as prenatal care programs; maternal mental health services; well-child services; screening programs, eg, maternal depression screening, screening for developmental delays in children; WIC; immunization services; early childhood education programs, eg, Head Start; parent education/skills training programs; shaken baby prevention programs; and home visitation services. These programs and services provide opportunities for preventing child maltreatment before it occurs, and the public health system is uniquely positioned to provide these preventive services at a population level. Public health plays a critical role in helping children start on the right path so that they can reach their full potential.[99] Because many health and social problems arise as a consequence of adverse childhood experiences, CDC, as the nation's lead public health agency, must continue to improve the science base for effective child maltreatment prevention and support the dissemination, implementation, and utilization of these prevention strategies in state and local public health systems. Every child in America should have the opportunity to reach his or her full potential, and a public health approach to the prevention of child maltreatment will yield valuable returns to the nation's health and quality of life for its people.

References

1. Mercy JA, Rosenberg ML, Powell KE, Broome CV, Roper WL. Public health policy for preventing violence. *Health Aff (Millwood).* 1993;12:(4):7-29.

2. United States Department of Health and Human Services, Administration for Children and Families, Children's Bureau. Child maltreatment 2008. Administration for Children and Families Web site. http://www.acf.hhs.gov/programs/cb/research-data-technology/statistics-research/child-maltreatment. Accessed February 14, 2013.

3. United States Advisory Board on Child Abuse and Neglect. *Child Abuse and Neglect: Critical First Steps in Response to a National Emergency.* Washington, DC: Government Printing Office; 1990.

4. Finkelhor D, Turner H, Ormrod R, Hamby S, Kracke K. Children's exposure to violence: a comprehensive national survey. National Institute of Corrections Web site. http://nicic.gov/Library/024077. Published 2009. Accessed October 13, 2009.

5. National Scientific Council on the Developing Child. The timing and quality of early experiences combine to shape brain architecture: working paper no. 5. Harvard University Center on the Developing Child Web site. http://developingchild.harvard.edu/index.php/resources/reports_and_working_papers/working_papers/wp5/. Published December 2007. Accessed February 18, 2013.

6. Nelson CA. The neurobiological bases of early intervention. In: Shonkoff JP, Meisels SJ, eds. *Handbook of Early Childhood Intervention.* 2nd ed. New York, NY: Cambridge University Press; 2000:204-227.

7. Carrion V, Weems C, Reiss A. Stress predicts brain changes in children: a pilot longitudinal study on youth stress, posttraumatic stress disorder, and the hippocampus. *Pediatrics.* 2007;119(3):509-516.

8. Shonkoff JP, Boyce WT, McEwen B. Neuroscience, molecular biology, and the childhood roots of health disparities: building a new framework for health promotion and disease prevention. *JAMA.* 2009;301(21):2252-2259.

9. Nelson CA III, McCleery JP. Use of event-related potentials in the study of typical and atypical development. *J Am Acad Child Adolesc Psychiatry.* 2008;47(11):1252-1261.

10. Anda RF, Croft J, Felitti V, et al. Adverse childhood experiences and smoking during adolescence and adulthood. *JAMA.* 1999;282(17):1652-1658.

11. Edwards VJ, Anda RF, Gu D, Dube SR, Felitti VJ. Adverse childhood experiences and smoking persistence in adults with smoking-related symptoms and illness. *Perm J.* 2007;11:5-7.

12. Dong M, Giles WH, Felitti VJ, et al. Insights into causal pathways for ischemic heart disease: Adverse Childhood Experiences study. *Circulation.* 2004;110:1761-1766.

13. Felitti VJ, Anda RF, Nordenberg D, et al. Relationship of childhood abuse and household dysfunction to many of the leading causes of death in adults: the Adverse Childhood Experiences (ACE) study. *Am J Prev Med.* 1998;14(4):245-258.

14. Williamson DF, Thompson TJ, Anda RF, Dietz WH, Felitti VJ. Body weight, obesity, and self-reported abuse in childhood. *Int J Obes Relat Metab Disord.* 2002;26(8):1075-1082.

15. Brown L, Kessel S, Lourie K, Ford H, Lipsitt L. Influence of sexual abuse on HIV-related attitudes and behaviors in adolescent psychiatric inpatients. *J Am Acad Child Adolesc Psychiatry.* 1997;36(3):316-322.

16. Dietz PM, Spitz AM, Anda RF, et al. Unintended pregnancy among adult women exposed to abuse or household dysfunction during their childhood. *JAMA.* 1999;282(14):1359-1364.

17. Hillis SD, Anda RF, Dube SR, Felitti VJ, Marchbanks PA, Marks JS. The association between adverse childhood experiences and adolescent pregnancy, long-term psychosocial consequences and fetal death. *Pediatrics.* 2004;113(2):320-327.

18. Hillis SD, Anda RF, Felitti VJ, Marchbanks PA. Adverse childhood experiences and sexual risk behaviors in women: a retrospective cohort study. *Fam Plann Perspect.* 2001;33(5):206-211.

19. Anda RF, Brown D, Dube S, Bremner J, Felitti V, Giles W. Adverse childhood experiences and chronic obstructive pulmonary disease in adults. *Am J Prev Med.* 2008;34(5):396-403.

20. Kendall-Tackett KA, Marshall R. Victimization and diabetes: an exploratory study. *Child Abuse Negl.* 1999;23(6):593-596.

21. Kendall-Tackett KA. Chronic pain syndromes as sequelae of childhood abuse. In: Kendall-Tackett KA, Giacomoni SM, eds. *Child Victimization.* Kingston, NJ: Civic Research Institute, Inc.; 2005:9-1–9-17.

22. Dube SR, Fairweather D, Pearson WS, Felitti VJ, Anda RF, Croft JB. Cumulative childhood stress and autoimmune diseases in adults. *Psychosom Med.* 2009;71(2):243-250.

23. Hillis SD, Anda RF, Felitti VJ, Nordenberg D, Marchbanks PA. Adverse childhood experiences and sexually transmitted diseases in men and women: a retrospective study. *Pediatrics.* 2000;106(1):E11.

24. Dong M, Dube SR, Felitti VJ, Giles WH, Anda RF. Adverse childhood experiences and self-reported liver disease: new insights into the causal pathway. *Arch Intern Med.* 2003;163(16):1949-1956.

25. Brown DW, Anda RF, Felitti VJ, et al. Adverse childhood experiences are associated with the risk of lung cancer: a prospective cohort study. *BMC Public Health.* 2010;10:311.

26. Fuller-Thomson E, Brennenstuhl S. Making a link between childhood physical abuse and cancer: results from a regional representative survey. *Cancer.* 2009;115(14):3341-3350.

27. Brown DW, Anda RF, Tiemmeir H. Adverse childhood experiences and the risk of premature mortality. *American J Preventative Med.* 2009;37(5):389-396.

28. Anda RF, Chapman DP, Felitti VJ, et al. Adverse childhood experiences and risk of paternity in teen pregnancy. *Obstet Gynecol.* 2002;100(1):37-45.

29. Delaney-Black V, Covington C, Ondersma SJ, et al. Violence exposure, trauma, and IQ and/or reading deficits among urban children. *Arch Pediatr Adolesc Med.* 2002;156(3):280-285.

30. Eckenrode J, Laird M, Doris J. School performance and disciplinary problems among abused and neglected children. *Dev Psychol.* 1993;29(1):53-62.

31. Perez C, Widom C. Childhood victimization and long-term intellectual and academic outcomes. *Child Abuse Negl.* 1994;18(8):617-633.

32. Chapman DP, Whitfield CL, Felitti VJ, Dube SR, Edwards VJ, Anda RF. Adverse childhood experiences and the risk of depressive disorders in adulthood. *J Affect Disord.* 2004;82(2):217-225.

33. Fergusson D, Boden J, Horwood L. Exposure to child sexual and physical abuse and adjustment in early adulthood. *Child Abuse Negl.* 2008;32(6):607-619.

34. Dube SR, Felitti VJ, Dong M, Chapman DP, Giles WH, Anda RF. Childhood abuse, neglect, and household dysfunction and the risk of illicit drug use: the Adverse Childhood Experiences study. *Pediatrics.* 2003;111(3):564-572.

35. Dube SR, Miller JW, Brown DW, et al. Adverse childhood experiences and the association with ever using alcohol and initiating alcohol use during adolescence. *J Adolesc Health.* 2006;38(4):444e1-444.e10.

36. Afifi TO, Boman J, Fleisher W, Sareen J. The relationship between child abuse, parental divorce, and lifetime mental disorders and suicidality in a nationally representative adult sample. *Child Abuse Negl.* 2009;33(3):139-147.

37. Dube SR, Anda RF, Felitti VJ, Chapman DP, Williamson D, Giles WH. Childhood abuse, household dysfunction, and the risk of attempted suicide throughout the life span: findings from the Adverse Child Experiences study. *JAMA.* 2001;286(24):3089-3096.

38. Duke NN, Pettingell SL, McMorris BJ, Borowsky IW. Adolescent violence perpetration: associations with multiple types of adverse childhood experiences. *Pediatrics.* 2010;125(4):e778-e786.

39. Wolfe DA, Wekerle C, Scott K, Straatman A, Grasley C. Predicting abuse in adolescent dating relationships over 1 year: the role of child maltreatment and trauma. *J Abnorm Psychol.* 2004;113(3):406-415.

40. Bensley L, Van Eenwyk J, Wynkoop Simmons K. Childhood family violence history and women's risk for intimate partner violence and poor health. *Am J Prev Med.* 2003;25(1):38-44.

41. Gómez AM, Speizer IS. Intersections between childhood abuse and adult intimate partner violence among Ecuadorian women. *Matern Child Health J.* 2009;13(4):559-566.

42. Knudsen E, Heckman J, Cameron J, Shonkoff J. Economic, neurobiological, and behavioral perspectives on building America's future workforce. *Proc Natl Acad Sci USA.* 2006;103(27):10155-10162.

43. Miller TR, Cohen MA, Wiersema B. *Victim Costs and Consequences: A New Look.* NIJ Research Report 90-IJ-CX-0050. Washington, DC: National Institute of Justice, US Department of Justice; 1996.

44. Centers for Disease Control and Prevention. Strategic direction for child maltreatment prevention: preventing child maltreatment through the promotion of safe, stable, and nurturing relationships between children and their caregivers. Centers for Disease Control and Prevention Web site. http://www.cdc.gov/ViolencePrevention/pdf/CM_Strategic_Direction--Long-a.pdf. Published 2008. Accessed September 2, 2009.

45. Dahlberg LL, Mercy JA. History of violence as a public health problem. *Virtual Mentor*. 2009;11(2):167-172.

46. Bronfenbrenner U. Toward an experimental ecology of human development. *Am Psychol.* 1977;32(7):513-531.

47. Dahlberg LL, Krug EG. Violence—a global public health problem. In: Krug E, Dahlberg LL, Mercy JA, Zwi AB, Lozano R, eds. *World Report on Violence and Health*. Geneva, Switzerland: World Health Organization; 2002:3-21.

48. Allegrante J, Marks R, Hansen DW. Ecological models for the control and prevention of unintentional injury. In: Gielen AC, Sleet DA, Diclemente R, eds. *Injury and Violence Prevention: Behavioral Science Theories, Methods, and Applications*. San Francisco, CA: Jossey Bass; 2005:105-128.

49. Belsky J. Child maltreatment: an ecological integration. *Am Psychol.* 1980;35(4):320-355.

50. Cicchetti D, Rizley R. Developmental perspectives on the etiology, intergenerational transmission, and sequelae of child maltreatment. *New Dir Child Adolesc Dev.* 1981;1981(11):31-53.

51. Cicchetti D, Lynch M. Toward an ecological/transiactional model of community violence and child maltreatment: consequences for children's development. *Psychiatry*. 1993;56(1):96-118.

52. Garbarino J. The human ecology of child maltreatment: a conceptual model for research. *J Marriage Fam.* 1977;39(4):721-735.

53. Stokols D. Establishing and maintaining healthy environments. *Am Psychol.* 1992;47(1):6-22.

54. Stokols D. Translating social ecological theory into guidelines for community health promotion. *Am J Health Promot.* 1996;10(4):282-298.

55. Centers for Disease Control and Prevention. The social-ecological model: a framework for prevention. Centers for Disease Control and Prevention Web site. http://www.cdc.gov/violenceprevention/overview/social-ecologicalmodel.html. Published September 9, 2009. Accessed January 15, 2015.

56. National Scientific Council on the Developing Child. Young children develop in an environment of relationships: working paper no. 1. Harvard University Center on the Developing Child Web site. http://developingchild.harvard.edu/index.php/resources/reports_and_working_papers/working_papers/wp1/. Published 2004. Accessed August 10, 2006.

57. National Research Council and Institute of Medicine. *From Neurons to Neighborhoods: The Science of Early Childhood Development.* Committee on Integrating the Science of Early Childhood Development. In: Jack P. Shonkoff and Deborah A. Phillips, eds. Board on Children, Youth, and Families, Commission on Behavioral and Social Sciences and Education. Washington, D.C.: National Academy Press, 2000.

58. Mercy JA, Saul J. Creating a healthier future through early interventions for children. *JAMA.* 2009;301(21):2262-2264.

59. Barnard KE, Solchany JE. Mothering. In: Bornstein MH, ed. *Handbook of Parenting: Volume 3: Being and Becoming a Parent.* 2nd ed. Mahwah, NJ: Lawrence Erlbaum Associates, Inc; 2002:3-25.

60. Ainsworth M. Patterns of infant-mother attachments: antecedents and effects on development. *Bull N Y Acad Med.* 1985;61(9):792-812.

61. Bowlby J. Developmental psychiatry comes of age. *Am J Psychiatry.* 1988;145(1):1-10.

62. Antonovsky A. How the sense of coherence develops over the lifespan in unraveling the mystery of health. In: Antonovsky A, ed. *How People Manage Stress and Stay Well.* San Francisco, CA: Jossey-Bass; 1987:89-127.

63. Widom CS, Maxfield MG. An update on the "cycle of violence." National Criminal Justice Reference Service Web site. https://www.ncjrs.gov/pdffiles1/nij/184894.pdf. Published February 2001. Accessed February 18, 2013.

64. Sidebotham P, Heron J. Child maltreatment in the "children of the nineties:" a cohort study of risk factors. *Child Abuse Negl.* 2006;30(5):497-522.

65. Stith SM, Lui T, Davies LC, et al. Risk factors in child maltreatment: a meta-analytic review of the literature. *Aggress Violent Behav.* 2009;14(1):13-29.

66. Seagull EAW. Social support and child maltreatment: a review of the evidence. *Child Abuse Negl.* 1987;11(1):41-42.

67. Seeman TE, Singer B, Horwitz R, McEwen BS. The price of adaptation—allostatic load and its health consequences: MacArthur studies of successful aging. *Arch Intern Med.* 1997;157(19):2259-2268.

68. Waters E, Kondo-Ikemura K, Posada G, Richters JE. Learning to love: mechanisms and milestones. In: Gunnar M, Sroufe L, eds. *Self Processes and Development.* Mahwah, NJ: Lawrence Erlbaum Associates, Inc; 1991:217-255. *Minnesota Symposium on Child Psychology*; vol 23.

69. Shaw DS, Gilliom M, Ingoldsby EM, Nagin DS. Trajectories leading to school age conduct problems. *Dev Psychol.* 2003;39(2):189-200.

70. Dawson G, Asman DB. On the origins of a vulnerability to depression: the influence of the early social environment on the development of psychobiological systems related to risk of affective disorder. In: Nelson CA, ed. *The Effects of Early Adversity on Neurobehavioral Development.* Vol 9. *Minnesota Symposia on Child Psychology.* Mahwah, NJ: Lawrence Erlbaum Associates Inc; 2000:245-279.

71. Dawson G, Frey K, Panagiotides H, Yamada E, Hessl D, Osterling J. Infants of depressed mothers exhibit atypical frontal electrical brain activity during interactions with mother and with a familiar nondepressed adult. *Child Dev.* 1999:70(5):1058-1066.

72. Garbarino J, Crouter A. Defining the community context of parent-child relations: the correlates of child maltreatment. *Child Dev.* 1978;49(3):604-616.

73. Garbarino J, Kostelny K. Child maltreatment as a community problem. *Child Abuse Negl.* 1992;16(4):455-464.

74. Hashima PY, Amato PR. Poverty, social support, and parental behavior. *Child Dev.* 1994;65(2 spec no):394-403.

75. Kotch JB, Browne DC, Ringwalt CL, Dufort V, Ruina E. Stress, social support, and substantiated maltreatment in the second and third years of life. *Child Abuse Negl.* 1997;21(11):1025-1037.

76. Lundahl B, Risser HJ, Lovejoy MC. A meta-analysis of parent training: moderators and follow-up effects. *Clin Psychol Rev.* 2006;26(1):86-104.

77. Reynolds AJ, Temple JA, Ou SR. School-based early intervention and child well-being in the Chicago Longitudinal Study. *Child Welfare.* 2003;82(5):633-658.

78. Taylor TK, Biglan A. Behavioral family interventions for improving child-rearing: a review of the literature for clinicians and policy-makers. *Clin Child Fam Psychol Rev.* 1998;1(1):41-60.

79. Dias MS, Smith K, deGuehery K, Mazur P, Li V, Shaffer ML. Preventing abusive head trauma among infants and young children: a hospital-based, parent education program. *Pediatrics.* 2005;115(4):470-477.

80. Chaffin M, Silovsky JF, Funderburk B, et al. Parent-child interaction therapy with physically abusive parents: efficacy for reducing future abuse reports. *J Consult Clin Psychol.* 2004;72(3):500-510.

81. Kaufman J, Yang B, Douglas-Palumberi H, et al. Social supports and serotonin transporter gene moderate depression in maltreated children. *Proc Natl Acad Sci USA.* 2004;101(49):17316-17321.

82. MacMillan HL, Wathen CN, Barlow J, Fergusson DM, Leventhal JM, Taussig HN. Interventions to prevent child maltreatment and associated impairment. *Lancet.* 2009;373(9659):250-266.

83. Hill P, Uris P, Bauer T. The Nurse-Family Partnership: a policy priority: in-home nurse visits are cost-effective and evidence based. *Am J Nurs.* 2007;107(11):73-75.

84. Council on Community Pediatrics. The role of preschool home-visiting programs in improving children's developmental and health outcomes. *Pediatrics.* 2009;123(2):598-603.

85. Prinz RJ, Sanders MR, Shapiro CJ, Whitaker DJ, Lutzker JR. Population-based prevention of child maltreatment: the US Triple P system population trial. *Prev Sci.* 2009;10(1)1-12.

86. Nowak C, Heinrichs N. A comprehensive meta-analysis of Triple P-Positive Parenting Program using hierarchical linear modeling: effectiveness and moderating variables. *Clin Child Fam Psychol Rev.* 2008;11(3):114-144.

87. Runyan D, Wattam C, Ikeda R, Hassan F, Ramiro L. Child abuse and neglect by parents and other caregivers. In: Krug E, Dahlberg LL, Mercy JA, Zwi AB, Lozano R, eds. *World Report on Violence and Health.* Geneva, Switzerland: World Health Organization; 2002:59-86.

88. Freisthler B, Merritt DH, LaScala EA. Understanding the ecology of child maltreatment: a review of the literature and directions for future research. *Child Maltreat.* 2006;11(3):263-280.

89. Runyan DK, Hunter WM, Socolar RRS, et al. Children who prosper in unfavorable environments: the relationship to social capital. *Pediatrics.* 1998;101(1 part 1):12-18.

90. Coulton CJ, Crampton DS, Irwin M, Spilsbury JC, Korbin JE. How neighborhoods influence child maltreatment: a review of the literature and alternative pathways. *Child Abuse Negl.* 2007;31(11-12):1117-1142.

91. Runyan DK, Curtis PA, Hunter WM, et al. LONGSCAN: a consortium for longitudinal studies of child maltreatment and the life course of children. *Aggress Violent Behav.* 1998;3(3):275-285.

92. Black MM, Oberlander SE, Lewis T, et al. Sexual intercourse among adolescents maltreated before age 12: a prospective investigation. *Pediatrics.* 2009;124(3):941-949.

93. Hammond WR. Public health and child maltreatment prevention: the role of the Centers for Disease Control and Prevention. *Child Maltreat.* 2003;8(2):81-83.

94. Mercy JA, Barker L, Frazier L. The secrets of the National Violent Death Reporting System. *Inj Prev.* 2006;12(suppl 2):ii1-ii2.

95. Anda RF, Dong M, Brown DW, et al. The relationship of adverse childhood experiences to a history of premature death of family members. *BMC Public Health.* 2009;9:106.

96. Corso PS, Edwards VJ, Fang X, Mercy JA. Health-related quality of life among adults who experienced maltreatment during childhood. *Am J Public Health.* 2008;98(6):1094-1100.

97. Schene P. Child abuse and neglect policy: history, models, and future directions. In: Briere J, Berliner L, Bulkley JA, Jenny C, Reid T, eds. *The APSAC Handbook on Child Maltreatment.* Thousand Oaks, CA: Sage; 1996:385-397.

98. Beitsch L, Brooks R, Menachemi N, Libbey P. Public health at center stage: new roles, old props. *Health Aff (Millwood).* 2006;25(4):911-922.

99. Friedan T. CDC priorities and challenges. Paper presented at: the Center Leadership Council Retreat: Atlanta, GA; 2009.

Additional Reading/Resources

Centers for Disease Control and Prevention. Injury prevention and control: data and statistics. Web-based Injury Statistics Query and Reporting System (WISQARS) Web site. http://www.cdc.gov/ncipc/wisqars. Updated December 17, 2012. Accessed April 5, 2006.

Centers for Disease Control and Prevention. *Third National Report on Human Exposure to Environmental Chemicals.* NCEH publication 05-0570. Atlanta, GA: Centers for Disease Control and Prevention; 2006.

Chapman DP, Whitfield CL, Felitti VJ, Dube SR, Edwards VJ, Anda RF. Adverse childhood experiences and the risk of depressive disorders in adulthood. *J Affect Disord.* 2004;82(2):217-225.

Danese A, Pariante C, Caspi A, Taylor A, Pulton R. Childhood maltreatment predicts adult inflammation in a life-course study. *Proc Natl Acad Sci USA.* 2007;104(4):1319-1324.

DePrince AP, Weinzierl KM, Combs MD. Executive function performance and trauma exposure in a community sample of children. *Child Abuse Negl.* 2009;33(6):353-361.

Dube SR, Anda RF, Felitti VJ, Edwards VJ, Williamson DF. Exposure to abuse, neglect and household dysfunction among adults who witnessed intimate partner violence as children: implications for health and social services. *Violence Vict.* 2002;17(1):3-17.

Eigsti IM, Ciccheti D. The impact of child maltreatment on expressive syntax at 60 months. *Dev Sci.* 2004;7(1):88-102.

Finkelstein EA, Corso PS, Miller TR. *Incidence and Economic Burden of Injuries in the United States.* New York, NY: Oxford University Press; 2006.

Kendall-Tackett KA. *Treating the Lifetime Health Effects of Childhood Victimization.* Kingston, NJ: Civic Research Institute, Inc.; 2003.

Langlois JA, Rutland-Brown W, Thomas KE. *Traumatic Brain Injury in the United States: Emergency Department Visits, Hospitalizations, and Deaths.* Atlanta, GA: Centers for Disease Control and Prevention, National Center for Injury Prevention and Control; 2004.

Litovitz TL, Klein-Schwartz W, White S, et al. 2000 Annual report of the American Association of Poison Control Centers Toxic Exposures Surveillance System. *Am J Emerg Med.* 2001;19(5):337-396.

McGowan PO, Sasaki A, D'Alessio AC, et al. Epigenetic regulation of the glucocorticoid receptor in human brain associates with childhood abuse. *Nat Neurosci.* 2009;12(3):342-348.

NHTSA's National Center for Statistics and Analysis. *Traffic Safety Facts 2004 Data: Children.* Washington, DC: NHTSA; 2005. http://www-nrd.nhtsa.dot.gov/Pubs/809906.pdf. Accessed December 30, 2005.

Putnam FW. Ten-year research update review: child sexual abuse. *J Am Acad Child Adolesc Psychiatry.* 2003;42(3):269-278.

Repetti RL, Taylor SE, Seeman TE. Risky families: Family social environments and the mental and physical health of offspring. *Psychol Bull.* 2002;128(2):330-366.

Shonkoff JP, Phillips DA, eds. *From Neurons to Neighborhoods: The Science of Early Childhood Development.* Washington, DC: National Academy Press; 2000.

US Department of Health and Human Services, Administration on Children, Youth, and Families. *Child Maltreatment 2003.* Washington, DC: Government Printing Office; 2005. http://www.acf.hhs.gov/programs/cb/pubs/cm03/index.htm. Accessed April 5, 2005.

US Department of Health and Human Services, Administration for Children and Families, Children's Bureau. Child maltreatment 2007. Administration for Children and Families Web site. http://www.acf.hhs.gov/programs/cb/research-data-technology/statistics-research/child-maltreatment. Accessed February 14, 2013.

Walker EA, Gelfand A, Katon WJ, et al. Adult health status of women with histories of childhood abuse and neglect. *Am J Med.* 1999;107(4):332-339.

Weems CF, Saltzman KM, Reiss AL, Carrion VG. A prospective test of the association between hyperarousal and emotional numbing in youth with a history of traumatic stress. *J Clin Child Adolesc Psychol.* 2003;32(1):166-171.

The findings and conclusions in this chapter are those of the authors and do not necessarily represent the official position of the Centers for Disease Control and Prevention.

Chapter 5

Economic Burden of Child Maltreatment

Phaedra Corso, PhD, MPA
Alexandria R. Chambers, MPH
Nathaniel H. Taylor, MPH

Introduction

Estimates of the burden of disease or injury for any health outcome, notwithstanding child maltreatment, have typically relied on epidemiologic evidence of morbidity and mortality as the first step in describing the magnitude of the health problem in the public health model for prevention. However, in this era of limited public resources to devote to any one health or nonhealth area of concern, burden of disease estimates are increasingly being supplemented with the economic impact of the disease or injury on society. In this way, economic burden estimates serve a number of useful purposes for practitioners, researchers, and policymakers alike. First, these estimates allow one to argue effectively for more funding to prevent and treat the consequences of child maltreatment. Second, these data describe the burden that child maltreatment places on society relative to other health outcomes under consideration, thus defining relative economic importance. Third, economic burden estimates can be used in future economic evaluations of interventions to prevent or treat the consequences of child maltreatment as an estimate of the potential savings should effective and cost-effective preventions be implemented. Assessment of the economic burden of child maltreatment is therefore essential in the dialogue about child maltreatment and its prevention.

Defining Economic Burden

Economic burden or economic impact analyses typically quantify burden by aggregating the direct medical expenditures resulting from a condition, the direct nonmedical expenditures associated with a condition, and the subsequent indirect losses in productivity potential for society (**Figure 5-1**). These analyses are often called cost of illness/injury (COI) analyses, although frequently COI analyses are limited to medical costs and productivity losses only.

Examples of direct medical expenditures include inpatient and outpatient hospital care, mental health care, medical transport required in the event of an emergency, medications and medical devices, and the medical treatment of chronic conditions resulting from the abuse. In general, any use of health care that would generate a medical claim or result in out-of-pocket expenses is considered in the estimates of medical costs associated with child maltreatment. Data sources for information on medical costs include, but are not limited to, medical chart review, national datasets (Medical Expenditure Panel Survey, Agency for Healthcare Research and Quality), self-report, and the literature. Direct non-medical expenditures include utilization of the child welfare services, law enforcement, and the criminal justice system. Sources for these unit cost estimates can include the literature, personal communication, and government records. Productivity losses are of 3 types: (1) the child missing school or performing at subpar levels in school because of

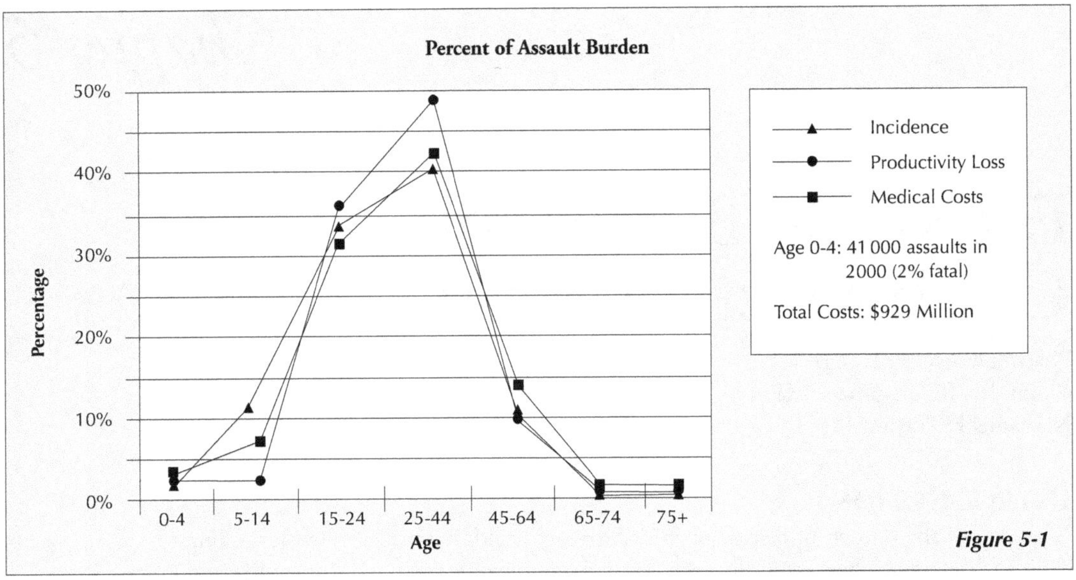

Figure 5-1. *Percent of assault burden by age in years.*

the abuse, (2) the parent missing work or performing at subpar levels at work because of the abuse situation or having to deal with child welfare and criminal justice services, and (3) permanent losses in lifetime productivity potential because of premature death. In most economic impact analyses, productivity losses are based on average employment wages (including fringe benefits) for the parent, with some adjustments for household productivity. These average employment wages are also used as a proxy for the child productivity losses. Premature death is valued at the average annual expected earnings based on gender, age, and remaining life expectancy.[1-6]

Three Approaches for Isolating Direct Medical Costs in Economic Burden Estimates

In assessing the direct medical costs for a health outcome of interest, such as violence, there are 3 general approaches. One approach is to first identify the population that has experienced the abuse, and then to sum the costs for all utilization of medical care services for that population. With this approach, the sum of all medical costs for one population, the "abused," is compared to the sum of all medical costs for a comparator population, the "nonabused," for example. The marginal difference in costs between the abused and nonabused group is, therefore, considered the excess utilization and costs of medical care associated with abuse. Following this approach, Bonomi et al[7] found that the average annual costs of health care for a group of women with no history of child maltreatment was $2413, compared to $2915 in average annual costs of health care for a group of women reporting a history of child maltreatment. The difference in costs between the 2 groups (multiplied by the number reporting abuse, or the incidence of abuse for the entire population) thus represents the excess burden on the health care system because of child maltreatment. The advantages of this method for assessing direct medical costs associated with maltreatment include the ability to conduct relative comparisons between populations and across time and to understand the incremental impact that specific diseases and injuries have on the health care system. The disadvantages of this approach are that it does not isolate the medical costs specifically tied to the illness or injury under consideration and this approach provides no understanding of the costs that comorbid health conditions, such as depression, may have on total costs of violence.

To address the disadvantages of summing all medical costs, a more conservative approach is to include only those health care costs that can be explicitly linked to the condition of interest. This method requires identifying diagnosis-specific health care utilization (and costs) through the use of diagnosis and external cause codes used in inpatient settings and/or self-reports of health care utilization that are identified as related to the abuse. For example, a broken arm treated in the emergency room would be identified as caused by violence through the use of an external cause code. The major advantages of this approach are that diagnosis-specific costs allow one to determine the percentage of total health care costs that are violence-related and costs are unlikely overinflated as in the previous approach. However, the major disadvantage of this approach is that many violence-related events are under-reported by the victim or incorrectly coded in health care settings for a number of reasons, including lack of proper screening protocols or training for health care providers and no health insurance reimbursement options. Thus, these estimates almost always yield a lower-bound estimate of violence-related costs, resulting in an under-inflated estimate of the true economic impact of violence.

A third approach attempts to supplement either of the 2 previously mentioned approaches by including the costs of the fraction of other health conditions attributed to child maltreatment. For example, if it is the case that child maltreatment is a significant contributor to poor mental health outcomes, then one would want to calculate the fraction of total mental health care costs that are attributable to child maltreatment and add those costs to the costs of health care directly attributable to child maltreatment. Defining costs this way includes the indirect health care expenditures associated with the violence through other diseases and conditions resulting from the maltreatment. The attributable fraction is added to the total diagnosis-specific costs, providing a total cost that deals directly with comorbidities. Although this method is adept at isolating all of the costs related to child maltreatment, it is often difficult to obtain the appropriate epidemiologic data. For example, epidemiologic data on attributable fraction from one study may not translate well to population-level attributable fraction; that is, the attributable fraction for one population may not hold for other populations.

Short-term and Long-term Economic Burden Estimates

Although it is useful to characterize economic burden by direct (medical and nonmedical) expenditures and productivity losses, one may also define economic burden of child maltreatment by its association with short- and long-term consequences of abuse. In order to define the economic burden this way, epidemiologic evidence on the negative short- and long-term consequences of the physical and mental health of its victims must be used to inform the COI estimates. Short-term medical costs are typically defined as the utilization of health care associated with the acute phases of the abuse that result in injury. These costs would include the use of medical transport, inpatient hospitalization, and any short-term follow-up in an outpatient setting, including medication or medical device use. Short-term productivity losses include the child missing school and the parent missing work because of the immediate abuse or the short-term follow-up with nonmedical entities.

A number of studies in the United States provide estimates of the cost per case of child maltreatment for these short-term costs and productivity losses. Hospitalization of child maltreatment victims is associated with significant and varied costs,[8] with one study finding average hospital charges per case of child abuse to be $5776 (1995 USD)[9] and another having charges of $35 461 (1994 USD)[10] for severe cases of abuse, many resulting in death. The length of stay required for inpatient care ranged from 8.2 days to 9.8 days.[10-13] Costs per case of child maltreatment differed based on type of abuse, with physical abuse being the most expensive at an average cost of $17593 (1999 USD), followed by neglect at $14292, sexual abuse at $11 285, and emotional/psychological abuse at $9875.[14] One study found that traumatic brain injury due to child abuse resulted in average hospital charges of $40 082 (1999 USD),[12] while another study estimated costs per case of head trauma at $25 481 (1993-2000 USD).[13] Finally, another study determined that burned victims of child maltreatment had total inpatient and outpatient costs of $23 253 per case (1990-1994 USD).[15]

Outside the United States, several similar studies of the short-term costs of child maltreatment have been conducted. For example, abused children seeking treatment in the emergency room of a Liverpool hospital had annual costs of $128 758 per case (2001 USD) for assessment and primary treatment only.[16] In a state in Brazil, average hospital costs for child and adolescent victims of violence were found to be $184 (1999 USD).[16]

Beyond medical costs and productivity losses, other short-term costs include those direct costs associated with law enforcement to investigate child abuse claims, with criminal justice to adjudicate abuse claims, and with child protective services for investigation, child welfare services, foster care, and in-home treatments, for example.

In addition to the deleterious effects of child maltreatment on short-term medical and nonmedical costs and productivity losses, there is increasing evidence that abuse leads to lifelong susceptibility to physical and mental health problems such as cardiovascular disease, hypertension, diabetes, anxiety disorders, depression, and substance abuse.[17-23] Related evidence indicates that early childhood maltreatment also has a profound effect on a range of cognitive, social, and emotional competencies that lay the foundation for negative impacts on education and future economic productivity.[24-26] Maltreatment may therefore hinder an individual's skill development so that they are unable to maintain or better their socioeconomic status, making maltreatment a causal factor in perpetuating social inequities strongly associated with long-term poor health and premature mortality.[25,27,28] Data to estimate long-term costs of child maltreatment are relatively scarce, but sources for these data include self-reports, medical record review, and the literature.[29]

Therefore, important long-term medical costs to consider include marginal increases in the utilization of physical and mental health care due to chronic sequelae, such as depression, drug/alcohol abuse, obesity, and other persistent conditions. Long-term productivity losses would include sustained deficits in future educational and occupational attainment and losses in future earnings associated with premature mortality. Special education for temporary or permanent cognitive disabilities represents another category of long-term costs, along with the increased utilization of social welfare services. Increased violence victimization and violence perpetration add to these costs by leading to increases in medical utilization and criminal justice system costs, decreases in productivity, and incarceration.[30] However, evidence on the costs of law enforcement and the judicial system is inconsistent and incomplete. These costs include utilization of the criminal justice system at the time of the crime as well as increased violence resulting from child maltreatment, including juvenile delinquency and adult criminality. Longitudinal studies of child maltreatment victims sponsored by the National Institute of Justice show increases in future violence perpetration and incarceration.[31] However, these findings have not been conclusively supported when the relationships were mediated by type of abuse and the role of child welfare services.[32-34] Even if conclusive evidence does link child maltreatment to longer-term criminal justice outcomes, those linkages still need to be adequately quantified in economic terms.[35] Furthermore, there is a lack of data on the losses in productivity for the perpetrator of the crime.

Defining Economic Burden as Prevalence- or Incidence-Based

Another way to consider the economic burden of child maltreatment is to consider prevalence- or incidence-based estimates. Prevalence-based estimates are cross-sectional estimates of costs that include all costs within a specific time period (usually a year), regardless of when the abuse occurred. For example, a prevalence-based estimate of child maltreatment costs occurring in 2006 would not only include the costs of new child maltreatment cases occurring in 2006 but also the follow-up costs for victims of child maltreatment that happened prior to 2006.

The advantage of prevalence-based estimates of the economic burden of child maltreatment is that because these estimates encompass all of the costs for child maltreatment in one specific time period, they are useful for thinking about the resources required for treatment within that time period. Data for prevalence-based estimates may also be more readily available from national health accounts or other national epidemiologic or economic data collection systems. For example, researchers from the National Commission of Inquiry into the Prevention of Child Abuse estimate that child abuse and neglect in England and Wales costs the government over 1 billion pounds annually ($1.7 billion 1996 USD).[36] In another study, it was estimated that the annual costs of welfare and legal services associated with child maltreatment in the UK is $1.2 billion annually (1996 USD).[16] Child maltreatment was responsible for 65.1% of hospital admissions and 77.9% of hospital costs per year in a major city of a state in Brazil.[37]

In the United States, the Bonomi et al study[7] described previously is also an example of a prevalence-based approach to assessing the economic burden of child maltreatment because claims data were analyzed for a cross-section of women over a 1-year time period. The authors found that women with a childhood history of physical and sexual abuse had annual health care costs that were 36% higher than those women who did not experience child abuse at all. Those women who had experienced physical or sexual abuse only had annual health care costs that were 22% and 16% higher, respectively, than those women who were not abused as children. Similarly, Hulme[38] found that women who had a history of childhood sexual abuse visited a primary care clinic 1.33 more times than women who were not sexually abused and their primary care costs were an average of $150 more over a 2-year period. In another prevalence-based study, women who self-reported as victims of child maltreatment had median annual health care costs that were $97 greater than women who did not report abuse or neglect.[39] Those cost differences increase to $245 when comparing women who were sexually abused to those who were not abused at all.

The disadvantage of prevalence-based estimates is that they do not account for the full, lifetime costs associated with a disease or injury, which has particular relevance for child maltreatment given the epidemiologic evidence of long-term effects. In comparison, incidence-based estimates are longitudinal analyses that measure the lifetime costs for all new illness and injury cases that occur during a particular time frame. For example, an incidence-based estimate of child maltreatment costs from the base year of 2006 would include all lifetime expenditures associated with all new cases of child maltreatment occurring in that year. The advantage of incidence-based estimates is that these data can be used to define the cost per case prevented in order to conduct full economic evaluations. These estimates provide a more complete picture of total costs, which may be a more powerful tool for lobbying for more resources to prevent child maltreatment. The disadvantages of incidence-based estimates are that they are the most difficult to assess because they require longitudinal data on epidemiologic outcomes and economic costs and the resources (in labor, expertise, and time) required to develop methodologically sound estimates are usually cost prohibitive. Thus, national incidence-based estimates of child maltreatment are scarce.

Corso and Fertig[40] provide a summary of all national incidence-based cost estimates of child maltreatment in the United States. The first comprehensive study providing a US estimate of the economic burden of child maltreatment was conducted by Daro in 1988.[41] The calculations of economic burden in that study included both short-term costs (hospitalization, foster care, and juvenile court and detention) and long-term costs (medical rehabilitation, special education, extended foster care, and productivity losses of future earnings). Total short-term and long-term costs associated with child maltreatment were found to be at a minimum of $3.3 billion in 1982 USD.

The next attempt to determine the US national estimate of the economic burden of child maltreatment was the Miller et al study in 1996.[42] By including an estimate of the reduced quality of life with a value for pain and suffering, the authors calculated a much larger estimate of the total cost of child maltreatment. In addition to the quality of life reduction estimates, medical costs, lost earning, and the cost of public programs for victims were also included in the estimation. Their main finding was that the national economic burden of child maltreatment in the United States was $56 billion in 1993 USD.

Two separate studies have been conducted by Prevent Child Abuse America (PCAA) to estimate the national cost of child maltreatment. The first study, published in 2001, included such costs as hospitalizations, long-term chronic health problems, mental health, child welfare, law enforcement, the judicial system, special education, juvenile delinquency, adult mental health and health care, productivity losses to society, and adult criminality.[43] Direct costs were estimated to be $24.4 billion (1993 USD) and indirect costs were estimated at $69.7 billion (1993 USD). The 2001 estimate was updated by PCAA in 2007 to $103.7 billion (2007 USD).[44] In the 2007 estimate, the set of cost categories was smaller than the 2001 report because of the removal of the costs of chronic health conditions and the costs of the judicial system.

More recently, Fang et al[45] estimated the aggregate lifetime costs for all new child maltreatment cases and the average lifetime costs per child maltreatment victim occurring in 2008 using an incidence-based approach from the societal perspective. Included in the analysis were long- and short-term health care costs (including physical and mental health), child welfare costs, special education costs, productivity losses, and criminal justice costs. The authors estimated the lifetime economic burden of new cases of child maltreatment in the United States in 2008 at $124 billion (2010 USD). These estimates resulted from over 570 000 new nonfatal cases and more than 1700 new fatal cases of child maltreatment. Per-victim costs of child maltreatment were estimated at over $200 000 for nonfatal and $1.2 million for fatal cases.

Defining Burden Using Other Measures of Relevance to Economics

Cost of illness/injury (COI) analyses are obviously important to policymakers and those lobbying for more prevention funding. However, COI estimates lack information on other important individual and societal costs such as losses in quality of life, functional capacity, harm to the family, intergenerational harm, and pathways to other forms of violence due to child maltreatment like youth violence, adult-perpetrated violence, partner violence, and suicide risks.[16,46]

For example, adult socioeconomic well-being is one type of information that is often neglected in measures of the economic burden of child maltreatment. A study by Zelinski[47] addressed this oft-overlooked measure and found several interesting implications for the impact of child maltreatment on adult socioeconomic well-being. Victims of any maltreatment, sexual abuse, and severe neglect were all nearly twice as likely as those not victimized to have incomes that fell below the federal poverty line and into the lowest quartile of the income distribution. Those adults who had experienced multiple types of child maltreatment were found to be at the greatest risk for income shortfalls and were 2 times as likely to have a low family income and 3 times as likely to be in poverty. Employment status was also dependent on the experience of maltreatment. Overall, adults who had experienced maltreatment as children were twice as likely as those not victimized to be unemployed, thus resulting in substantial losses of productivity to society. This effect was mainly driven by those adults who had been physically abused or experienced multiple types of maltreatment, with higher rates of risk of being unemployed at 140% and 190%, respectively. Maltreatment was also shown to be associated with lower rates of health care coverage and a greater dependence on Medicaid, especially for victims experiencing sexual abuse. This finding suggests that taxpayers pay an incrementally higher share of health care costs for victims of abuse. Zelinski also found that parents who had been maltreated as children were themselves more likely to abuse and neglect their own children, indicating the often intergenerational nature of child maltreatment and family violence.[47] The author posits that the relationship between maltreatment and socioeconomic well-being may be a significant mechanism in understanding this intergenerational cycle of violence, not unlike the findings of others.[46]

Another measure of burden of disease/injury of relevance to the field of health economics is the impact on health-related quality of life (HRQoL). One commonly used HRQoL index for use in measuring burden of disease/injury is the quality-adjusted life year (QALY), which combines the disease/injury impact on length of life (survival) and quality of life.[48,49] Child maltreatment may largely influence its victims' life expectancy and long-term health-related quality of life (HRQoL), given the epidemiologic evidence on the long-term effects of abuse, and therefore the QALY is an appropriate burden measure to consider. Looking at these 2 outcomes together, therefore, allows one to assess the impact that child maltreatment has on the victims' remaining quality-adjusted life expectancy.

QALYs have relevance in the field of health economics for its use as an outcome measure in economic evaluations of health interventions, especially cost-effective analyses (CEAs)—whereby an intervention's costs are compared to its effects. For CEAs that use QALYs as the outcome measure, one compares the intervention's costs with the intervention's impact on life expectancy (survival) and HRQoL, or combined as cost per QALY saved relative to a comparator intervention. A distinct advantage in using QALYs as a measure of disease burden is that it allows one to compare interventions that affect disparate health outcomes and populations, such as child maltreatment versus pediatric cancer screening interventions.

Other health indices have been developed for more narrowly defined concepts of health and specific to the field of injury and violence. For example, the Functional Capacity Index (FCI) is a measure of disease/injury burden that incorporates death and functional loss (eg, excretory function, sexual function, ambulation, hand/arm movement) typically resulting from an injury into a single metric that can be used to adjust potential years of life and produce a measure of function-adjusted life years.[50,51] The resulting measure is similar to QALYs, but it is designed to measure physical function only (not mental/emotional and physical well-being) and the capacity of individuals to perform certain everyday tasks (and not the capacity to perform socially defined roles such as working or going to school). The FCI is potentially useful for comparing the impact that certain interventions, such as the prevention of shaken baby syndrome, have on multiple trauma in terms of reduced physical capacity.

Regardless of the health index selected, it may be quite challenging to assess the effects that child maltreatment may have on HRQoL. Prosser & Corso summarize the HRQoL literature relevant to child maltreatment.[52] The authors did not identify any studies that directly evaluated HRQoL in maltreated children, although several studies assessed HRQoL in adult survivors of child maltreatment. In general, the authors found that HRQoL instruments designed specifically for use in cost-effectiveness analyses have been developed for adults only and do not include many of the domains of health identified as being important in capturing changes in quality of life for child maltreatment, such as potential for growth and development or psychological sequelae specific to maltreatment.

Some of the challenges in assessing HRQoL for child maltreatment outcomes include problems in defining an average health state for acute or continuing violent episodes, the cognitive difficulties in determining impacts on health from the children themselves,[53] proxy issues concerning parents or caregivers who are likely the perpetrators of violence, and other reasons associated with research priorities and the development of the field of child maltreatment prevention.[54] Although it is often difficult to assess the impact of child maltreatment or its prevention on a person's quality of life after the maltreatment has ended, it proves even more challenging to determine that impact on a child's quality of life while the abuse is ongoing. A major reason for these challenges is that the measures used to evaluate changes in the HRQoL (see Gold et al[49] for a thorough examination of these measures) for different health states are often developmentally inappropriate to administer to children. To get at the child's HRQoL another way, parents often act as a proxy for assessing the child's quality of life and adjustments to it in response to changes in the child's life.[55-57] While this method is beneficial for valuing the impact on HRQoL of some interventions for other health states experienced by children (such as asthma, diabetes, cancer), parents are the most common perpetrators of child maltreatment and are therefore unreliable sources of information on their child's quality of life. Also, though it is already difficult to determine preferences for different health states from children, few generic elicitation instruments exist that have been validated in children and, until recently, no instruments had been developed or validated for children under the age of 10. In 2010, Wille et al[58] developed the European Quality of Life 5 Dimensions Youth (EQ-5D-Y) survey and it was validated by Ravens-Sieberer et al[59] for children and adolescents aged 7 to 12 years. However, further evaluations of EQ-5D-Y show that the survey is only reliable for self-assessment in children aged 9 to 12 years.[57]

One study that did assess the long-term impact of child maltreatment on HRQoL identified in the Prosser and Corso review[52] was conducted by Edwards et al[60] from the Adverse Childhood Experiences (ACE) Study.[17] The authors compared self-reports of HRQoL in an adult population to an index measure of the number of adverse exposures, including child maltreatment, experienced during childhood (the ACE score). One of this study's main findings was an inverse relationship between the ACE score (where the more adverse experiences, the higher the score) and the HRQoL summary measure. Expanding on Edwards' original study design and data, Corso et al[61] found a yearly loss of 0.03 QALYs, or 11 days per year, for adults self-reporting any form of maltreatment during childhood. Additionally, significant differences between the child maltreatment group and a no child maltreatment group were found for all age groups on HRQoL. The youngest age group showed the highest differential losses in HRQoL (0.04 QALYs, or 15 days per year). As age increased, the differential losses decreased, until 70+ years, at which time the marginal difference in utility losses between the child maltreatment and no child maltreatment groups increased.

Implications for Future Research

Compared to other fields in public health, there is a paucity of literature on the economic burden of child maltreatment. One reason for this lack of data is the challenge involved in placing a monetary value, or value of HRQoL, on possible outcomes associated with child maltreatment. For example, how does one calculate the dollar value of improved parental interpersonal relationships or enhanced children's social and character development? In addition, ethical issues arise with putting a monetary value on a person's life. To address this concern, one can view these estimates in light of cost per case of child maltreatment prevented based on these economic impact analyses. Another way to look at economic analyses of child maltreatment is society's willingness to pay to prevent child maltreatment. Taking this angle in evaluating the economic burden of child maltreatment is a possible area of research in the future and may be useful in assisting policymakers' decisions for allocating public health resources to improve the lives of children.[62]

Even after addressing the difficulty of placing a monetary value on life outcomes, investigators must further explore several research areas to have credible estimates of the economic impact of child maltreatment. First, as described in the previous section, more research is needed on the influence that child maltreatment has on HRQoL during childhood and its lasting impacts on HRQoL in adulthood. Second, an incidence-based model of long-term costs of child maltreatment needs to be developed in a methodologically rigorous way. Finally, another area of the cost estimates that needs to be explored is those costs associated with mortality and reduced life expectancy. To be able to precisely assess the economic impact of child maltreatment, dynamic epidemiological models must be developed to ascertain decreases in life expectancy associated with abuse, increases in long-term chronic disease as a result of the violence, and decreases in quality of life related to the medical and nonmedical costs of child maltreatment to the individual. Creating these models is a demanding undertaking, however. Establishing causal links to specific enduring injurious effects of child maltreatment, such as increased risky behaviors, criminal activity, and chronic victimization and perpetration of violence, is a complicated endeavor. Longitudinal studies comparing the maltreated to a control group are required to determine these causal links, a design that is often not possible. Arguments have also been made that one should not look at child maltreatment in isolation of other adverse childhood experiences that impact children, such as poverty, divorce, and exposure to parental alcohol and substance abuse,[17] but attempting to cost out the impacts of child maltreatment in respect to these other experiences is even more difficult.

By creating initial estimates of the economic impact of child maltreatment, research has taken the first step in preventing child maltreatment. The next step is to conduct economic evaluations of interventions designed to prevent violence to evaluate the efficiency of scarce resources and assess returns on investments in prevention of child maltreatment. The challenges inherent in this type of research are difficult to overcome but well worth the benefit to the victims of child maltreatment as well as the researchers, policymakers, and practitioners involved in drawing attention to the economic impact of child maltreatment and influencing the public health policy debates about the need for prevention.

References

1. Hodgson TA, Meiners MR. Cost-of-illness methodology: a guide to current practices and procedures. *Millbank Mem Fund Q Health Soc.* 1982;60(3):429-462.
2. Rice DP. Estimating the cost of illness. *Am J Public Health Nations Health.* 1967;57(3):424-440.
3. Rice DP, Hodgson T, Kopstein A. The economic cost of illness: a replication and update. *Health Care Financ Rev.* 1985;7(1):61-68.
4. Larg A, Moss JR. Cost-of-illness studies: a guide to critical evaluation. *Pharmacoeconomics.* 2011;29(8):653-671.
5. Clabaugh G, Ward MM. Cost-of-illness studies in the United States: a systematic review of methodologies used for direct cost. *Value Health.* 2008;23(3):294-299.
6. Akobundu E, Ju J, Blatt L, Mullins CD. Cost-of-illness studies – a review of current methods. *Pharmacoeconomics.* 2006;24(9):869-890.
7. Bonomi A, Anderson M, Rivara F, et al. Health care utilization and costs associated with childhood abuse. *J Gen Intern Med.* 2008;23(3):294-299.
8. Brown DS, Fang X, Florence CS. Medical costs attributable to child maltreatment: a systematic review of short- and long-term effects. *Am J Prev Med.* 2011;41(6):627-635.
9. Forjuoh SN. Child maltreatment related injuries: incidence, hospital charges, and correlates of hospitalization. *Child Abuse Negl.* 2000;24(8):1019-1025.
10. Irazuzta JE, McJunkin JE, Danadian K, Arnold F, Zhang J. Outcome and cost of child abuse. *Child Abuse Negl.* 1997;21(8):751-757.
11. DiScala C, Sege R, Li G, Reece RM. Child abuse and unintentional injuries: a 10-year retrospective. *Arch Pediatr Adolesc Med.* 2000;154(1):16-22.

12. Ettaro L, Berger RA, Songer T. Abusive head trauma in young children: characteristics and medical charges in a hospitalized population. *Child Abuse Negl.* 2004;28(10):1099-1111.

13. Libby AM, Sills MR, Thurston NK, Orton HD. Costs of childhood physical abuse: comparing inflicted and unintentional traumatic brain injuries. *Pediatrics.* 2003;112(1 part 1):58-65.

14. Rovi S, Chen P, Johnson MS. The economic burden of hospitalizations associated with child abuse and neglect. *Am J Public Health.* 2004;94(4):586-590.

15. Evasovich M, Klein R, Muakkassa F, Weekley R. The economic effect of child abuse in the burn unit. *Burns.* 1998;24(7):642-645.

16. Krug EG, Dahlberg LL, Mercy JA, Zwi AB, Lozano R, eds. *World Report on Violence and Health.* Geneva, Switzerland: World Health Organization; 2002.

17. Felitti VJ, Anda RF, Nordenberg D, et al. Relationship of childhood abuse and household dysfunction to many of the leading causes of death in adults. The Adverse Childhood Experiences (ACE) Study. *Am J Prev Med.* 1998;14(4):245-258.

18. Kendall-Tackett KA. *Treating the Lifetime Health Effects of Childhood Victimization.* Kingston, NJ: Civic Research Institute; 2003.

19. Kolko DJ. Child physical abuse. In: Myers JEB, Berliner L, Briere J, Hendrix CT, Reid TA, Jenny CA, eds. *The APSAC Handbook on Child Maltreatment.* 2nd ed. Thousand Oaks, CA: Sage Publications Inc; 2002.

20. Malinosky-Rummell R, Hansen DJ. Long-term consequences of childhood physical abuse. *Psychol Bull.* 1993;114(1):68-79.

21. Paolucci EO, Genuis ML, Violato C. A meta-analysis of the published research on the effects of child sexual abuse. *J Psychol.* 2001;135(1):17-36.

22. Putnam FW. Ten-year research update review: child sexual abuse. *J Am Acad Child Adolesc Psychiatry.* 2003;42(3):269-278.

23. Young JC, Widom CS. Long-term effects of child abuse and neglect on emotion processing in adulthood. *Child Abuse Negl.* 2014;38(8):1369-1381.

24. Hekman JJ. Skill formation and the economics of investing in disadvantaged children. *Science.* 2006;312(5782):1900-1902.

25. Repetti RL, Taylor SE, Seeman TE. Risky families: family social environments and the mental and physical health of offspring. *Psychol Bull.* 2002;128(2):330-366.

26. Corso PS, Taylor NH. The economic costs of violence. In: Ward C, Donnelly P, eds. *Oxford Textbook of Violence Prevention: Epidemiology, Evidence, and Policy.* Oxford, UK: Oxford University Press; 2015.

27. Taylor SE, Lerner JS, Sage RM, Lehman BJ, Seeman TE. Early environment, emotions, responses to stress, and health. *J Pers.* 2004;72(6):1365-1394.

28. Williams DR, Collins C. US socioeconomic and racial differences in health: patterns and explanations. *Annu Rev Sociol.* 1995;21:348-386.

29. Franey K, Geffner R, Falconer R, eds. *The Cost of Child Maltreatment: Who Pays? We All Do.* San Diego, CA: Family Violence & Sexual Assault Institute; 2001.

30. Greenwood PW, Model KE, Rydell CP, Chiesa J. *Diverting Children from a Life of Crime.* Santa Monica, CA: RAND; 1996.

31. Widom CS, Maxfield MG. An update on the "cycle of violence." National Criminal Justice Reference Service Web site. https://www.ncjrs.gov/pdffiles1/nij/184894.pdf. Published February 2001. Accessed February 18, 2013.

32. Jonson-Reid M, Barth RP. From maltreatment report to juvenile incarceration: the role of child welfare services. *Child Abuse Negl.* 2000;24(4):505-520.

33. Runyan DK, Gould CL. Foster care for child maltreatment: impact on delinquent behavior. *Pediatrics.* 1985;75(3):562-568.
34. Widom CS. Childhood victimization: risk factor for delinquency. In: Colten ME, Gore S, eds. *Adolescent Stress: Causes and Consequences.* New York, NY: Aldine de Gruyter; 1991:201-221.
35. Perez CM, Widom CS. Childhood victimization and long-term intellectual and academic outcomes. *Child Abuse Negl.* 1994;18(8):617-633.
36. Browne KD, Lynch MA. The cost of child abuse and neglect. *Child Abuse Rev.* 1997;6(4):237-240.
37. Waters H, Hyder A, Rajkotia Y, Basu S, Rehwinkel JA, Butchart A. *The Economic Dimensions of Interpersonal Violence.* Geneva, Switzerland: Department of Injuries and Violence Prevention, World Health Organization; 2004.
38. Hulme PA. Symptomatology and health care utilization of women primary care patients who experienced childhood sexual abuse. *Child Abuse Negl.* 2000;24(11):1471-1484.
39. Walker EA, Unutzer J, Rutter C, et al. Costs of health care use by women HMO members with a history of childhood abuse and neglect. *Arch Gen Psychiatry.* 1999;56(7):609-613.
40. Corso PS, Fertig AR. The economic impact of child maltreatment in the United States: are the estimates credible? *Child Abuse Negl.* 2010;34(5):296-304.
41. Daro D. *Confronting Child Abuse Research for Effective Program Design.* New York, NY: Free Press; 1988:149-198.
42. Miller TR, Cohen MA, Weirsema B. *Victim Costs and Consequences: A New Look.* NCJ 155282. Washington, DC: US Department of Justice, National Institute of Justice; 1996.
43. Fromm S. *Total Estimated Cost of Child Abuse and Neglect in the United States—Statistical Evidence.* Chicago, IL: Prevent Child Abuse America; 2001.
44. Wang CT, Holton J. *Total Estimated Cost of Child Abuse and Neglect in the United States.* Chicago, IL: Prevent Child Abuse America; 2008.
45. Fang X, Brown D, Florence C, Mercy J. The economic burden of child maltreatment in the United States and implications for prevention. *Child Abuse Negl.* 2012;36(2):156-165.
46. Fang X, Corso PS. Child maltreatment, youth violence, and intimate partner violence: developmental relationships. *Am J Prev Med.* 2007;33(4):281-290.
47. Zielinski DS. Child maltreatment and adult socioeconomic well-being. *Child Abuse Negl.* 2009;33(10):666-678.
48. Haddix A, Teutsch S, Corso PS, eds. *Prevention Effectiveness: A Guide to Decision Analysis and Economic Evaluation.* New York, NY: Oxford University Press; 2003.
49. Gold MR, Siegel JE, Russell LB, Weinstein MC, eds. *Cost-Effectiveness in Health and Medicine.* New York, NY: Oxford University Press; 1996.
50. MacKenzie EJ, Damiano A, Miller T, Luchter S. The development of the Functional Capacity Index. *J Trauma.* 1996;41(5):799-807.
51. MacKenzie EJ, Sacco WJ, Luchter S, et al. Validating the Functional Capacity Index as a measure of outcome following blunt multiple trauma. *Qual Life Res.* 2002;11(8):797-808.
52. Prosser LA, Corso PS. Measuring preference-based quality of life for child maltreatment: a systematic literature review. *Health Qual Life Outcomes.* 2007;42(5):1-10.

53. Matza LS, Swensen AR, Flood EM, Secnik K, Leidy NK. Assessment of health-related quality of life in children: a review of conceptual, methodological, and regulatory issues. *Value Health.* 2004;7(1):79-92.

54. Corso PS, Lutzker JR. The need for economic analysis in research on child maltreatment. *Child Abuse Negl.* 2006;30(7):727-738.

55. Petrou S. Methodological issues raised by preference-based approaches to measuring the health status of children. *Health Econ.* 2003;12(8):697-702.

56. Keren R, Pati S, Feudtner C. The generation gap: differences between children and adults pertinent to economic evaluations of health interventions. *Pharmacoeconomics.* 2004;22(2):71-81.

57. Noyes J, Edwards RT. EQ-5D for the assessment of Health-Related Quality of Life and resource allocation in children: a systematic methodological review. *Value Health.* 2011;14(8):1117-1129.

58. Wille N, Badia X, Bonsel G, et al. Development of the EQ-5D-Y: a child-friendly version of the EQ-5D. *Qual Life Res.* 2010;19(6):875-886.

59. Ravens-Sieberer U, Wille N, Badia X, et al. Feasibility, reliability, and validity of the EQ-5D-Y: results from a multinational study. *Qual Life Res.* 2010;19(6):887-897.

60. Edwards VJ, Anda RF, Felitti VJ, Dube SR. Adverse childhood experiences and health-related quality of life as an adult. In: Kendall-Tackett K, ed. *Health Consequences of Abuse in the Family: A Clinical Guide for Evidence-Based Practice.* Washington, DC: American Psychological Association; 2003:81-94.

61. Corso PS, Edwards VJ, Fang X, Mercy JA. Health-related quality of life in adults who experienced maltreatment during childhood. *Am J Public Health.* 2008;98(6):1094-1100.

62. Corso PS, Ingels JB, Roldos MI. A comparison of willingness to pay to prevent child maltreatment deaths in Ecuador and the United States. *Int J Environ Res Public Health.* 2013;10(4):1342-1355.

Additional Reading/Resources

Agency for Healthcare Research and Quality. Medical expenditure panel survey. Agency for Healthcare Research and Quality Web site. http://www.meps.ahrq.gov/mepsweb. Accessed February 25, 2013.

Filene JM, Lutzker JR, Hecht D, Silovsky J. Project SafeCare: issues in replication of an ecobehavioral model of child maltreatment prevention. In: Kendall-Tackett KA, Giacomoni SM, eds. *Child Victimization: Maltreatment, Bullying and Dating Violence, Prevention and Intervention.* Kingston, NJ: Circle Research Institute; 2005:18-1–18-21.

Walker EA, Gelfand A, Katon WJ, et al. Adult health status of women with histories of childhood abuse and neglect. *Am J Med.* 1999;107(4):332-339.

Section II

The Science of Prevention

Chapter 6

Expanding the Definition of Evidence in Child Maltreatment Prevention

Richard W. Puddy, PhD, MPH
Natalie Wilkins, PhD
Sally Thigpen, MPA
Helen Singer, MPH
John Donovan, MPH

Introduction

Prevention practitioners, researchers, and policymakers in public health and other related fields are increasingly recognizing the importance of evidence-based decision-making (EBDM) in their work. Questions remain, however, about how evidence should be defined. Is information gathered from randomized controlled trials (RCTs) the sole form of evidence that should be considered? What role does context play in EBDM? How is practice-based knowledge relevant to successful adoption of evidence? These questions pose a challenge to EBDM processes in public health, including the field of child maltreatment prevention.[1-3] This chapter will first provide an overview of a comprehensive framework for expanding the definition of evidence and will then describe each type of evidence and its use in decision-making. Examples from home visitation will be used to illustrate the application of each type of evidence. Finally, implications for the broader child maltreatment prevention field will be discussed.

Definitions of evidence have ranged from the very specific (ie, findings from RCTs and other forms of rigorous, empirical research) to the very broad (ie, sound theory and practical, ethical and expert knowledge).[4] In 1992, the concept of evidence-based medicine was introduced in the *Journal of the American Medical Association* with a focus on decision-making rooted in the best available research.[5] Used in this way, the best available research evidence included data from patient populations both in the lab and in the field, as well as results related to assessment, clinical issues, and various intervention approaches. Systematic reviews of clinical RCTs were identified as the preferred method for establishing evidence of effectiveness.[5-7] Selection criteria for most existing registries of evidence-based programs, practices, and policies also focus almost exclusively on research evidence of effectiveness, particularly evidence from studies with strong research designs (ie, experimental studies with random assignment or quasi-experimental studies with matched comparison groups).[8-10]

Many areas of public health (including child maltreatment prevention) are still developing the research evidence base for specific strategies, which limits practitioners' options for implementing evidence-based preventive interventions.[11] While initial RCTs and other rigorous research studies conducted on specific strategies may reveal which prevention programs, practices, or policies work for specific types of individuals, under specific conditions, in unique settings, they often do not necessarily show whether or not these prevention strategies will generalize to other settings and populations.[3,12-14] It is important to note that there are some prevention strategies that have been replicated, rigorously evaluated in multiple applied settings, and found to be effective (eg, Hahn et al,[15] Wilson et al[16]). In these cases, there is stronger research evidence indicating the generalizability of these prevention strategies across different contexts and populations. As mentioned previously, however, in many areas of public health (including child maltreatment prevention), the research evidence is still being developed, and even in those areas with stronger research evidence, more information is still often required to understand how a decision should be made in a local community.[17] Thus, the best available research evidence, contextual evidence, and experiential evidence are all important components of an EBDM process.[18(p56)]

In line with this thinking, Brownson and colleagues[12,19] suggest that in public health, evidence includes epidemiologic (quantitative) data, results of program or policy evaluations, and/or qualitative data used for making judgments or decisions. They also explain that public health decision-making must take into account the best available research evidence, contextual factors related to settings and populations, as well as practitioner expertise.[12] Furthermore, both the American Psychological Association and Institute of Medicine have called for a greater emphasis on the importance of context and experience/expertise in making informed decisions.[6,20] These additional forms of evidence can complement the best available research evidence (and vice versa) in an informed decision-making process.[13] With this in mind, the Division of Violence Prevention (DVP) at the Centers for Disease Control and Prevention (CDC) has created an EBDM framework called The Framework for Thinking About Evidence.

Background on the Development of the Framework

In 2004, CDC funded 3 national organizations in the child maltreatment prevention field through the BECAUSE Kids Count! initiative. These organizations, namely the National Alliance of Children's Trust and Prevention Funds, Parents Anonymous, Inc., and Prevent Child Abuse America, collaborated to expand their national, state, and local capacity to effectively address the prevention of child abuse and neglect. The BECAUSE initiative identified that there was limited use of the best available research evidence on effective strategies in the field. Furthermore, this group also noted that there was slow uptake of evidence-based practice with limited fidelity to the practice when evidence-based models were used. Increasing the knowledge, understanding, and use of evidence in decision-making became a joint priority of all 3 of the BECAUSE child maltreatment prevention organizations. Concurrently, CDC's Division of Violence Prevention was engaged in a process to provide coherent and consistent language around its use of the word "evidence" in programmatic activities. To support this effort, key stakeholder and small group discussions were completed along with an extensive literature review to define the term evidence, identify the limits of what it did and did not encompass, and to place parameters on its usage. This systematic inquiry led to intensive thinking about the application of the best available research evidence as well as other types of evidence (experiential and contextual evidence) that appeared necessary when faced with decision-making. Thus, out of the interactions between CDC, the BECAUSE grantees, and their national advisory boards, who were deeply steeped in decades of work in bridging science and practice, the Framework for Thinking About Evidence was originally conceptualized.

After this initial conceptualization, further review included compiling and analyzing existing evidence theories and registries such as Blueprints for Violence Prevention,[9] the Substance Abuse and Mental Health Services Adminstration (SAMHSA) National Registry of Evidence Based Programs and Practices,[10] the California Evidence-Based Clearinghouse,[22] and *Guide to Community Preventive Services.*[23] In total, over 42 registries, frameworks, or classification systems were reviewed from fields as diverse as psychology, epidemiology, human services, policy, medicine, child welfare, violence, juvenile justice, substance abuse, and education. A guidance document, *Understanding Evidence Part I: Best Available Research Evidence - A Guide to the Continuum of Evidence of Effectiveness*, was created to facilitate a common understanding and language of what is meant by the best available research evidence. The 6 vertical dimensions making up the continuum include effect, internal validity, research design, independent replication, implementation guidance, and external/ecological validity. There are 4 broad horizontal areas (well supported, supported/promising direction, emerging, undetermined/unsupported/harmful) used to place the 6 dimensions along a continuum of higher to lower effectiveness.[24] Similar guidance documents were being developed for both experiential and contextual evidence. In developing the Framework, CDC intended to resolve inconsistencies in defining evidence and to further illustrate and clarify the process behind EBDM.

The Framework for Thinking About Evidence

The Framework includes evidence from both research and practitioners 'to provide a more comprehensive view of evidence that is appropriate and necessary for decision-making. To inform public health decision-making, the Framework is composed of 3 dimensions that complement one another (**Figure 6-1**):

— ***Best available research evidence***: Information derived from scientific inquiry that assists in determining whether or not a prevention program, practice, or policy is actually achieving its intended outcomes.

— ***Contextual evidence***: A collection of measurable factors in the community that are likely to influence whether or not a strategy fits with the setting in which it is to be implemented.

— ***Experiential evidence***: The collective lived experience and expertise drawn from the community about whether a prevention strategy is appropriate or acceptable for their community.

The Framework for Thinking About Evidence

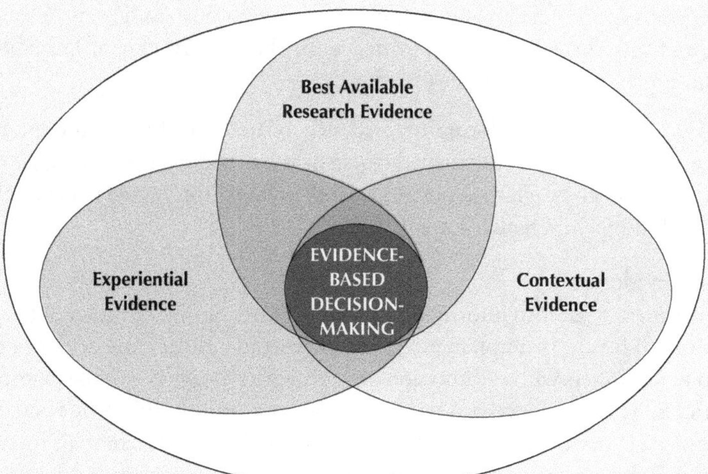

Figure 6-1

Figure 6-1. *The Framework for Thinking About Evidence prescribes evidence-based decision-making informed by a combination of best available research evidence, contextual and experiential evidence from community data, and field-based expertise. Reprinted from Centers for Disease Control and Prevention.*[21]

EBDM occurs where these 3 forms of evidence intersect. These intersections allow each type of evidence to complement one another, adding layers of knowledge and leading to a more informed decision. In instances where one or more types of evidence are lacking, the Framework can highlight the need to address gaps in a particular form(s) of evidence. The overall intention of the Framework is to integrate the best available research evidence, contextual evidence, and experiential evidence to make the most informed decision that provides a community with the best opportunity to prevent violence before it occurs.

The remainder of this chapter will take a closer look at the 3 forms of evidence in The Framework for Thinking About Evidence and how they intersect in the EBDM process. In addition, the chapter will look at EBDM through a child maltreatment prevention lens with a focus on building Safe, Stable, Nurturing Relationships (SSNRs) for children across the social ecology, CDC's strategic direction for preventing child maltreatment. Currently, early childhood home visitation is widely recognized as having strong research evidence of effectiveness for preventing child maltreatment[8,25] and for promoting SSNRs. As such, home visitation will be woven throughout the remainder of the chapter as a case example of a child maltreatment prevention strategy that could be considered when making evidence-based decisions.

Best Available Research Evidence

Best available research evidence is information that enables researchers, practitioners, and policymakers to determine whether or not a program, practice, or policy is actually achieving its intended outcomes. The more rigorous a study (eg, true or quasi-experimental design, independent replication), the more compelling the research evidence is indicating whether or not a program, practice, or policy is effective. The extent to which a prevention strategy has been replicated in multiple, applied settings with diverse populations (external/ecological validity), and the availability and accessibility of implementation supports (implementation guidance) are also important aspects of best available research evidence.

Best available research evidence has long been the primary form of evidence considered when making decisions about preventing a problem for the majority of science-based fields, including public health. For example, in the field of child maltreatment prevention, there is a strong body of research evidence indicating the effectiveness of home visitation programs in preventing child maltreatment. The *Guide to Community Preventive Services* conducted a systematic review of rigorous studies on home visiting programs, and found strong research evidence for the effectiveness of home visitation programs in preventing child maltreatment.[25,26]

Increasingly, however, other forms of evidence related to clinical and practitioner expertise, and setting and contextual factors, have been recognized as crucial to the success of prevention programs, practices, and policies for many behavioral health problems, including child maltreatment.[2,6,19-20,27]

Contextual Evidence

Contextual evidence refers to information about whether or not a strategy "fits" with the context in which it is to be implemented. In other words, contextual evidence provides prevention practitioners with information on whether a strategy is feasible to implement, is useful, and is likely to be accepted by a particular community.[3,28,29] While best available research evidence answers questions about whether and to what extent an intervention is effective in achieving specific outcomes, contextual evidence can answer questions about the meaning a strategy may have for a particular community and whether that strategy is a good fit given the community's characteristics and specific circumstances. The types of questions that contextual evidence can be useful in answering include, but are not limited to:

— Does the community have the resources and/or capacity to implement the prevention strategy effectively?

— Do the strengths documented in the research evidence match well with the needs of the community?

— What are the characteristics of the population to be served by the prevention strategy?

— Who are the people and organizations that will implement the prevention strategy?

— What are the characteristics of the setting for the proposed program, policy, or practice that could affect its implementation?[11,30]

Most of the major proponents of EBDM, including the American Psychological Association, Institutes of Medicine - Committee on Quality of Health Care in America, and the World Health Organization, agree that information on context is important for interventions to be successful. These groups currently acknowledge the necessity of information on context in their official guidance about EBDM.[2,27,31] Also, in the dissemination and implementation research field, researchers recognize the importance of adapting interventions to better "fit" the contexts within which they are being implemented to ensure strong uptake. These adaptations are important for increasing the feasibility, utility, and acceptability of interventions, so long as they do not disrupt any of the intervention's core causal components.[32] If contextual evidence, such as the resources, time, infrastructure, capacity, values, and historical experiences of a given setting and population, are not taken into account in decision-making processes, it is unlikely an intervention will be successfully implemented.[19,33]

The variety of information that can be collected on the context of a given setting is near limitless, and includes social, political, economic, organizational, and cultural factors. Many, but not all, of these contextual factors have the potential to influence how a prevention strategy is received and used by a particular community.[3,11] Contextual evidence is the situational information that is specifically relevant and useful for EBDM and the selection, implementation, and sustainability of a prevention strategy. The contextual factors that are considered to be evidence will vary based on the circumstances and prevention goals of a particular community.[11] For example, some of the relevant contextual evidence for a community considering implementing a home visitation program for child maltreatment prevention might include the number of first-time parents in the community, the number of households in the community with children in the intended age group, the cultural norms related to parents seeking child-rearing advice, and the availability/accessibility of qualified professionals to implement the selected program. Each of these pieces of contextual evidence will have implications about which program is selected and how it will be implemented. However, other community contextual factors may not be as relevant to the decision regarding implementing this particular strategy. Examples of nonrelevant contextual factors in this situation might include data on the number and size of school districts in the area, as this information would not be likely to directly impact a home visitation intervention.

In EBDM, contextual evidence is used in conjunction with best available research evidence and experiential evidence to make strategic decisions about prevention. As mentioned earlier, the role that contextual evidence plays in the EBDM process is to determine the extent that the prevention strategies that are being considered for adoption and implementation are a good "fit" for the particular setting in question.[3] For example, consider a community that is looking to implement a home visitation program. This community has many multi-child families. In reviewing the best available research evidence on home visitation programs, the programs which have been found to be effective through rigorous evaluation with multiple RCTs are specifically geared toward first-time parents, and in these programs, effectiveness is contingent on the services being delivered by certified nurse practitioner.[34] While there is strong research evidence to suggest that these programs can be effective, there may be a mismatch with the values and fit for this particular community.

There are examples of other home visitation programs that are intended for multi-child families and use trained paraprofessionals for service delivery.[35] While these programs may not have the same effects as programs using certified nurse practitioners, the contextual evidence suggests that they may be a better fit with the need for a program that addresses multi-child families. In this situation, evidence from research and context (plus experience, which will be discussed in the next section) can be integrated into choosing a program that would also be acceptable, and thus more likely to have better uptake in this setting.

There are many potential sources of contextual evidence at each level of the social ecology.[19] **Figure 6-2** illustrates specific examples of contextual evidence that can be gathered and measured at each of these levels. Sources of and methods for gathering contextual evidence can be both quantitative (census, economic analyses) and qualitative (focus groups, interviews).[3,11] Continuing the home visitation example, census records could provide information about family size and ages of children, economic indices from the local chamber of commerce might be a source for estimating the number of qualified professionals in the area, and community-based focus groups could provide information about help-seeking behaviors/attitudes to provide insight into the specific cultural norms of the target population.

Figure 6-2. *Examples of contextual factors across the social ecology. Adapted from Brownson RC, Fielding JE, Maylahn CA.*[19]

Examples of Contextual Factors Across the Social Ecology

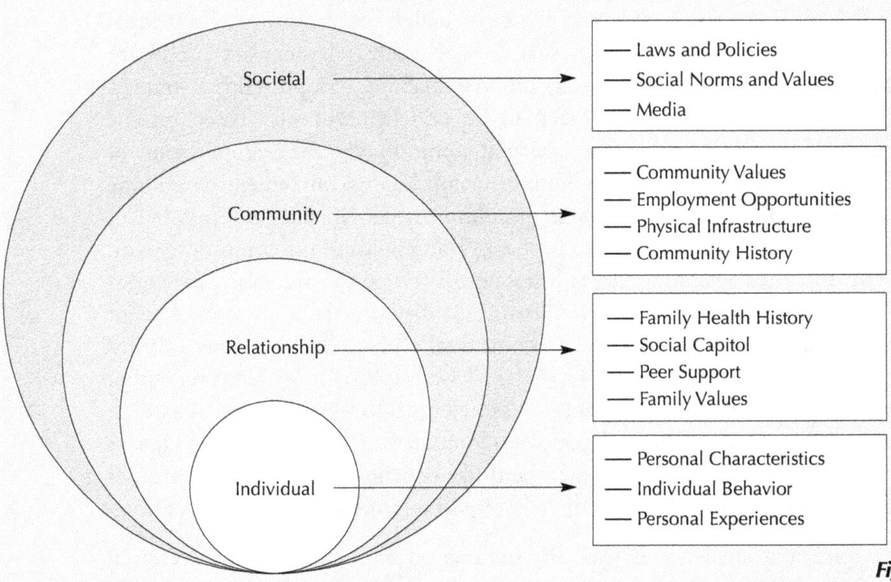

Figure 6-2

In other words, by taking contextual evidence into account, decision-makers will be able to determine which home visitation program is a better fit for the specific situation in which it will be implemented. In this case, it is likely that the program that addresses the needs of multi-child families with trained paraprofessional home visitors will fit the needs of, and be more acceptable to this particular community. The alternative of selecting and implementing a program that does not fit with the characteristics of the community could result in the desired child maltreatment prevention outcomes not being realized. Additionally, while "fit" between a prevention strategy and the local community context is not the sole consideration for effective implementation, it is an important component of implementation success.[36,37] Each specific program or policy decision will have a unique combination of evidence for decision-makers to weigh and consider in this deliberative manner.

Experiential Evidence

Best available research evidence can show how effective an intervention has been in specific settings. Contextual evidence can show whether or not an intervention may fit with the setting in which it is to be implemented. However, only the collective experience and expertise of those who have practiced or lived in that setting can show how appropriate or acceptable an intervention may be received by the community, thus balancing both the best available research evidence and the contextual evidence for a given intervention.

There are several types of knowledge or experience that are relevant when choosing and implementing a prevention strategy. This includes knowledge about the problem (eg, child maltreatment), what works to solve this problem (best available research evidence on interventions), and knowledge about how to put an intervention into practice, who to involve, and why this intervention is necessary. Experiential knowledge provides a unique perspective to the decision-making process and provides answers to the "how," "who," and "why" of choosing and implementing a prevention strategy.[13,38]

Experiential evidence has been used by many disciplines as a critical piece of the decision-making process. McCracken and Marsh[39] describe 3 types of practitioner expertise that are important to the ways clinical decisions are made: (1) clinical expertise (ie, understanding one's patient), (2) technical expertise (ie, determining whether an intervention can be adapted to contextual realities), and (3) organizational expertise (ie, knowledge and skills related to organizational design). The combination of these 3 types of clinical (or practitioner in the world of public health) expertise leads to more reliable and almost instantaneous responses in clinical settings.

Clinical expertise, for example, includes the understanding that some individuals prefer detailed information about options, while others may be overwhelmed by too much information. This expertise is deeply rooted in experiences gained by practice and forming relationships with patients.[40] Particular decisions for patient care depend on practitioner expertise in subject matter, lessons learned through practice, and an understanding of each particular patient's preferences.[41] Organizational expertise and influences also impact the uptake of evidence. For example, the fact that an intervention is evidence based does not mean that staff, regardless of expertise, will want to use it. Preparing staff prior to introduction of a new guideline or procedure to ensure buy-in and knowledge-sharing can increase the likelihood of positive impact of a practice supported by evidence.[42-44]

Another example of the value and use of experiential evidence comes from the field of athletic coaching. Athletic coaching education often includes, as a core component of training, apprenticeships with more experienced coaches. Expert athletic coaches value experiential evidence for instant decision-making in highly charged, stressful situations. Expert coaches rely on what they learn through formal education (physiology, psychology, biology, etc.), as well as what they learn from the practice of coaching (sport-specific processes and techniques, teaching methods/pedagogy, etc.) to develop well-seasoned and successful coaching decisions (eg, calling an opportune "timeout"). As a result, effective athletic coaches are better able to use past experiences in formulating game time decisions, separating relevant from irrelevant information, recognizing patterns, and best utilizing their players during a game.[45] Effective coaches are also able to use past experiences and knowledge to successfully groom and develop players, utilizing communication and training drills that integrate fitness, motor memory, and mental skills. These preparatory actions allow the reinforcement of proper technique and allow the players to make quicker decisions during game play.[46,47]

Like athletic coaching, the military also values the experience of leaders as a critical component to making good decisions under stressful situations. Leaders in various levels of military ranking base decisions on both data and experience in the field and perform 3 basic tasks that call upon varying levels of experiential knowledge: (1) maintaining operations already in place, (2) sustaining the institution (training additional troops, aiding in research/development), and (3) interacting with external agencies.[48,49] These 3 main duties are reflected at different levels of military service, with important nuances. Platoon leaders have limited experience, and as such, they have the responsibility of managing troops, monitoring performance, and seeking feedback. Company commanders, who have more experience, tend to have a more broad range of expert knowledge from directing and managing subordinates to strategically balancing mission and troop responsibilities. Battalion commanders, who have the most experience, offer a systems-level expertise that shapes organizational structure.[48] In addition, Hedlund and colleagues found that military leaders, regardless of rank, who possessed higher tacit/experiential knowledge ratings were identified as more effective leaders by other military personnel, illustrating the overall importance of this form of knowledge.[48]

The field of medicine also places a high value on the development of experiential knowledge through a process of procedural learning, commonly referred to as "see one, do one, teach one."[50] Most medical training programs in the United States require completion of academic coursework followed by years of ongoing experiential learning through internships and residency positions.[51] During this procedural learning process, medical students learn both by "doing" during their internships and by teaching during their residencies. The opportunity to combine formal academic knowledge with practical procedural know-how results in practices that are far more relevant than academic learning in isolation. The accumulated experience of working with diverse groups of people—both patients and other medical professionals—helps learners develop the practical ability to apply nuanced, highly technical scientific knowledge in often ambiguous real-world situations.[50,52]

Building experiential knowledge is a key feature of successfully putting research, learned material, and other abstract information into practice. In the field of child maltreatment prevention, for example, practicing parenting skills/roleplaying is a core component of many home visitation programs, and is a method of building parents' experiential knowledge by "learning in context." By putting information they have learned about successful parenting into practice, parents build the more intuitive knowledge and skills needed to effectively deliver these parenting practices later on.[53]

The role of experiential evidence in EBDM is to provide information on some of the less explicit factors that are important to consider when choosing or adapting a prevention strategy like home visitation for a particular setting and population. Many prevention practitioners, clinicians, service providers, and consumers have knowledge about "what works" at the ground level for preventing child maltreatment. This knowledge is often not easy to make explicit as it consists of intuition and other forms of intangible knowledge developed through an accumulation of hands-on experience and knowledge.[54-56] In home visitation, less explicit knowledge may include cultural facilitators to successful implementation like a culture that values the extended family in caregiving. A home visitation program in such a community might include the extended care givers into the interventions to not only support the primary parent, but give consistency in parenting skills development to all caregivers of the child. By gathering and examining information on patterns of experience[50,57-59] and engaging in processes that build consensus around practitioners' knowledge and experiences,[4,60,61] these less tangible ideas contribute to "what works" and become more concrete, robust pieces of evidence to incorporate into an EBDM process.

Implications for Child Maltreatment Prevention Practitioners

"It is not enough for scholars and program evaluators, on the one hand, to learn how maltreatment develops and what interventions are effective and for practitioners, on the other, to implement innovative interventions in their work with families. Instead, initiatives must be implemented and assessed in such a way as to maximize both the ability of program managers and policy makers to draw on these data to shape their practice and policy decisions."[62(p88)]

Daro and Dodge[62] make clear the value of expanding the framework for how we define evidence when making decisions about prevention strategies intended to have impact in a complex world. Similarly, Schorr and Farrow state that the "framework for what is conventionally considered credible evidence is constructed too narrowly."[63(p1)] They report that in attempts to draw tight boundaries around what evidence is acceptable, we have significantly limited the knowledge base and diminished our capacity to assemble and make it available to policymakers, program designers, and evaluators to solve complex social problems affecting children and youth. Additionally, the lack of available supports for dissemination and implementation for some evidence-based prevention strategies has hampered the expansion and widespread adoption of effective child maltreatment prevention interventions.[64] To increase success, prevention efforts must include a wide variety of stakeholders who can (1) assess the scope of child maltreatment in their community, (2) identify effective prevention strategies, and (3) identify delivery mechanisms that are compatible with local realities.[65]

With a more comprehensive understanding of evidence, decision-makers are better equipped to make the best choices for their organizations and communities. Careful consideration of the best available research evidence, as well as both contextual and experiential evidence, can lead to decisions that will assure more successful, sustainable prevention strategies that are congruent with community needs and norms.[12,33]

Next Steps: The Decision-making Process

Combining best available research evidence on effectiveness with contextual and experiential evidence in order to make programmatic or policy decisions is a multi-faceted process that will require adequate preparation, ample time, and inclusive participation. As the nature of this type of decision-making is a uniquely human endeavor, it requires assessing complex information and considering input from a variety of stakeholders. It will most likely be a collaborative process of weighing factors and will vary according to local circumstance.[3] EBDM tools and accompanying support materials are being developed and refined by CDC along with a variety of external researchers and violence prevention practitioners. These resources will be relevant for the field of child maltreatment prevention in that they will be both practical and useful for groups and individuals charged with making primary prevention programmatic and/or policy decisions. This decision-making process must involve the identification and distillation of the relevant pieces of each of the 3 types of evidence. In addition, it will involve some form of deliberation or thoughtful debate to which key stakeholders would contribute and learn how those pieces of evidence best fit together to guide decisions.[3,11,66]

Caveats/Limitations

Acknowledging and exploring other forms of evidence besides best available research evidence is not intended to devalue the role of research evidence on effectiveness in programmatic and policy decisions. Rather, this work encourages the use of the best available research, contextual, and experiential evidence in decision-making, so that communities can leverage the unique strengths of each form of evidence to make the most informed prevention decision for their setting and population. Moreover, this work is meant to bolster the use of best available research evidence and strengthen the likelihood that decisions will lead to success by taking a systematic approach to assessing the important role of context and experience.

Implementation, adaptation, and evaluation of any strategy are also important issues that are obviously related to EBDM, however, a detailed explanation of those features are beyond the scope of this chapter. Still, part of the longer-term vision of this work is to link EBDM to resources that provide guidance on these critical issues.

The Framework for Thinking About Evidence that is described in this chapter is meant to represent a comprehensive approach to considering evidence for decision-making, while recognizing that many decisions are required to be made with less than ideal time, resources, and participation. Thus, the purposeful intention is that the tools and templates developed to support EBDM will be modified and utilized in a variety of circumstances with the Framework serving as a guide toward which to direct future efforts. The role of an iterative and recursive evaluation process seems critical here to continue to refine and update the Framework as knowledge of evidence continues to grow and evolve.

Conclusion

In developing the Framework for Thinking About Evidence and the supporting tools, CDC hopes to offer the field of child maltreatment prevention a guide for understanding evidence in its various forms. It is also hoped that this framework and supporting tools will provide knowledge about how these different forms of evidence can be collected and used to make strategic and practical evidence-based decisions for programming and policy that, followed up with strong implementation, will result in preventing violence before it occurs. Combining best available research evidence on effectiveness, contextual evidence, and experiential evidence for decision-making is a complex process. A thorough understanding of the unique contributions of each type of evidence as well as a clear articulation of the specific circumstances associated with each decision-making opportunity will enable practitioners to more confidently, efficiently, and successfully use evidence in their work to prevent child maltreatment.

References

1. Canadian Health Services Research Foundation. *Weighing Up the Evidence: Making Evidence-informed Guidance Accurate, Achievable, and Acceptable.* Ottawa, ON: Canadian Health Services Research Foundation; 2006.

2. Clements D; Canadian Health Services Research Foundation. *Annual Invitational Workshop. What Counts? Interpreting Evidence-based Decision-making for Management and Policy.* Ottawa, ON: Canadian Health Services Research Foundation; 2004.

3. Lomas J; Canadian Health Services Research Foundation; Provincial/Territorial Conference of Deputy Ministers of Health; et al. *Conceptualizing and Combining Evidence For Health System Guidance: Final Report.* Ottawa, ON: Canadian Health Services Research Foundation; 2005.

4. Buetow S, Kenealy T. Evidence-based medicine: the need for a new definition. *J Eval Clin Pract.* 2000;6(2):85-92.

5. Evidence-Based Medicine Working Group. Evidence-based medicine: a new approach to teaching the practice of medicine. *JAMA.* 1992;268(17):2420-2425.

6. American Psychological Association. *Policy Statement on Evidence-Based Practice in Psychology.* Washington, DC: American Psychological Association; 2005.

7. Sackett DL. The Cochrane Collaboration. *ACP J Club.* 1994;120 suppl 3:A11.

8. Coalition for Evidence-Based Policy. Top Tier Evidence Web site. http://toptierevidence.org/wordpress/. Updated 2012. Accessed March 4, 2013.

9. Mihalic S, Irwin K, Elliot D, Fagan A, Hansen D. *Blueprints for Violence Prevention.* Washington, DC: Office of Juvenile Justice and Delinquency Prevention; 2001.

10. About NREPP. SAMHSA's National Registry of Evidence-based Programs and Practices Web site. http://www.nrepp.samhsa.gov/AboutNREPP.aspx. Updated June 19, 2012. Accessed March 13, 2013.

11. Rychetnik L, Frommer M, Hawe P, Shiell A. Criteria for evaluating evidence on public health interventions. *J Epidemiol Community Health.* 2002;56(2):119-127.

12. Brownson RC, Chriqui JF, Stamatakis KA. Understanding evidence-based public health policy. *Am J Public Health.* 2009;99(9):1576-1583.

13. Kitson A. Recognising relationships: reflections on evidence-based practice. *Nurs Inq.* 2002;9(3):179-186.

14. Nutley S, Walter I, Davies HTO. From knowing to doing: a framework for understanding the evidence-into-practice agenda. *Evaluation.* 2003;9(2):125-148.

15. Hahn R, Fuqua-Whitley D, Wethington H, et al. Effectiveness of universal school-based programs to prevent violent and aggressive behavior: a systematic review. *Am J Prev Med.* 2007;33(2 suppl):S114-S129.

16. Wilson SJ, Lipsey MW, Derzon JH. The effects of school-based intervention programs on aggressive behavior: a meta-analysis. *J Consult Clin Psychol.* 2003;71(1):136-149.

17. Rychetnik L, Hawe P, Waters E, Barratt A, Frommer M. A glossary for evidence based public health. *J Epidemiol Community Health.* 2004;58(7):538-545.

18. Korsen N, Pietruszewski P. Translating evidence to practice: two stories from the field. *J Clin Psychol Med Settings*. 2009;16(1):47-57.

19. Brownson RC, Fielding JE, Maylahn CA. Evidence-based public health: a fundamental concept for public health practice. *Annu Rev Public Health*. 2009;30:175-201.

20. Centers for Disease Control and Prevention. *The Evidence Project Overview*. Atlanta, GA: Centers for Disease Control and Prevention; 2013. Centers for Disease Control and Prevention Web site. http://www.cdc.gov/violenceprevention/pdf/evidence_project_overview2013-a.pdf. Accessed September 15, 2016.

21. Institute of Medicine, Committee on Quality of Health Care in America. *Crossing the Quality Chasm: A New Health System for the 21st Century*. Washington, DC: National Academy Press; 2001. National Academy Press Web site. http://www.nap.edu/books/0309072808/html/. Published March 2001. Accessed September 16, 2016.

22. Gambrill E. Evidence-based practice and policy: choices ahead. *Res Soc Work Pract*. 2006;16(3):338-357. doi:10.1177/1049731505284205.

23. Systematic review methods. The Community Guide to Preventative Services Web site. http://www.thecommunityguide.org/about/methods.html. Updated February 19, 2013. Accesed March 4, 2013.

24. Puddy R, Wilkins N. *Understanding Evidence Part I: Best Available Research Evidence: A Guide to the Continuum of Evidence of Effectiveness*. Atlanta, GA: Centers for Disease Control and Prevention; 2011.

25. Violence prevention focused on children and youth: early childhood home visitation. The Guide to Community Preventative Services Web site. http://www.thecommunityguide.org/violence/home/index.html. Updated September 21, 2010. Accessed March 4, 2013.

26. Bilukha O, Hahn RA, Crosby A, et al. The effectiveness of early childhood home visitation in preventing violence: a systematic review. *Am J Prev Med*. 2005;28(2):11-39.

27. American Psychological Association. *Report of the 2005 Presidential Task Force on Evidence-Based Practice*. Washington, DC: American Psychological Association; 2005.

28. Substance Abuse and Mental Health Services Administration. Identifying and Selecting Evidence-Based Interventions. Washington, DC: US Department of Health and Human Services; 2007. http://fcpr.fsu.edu/sarg/tools/docs/CSAP4p56_Guidance_Jan04_2007.pdf. Published January 2007. Accessed March 4, 2013.

29. Victora CG, Habicht JP, Bryce J. Evidence-based public health: moving beyond randomized trials. *Am J Public Health*. 2004;94(3):400-405.

30. Green J, Britten N. Qualitative research and evidence based medicine. *BMJ*. 1998;316(7139):1230-1232.

31. World Health Organization. *Violence Prevention: The Evidence: Overview*. Geneva: World Health Organization; 2009.

32. Baker EA, Brennan Ramirez LK, Claus JM, Land G. Translating and disseminating research- and practice-based criteria to support evidence-based intervention planning. *J Public Health Manag Prac*. 2008;14(2):124-130.

33. Green LW, Glasgow RE. Evaluating the relevance, generalization, and applicability of research: issues in external validation and translation methodology. *Eval Health Prof.* 2006;29(1):126-153.

34. Olds DL, Robinson J, O'Brien R, et al. Home visiting by paraprofessionals and by nurses: a randomized, controlled trial. *Pediatrics.* 2002;110(3):486-496.

35. Duggan AK, McFarlane EC, Windham AM, et al. Evaluation of Hawaii's Healthy Start Program. *Future Child.* 1999;9(1):66-90.

36. Klein KJ, Conn AB, Sorra JS. Implementing computerized technology: an organizational analysis. *J Appl Psychol.* 2001;86(5):811-824.

37. Klein KJ, Sorra JS. The challenge of innovation implementation. *Acad Manag Rev.* 1996;21(4):1055-1080.

38. Tanenbaum SJ. Evidence and expertise: the challenge of the outcomes movement to medical professionalism. *Acad Med.* 1999;74(7):757-763.

39. McCracken SG, Marsh JC. Practitioner expertise in evidence-based practice decision making. *Res Soc Work Pract.* 2008;18(4):301-310.

40. Comas-Díaz L. Cultural variation in the therapeutic relationship. In: Goodheart C, Kazdin A, Sternberg R, eds. *Evidence-based Psychotherapy: Where Practice and Research Meet.* Washington, DC: American Psychological Association; 2006:81-105.

41. Proctor E, Rosen A. Concise standards for developing evidence-based practice guidelines. In: Roberts A, Yeager K, eds. F*oundations of Evidence-Based Social Work Practice.* New York, NY: Oxford University Press; 2006:93-102.

42. Corrigan P, McCracken S. *Interactive Staff Training: Rehabilitation Teams That Work.* New York, NY: Plenum; 1997.

43. Fixsen D, Naoom S, Blasé K, Friedman R, Wallace F. *Implementation Research: A Synthesis of the Literature.* Tampa, FL: University of South Florida, Louis de La Parte Florida Mental Health Institute; 2005.

44. McCracken S, Corrigan P. Staff development in mental health. In: Briggs H, Rzepnicki T, eds. *Using Evidence in Social Work Practice: Behavioral Perspectives.* Chicago, IL: Lyceum Books; 2004.

45. Nash C, Collins D. Tacit knowledge in expert coaching: science or art? *Quest.* 2006;58(4):465-477.

46. Abraham A, Collins D, Martindale R. The coaching schematic: validation through expert coach consensus. *J Sports Sci.* 2006;24(6):549-564.

47. Thompson A, Bezodis IN, Jones RL. An in-depth assessment of expert sprint coaches' technical knowledge. *J Sports Sci.* 2009;27(8):855-861.

48. Hedlund J, Forsythe GB, Horvath JA, Williams WM, Snook S, Sternberg RJ. Identifying and assessing tacit knowledge: understanding the practical intelligence of military leaders. *Leadersh Q.* 2003;14(2):117-140.

49. Ulmer W Jr. Military learnings: a practitioner's perspective. In: Sternberg RJ, Horvath JA, eds. *Tacit Knowledge in Professional Practice: Researcher and Practitioner Perspectives.* Mahwah, NJ: Lawrence Erlbaum Associates; 1999:59-72.

50. Irby DM. What clinical teachers in medicine need to know. *Acad Med.* 1994;69(5):333-342.

51. Deraci W, Vassev P, eds. *AAMC Data Book 2009: Medical Schools and Teaching Hospitals by the Numbers*. Washington, DC: Assn of American Medical Colleges; 2009.

52. Hilton SR, Slotnick HB. Proto-professionalism: how professionalisation occurs across the continuum of medical education. *Med Educ*. 2005;39(1):58-65.

53. Centers for Disease Control and Prevention. *Parent Training Programs: Insight for Practitioners*. Atlanta, GA: Centers for Disease Control and Prevention; 2009.

54. Ambrosini V, Bowman C. Tacit knowledge: some suggestions for operationalization. *J Manag Stud*. 2001;38(6):811-829.

55. Herschel RT, Nemati H, Steiger D. Tacit to explicit knowledge conversion: knowledge exchange protocols. *J Knowledge Manag*. 2001;5(1):107-116.

56. Porter S. Fundamental patterns of knowing in nursing: the challenge of evidence-based practice. *ANS Adv Nurs Sci*. 2010;33(1):3-14.

57. Carper B. Fundamental patterns of knowing in nursing. *ANS Adv Nurs Sci*. 1978;1(1):13-23.

58. Hussain F, Raza SA. A knowledge management framework to operationalize experiential knowledge: mapping tacit medical knowledge with explicit practice guidelines. Paper presented at: National Conference on Emerging Technologies; 2004; Pakistan.

59. Popay J, Williams G. Public health research and lay knowledge. *Soc Sci Med*. 1996;42(5):759-768.

60. Black N, Murphy M, Lamping D, et al. Consensus development methods: a review of best practice in creating clinical guidelines. *J Health Serv Res Policy*. 1999;4(4):236-248.

61. Veatch RM. Consensus of expertise: the role of consensus of experts in formulating public policy and estimating facts. *J Med Philos*. 1991;16(4):427-445.

62. Daro D, Dodge KA. Creating community responsibility for child protection: possibilities and challenges. *Future Child*. 2009;19(2):67-93.

63. Schorr LB, Farrow F. Expanding the evidence universe: doing better by knowing more. Paper presented at: Center for the Study of Social Poilcy, Harold Richman Public Policy Symposium; July 2011. http://lisbethschorr.org/doc/ExpandingtheEvidenceUniverseRichmanSymposiumPaper.pdf. Accessed March 4, 2013.

64. Saul J, Wandersman A, Flaspohler P, Duffy J, Lubell K, Noonan R. Research and action for bridging science and practice in prevention. *Am J Community Psychol*. 2008;41(3-4):165-170.

65. Daro D, Donnelly AC. Charting the waves of prevention: two steps forward, one step back. *Child Abuse Negl*. 2002;26(6-7):731-742.

66. Brownson RC, Jones E. Bridging the gap: translating research into policy and practice. *Prev Med*. 2009;49(4):313-315.

The findings and conclusions in this chapter are those of the authors and do not necessarily represent the official position of the Centers for Disease Control and Prevention.

Chapter 7

Does the Intervention Work?: Research Designs in Prevention

Caroline J. Kistin, MD
Robert Sege, MD, PhD

Introduction

Victims of child maltreatment suffer significant physical and psychological consequences, many of them long-term. Thus, effective prevention of maltreatment is a public health priority. Over the past decades, many child abuse and neglect prevention programs have been developed in an effort to reduce risk factors for maltreatment or increase protective factors. High quality research and evaluation, now possible through methodological advances and better data sources, can help estimate program impact, identify key components of effectiveness, and improve program implementation and dissemination. Rigorous evaluation results should be marshaled to justify distribution of resources toward cost-effective prevention programs. This chapter reviews examples of methods used to study child abuse prevention programs in the past, discusses additional study designs that should be considered for prevention initiatives in the future, and describes the application of theoretical frameworks for the evaluation and implementation of prevention evidence.

In general, child abuse prevention efforts face measurement challenges. Reported cases of child abuse, as measured by state child welfare agencies and collated by the National Center on Child Abuse and Neglect data system,[1] report a lower incidence of abuse then the more thorough National Incidence Study[2]; both are lower than suggested by adult recall of child maltreatment.[3] Put simply, although the effectiveness of prevention efforts may be most readily measured using reporting rates, there are inherent uncertainties in this measure that must be accounted for in study, design, and analysis.

Taxonomy of Prevention: Universal, Selected, and Indicated Public Health Activities

According to the World Health Organization (WHO), prevention efforts fall into 3 general categories: (1) universal prevention programs, which target the general population; (2) selective prevention programs, which target a high-risk subset of the population; and (3) indicated prevention programs, in which targeted individuals have demonstrably high risk, such as prior history of maltreatment.[4] Each level of public health prevention requires specific tailored research and evaluation methods. The following sections detail examples of universal, selective, and indicated child maltreatment interventions in an effort to highlight the different methods that have been used in child abuse prevention research. These examples are not intended to represent a definitive list of evidence-based programs.

Universal Prevention: Shaken Baby Prevention

Dias et al[5] conducted a pre-post community intervention trial with a concurrent control group to evaluate a program aimed at preventing abusive head injuries in infants and children. The intervention consisted of a hospital newborn nursery-based education program on infant shaking. This program was provided to all parents, regardless of risk factors, at the time of the infant's birth. The program was evaluated using a simple pre-post design, using a neighboring state as a concurrent control. The primary outcome of interest was the regional incidence of abusive head injuries in children less than 36 months of age. The incidence after the universal adoption of the intervention was compared to the incidence in the same region during the 60 months before the program began, and was also compared to incidence rates of abusive head injuries during the same time period in a neighboring state with no intervention program. The study demonstrated a 47% decrease in the incidence of abusive head trauma in the region during the study period with no comparable decrease seen in the neighboring state that did not have the intervention.

The Period of PURPLE Crying program is a second example of universal maltreatment prevention program. Barr et al[6,7] used a randomized controlled trial design to study whether parent education materials on infant crying (the Period of PURPLE Crying program) change knowledge or behavior related to infant shaking. Mothers were recruited at prenatal classes, maternity wards, and pediatric offices and were assigned to either the PURPLE intervention, consisting of a booklet and DVD with information related to infant crying, or to a control group who received other injury prevention materials. Telephone interviews were conducted 2 months later and measured knowledge around infant crying and shaking and self-reported behaviors. Mothers in the intervention group knew more about infant crying and shaking than mothers in the control group. Behaviors related to infant crying were similar in the 2 groups, but more mothers in the intervention group reported telling other caregivers about the danger of infant shaking and about the option of walking away when frustrated.

Selective Prevention: The Nurse Home Visiting Model

Selective prevention programs are directed at high-risk populations. Olds et al[8-10] used a randomized controlled trial design to evaluate the impact of the Nurse-Family Partnership, a program in which first-time mothers receive home visits from registered nurses both prenatally and for 2 years after the birth of their child. The program's goals were to improve pregnancy outcomes, improve child care, decrease intentional and unintentional child injuries, and improve parental self-sufficiency. The program was initially tested as a universal prevention model, recruiting all first-time mothers, but became a selective prevention initiative after initial studies showed a greater impact of the program on mothers who were unmarried or low-income. Three large-scale randomized controlled trials were performed in different populations. Participants were randomized to receive either home visitation services or comparison services. Outcomes were measured with periodic maternal interviews, up to 15 years after the intervention, as well as by medical record review, social service records review, and observations of parenting practices and the home environment. Overall, the mothers in the intervention group had improved prenatal health, fewer preterm deliveries, fewer child injuries, fewer subsequent pregnancies, and higher levels of maternal employment when compared to mothers in the control group. Importantly, a trial examining the impact of using paraprofessionals instead of nurses to do the home visits showed smaller improvements in all the outcomes. This program has been so successful that the Affordable Care Act of 2010 included funding for rapid expansion of evidence-based home visiting. Within 3 years, the federal government committed to spending $450 million per year on evidence-based home visiting.

Indicated Prevention: Project 12-Ways

Indicated prevention programs target situations in which maltreatment has already occurred with the goal of preventing recurrence or minimizing consequences. Lutzker and Rice[11] used a quasi-experimental design to evaluate Project 12-Ways, a program that works with families in rural Illinois who have abused or neglected their children. The program provides a number of in-home services to families, such as training in stress reduction, job skills, money management, and parenting skills. In this study, families who received the Project 12-Ways services were compared to families in the same region who received child protective services but were not enrolled in Project 12-Ways. The outcome of interest was the number of subsequent child abuse or neglect reports on the families. Overall, the families who received Project 12-Ways services had fewer subsequent reports of child abuse or neglect compared to the families who did not receive the services, but the number of reports in the families who received services rose steadily each year following completion of the program, suggesting that the benefits of Project 12-Ways decreased with time.

Research Design and Methods

This brief review of the 3 types of intervention—universal, selective, and indicated—demonstrates the range of activities that have been undertaken for the prevention of child abuse and neglect. In clinical research, the "evidence pyramid" has been used to depict the hierarchy of evidence based on study design (**Figure 7-1**). In this framework, systematic reviews and randomized controlled trials have traditionally been considered the highest quality study designs in medical research. Randomization offers high internal validity by accounting for most sources of bias that might confound the results.

Figure 7-1. *Systematic reviews and randomized controlled trials (at the top of the pyramid) have traditionally been considered the highest quality study designs in medical research.*

Randomized controlled trials were successfully used by Olds et al to demonstrate the effectiveness of the Nurse-Family Partnership. The success of this program and its wide dissemination illustrates some of the strengths and challenges of randomized controlled trials. When applied to prevention programs, however, randomized controlled trials can become complex and expensive. In addition, experimental conditions may be difficult to reproduce when the intervention goes to scale. Approaches to these limitations are discussed in more detail below. There is no doubt, however, that the conduct of rigorous clinical trials has supported the large-scale application of the Nurse-Family Partnership and other interventions.

The Traditional Evidence Pyramid

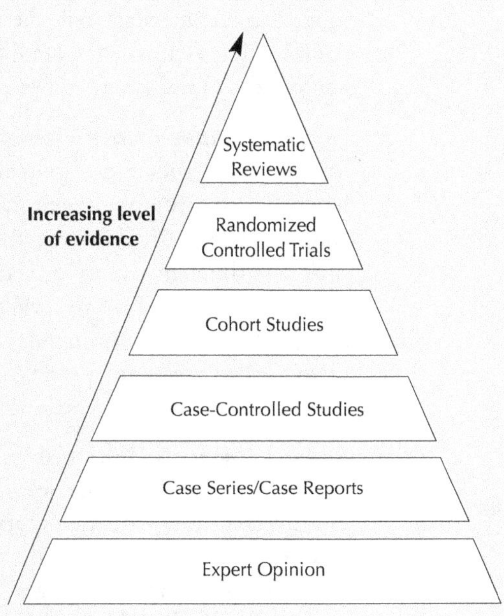

Figure 7-1

Traditional randomized controlled trials are particularly well suited for studying treatment interventions in individuals, especially when there are frequent short-term outcomes that can be accurately measured. A randomized controlled trial of a universal prevention program, however, requires the enrollment of a large numbers of subjects each with a relatively low risk of an adverse outcome, which translates into increased study complexity and significant study cost.[12,13] In addition, many of the effects of prevention programs may not be seen for some time, requiring long-term follow-up.

In addition, as described below, there are additional nonrandomized research and evaluation paradigms that may prove useful in assessing the effectiveness of child maltreatment prevention programs. When community and population-based interventions in particular may not be readily studied using randomized controlled trials, other methods of evaluation should be considered. The Evidence for Practice (E4P) Matrix[14] provides a framework to guide study design selection based on both the goal of the intervention of interest as well as on the intended target of the intervention. In prevention research, the intervention can again be conceptualized as either universal prevention, corresponding to "Health Promotion/Optimization" in the matrix; selective prevention, corresponding to "Risk Reduction/Asset Promotion" in the matrix; or indicated prevention, corresponding to "Deficit Mitigation" in the matrix. The target of the intervention can be the individual, the family, or the systems/community. Within the framework, an intervention designed to reduce or treat an existing problem in an individual patient is well suited for evaluation using a randomized controlled trial design, while an intervention designed to promote protective factors within a community may be more effectively and efficiently studied using an alternative approach.

The methods used for the evaluation of prevention interventions not well suited for investigation by randomized controlled trials are central to the new field of evidence-based public health[15]; a few examples are offered here.

Longitudinal cohort study designs can be used to follow a target population over time and evaluate for the development of outcomes of interest. Treatments may be assessed retrospectively by comparing outcomes among those who did or did not receive services, using statistical testing to correct for confounding factors.

Quasi-experimental/cluster randomized trials randomly assign treatment or control conditions on a group basis (eg, health care center may be randomly assigned, with measurements of individual outcomes among patients seen at each center). This study design is used to evaluate site-level interventions that either preclude individual randomization, or raise for cross-contamination between individuals.[16,17] The cluster design also has the potential to increase efficiency and decrease study cost. Unlike a randomized controlled trial, the intervention group is assigned. Known or suspected confounding factors can be adjusted for in the statistical analysis, but unidentified confounding factors may still be present.

Interrupted time-series designs are useful for the evaluation of prevention initiatives that are more widely distributed, such as on a county or statewide level. Outcomes before the prevention program starts can be compared to outcomes after the program is adopted. This method is strengthened by the inclusion of a concurrent control group, such as a different county or state, where the same outcome can be followed during the study period. Similarly, when a prevention initiative is rolled out on a stepwise basis, the outcome in the population in the health center, neighborhood, or other group receiving the intervention can be compared to the outcome in the population where the intervention has not yet been introduced.

Research methods developed in the field of quality improvement should also be considered for the study of child maltreatment prevention programs. Quality improvement study methods typically incorporate process measures into evaluation and focus on measuring program impact over time while conducting a series of short-term experiments to evaluate changes.[18,19] The Plan-Do-Study-Act cycle,[20] which highlights steps for evaluating change quickly and repeatedly in "real world" conditions, could easily be adapted to evaluate a new maltreatment prevention initiative.[21]

Often, public health or administrative data may be available. In those cases, additional epidemiological methods can be used. Case-control studies, which are often retrospective, can be performed using the information in an existing database to compare past risk and protective factors in subjects with and without an outcome of interest. An existing database may also be used to perform cross-sectional or ecological studies to examine correlations between an intervention and either individual or population-level outcomes respectively at one point in time. While these study designs can help describe associations between interventions and outcomes, they cannot determine causation.

In some cases, data collected related to an intervention or study can be combined with preexisting public health or population data that are already available. In the field of child development, for instance, investigators in Canada developed a tool known as the Early Development Inventory to assess school readiness at the community level.[22] The survey, completed by teachers, provides population-level data on children's level of preparedness for learning. The results can be analyzed in the context of other available community-level data, such as municipal spending on resources for young children and families, and can be followed over time to track changes that occur after an intervention is initiated. This can be an effective means of evaluating community and societal approaches to prevention.

Evaluating the Evidence

Independent of the research method used, the study quality and validity must be evaluated to determine the usefulness of the prevention initiative. Internal validity refers to the strength of the design—was the study performed in a fashion that allows one to determine the outcomes of interest within the study group? External validity, the generalizability of the study, refers to the ability to apply the study results to the larger population of interest. The ultimate impact of the research in the "real world" depends on the potential for successful implementation and dissemination of the findings. Conceptual frameworks, including the RE-AIM framework,[23] developed by Glasgow et al; the LEAD framework,[24] developed by the Institute of Medicine; and the Consolidated Framework For Implementation Research (CFIR)[25] are helpful in guiding program evaluation and subsequent policy and implementation decision-making.

The RE-AIM framework was developed for the purpose of comprehensively evaluating the public health impact of an intervention by taking into account factors related to the internal and external validity of study results, as well as the potential for dissemination and sustainability. The acronym RE-AIM stands for **R**each, **E**fficacy, **A**doption, **I**mplementation, and **M**aintenance, which are all dimensions of the intervention of interest that should be evaluated to determine its public health impact.

Reach refers to the proportion of people within the population of interest who participate in or are impacted by the program. It also looks at the characteristics of the participants in an effort to evaluate the representativeness of the study population. ***Efficacy*** identifies and evaluates both positive and negative outcomes of the program, while ***Adoption*** looks at the proportion and representativeness of the settings (such as postpartum departments or Head Start programs) where the intervention is adopted. ***Implementation*** measures whether the intervention is performed as designed, including a description of the resources needed for implementation, and ***Maintenance*** evaluates whether the intervention results in long-term sustained change. Taken together, RE-AIM can be used to compare the impact of different interventions and to evaluate changes in the effect of an intervention over time.

In April of 2010, the Institute of Medicine published the LEAD framework as part of a guide to both the use of evidence in decision-making about obesity prevention, as well as the development of new and relevant evidence for public health interventions in complex arenas. The framework emphasizes a systems approach to evaluation that takes into account the practical, real-word context of the prevention initiatives.

The LEAD acronym stands for **L**ocate evidence, **E**valuate it, **A**ssemble it, and inform **D**ecisions. Child maltreatment, similar to obesity, is a complicated public health problem with complex risk and protective factors. As a result, there are many potential approaches to prevention. The LEAD framework starts by specifying the questions that need to be answered in order to make a policy or program-related decision. "Locate evidence" employs a multidisciplinary approach by searching for relevant information within the medical literature and public health databases, but also from other sources, such as the economic, educational, and legal disciplines. In addition, this step includes gathering of specific local wisdom, including cultural beliefs and values that may influence implementation. The next step, "evaluate it" emphasizes study quality. Each type of evidence is evaluated on its own terms. Medical decision-makers are familiar with the characteristics of a well-conducted randomized trial. Similarly, other epidemiologic evaluation techniques may be assessed for quality. In this step, the evaluation of evidence includes the evaluation of external validity, as suggested by the RE-AIM model. "Assemble it" refers to the need for a clear summary of the evidence in the context of the questions asked at the beginning of the process. "Inform decisions" follows, based on the evidence available, the level of certainty needed about a particular intervention and the timing in which a decision needs to be made. Often, decisions need to be made in the absence of perfect evidence. For policymakers, the framework provides a reasonable model for obtaining as much evidence as is available, identifying the strengths and weaknesses of that evidence, and making a decision that is most likely to be the correct one given the current state of information. Finally, the framework emphasizes a focus on generating new, relevant evidence, particularly if, as typically happens, the process highlighted above reveals gaps in the evidence needed to answer important questions about prevention initiatives or approaches.

The Consolidated Framework for Implementation Research (CFIR) is a validated approach to assessing barriers and facilitators to individual and organizational behavior change needed for the successful implementation and dissemination of research findings. The CFIR is composed of 5 domains: characteristics of the intervention, inner setting (eg, the structural organization of a clinic practice, outer setting (ie, the economic, political, and social context within which an innovation is implemented), characteristics of the individuals involved in the work; and the overall process of implementation. Like RE-AIM and LEAD, the CFIR can be used to evaluate existing research but also to prospectively inform study design with a goal of maximizing intervention effectiveness.

Conclusion

In the field of child maltreatment prevention, there is a need for more robust data on universal, selective, and indicated prevention programs to help inform policy decisions and guide effective implementation and dissemination of successful interventions. Broadening the approach to program evaluation and adopting research models that have been successfully used in other disciplines provides a promising framework for increased evidence-based evaluation.

References

1. Child Maltreatment 2012. http://www.acf.hhs.gov/programs/cb/resource/child-maltreatment 2012 Accessed October 1, 2014.

2. National Incidence Study of Child Abuse and Neglect (NIS-4), 2004-2009. http://www.acf.hhs.gov/programs/opre/research/project/national-incidence-study-of-child-abuse-and-neglect-nis-4-2004-2009. Accessed October 1, 2014.

3. Centers for Disease C, Prevention. Adverse childhood experiences reported by adults --- five states, 2009. *MMWR. Morbidity and mortality weekly report.* Dec 17 2010;59(49):1609-1613.

4. Gordon R. An operational classification of disease prevention. In: Steinberg A, Silverman M, eds. *Preventing Mental Disorders: a Research Perspective.* Rockville, MD: Department of Health and Human Services; 1987:20-26.

5. Dias MS, Smith K, DeGuehery K, Mazur P, Li V, Shaffer ML. Preventing abusive head trauma among infants and young children: a hospital-based, parent education program. *Pediatrics.* Apr 2005;115(4):e470-477.

6. Barr RG, Barr M, Fujiwara T, Conway J, Catherine N, Brant R. Do educational materials change knowledge and behaviour about crying and shaken baby syndrome? A randomized controlled trial. *CMAJ : Canadian Medical Association journal = journal de l'Association medicale canadienne.* Mar 31 2009;180(7):727-733.

7. Barr RG, Rivara FP, Barr M, et al. Effectiveness of educational materials designed to change knowledge and behaviors regarding crying and shaken-baby syndrome in mothers of newborns: a randomized, controlled trial. *Pediatrics.* Mar 2009;123(3):972-980.

8. Olds DL, Henderson CR, Jr., Chamberlin R, Tatelbaum R. Preventing child abuse and neglect: a randomized trial of nurse home visitation. *Pediatrics.* Jul 1986;78(1):65-78.

9. Olds DL, Eckenrode J, Henderson CR, Jr., et al. Long-term effects of home visitation on maternal life course and child abuse and neglect. Fifteen-year follow-up of a randomized trial. *JAMA.* Aug 27 1997;278(8):637-643.

10. Izzo CV, Eckenrode JJ, Smith EG, et al. Reducing the impact of uncontrollable stressful life events through a program of nurse home visitation for new parents. *Prev Sci.* Dec 2005;6(4):269-274.

11. Lutzker JR, Rice JM. Project 12-ways: measuring outcome of a large in-home service for treatment and prevention of child abuse and neglect. *Child Abuse Negl.* 1984;8(4):519-524.

12. Briss PA, Zaza S, Pappaioanou M, et al. Developing an evidence-based Guide to Community Preventive Services--methods. The Task Force on Community Preventive Services. *Am J Prev Med.* Jan 2000;18(1 Suppl):35-43.

13. Truman BI, Smith-Akin CK, Hinman AR, et al. Developing the Guide to Community Preventive Services--overview and rationale. The Task Force on Community Preventive Services. *Am J Prev Med.* Jan 2000;18(1 Suppl):18-26.

14. Sege RD, De Vos E. Evidence-based health care for children: what are we missing? *Issue brief.* Apr 2010;85:1-14.

15. *Evidence-Based Public Health*. Oxford, UK: Oxford University; 2003.

16. DiGuiseppi C, Coupland C. The design and use of cluster randomised controlled trials in evaluating injury prevention interventions: part 1. Rationale, design and informed consent. *Inj Prev*. Feb 2010;16(1):61-67.

17. Coupland C, DiGuiseppi C. The design and use of cluster randomised controlled trials in evaluating injury prevention interventions: part 2. Design effect, sample size calculations and methods for analysis. *Inj Prev*. Apr 2010;16(2):132-136.

18. Berwick DM. Broadening the view of evidence-based medicine. *Quality & safety in health care*. Oct 2005;14(5):315-316.

19. Berwick DM. The science of improvement. *JAMA*. Mar 12 2008;299(10):1182-1184.

20. Langley GJ, Moen R, Nolan KM, Nolan TW, Norman CL, Provost LP. *The Improvement Guide: a practical approach to enhancing organizational performance*. San Francisco: Jossey-Bass; 1996.

21. Deming WE. *The New Economics for Industry, Government, and Education*. Cambridge, MA: MIT Press; 2000.

22. Hymel S, Le Mare L, McKee W. The Early Development Inventory (EDI): An Examination of Validity. American Educational Research Association. 2006; San Francisco, CA.

23. Glasgow RE, Vogt TM, Boles SM. Evaluating the public health impact of health promotion interventions: the RE-AIM framework. *Am J Public Health*. Sep 1999;89(9):1322-1327.

24. Institute of Medicine. Bridging the Evidence Gap in Obesity Prevention: A Framework to Inform Decision Making. Washington, DC: The National Academies Press; 2010.

25. Damschroder LJ, Aron DC, Keith RE, Kirsh SR, Alexander JA, Lowery JC. Fostering implementation of health services research findings into practice: a consolidated framework for advancing implementation science. *Implement Sci*. 2009;4:50.

Chapter 8

Complexity Science Applications in Child Maltreatment Prevention

Richard W. Puddy, PhD, MPH
Beverly A. Parsons, PhD
Melissa L. Brodowski, PhD MSW, MPH
Jacqueline M. Counts, PhD, MSW

Introduction

This chapter unpacks the concepts of complexity science so they are accessible to researchers, practitioners, and policymakers as they enact the social-ecological model of child maltreatment (CM) prevention. The complexity science framework transforms how the multifaceted phenomena of CM prevention is conceptualized and viewed and offers unique opportunities for application. This chapter is organized into 3 sections: The first grounds the reader and reframes existing thinking to look at CM prevention in new ways; the second addresses computer modeling techniques; the third describes examples of the use of complexity science in CM prevention and evaluation. These examples illustrate the usefulness of these concepts and their ability to shift current thinking and approaches to CM prevention to better fit reality and address intractable social problems.

Complexity Science Framework

Complexity science studies the common features of systems that are considered fundamentally complex. Initially in this field, scientists used complexity, as derived from the work of mathematicians and physicists, to model biological and physical systems. Their work has spread and joined forces with economists and social scientists working in many disciplines.

Figure 8-1. *Social-ecological model.*

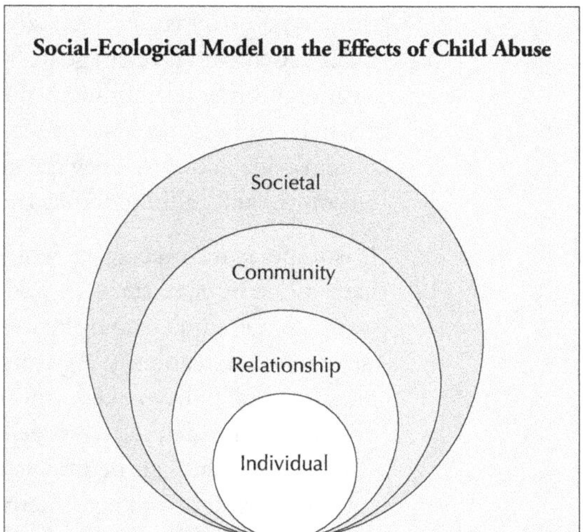

Figure 8-1

The concepts of complexity science are in contrast to the long-standing scientific approaches that have focused on seeking order, control, and regularity within nature. The bringing together of both of these lines of scientific endeavor provide an expanded range of ways to study complex social systems such as those that exist within the field of CM prevention. In addition to expanding ways of studying systems, complexity science provides a greater range of ideas of how to influence complex systems.

To understand the benefits of complexity science, it is useful to first consider that the field of CM prevention has adopted the social-ecological model (SEM) (**Figure 8-1**) as an organizing conceptual framework for its work.[1-3] The SEM is a systems perspective, meaning that attention should be directed both to distinguishable parts and interconnections. Factors at the individual level are related to factors at the community and societal levels. Strategies need to be targeted at all 4 levels of the social ecology (individual, relationship, community, societal) to ultimately impact the rate of CM at a population level.

However, this conceptual understanding has resulted in only small shifts in CM prevention study and programs operation. It is still typical for programs to only focus on one level or one part of the social ecology at a time.[4,5] Those programs are predominately at the individual and relationship levels.[6]

Complexity science provides additional tools and perspectives that promise to move forward the study of and implementation of practices that truly take a systemic perspective. An expanded systemic perspective can aid investigation of the myriad of interconnections among each level of the SEM. This would support more complete implementation of the SEM through new pathways for practice and research.

Traditional research perspectives have either focused solely on the parts rather than the interconnections or have used models and methods that have treated systems mechanistically, like a machine that is simply the sum of its parts. It assumes that if we could only understand the individual parts, then we would be able to understand the complete whole of the system—a reductionist approach.

By taking into account interconnections among multiple dynamic, nonlinear parts, complexity science helps move the field toward understanding the world in terms of the whole being more than the sum of its parts. This view of systems thinking looks at the types and patterns of relationships that bring about system-wide change.[7-9]

Complex systems are a combination of multiple dynamics occurring simultaneously. These dynamics can be thought of as 3 types: organized, adaptive, and random. ***Organized dynamics*** are deterministic where stability is sought. When thinking in terms of human situations, these dynamics may be intentionally organized and/or controlled by people (usually those who are in organizational positions of power), are often standardized (such as an accounting system), and/or are considered to move according to fixed laws.[10] From the perspective of scientific models that focus solely on organized dynamics, dynamics that are completely disorganized and appear to have no definable patters are considered ***random dynamics***. Complexity science, however, introduces a third type of dynamic, ***adaptive dynamics***. These dynamics result from many semi-independent and diverse agents free to act in unpredictable ways, continually interacting with each other.[11,12] Simultaneously, they adapt to each other and the environment as a whole, as both the environment and the agents change. This can create influential system-wide patterns. They are not necessarily moving toward stability and tend not to be controllable, although they can be influenced.

It is important to recognize which type of dynamics one is working with because they have different characteristics and consequently are influenced and studied in different ways. To help understand the dynamics, consider 2 factors present in many situations: agreement and certainty. Agreement refers to current degree of accord (eg, that among practitioners, policymakers, and researchers in CM prevention regarding fundamental principles on which related systems are built and which activities will ultimately prevent CM). Agreement can be understood as existing on a continuum, from being close to agreement to far from agreement about what is likely to prevent CM. Certainty refers to how predictably cause-and-effect relationships exist among actions, conditions, and consequences. Certainty can be conceptualized as existing on a continuum, ranging from being close to certainty of knowing the cause-and-effect relationship in terms of a short causal chain (effect of a well-established medicine for a particular ailment) to being far from certainty by not knowing the cause-and-effect relationship in terms of a long complex or complicated causal chain (effect of poverty on CM).

Figure 8-2 illustrates the relationship among these dynamics on these 2 dimensions—agreement and certainty. When agreement and certainty are extremely low, one finds random dynamics. That is, relationships and events appear to have no order or patterns. When agreement and certainty are moderate and/or imbalanced, one tends to find self-organizing, adaptive dynamics to be prominent. When agreement and certainty are high, organized dynamics tend to dominate.

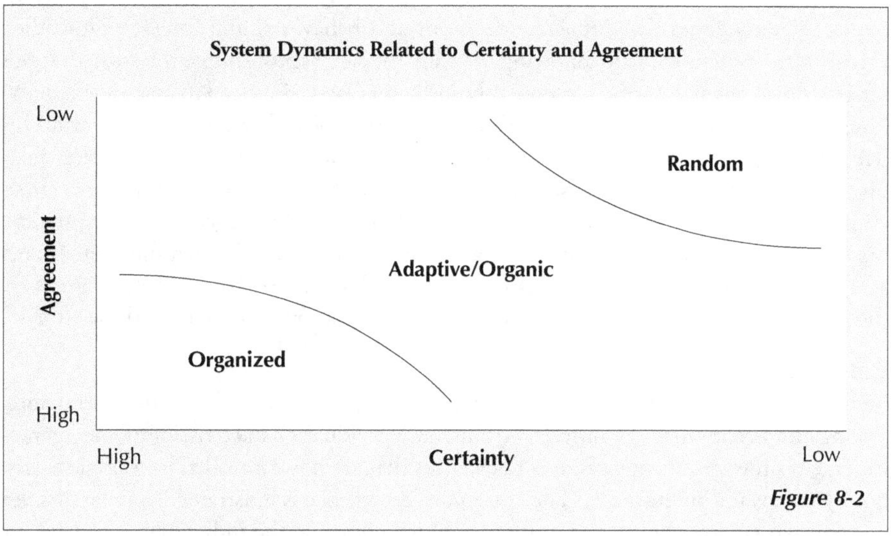

Figure 8-2. *System dynamics related to certainty and agreement. Adapted from Stacey R,[10] Zimmerman B,[13] Holladay R,[14] Parsons B.[15]*

Aligning Research Methods and Finding Leverage Points in Complex Systems

The reason for distinguishing the dynamics within complex systems is that organized dynamics and adaptive dynamics are researched and influenced differently. As noted earlier, organized dynamics are aligned with traditional linear research methods and deterministic system models that build on concepts or order, control, standardization, and hierarchical/nested organizations. Such dynamics assume a linear or a nonlinear, yet predictable, cause-and-effect relationship. They are based on the intention to stabilize and balance a system. Networked systems are more characteristic of systems with a high extent of adaptive dynamics rather than hierarchical systems. Adaptive dynamics, which to date have received the least attention in CM prevention, are characterized by different features. The following are important features that exist in tandem and interact with one another.

Agents Who Learn

As noted earlier, ***adaptive dynamics*** are the result of many semi-independent and diverse agents, who are free to act in unpredictable ways, continually interacting with each other. They adapt to each other and the environment as a whole and create system-wide patterns. Unlike traditional approaches, when complexity science is the basis of understanding human behavior, there is an acknowledgement that individuals have a history that accompanies them and influences their current decisions (ie, learning is acknowledged). Learning implies that individual agents learn from past interactions with other agents and incorporate this new knowledge into decision-making. For example, agents in complex adaptive social systems learn from each other and develop new techniques for solving problems based on previous interactions with each other. Consider how at the national level rates of physical abuse have decreased over the last decade while rates of neglect have remained relatively stable. Individual agents (eg, researchers, practitioners, advocates) are separately applying their successful lessons learned from this occurrence and now focusing on understanding how to prevent neglect based on this new knowledge.

Self-Organization Based on Simple Rules

Individual agents both shape and adapt to system patterns in order to solve problems or accomplish some purpose through self-organization. That is, they are acting without being told exactly what to do or how to do it. Agents individually use a few simple rules (ie, simple guidelines that influence decisions and behaviors) and interact with other agents in the system who are following basically the same set of simple rules whether the other agents know it or not. Consequently, individual behaviors lead to macro or system-level patterns of behavior and effects through this type of self-organization. Continuing with the neglect example, as individual researchers, practitioners, and advocates take up the charge to prevent, study, and measure neglect, a structure and order to these efforts begins to form out of the individual work of each of the agents. No hierarchical organizing may go into the efforts, yet a national formation of varied individuals and agencies working on this issue gets generated. A hidden structure may surface even though there was no distinct and separate lead organization coordinating these efforts.

Emergence

System-level patterns of behaviors gradually emerge over time from the interactions among the agents that are different from the individual characteristics of the agents. Emergent order results in patterns of behaviors that are not controlled by a single entity but by the agents' interactions. The concept of emergence is illustrated by a macro-level pattern that emerges as a result of the combined efforts of the individual agents (ie, in this illustration, it could be a pattern resulting in decreases in national rates of neglect). This macro-level pattern emerges out of the interactions between the constituent parts of the system at the micro level. A recent example of emergence involves the Network for Action Meeting that was sponsored by the Office of Child Abuse and Neglect (OCAN) and the Division of Violence Prevention at the Centers for Disease Control and Prevention. As the result of individual agents working and interacting with each other to prevent child maltreatment and promote well-being, a network of those directly and indirectly involved in 16 separate projects emerged and came together for 2 separate meetings, one year apart, to share and learn together at a national level what each was not able to simply accomplish by remaining in isolation of the others.

Coevolution

Agents (eg, humans) exist within a system and interact with it. Through the interactions of the agent with the system, the agent changes over time and the system changes as a result of the interaction of the agent. Both coevolve and change with each other to shift patterns. Observing these coevolutionary changes is a rich opportunity for gaining insight into the dynamics of the system.[16] Imagine networks of individual groups working on the primary prevention of child maltreatment in the form of neglect and their collective efforts impacting the environment and prompting legislation setting funds aside for this work. These funds further propel the amount of work that can be done in preventing neglect and soon social norms about neglect begin to shift as well, thus further accelerating the reduction in national rates of neglect. This illustrates the coevolution of the agents with their environment.

These principles illustrate how complexity science goes beyond traditional ways of viewing the world. In terms of the example of the SEM, complexity science provides a lens for us to view not only the interactions from level to level from a nonlinear, organized perspective, but also how each level coevolves with the others in a self-organizing way for new patterns to emerge.

Modeling/Simulation

Imagine a technique that can describe a range of plausible futures that might result from policy or program decisions. One of the promising aspects of applying complexity science to the work of CM prevention is discovering the counterintuitive nature of the behavior of systems in situations where there is no way to literally predict the unanticipated consequences that might arise from policy and program decisions. This is somewhat similar to the way a light emitted from a flashlight illuminates a limited portion of the pathway ahead and only in the direction it is facing. This band of light provides more clarity on objects closer to the source of the light but less clarity on those things at the far end of its reach. Complexity science provides the field with a tool that illuminates a range of possible outcomes contained within a band, similar to the band of light emitted from the flashlight. This tool is known as simulation and can be used to visualize and examine the counterintuitive nature of complex systems which arise from the many reinforcing and balancing loops and time delays that exist as well as the movement of semi-independent agents. To illustrate this concept, consider an image of a prototypical generic community in the United States. This could be anywhere and is unremarkable. Now imagine what would happen to the child maltreatment rates in that community if you could turn up or down (like dials on a radio) a multitude of factors affecting child maltreatment (ie, parenting skills, family stress, resiliency, neighborhood conditions, neighborhood erosion, social capital). When various factors are turned up, down, or held constant, a range of plausible futures in terms of child maltreatment rates are created for this community. An example of discovering a counterintuitive tendency may be one where the underlying assumption driving the behavior of the system is that if everyone had near-perfect parenting skills, then child maltreatment rates would drop considerably. However, when the experiment is run a thousand times over using the simulation, family stress, neighborhood conditions, and social capital are seen to play a considerable role in decreasing child maltreatment rates. In this simulation, just improving parenting skills, albeit to near-perfect levels, does not decrease the long-term occurrence of child maltreatment as there are other factors that can be at play.

The ability to engage in computerized modeling/simulation has become an especially useful application of complexity science. Recent advances in computer processing power have done for complexity science (via modeling and simulation) what the PC has done for modernizing desktop publishing over using a typewriter. In short, the computer revolution has allowed discussion to move from mental maps and the abstract to specification of individual agents who follow simple rules and interact with each other and their environment over time resulting in macro-level effects emerging from these interactions.[9]

Simulation science provides a method to experimentally manipulate variables that could not be done in the real world. Limitations dictated by ethics, finances, and time[17] often prevent the study of complex societal problems such as violence, suicide, and CM. However, studying those issues in a simulation offers a promising solution that has successfully been applied in several fields including diabetes,[18] cardiovascular diseases,[19] tobacco,[20] heroin epidemics,[21] mental health,[22] and crowd behavior.[23]

Until recently, formal models in the field did not adhere to the basic properties of complex systems but instead relied on a statistical regression approach that tends to model only linear organized dynamics. They do not capture the causal feedback, time delays, and unintended consequences or the adaptive dynamics of semiautonomous agents that make CM resistant to change.

The dynamics and complexity of CM can be approached from 2 simulation techniques: systems dynamic modeling and agent-based modeling. Both techniques can be employed as a tool for enhancing both learning and action in the prevention of CM.

Systems Dynamic Modeling

Considered a top-down approach (or one that emphasizes nonlinear, organized dynamics), systems dynamic modeling (SDM) characterizes the rates at which the population as a whole moves (flows) from one state of being (stock) to another within the system. The increases or decreases in these stocks are impacted by feedback loops that affect the flows. The dynamics of how the population behavior changes over time are captured visually.

SDM is iterative, evolving in response to new insights gained by those interacting with the model and changing conditions or goals.[24] It enables diverse stakeholders to combine their knowledge of a problematic situation into a visible dynamic hypothesis and then, using computer simulation, to formally compare various scenarios for how to facilitate change.[25] Often the process reveals critical leverage points, new areas to intervene in the system, that take into account a system's counterintuitive tendencies, opening new avenues for fundamental improvement.[26,27] For example, in the diabetes modeling project, a major finding was the inability of management and control efforts alone to reduce diabetes.[28] System dynamics modeling focuses on reinforcing and balancing loops and time delays.

Agent-Based Modeling

Agent-based modeling (ABM) offers another framework to explore complex adaptive systems. It is "agent-based" because it takes a model of the autonomous decision-making entities, called agents (the modeling of adaptive dynamics), to create the social system as a theoretical starting point. ABM is a formal method that deduces, in a systematic and rigorous way, macro-level implications from assumptions about micro-level behavior.[29] The ABM framework consists of describing a system from the viewpoint of its constituent units. This type of 'bottom-up' modeling begins by capturing, in the form of simple algorithms, the essential behavior (ie, simple rules) of the key agents in the system under investigation. Each simulated agent individually assesses its situation and makes decisions on the basis of these simple rules. Agents may then execute various behaviors appropriate for the system in which they belong. Next, these simulated agents are allowed to interact with one another, exploring a new model system (environment). Each of these agents can perform their own computations and have their own local knowledge as they exchange information with each other and react to input from other agents. In addition, agents are capable of evolving, allowing unanticipated behaviors to emerge.[30]

ABM is different from SDM because it simulates the behaviors of individuals interacting over time. These interactions lead to a variety of patterns at the system level. However, SDM starts off by modeling the behavior of the whole population at the systems level resulting in changes in population-level states of behavior. The modeling process begins by deciding what kind of model to generate to account for CM fatalities—a system dynamic model or an agent-based model. The SDM approach might account for how a whole population of children move from various states of risk (eg, noninjured, at-risk, abused, fatal) and the factors that influence that movement. The ABM approach might account for the simple rules of how the caregiver-child dyad (agent) interacts with each other, other family, community, and societal members and the influences on those interactions that ultimately result in fatality.

To apply either SDM or ABM to understanding CM fatalities, an interactive, simulation-based in-person "learning lab" can be created that enables multiple stakeholders design and formally evaluate CM-related policies. For example, a learning lab could engage multiple stakeholders in a facilitated process designed to explore the structural reasons for CM fatality trends that have remained resistant to reduction over the past 10 years.[28] Integrating research findings from the literature and insights from practical experience is the goal of this first step.

Next, these system characteristics (SDM) or agent characteristics (ABM) are translated into a formal simulation model using a set of differential equations and specialized modeling software. The model is then calibrated based on existing data. The model creates a simulated world for learning in which structured experiments (ie, simulated policy actions, can be conducted as a prelude to introducing policies in the real world). CM stakeholders could use the model to propose and test policies that deliver long-term impacts while simultaneously assessing risk for unintended challenges or negative effects. Users can also formally compare and evaluate CM prevention policies or interventions that would otherwise have to be tested over decades through trial and error in real populations.[31]

Results of such modeling of a range of plausible futures has implications for both program and policy interventions. Now policymakers can better understand the factors that influence CM fatalities at a systems level and can experiment in a simulated setting to determine the types of strategies that will have the greatest impact and/or least negative unintended consequences. Results of simulation modeling can also reveal new leverage points that have not been previously identified.

This speculative illustration, patterned after the diabetes modeling project,[32] allows one to see the potential benefits of conducting simulations that project forward over time, rather than real-world, multi-year experiments. Without the checks available through formal simulation modeling experiments, long-range target-setting and policy-making may succumb to the weakness of failing to recognize the system's counterintuitive tendencies, unintended consequences, and time delays.[32]

Simulation modeling, in the form SDM or ABM, puts mental models and causal maps into motion by modeling different dynamics. The modeling compresses decades into seconds and allows analysts to play out long-term scenarios of various policy options. This tool helps planners better understand the connection between structure and behavior in the dynamically complex world by providing a way to explore a wide set of plausible futures. It also gives policymakers the opportunity to assemble additional support for a desired course of change and to rehearse how they may handle periods of escalating social problems. The Collaborative Systems Inquiry Model for Childhood Obesity, developed in 2008 by the Georgia Health Policy Center, provides an example of building state legislators' capacity for decision-making by applying a systemic framework to understand childhood obesity as a complex health policy issue. Legislators explored 6 policy interventions, such as school, community, and health care–based approaches, to reduce childhood obesity. Computer simulation was used to translate evidence, making research easily understood by legislators and shift the policy debate from ideological issues to the systemic structure. Individual legislators commented that modeling took politics out of the issue, allowed them to see all of the information at one time, in one place, and talk with each other about it and that the fast turnaround time in rerunning the model was helpful.[33]

Applying Complexity Science to Evaluation of Large-scale CM Prevention Initiatives

The next 2 examples show how understanding differences in dynamics within complex systems can help determine how to bring about desired change and study the change process. In the first example—Strengthening Families—existing programs, services, communities, and policymakers are engaged in building a new paradigm (ie, a different set of "simple rules") for their actions/behaviors. It is not about using a particular model or starting a new program. In the second example—Evidence-based Home Visitation programs—the approach is to put in place specific evidence-based programs and build a supporting infrastructure. Both initiatives are happening within highly complex systems. The approaches used to study the change process are different because of the differences in attention to the system dynamics shown in **Figure 8-2** and the difference in the type of change sought (ie, changing general rules of behavior versus implementing specific programs). These examples illustrate how application of complexity science principles can enrich research or evaluation designs to provide practical knowledge about actions to enhance ways to prevent CM and promote optimal child development (**Box 8-1**).

Box 8-1. Complexity Science Concepts Applied to CM Prevention

The Strengthening Families and Evidence-based Home Visitation initiatives show that when seeking to change complex systems, it is useful to:

— Think of complex systems as heavily entwined subsystems with different balances of organized and adaptive dynamics.

— View the evaluation of change as multiple feedback loops within the change process.

— Work with and across multiple subsystems to build coherence across scale and location and encourage coevolution among subsystems.

— Recognize that adaptive dynamics are influenced and leveraged differently than organized dynamics in complex systems.

— Recognize that some desirable outcomes are not fixed, static, or even knowable in advance in complex adaptive systems.

Strengthening Families

Background

Building protective factors within families has become a focus of considerable attention in efforts to prevent CM. This orientation has gained momentum from the research synthesis and framing of "Strengthening Families" by the Center for the Study of Social Policy (CSSP). (*See Volume 1, Chapter 10, "Stengthening Families Through Early Care and Education," for more information on the Strengthening Families initiative.*) Strengthening Families is designed around 5 protective factors that are important within families: (1) parental resilience, (2) social connections, (3) concrete support in time of need, (4) knowledge of parenting and child development, and (5) social and emotional competence of children. Strengthening Families is about engaging existing programs, services, and other entities as partners around the use and promotion of these protective factors as their rules for action and behavior. It is not about using a particular model or necessarily starting a new program.

The 5 protective factors can be thought of as being the simple rules that fundamentally shape the actions of agents in a complex adaptive system. Simple rules are straightforward and can be applied to action in multiple settings. They are not necessarily easy to follow. These simple rules, focused on protective factors, stand in contrast to those that implicitly or explicitly guide the behavior of families in which CM occurs. They also may be in contrast to the dominate factors influencing policymakers or social service agencies as they seek to help prevent maltreatment. For example, risk factors rather than protective factors may be the primary focus of attention (implicitly or explicitly) of agency personnel and policymakers. Moving to an emphasis on protective factors is a shift in the mental model or paradigm that is guiding one's actions. Shifting paradigms is a powerful leverage point for changing a system.[34]

Mapping Patterns of Change in a Complex System

Because there is no one right way to implement a paradigm shift in a complex system, it is challenging to determine how to frame the situation for multiple stakeholders to leverage both the organized and adaptive dynamics of the multiple subsystems at play and determine if they are making progress. Creating a visual depiction of the subsystems involved in change along with attention to simple rules, multiple system dynamics, and a tipping point can be a useful communication tool as multiple stakeholders engage in simultaneous and independent shifts to a new paradigm.[15]

Table 8-1 presents an example of how those involved in implementing and/or studying the evolution of patterns within relevant subsystems can track and leverage multiple system dynamics. The statements within the framework provide practical descriptions that help communicate what patterns of change might look like.

Table 8-1. Patterns of Change in Complex Systems: Strengthening Families Example

Points of Influence	Baseline Analysis of Fundamentals and System Dynamics To What Extent	Testing Applications of New Fundamentals and System Dynamics	Tipping Point to New Fundamentals and System Dynamics Balance	Sustainable Adaptive Balance
Families	Are families aware of practicing protective factors? Are parents engaged with their child in supportive ways? Do parents use both organized and adaptive dynamics?	Families test use of protective factors and determine changes in relationships and boundaries in daily life. Families learn to self-assess use of protective factors.	Enough families are habitually using and self-assessing protective factors that community norms are shifting in support of protective factors.	Families are connected with other families who are skilled at using and building protective factors. Evidence of well-being of families and levels of child maltreatment are regularly monitored in communities.

(continued)

Table 8-1. Patterns of Change in Complex Systems: Strengthening Families Example *(continued)*

Points of Influence	Baseline Analysis of Fundamentals and System Dynamics To What Extent	Testing Applications of New Fundamentals and System Dynamics	Tipping Point to New Fundamentals and System Dynamics Balance	Sustainable Adaptive Balance
Programs	Are programs designed around building protective factors? Do programs encourage adaptive dynamics between workers and families that support protective factors?	Programs pilot new ways of operating that are grounded in protective factors. They determine cost implications.	Programs commit to redesigned programs that incorporate protective factors. Programs leverage organized and adaptive dynamics.	Programs use outcomes and other data to adjust to social conditions in community with emphasis on supporting protective factors. Programs put high priority on leveraging both adaptive and organized dynamics.
Professional Development (practitioners)	Do professional development activities address protective factors? Are professional development activities designed to model adaptive dynamics/organized dynamics?	Professional development redesigned and tested with greater attention to protective factors and use of more interactive, peer-to-peer learning and learning from families.	Communities of practice grounded in peer-to-peer learning and application are common; include reflective practices for critical analysis of balance of protective and risk factor attention in different contexts.	Learning and teaching becomes woven into all aspects of practice with structured professional development sessions and communities of practice strategically used to shore up challenging areas. Practitioner knowledge and practice regularly assessed.

(continued)

Table 8-1. Patterns of Change in Complex Systems: Strengthening Families Example *(continued)*

Points of Influence	Baseline Analysis of Fundamentals and System Dynamics To What Extent	Testing Applications of New Fundamentals and System Dynamics	Tipping Point to New Fundamentals and System Dynamics Balance	Sustainable Adaptive Balance
Organizational Connections	Are connections built to encourage protective factors? Do connections support adaptive dynamics/organized dynamics?	Entities, including ones not formerly involved, explore formal and informal connections to build attention to protective factors.	Key organizations have multiple interconnections that encourage attention to protective factors on a micro and macro level. Attention to protective factors is fundamental to connections.	Organizations use data feedback to strategically shift connections to respond to contextual changes to ensure primary attention to protective factors. Shifts are based on attention to boundaries, relationships, and perspectives.
Policy Context (State, Organizational)	Are policies based on encouraging protective factors? Are policies attentive to both organized and adaptive dynamics?	Policies adjusted with engagement of multiple voices, perspectives, valuing of protective factors.	Policies overall predominantly encourage building of protective factors. Policies leverage both organized and adaptive dynamics.	Policymakers balance attention to risk and protective factors tailored to microcontexts. They adjust policy features that affect system fundamentals and dynamics over time based on data systems to maintain grounding in protective factors and related new knowledge.

Identifying Points of Influence (Subsystems)

The first step in developing the framework is to identify subsystems within the overall complex system that span the full range of stakeholders who can influence CM. Such subsystems have coherence of their own, are likely to change in different ways and/or at different rates, and interact with other subsystems. They are important leverage points for systemic change. Multiple stakeholders are engaged simultaneously in these multiple parts of the system. Different patterns of change are likely for each subsystem because they have different system dynamics, especially differences in the extent and nature of organized and adaptive dynamics.

The example in **Table 8-1** uses 5 subsystems (Points of Influence) identified as being particularly significant by those involved with Strengthening Families: (1) families (the most fundamental subsystem), (2) organization programs and activities, (3) professional development for practitioners, (4) formal and informal organizational connections, and (5) governmental and organizational policy. Each subsystem is coevolving with the other subsystems as they interface with one another.

Although the subsystems are displayed separately, recognize that the boundaries between the subsystems are fuzzy and permeable. Furthermore, although all subsystems need to progress, it is not expected that they will change at the same rate or in the same time frame.

Determiners of Patterns of Change in Complex Systems

The second step in developing the framework is to identify aspects of change over time for each subsystem. In **Table 8-1** these are the headings across the top of the figure. The assumption underlying this progression of change is that stakeholders are seeking a long-term predominance of the new paradigm (ie, emphasis on protective factors). However, this is not a stable fixed state of being; rather, the use of the new paradigm continues to occur in a dynamic changing context. Thus the final state of change (far right side of the diagram) is a dynamic one: "Sustainable Adaptive Balance." The descriptors in the body of the diagram under this heading illustrate a continual dynamic balance of the new fundamentals (ie, the 5 protective factors) and both organized and adaptive system dynamics in a continually shifting context. The intention is to maintain a balance (not a fixed state) where the protective factors are the main driver of people's behaviors within the dynamic context. The expectation is that there will be an oscillation over time of CM rates. The "long-term outcome" is a situation in which multiple agents across subsystems of the overall complex system have ongoing feedback about outcome levels and key system dynamics and elements. Using this knowledge, they can be vigilant about how they are interacting and maintaining a dynamic balance that is continually adjusted in light of changing conditions to keep the CM rates as close to zero as possible.

The progression toward this state of sustainable balance involves an interactive process of assessing the current status of the systems dynamics and the extent of use of the protective factors within each subsystem until a tipping point is reached. Each subsystem is observed first in regard to a baseline analysis (labeled in **Table 8-1** as "Baseline Analysis of Fundamentals and Systems Dynamics") of the subsystems. Whenever attention is directed to a given subsystem by those involved in implementation or evaluation, the first task is to develop an understanding of what current "simple rules" implicitly underlie behavior in regard to the subsystem and the extent to which the protective factors might already be part of the underlying simple rules. The analysis also looks at system dynamics to understand the balance and nature of organized and adaptive dynamics. (See **Box 8-2**.)

Moving to the right in the diagram from the baseline assessment, attention is paid to the nature and extent of how people test ways to change each subsystem ("Testing Applications of Fundamentals and System Dynamics"). To move to a tipping point,

Box 8-2. Zooming in on Parental Involvement for Data Collection and Analysis

The Center for Public Partnerships (formerly the Institute for Educational Research and Public Service, University of Kansas) conducted an agency survey with over 90 agencies to identify systems components that support parent involvement as a CM prevention strategy. The Center also conducted focus groups with over 100 parents from diverse backgrounds. When viewed through a complexity lens, the researchers saw factors that may have been previously overlooked. Researchers learned as much from the process as the data themselves and begin to arrange the findings in a nonlinear, systematic fashion that is more than inputs, outputs, and outcomes.

Parents shared that they create their own support networks of family and friends. These systems of support are dynamic and operate outside of the formalized agency support structure. Agencies operate with high agreement and high certainty (organized), whereas parents are focused on the informal support networks that are adaptive systems dynamics. Results show that agencies are not maximizing family and friends as supports that could foster parent involvement in home environments and in agency activities. Conversely, agencies were seldom mentioned as primary contacts in times of need, creating boundaries that prevent parents from accessing available resources. Thus, sources of formal and informal social support (eg, neighborhood, community, churches) may be missed or underutilized by agencies.

Most agencies address and evaluate parent involvement as if it occurs in an organized, predictable system. Strategies to increase parent participation and parent input are highly structured and inflexible to changing parent roles and needs. Rather than concluding that parents do not want to help and blaming them,[35] complexity science adds value to a more traditional, static approach by leveraging different dynamics and identifying a potential avenue to enhance social networks as a protective factor against child maltreatment.

The availability of social networks may have been missed if the evaluators had not used a complex systems lens and paid attention to the adaptive dynamics evident in the focus group process and saw its implications for the overall strategy to build protective factors. The identification of patterns illuminated potential areas of influence to support strategies for positive change and address barriers to parent involvement and encouraged interventions at multiple levels of the ecological model. Had the divergent definitions of involvement and identification of family and friends as adaptive informal support networks not been acknowledged, agencies would have kept doing business as usual. Adaptive patterns are seen as additional resources within the system as another avenue to engage families. The thinking of agency staff is being broadened to acknowledge the organic nature of the system in which parents operate. Moving beyond token representation of parents on advisory boards to looking at how to encourage healthy adaptive networks that could result in big changes as to where agencies focus their work on present involvement.

iterative assessments and large- and small-scale changes are made, often on a pilot test basis, to shape and understand how to embed protective factors in people's actions and leveraging both organized and adaptive dynamics. Some pilot tests might be done in a coordinated fashion across subsystems or within a subsystem with attention to the other subsystems. (See W.K. Kellogg Foundation[36] for a discussion of pilot test designs.)

As iterative assessment and multiple small- and large-scale changes are undertaken, momentum builds to a tipping point ("Tipping Point to New Fundamentals and System Dynamics Balance"). It is much like getting a large, heavy flywheel moving. It can take great effort over a period of time to inch the flywheel forward. Eventually, the flywheel makes a complete turn and then another—each time moving a bit faster. Gradually, it builds momentum and at some point, there is a breakthrough and it is carried forward with its own momentum. The shift has occurred to the protective factors as the predominant underlying way in which people are working within and across subsystems. At this point, the role of those moving the wheel changes. It is time to consolidate successful actions and build ways of watching, reflecting, and making minor, but strategic, adjustments to sustain the dynamic balance.

The framework allows multiple stakeholders to engage in dialogue using an understanding of the features of complex systems to identify possible small changes that can have large impact in moving the system as a whole to the tipping point. (See Parsons[37,38] for more details on use of a similar tool in other settings.) It can also serve as the basis for evaluators and researchers to follow and map the pattern and rate of change within and among the subsystems. Such investigations are enhanced by carefully framed questions that direct attention to changes in boundaries, relationships, and differences in levels of energy.[39] Such questions help identify ways to leverage both organized and adaptive dynamics to shift patterns within the complex systems. As stakeholders engage in dialogue and evaluative inquiries proceed, the boundaries among the subsystems are likely to be even more permeable with the new knowledge about protective factors moving across boundaries and moving to a deeper level of understanding and integration.

Supporting Evidence-based Home Visiting Programs Example

The Supporting Evidence-based Home Visiting (EBHV) programs grant initiative funded by the Children's Bureau provides an example of using a complexity science approach in a national cross-site evaluation. Whereas the purpose of the Strengthening Families initiative is not about using a particular model or program, the primary purpose of EBHV initiative is focused on the use of particular programs. Yet it goes beyond the programs themselves to developing and supporting the infrastructure needed for the widespread adoption, implementation, and sustainability of evidence-based home visitation programs.

The Children's Bureau funded 17 projects in 15 states in October 2008, as well as a national cross-site evaluation. Thinking systemically, grantees are expected to implement (1) collaborative planning efforts to leverage other federal, state, and local investments of existing funding streams into EBHV programs and practices; (2) activities needed to build infrastructure systems that can fully adopt, implement, and sustain EBHV with fidelity; and (3) rigorous local evaluations that include process/implementation, outcome, and cost analysis components.[40]

EBHV National Cross-Site Evaluation

Mathematical Policy Research, Inc. was awarded the contract for the national cross-site evaluation. The Children's Bureau required that a participatory and utilization-focused evaluation framework be used to guide the design and implementation for the cross-site evaluation because of the congruence between such evaluation frameworks and the principles of complexity science. The discussion below focuses on how the national cross-site evaluation is carried out with systems thinking in mind and attention to the multiple types of dynamics within complex systems.

Within this context, complexity science principles drove the overall national evaluation design. The EBHV initiative is comprised of various complex systems with both organized and adaptive dynamics. The grantees function as agents in complex adaptive systems. They are interrelated and interdependent actors (both individuals and organizations) working in various contexts on activities that are directly or indirectly related to CM prevention.[8,36,41,42] These webs of interacting and interdependent agents form a complex whole, which is changed through the evolving interactions of its parts.[43,44]

In the EBHV cross-site evaluation, system-based evaluation methods are being used to understand how grantees are building various kinds of infrastructure capacity, alone and in combination, to achieve 3 goals: the implementation, scale-up, and sustainability of high-fidelity EBHV programs.[41] Accomplishment of these 3 related goals involves different degrees of emphasis on organized versus adaptive dynamics for each grantee's situation.

The evaluation methods used track grantees' plans and activities, the key system attributes of the environments in which they work, and interactions between grantees and their environments. Attributes include system boundaries and infrastructure levels and collaborative relationships and communication patterns among key players. Applying the concept of individual agents and self-organization within complex systems, each EBHV grantee was viewed as operating within a set of unique contacts and relationships with individuals and organizations at many levels each with its own set of infrastructure capacities, opportunities, and constraints.

The initial step in the national evaluation was to develop a detailed 'system map' with the grantees. This process entailed conducting in-depth conversations with each grantee to document a baseline pattern of infrastructure capacity and system attributes, including the boundaries and levels of grantee activities, key players and their relationships, and grantees' EBHV goals and associated infrastructure functions. **Table 8-2** provides an example of a baseline grantee system map that shows connections among activities, key players, and infrastructure features to serve as a starting point for understanding infrastructure changes over time.

The features of the infrastructure include both ones that exhibit predominantly organized dynamics (eg, planning, operations, and fiscal) as well as those that predominantly exhibit adaptive dynamics. Attending to the difference in the balance of dynamics within each of these infrastructure features helps the evaluators and grantees expand their thinking about how to leverage change in these complex settings. (See **Box 8-3**.)

EBHV Initiative Management

The overall EBHV initiative approach is heavily focused on building and enhancing relationships within and across the various participants in this process because the Children's Bureau recognize that coevolution and adaptation are powerful features of adaptive dynamics that can be leveraged for the overall success of the projects. They also recognize the power of ongoing feedback in complex systems. It is consequently a critical component of the EBHV initiative and the cross-site evaluation design. For example, a peer-learning community was established as a vehicle for planning and learning together across the grantee projects. As part of developing the cross-site evaluation plan, grantees were engaged in a number of workgroups which provided input and recommendations regarding the feasibility and level of burden on data collection requirements. The national evaluator has assigned grantee liaisons to work with a small number of grantee

Table 8-2. Evidence-based Home Visiting Cross-Site Evaluation: System Map of Selected Activities and Key Players

System Level	Activities	Key Players	Planning	Operations	Fiscal	Communication	Collaboration	Political Support	Workforce	Evaluation
Core Operations	Provide ongoing technical assistance for implementation and management of home visiting models.	National home visiting programs, local implementing agencies, EBHV grantee (state child welfare agency)	X	X			X		X	
	Monitor fidelity to the home visiting models.			X			X		X	X
Organizational Support	Draft and issue RFP for additional service providers; select providers.	EBHV grantee	X	X	X		X			
	Develop and issue RFP developing a uniform prenatal screening and central intake system.		X	X	X		X			
Community/County Level	Develop systems for community-level coordination and integration across home visiting models (NFP, HFA, PAT*).	National home visiting programs, local implementing agencies, EBHV grantee (state child welfare agency)	X	X	X		X			
	Advocacy at the community level to gain buy in from hospitals, federally funded health centers, clinics, social services, and county and city government.	Local implementing agencies	X	X	X		X			

**Nurse-Family Partnership, Healthy Families America, Parents as Teachers*

(continued)

Table 8-2. Evidence-based Home Visiting Cross-Site Evaluation: System Map of Selected Activities and Key Players ***(continued)***

System Level	Activities	Key Players	Planning	Operations	Fiscal	Communication	Collaboration	Political Support	Workforce	Evaluation
State Level	Solicit ongoing input and advice for planning from the Home Visitation Workgroup (formed prior to receiving the grant).	(32 different entities statewide)	X	X	X	X	X	X	X	X
	Develop a sustainability committee within the Home Visitation Workgroup.	EBHV grantee, Medicaid, managed care HMOs, provide foundations, advocacy groups	X		X	X	X	X		
	Develop a strong local evaluation and contract with an evaluator.	Evaluation committee, EBHV grantee								X
	Collect data to provide information about the result of screening families, to identify unmet needs, and to advocate for needed services.	Local lead agencies, EBHV grantee, Home Visitation Workgroup		X		X	X	X		X
	Develop a publicity materials and media strategy.	EBHV grantee, Home Visitation Workgroup	X			X		X		
National Level	Participate in EBHV grantee peer learning network and cross-site evaluation.	EBHV grantee, local evaluator	X			X	X			X
	Disseminate evaluation findings at conferences and other forums.					X		X		X

Box 8-3. Creating the Systems Map

The national evaluators worked with each of the grantees to create a baseline systems map for infrastructure change, which captured the various activities at multiple levels. (See **Table 8-1**.) Grantees will be asked to report on changes to the infrastructure capacity and goals over the life of the project. The national evaluators will conduct 2 site visits to each of the grantees to interview key stakeholders and collect additional data regarding the changes in patterns of system relationships, boundaries, perspectives, and other system attributes. Through this process, national evaluators will track the individual and system-level patterns of behavior among grantees that emerge over the course of the EBHV initiative. Complexity science principles offer a way to better understand how the individual behaviors from the grantees and their partners influence and shape both their own state/local effort and the national EBHV initiative.

Collaboration among EBHV grant partners is a central strategy for working toward infrastructure change goals. As such, the cross-site evaluation will include a partner/network survey of key players in grantees' projects, including staff, service providers, county and state government officials, and national model developers. The survey will examine grantee relationships with key partners and how these change over time, paying special attention to relationships, boundaries, and perspectives that are likely to have important system influences. The survey will be used to confirm and track not only the infrastructure areas in which partners are collaborating but also whether their ties become stronger or weaker and more or less collaborative over time—moving along the collaboration continuum from sharing information to sharing service referrals, training, technical assistance, and resources. The network survey will coincide with each round of site visits and at the end of the grant period. A network analysis will be used to create measures about each grantee system and its members, such as the size of the networks, the density of ties among network members, and the centrality of grantees and other partners in the network. The results of these analyses will be used in the cross-site and cross-domain analyses to understand the relationships between grantees' network structures, infrastructure changes, achievement of EBHV goals, grantee costs, and fidelity of grantee programs. Results will be shared with grantees and technical assistance will be provided to interpret and apply the network analysis to planning and implementation efforts.

sites as a way to build and foster those relationships. Because these projects are funded as cooperative agreements, federal project officers work collaboratively with the grantees and are highly involved in the project activities. The Children's Bureau is committed to creating transformative relationships with grantees and contractors that can truly result in lasting systemic change and positive outcomes for children and families. Complexity science offers a framework for guiding the interactions with grantees as well as several analytical approaches that helps explain how these systems change processes occur.

Conclusion

This chapter has emphasized 2 themes that were elaborated upon at the outset: (1) to reframe existing thinking with a complexity science lens so as to view CM prevention in a new way and (2) to demonstrate the added value that complexity science offers in advancing the work of CM prevention. Examples were presented that illustrated these themes. Simulation and modeling techniques were described that could advance the field's understanding of preventing CM fatalities. The Strengthening Families and Evidence-Based Home Visitation examples illustrated how differences in the dynamics (nonlinear organized, adaptive) influence 2 different approaches to studying the change process, thus illustrating how complexity science can advance the CM prevention fields' understanding of research and evaluation design.

The application of complexity science principles to preventing CM offers a unique, yet powerful, lens to address this entrenched problem. This chapter described both mathematically based simulation techniques and practical evaluation applications that offer new insights into the "business as usual" world of child maltreatment prevention. Complexity science is an alternative and complementary approach to traditional statistical equations and evaluation techniques. It provides researchers, practitioners, and policy makers with useful tools and insights that correspond more closely to the way the real world operates than existing approaches. By becoming informed by a complexity science lens in terms of evaluation application, modeling/simulation, and interdisciplinary collaborations investigators, practitioners, and decision makers can increase the likelihood of significant advances in the field of child maltreatment prevention.

References

1. Belsky J. Child maltreatment: an ecological integration. *Am Psychol.* 1980;35(4):320-335.
2. National Research Council, Panel on Research on Child Abuse and Neglect. *Understanding Child Abuse and Neglect.* Washington, DC: National Academy Press; 1993.
3. Dahlberg LL, Krug EG. Violence – a global public health problem. In: Krug EG, Dahlberg LL, Mercy JA, Zwi AB, Lozano R, eds. *World Report on Violence and Health.* Geneva, Switzerland: World Health Organization; 2002:1-24.
4. Kelly JG. *Becoming Ecological: An Expedition Into Community Psychology.* New York, NY: Oxford University Press; 2006.
5. Stokols D. Establishing and maintaining healthy environments. toward a social ecology of health promotion. *Am Psychol.* 1992;47(1):6-22.
6. Freisthler B, Merritt DH, LaScala EA. Understanding the ecology of child maltreatment: a review of the literature and directions for future research. *Child Maltreat.* 2006;11(3):263-280.
7. Trochim WM, Cabrera DA, Milstein B, Gallagher RS, Leischow SJ. Practical challenges of systems thinking and modeling in public health. *Am J Public Health.* 2006;96(3):538-546.
8. Foster-Fishman PG, Nowell B, Yang H. Putting the system back into systems change: a framework for understanding and changing organizational and community systems. *Am J Community Psychol.* 2007;39(3-4):197-215.
9. Parsons BA. The state of methods and tools for social systems change. *Am J Community Psychol.* 2007;39(3-4):405-409.
10. Stacey R. *Strategic Management and Organisational Dynamics.* 2nd ed. London: Pitman Publishing; 1996.
11. Dooley K. A complex adaptive systems model of organizational change. *Nonlinear Dynamics Psychol Life Sci.* 1997;1(1):69-97.
12. Eoyang G. *Conditions for Self-Organizing in Human Systems* [dissertation]. Cincinnati, OH: Union Institute and University; 2002.

13. Zimmerman BJ. Ralph Stacey's agreement & certainty matrix. Edgeware Web site. http://216.119.127.164/edgeware/archive/think/main_aides3.html. Published 2001. Accessed August 13, 2015.

14. Holladay R. Using human systems dynamics in supervisory relationships. In: Eoyang GH, ed. *Voices From the Field: An Introduction to Human Systems Dynamics*. Circle Pines, MN: Human Systems Dynamics Institute; 2003.

15. Parsons B. *Evaluating Patterns of Change in Complex Systems: Strengthening Families Example*. Fort Collins, CO: InSites; 2009.

16. Anderson RA, Crabtree BF, Steele DJ, McDaniel RR, Jr. Case study research: the view from complexity science. *Qual Health Res*. 2005;15(5):669-685.

17. Axelrod R. Advancing the art of simulation in the social sciences. In: Conte R, Hegselmann R, Terna P, eds. *Simulating Social Phenomena*. Berlin: Springer-Verlag; 1997:21-40.

18. Jones AP, Homer JB, Murphy DL, Essien JDK, Milstein B, Seville DA. Understanding diabetes population dynamics through simulation modeling and experimentation. *Am J Public Health*. 2006;96(3):488-494.

19. Homer J, Hirsch G, Minniti M, Pierson M. Models for collaboration: how system dynamics helped a community organize cost-effective care for chronic illness. *Syst Dyn Rev*. 2004;20(3):199-222.

20. Teng TO, Ahmad S, Savage JM, Moore R, Gage E. The AMA proposal to mandate nicotine reduction in cigarettes: a simulation of the population health impacts. *Prev Med*. 2005;40(2):170-180.

21. Agar MH, Wilson D. Drugmart: heroin epidemics as complex adaptive systems. *Complexity*. 2002;7(5):44-52.

22. Smith G, Wolstenholme EF, McKelvie D, Monk D. Using system dynamics in modeling mental health issues in the UK. Paper presented at: 22nd International Conference of the System Dynamics Society; July 25-29, 2004; Oxford, England.

23. Henein CM, White T. Agent-based modeling of forces in crowds. In: Davidsson P, Logan B, Takadama K, eds. *Multi-Agent and Multi-Agent-Based Simulation*. Berlin, Heidelberg: Springer-Verlang; 2005: 173-184.

24. Homer JB. Why we iterate: scientific modeling in theory and practice. *Syst Dyn Rev*. 1996;12(1):1-19.

25. Andersen DF, Richardson GP, Vennix JAM. Group model building: adding more science to the craft. *Syst Dyn Rev*. 1997;13(2):187-201.

26. Forrester JW. Counterintuitive behavior of social systems. *Tech Rev*. 1971;73(3):53-68.

27. Meadows D. Leverage points: places to intervene in a system. The Donella Meadows Institute Web site. http://www.donellameadows.org/archives/leverage-points-places-to-intervene-in-a-system/. Published December 1999. Accessed August 17, 2015.

28. Jones LM, Finkelhor D, Halter S. Child maltreatment trends in the 1990s: why does neglect differ from sexual and physical abuse? *Child Maltreat*. 2006;11(2):107-120.

29. Flache A, Macy MW. Social life from the bottom up: agent modeling and the new sociology. Paper presented at: Social Dynamics: Interaction, Reflexivity, and Emergence; 2004; Chicago, IL.

30. Bonabeau E. Agent-based modeling: methods and techniques for simulating human systems. *Proc Natl Acad Sci U S A*. 2002;99(suppl 3):7280-7287.

31. Homer J, Jones D, Seville D, Essien J, Milstein B, Murphy D. The CDC's diabetes systems modeling project: developing a new tool for chronic disease prevention and control. Paper presented at: 22nd International Conference of the System Dynamics Society; 2004; Oxford, England.

32. Milstein B, Jones A, Homer JB, Murphy D, Essien J, Seville D. Charting plausible futures for diabetes prevention in the United States: a role for system dynamics simulation modeling. *Prev Chronic Dis*. 2007;4(3):A52.

33. Minyard K. An applied example: systems thinking in the legislative health policy arena. Preconference workshop presented at: Society for Prevention Research on Participatory System Dynamics Modeling: Applications for Preventive Research; 2012; Washington, DC.

34. Meadows D. *Thinking in Systems: A Primer*. White River Junction, VT: Chelsea Green Publishing Company; 2008.

35. Gambrill E. *Social Work Practice: A Critical Thinker's Guide*. New York, NY: Oxford University Press; 1997.

36. WK Kellogg Foundation. *Designing Initiative Evaluation: A Systems-Oriented Framework for Evaluating Social Change Efforts*. Battle Creek, MI: WK Kellogg Foundation; 2007.

37. Parsons B. Using a systems change approach to building communities. In: *Implementation Tools*. Saint Louis, MO: The Danforth Foundation; 1998:F-1–F-63. *The Policymakers' Program: The First Five Years: Strategies for Improving the Well-Being of Children and Families*; vol 2.

38. Parsons B. *Evaluative Inquiry: Using Evaluation to Promote Student Success*. Thousand Oaks, CA: Corwin Press; 2002.

39. Parsons B, Jessup P. *Questions That Matter: A Tool for Working in Complex Situations*. Fort Collins, CO: InSites; 2009.

40. Koball H, Zaveri H, Boller K, et al. *Supporting Evidence-Based Home Visiting to Prevent Child Maltreatment: Overview of the Cross-Site Evaluation*. Washington, DC: US Department of Health and Human Services, Administration for Children and Families, Children's Bureau; 2009.

41. Mathematica Policy Research, Inc. *Proposed Evaluation Design for Systems Domain: Supporting Evidence-Based Home Visiting Programs National Cross-Site Evaluation Contract with the Children's Bureau, USDHHS*. Princeton, NJ: Mathematica-Policy Research, Inc; 2009.

42. Holland J. *Hidden Order: How Adaptation Builds Complexity*. Reading, MA: Helix Books; 1995.

43. Kauffman S. *At Home in the Universe: The Search for Laws of Self-Organization and Complexity*. New York, NY: Oxford University Press; 1995.

44. Coffman J. A framework for evaluating systems initiatives. BUILD Initiative Web site. http://www.buildinitiative.org/files/BuildInitiativefullreport.pdf. Published August 2007. Accessed March 9, 2013.

Additional Reading/Resources

Castellani B, Hafferty FW. *Sociology and Complexity Science: A New Field of Inquiry.* Berlin, Heidelberg: Springer-Verlag; 2009.

Gladwell M. *The Tipping Point: How Little Things Can Make a Big Difference.* Boston, MA: Little, Brown and Company; 2000.

Patton M. *Qualitative Research & Evaluation Methods.* 4th ed. Thousand Oaks, CA: Sage Publications; 2008.

Plsek P. Redesigning health care with insights from the science of complex adaptive systems. In: Institute of Medicine, Committee on Quality of Health Care in America, eds. *Crossing the Quality Chasm: A New Health System for the 21st Century.* Washington, DC: National Academy Press; 2001:322-335.

Ungar M. A deeper, more social ecological social work practice. *Soc Serv Rev.* 2002;76(3):480-497.

The findings and conclusions in this chapter are those of the authors and do not necessarily represent the official position of the Centers for Disease Control and Prevention.

Chapter 9

A Research Agenda to Accelerate the Adoption and Effective Use of Promising Child Maltreatment Prevention Strategies

Rita Noonan, PhD
Linda Anne Valle, PhD

Background

As noted elsewhere in this book, child maltreatment exacts an enormous burden on the public's health, resulting in more than 3 million reports of child maltreatment to state and local agencies and over 1500 child deaths each year in the United States.[1] The financial cost is significant as well with a total lifetime economic cost of fatal and nonfatal child maltreatment reaching $124 billion each year.[2] In order to help millions of children survive and live to their full potential, evidence-based interventions must be identified and packaged for use, disseminated broadly, supported with training and technical assistance, adopted widely, and implemented as designed. A number of promising child maltreatment prevention interventions have been identified through rigorous research, but too few have gained wide community acceptance, and little is known about the best ways to encourage their broader use. Therefore, as in many other fields, child maltreatment prevention suffers from a gap between scientific discoveries and their everyday use. This gap is not a mere scientific or programmatic puzzle—it contributes to unacceptably high rates of child injury, death, and disability.

A public health approach has been used successfully to address other health problems and is a promising approach to close the gap between research and practice in child maltreatment.[3] This systematic approach describes the problem, identifies risk and protective factors, develops and tests prevention interventions, and translates effective interventions into community-based programs to ensure widespread adoption. This method incorporates the continuum of research from basic and descriptive research to risk factor research, intervention development and testing, and translation, dissemination, adoption, and implementation research. The goal of this approach, theoretically, is to stimulate the movement from research into practice by sequentially following these 4 steps. Although much has been learned using the public health model to address child maltreatment prevention, gaps in knowledge remain. This chapter articulates the key activities embedded in Step 4 of the public health model—specifically, translation and dissemination to ensure widespread adoption and use—in order to illuminate critical research needs in child maltreatment prevention. These needs, if addressed, will help close the gap between research and practice.

The Importance of Moving From Research to Practice in Child Maltreatment Prevention

Relatively few child maltreatment prevention programs are considered well-supported by evidence (ie, as identified through a minimum of at least 2 independent randomized trials examining child maltreatment outcomes).[4] However, a number of promising evidence-based child maltreatment prevention interventions have been identified.[5-7] Currently, the evidence base for effective child maltreatment prevention involves interventions that work directly with parents. For example, the Nurse-Family Partnership home visitation model, the pediatric primary care-based Safe Environment for Every Kid (SEEK) model, and the Chicago Child-Parent Centers (a preschool/kindergarten approach with direct parental involvement) have all demonstrated preventive effects on incidents of child maltreatment in at least one rigorous evaluation.[8-11] In addition, a number of behaviorally-based parent training approaches have been shown to reduce initial occurrences or recurrences of child maltreatment (eg, parent-child interaction therapy or PCIT).[12-15] Research is clearly needed to replicate the results of early studies and to identify additional effective strategies, programs, and policies for child maltreatment prevention. In the meantime, encouraging broader use of programs with the strongest evidence is essential to prevention of child maltreatment and maltreatment-related injuries.

Despite a growing awareness in the field of the need to better understand the broad spectrum of factors influencing the flow from research to practice in child maltreatment, many of the existing empirical studies have focused on relatively small pieces of the puzzle (eg, identifying facilitators or barriers to adoption or implementation of evidence-based practices or on descriptive case studies describing implementation).[16-23] Although understanding facilitators and barriers and lessons learned during implementation are informative, relatively few empirical studies have focused on testing optimal methods of moving child maltreatment prevention from research to practice. In addition, as evidenced below, the majority of studies have focused on the 3 efficacious parent training models, primarily with respect to adaptation and fidelity during initial implementation. To address these shortcomings, this chapter provides examples from the research that has been conducted and highlights gaps in knowledge and research questions to be addressed.

Moving research into practice requires 4 steps: (1) translating an efficacious intervention into a practical prevention program, (2) building capacity to promote dissemination and use, (3) pursuing strategies to support successful adoption and implementation, and (4) disseminating widely based on known properties of the delivery channels and the intervention users or intended recipients.

Translation Research Needs

Interventions that have been shown to be effective using randomized controlled trials often require additional work before they can be implemented in community or clinical settings.[24] Interventions may lack identified delivery channels, training materials, and user manuals; others require modifications in order to reach new audiences or gain acceptance in implementation settings. Research is needed on approaches that could accelerate the translation of efficacious interventions into effective programs. Some states have required agencies to select and implement evidence-based programs and practices for addressing child maltreatment, but there is limited evidence to guide decision-making about selection and implementation.[25] Public health and child welfare systems may be appropriate venues for disseminating evidence-based child maltreatment approaches. For example, Chaffin and Friedrich[5] noted that the large-scale nature of programmatic activities in child welfare systems may transcend multiple efforts at the level of individual agencies and thus have a broad impact on uptake. Questions that need to be addressed include:

— "Which interventions require minimal translation for effective implementation?"

— "How can a program best be translated so it can be effectively incorporated into the infrastructure and/or delivery system?"

— "What interagency collaborations and characteristics will ensure an adequate client base for program use and sustainability?"

Another important area is determining how to best match efficacious interventions with delivery systems and implementers. For many promising child maltreatment approaches, there is limited information on the monetary or other resources needed to adopt, implement, and sustain a program, or information may be limited to specific cost categories, such as the costs of training.[26,27] Techniques have been developed to examine costs associated with different implementation approaches and stages of implementation, which could potentially be adapted and applied to child maltreatment prevention implementation and sustainability research.[28] Research questions include:

— "What resources are needed for successful implementation and integration of an intervention?"

— "What resources or tools are needed to help practitioners incorporate child maltreatment prevention assessment and referral into their clinical practices?"

— "How does an agency determine the costs and benefits of adopting a particular approach?"

— "Are some implementation approaches more efficient or better suited to certain implementation sites than others?"

A key issue in moving from effective programs to widespread use is how to package child maltreatment prevention to maximize adoption and use by organizations and practitioners. Research should address the effectiveness of communication approaches, marketing strategies, and tailored messages to reach potential adopting organizations and audiences. One example of a media-based communication approach is the Triple P "Stay Positive" campaign, but limited empirical information is available on the effectiveness of this approach in encouraging uptake.[29] Additionally, flexibility in implementing evidence-based practices to meet the needs of families has been identified as an important aspect related to practitioner acceptability and implementation.[30,31] For example, Baumann and colleagues interviewed service providers working with families who had experienced physical abuse; practitioners who thought manuals were important were more likely to use them, but most practitioners were unfamiliar with treatment manuals.[32] In addition, practitioners may express concerns that manuals would result in a rigid approach that could not meet the unique needs of families.[18,32] Important questions include:

— "What program format is most appealing to organizations working with parents and at-risk families?"

— "How does one promote ownership and buy-in for using evidence-based practices with fidelity?"

— "How can child maltreatment prevention be incorporated into practice?"

— "What is needed to facilitate the dissemination and implementation of evidence-based programs?"

Future studies also should clarify the best methods for engaging parents and promoting change. Attendance at parenting programs may be stigmatizing due to perceptions that such attendance is an indicator that one is an incompetent or abusive parent, and ways to enhance enrollment, participation, and retention should be explored.[33] For example, Metzler and colleagues examined parents' preferred formats for receiving parenting information.[34] Although no statistical tests were reported to determine if preferences for different methods were significantly different, parents more often selected self-administered formats, such as television, online, or workbook approaches, than more intensive face-to-face approaches, such as group or individual sessions. However, because the parent sample was largely middle-class and recruited online, the extent to which the results may generalize to parents in other income groups or who may be less comfortable with technology is not clear.[34]

With respect to engaging parents in more traditional approaches to service delivery, Ingoldsby and colleagues compared training Nurse-Family Partnership home visiting nurses in motivational interviewing and use of a tailored delivery approach to the standard delivery format and reported better retention and visit completion in the tailored format.[35] Incorporating motivational approaches in other evidence-based parenting programs also has been explored and been effective at increasing retention in child welfare populations.[33,36] Communication campaigns that normalize attendance at evidence-based parenting programs (eg, "Stay Positive" campaign for Triple P) may be promising.[29] Research questions that need to be addressed include:

— "What messages will resonate with parents and families?"

— "What barriers may need to be overcome for parents to participate in parenting approaches?"

— "What approaches will encourage parents to talk about parenting with their health care provider?"

— "What are the most effective ways to encourage parents to engage in programs and change behaviors?"

Capacity Building Research Needs

Translated programs need an appropriate infrastructure or delivery system in order to be adopted and used effectively. For successful dissemination, it is important to develop institutional capacities to understand and use new innovations. Shera and Dill described the Practice and Research Together (PART) initiative in Ontario as facilitating the use of evidence-informed practice in child welfare practitioner agencies.[37] PART member agencies pay an annual fee for access to conferences, webinars, user-friendly literature reviews, and an electronic library. In addition, representatives from the member agencies work within their organizations to facilitate organizational change. After 3 years of implementation, however, the authors concluded the program had only a modest impact on changing practice behaviors, suggesting the need for additional research to address institutional capacity.[37] Collaborations may be important and even critical in implementing evidence-based practices on a broad scale by allowing shared financial and informational resources and ensuring a sufficient population base with which to implement programs.[38] Adopting organizations may need additional training or technical assistance in order to incorporate child maltreatment prevention programs into their ongoing services. Limited research has been conducted regarding organizational capacities and how best to increase them. In a survey of Triple P providers, integration of the program with other responsibilities and supervision and consultation was related to greater use of Triple P, although an organizational climate favorable to innovation was not associated with use.[22] Similarly, Bronson suggested that intangible aspects of organizational support, such as recognition for practitioners using evidence-based practice and incorporating evidence-based practice into regular supervision, were essential to implementation and sustainability.[18]

In addition, individuals must be trained on how to use new programs or strategies. McHugh and Barlow note the difference between didactic training, which frequently occurs in the context of workshops or other mechanisms for transferring information, and competence training, which involves ongoing supervision or training to ensure competence and support ongoing implementation with fidelity and sustainability over time.[39] A systematic review concluded that didactic training alone is insufficient to promote changes in practice.[40] Many evidence-based models that have been shown to be effective at preventing child maltreatment have national organizations or accredited trainers that provide training according to specified training protocols (eg, Nurse-Family Partnership, SafeCare, PCIT, Triple P). However, only a few studies have empirically examined different training approaches to determine which are most effective. In training PCIT providers, Funderburk and colleagues compared the effects of a phone consultation approach with a live video model that permitted mentored co-therapy as typically conducted in traditional PCIT training on implementation and family outcomes.[41] Small, but significant, advantages in observed rates of change of parent-reported child behavior problems were reported for the live video condition.[41] Similarly, in a state-wide randomized trial comparing SafeCare with services as usual, Chaffin et al examined the effects on child maltreatment outcomes of coaching or not coaching service providers during implementation.[15] Although there were limited effects for coaching overall, the results suggested coaching increased effectiveness with more challenging, multi-problem cases that are frequently observed in the field.

Ways to improve training are important considerations.[30] However, having sufficient cases with which to practice new skills appears to be necessary to gaining competence and encouraging use of an evidence-based program.[42] For example, Whitaker et al reported that even when practitioners demonstrated mastery of SafeCare during training and implemented the program model with fidelity in the field when they used the model, only 25% of practitioners actually used the model following training. Similarly, Nelson, Shanley, Funderburk, and Bard reported a positive association between the number of cases therapists had and the therapists' attendance at and favorable evaluations of consultation sessions.[43]

In addition, self-efficacy and feelings of competence appear to be important predictors of practitioners' implementation of evidence-based practices. Shapiro, Prinz, and Sanders reported self-efficacy at the completion of training predicted practitioners' initial use of Triple P.[21] However, over a 2-year post-training interval, confidence scores decreased and were no longer predictive of use within the last year.[22] Similarly, implementing the SafeCare program with coaching, compared to SafeCare without coaching or services as usual with and without coaching, resulted in less staff turnover even after controlling for other work-related attitudes, perceived job autonomy, and turnover intentions.[44,45] In contrast, staff in the SafeCare without coaching condition were 2.6 times more likely to turn over than staff in the other conditions.[44,45] Consistent with many studies in implementation science, these results suggest ongoing consultation and support may be important to ensure self-efficacy and satisfaction with implementing evidence-based approaches.[46] However, additional research is needed to determine the most effective and efficient ways to provide implementation support to child maltreatment practitioners.

Specifically, research is needed to determine the capacities required by individuals, organizations, and systems to deliver a child maltreatment prevention program effectively (ie, with fidelity to the core programmatic and implementation components). To facilitate institutional and individual capacity building, a systematic approach is needed to enable organizations and individuals to effectively use "best practices" and to provide the training and resources needed to succeed. Research is also needed to determine how organizational factors relate to actual adoption, implementation, and sustainability of practices in child maltreatment prevention settings and how to increase those characteristics of organizations most conducive to adoption and implementation of evidence-based practices. For example, organizational and leadership support has been identified as important in implementing evidence-based practices.[30] Positive organizational climate has been associated with more positive attitudes toward adopting evidence-based practice in mental health settings.[47] In this area, research questions include:

— "What resources are needed to implement a program, and how can such capacities be developed most efficiently?"

— "How much training, technical assistance, and monitoring is required for a particular health care sector or professional group to effectively implement a program?"

— "How sustainable are efforts to build capacity and retain trained staff?"

Adoption and Implementation Research Needs

Adoption and implementation research can help provide what the necessary determinants of adoption and implementation are before we disseminate. Research suggests that the adoption and use of innovations are explained by a variety of factors ranging from individual preferences to organizational practices. Klein and Sorra's model condensed these factors into 2 related sets of variables: (1) ***innovation fit***, which refers to the antecedents that capture the extent to which an innovation is likely to fit well with the current needs and preferences of an organization and (2) ***climate for implementation***, which refers to the organizational culture, administrative support, training, and other reinforcements for implementing that innovation in the organization.[48]

Child maltreatment research should investigate methods to maximize both the fit of effective programs as well as the climate for implementing them. For example, the fit between the program and agency mission, provider, and families served has been identified as important in child welfare service provider acceptance and implementation.[30] Such questions would include:

— "What can be done to increase the fit of programs into practice settings?"

— "How can we increase leadership support for incorporating effective child maltreatment prevention programs in sectors such as public health, health care, and child welfare?"

— "How can policies (or enabling legislation) that encourages widespread use of effective strategies best be facilitated?"

— "What factors influence the long-term sustainability of child maltreatment prevention programs in particular settings?"

Finally, research should address the balance between program fidelity (the degree to which a program is implemented as it was originally designed) and adaptation.[46,49] Fidelity to parenting interventions has been associated with greater completion rates, as well as improved outcomes.[50] Research questions include, "What are the core or critical components that must be included to maintain program effectiveness and what elements can be changed?" and "What factors encourage implementation with fidelity of the core components?"

An underlying issue related to fidelity and adaptation balance is the assumption that there is a need to adapt programs for different populations and settings, and research is needed to examine programs to ensure that adaptation is necessary. For example, Self-Brown et al surveyed practitioners providing SafeCare to diverse families to assess the need for cultural adaptations to the program.[51] Practitioners saw limited usefulness to systematically adapting the program for different ethnic groups but reported making some case-by-case enhancements in practice while retaining the content of the original program, such as including scenarios that may be relevant to a particular group. In addition, systematic adaptation was perceived as essentially limiting the program's reach.[51] In child maltreatment prevention and parenting outcomes, most adaptation research has focused on cultural adaptations or adaptations to meet the special needs of high-risk populations. Although a recent meta-analysis reported a moderate effect size favoring culturally adapted mental health treatments, evidence suggesting that adaptation of parenting programs for different cultural groups results in more effective interventions is currently lacking.[52,53] In addition, evidence-based programs are not necessarily perceived as culturally irrelevant by their intended audience. In a randomized controlled trial comparing SafeCare to services as usual, families participating in SafeCare attained more treatment goals and reported higher perceived provider cultural competence and higher satisfaction with the intervention.[54] American Indian clients receiving SafeCare, compared to American Indian clients in services as usual, reported greater decreases in depression and better working alliances with their service providers and rated their services as of higher quality, more beneficial, and more culturally competent.[55]

Even when adaptations are done with great care to ensure cultural relevance to the target population, there may be limited changes in effectiveness on the outcomes of interest for the adapted program compared with the unadapted program.[56,57] In child maltreatment populations, which are often complicated by numerous comorbid risk factors, such as depression, substance abuse, or intimate partner violence, enhancements to address these problems may result in no benefits or in relatively small, circumscribed benefits.[12,58,59]

When adaptation is necessary, an understanding of how to best adapt different programs is needed. Fixsen et al suggest that adaptation should not occur until implementation with high fidelity is established.[46] It is unclear, however, how this establishment of high fidelity implementation can be ascertained.[49] Adaptation may be undertaken due to organizational needs or may be provider- or consumer-driven, and the way adaptation is approached (ie, planned versus ad hoc or "drift") and the level at which adaptation is undertaken may result in greater fidelity to and less drift from the core components of models.[60] A number of models or approaches for planned adaptation currently exist. These models specify varying degrees of involvement and collaboration by developers, agencies and practitioners, and representatives of the populations with which the program will be used, but most emphasize adherence to the core components related to program effectiveness.[24,31,61,62]

Research is needed to determine which approaches yield the most useful information for effective adaptation as different sources of information and approaches may result in different conclusions. For example, Kohl gathered data to assess African American fathers' perceptions of Triple P (a program developed in Australia), which included exposing fathers to the Triple P materials through focus groups and through attending a pilot group of the entire intervention.[33] Prior to exposure to the materials, fathers did not see the need for a parenting intervention or the relevance to their lives; however, after exposure to the materials, the fathers saw the potential benefits and asked to participate in the program. Final adaptations were minimal and involved enhancements using additional examples relevant to the fathers' unique circumstances, including a motivational orientation session to reinforce the benefits of participating and providing more opportunities for fathers to interact with each other.[33] Such tailoring approaches, involving input from the target population and minimal adaptation, have been used with success in other parenting programs.[63]

Dissemination Research Needs

Once the determinants of adoption and implementation are known and a feasible delivery system is established, dissemination may be accelerated by involving early implementers and other champions of an evidence-based approach to improve uptake.[21]

Dissemination studies of community-based programs need to include assessments of reach, adoption, feasibility, fidelity, acceptability, and adaptability. Questions to address include:

— "What dissemination factors influence a community-based organization's ability to involve families in parenting programs?"

— "Is it feasible to take a community program developed for one setting and implement it in another?"

— "What are the costs of delivering various community programs and how can these costs be minimized?"

Currently, the evidence base for effective child maltreatment prevention involves direct program delivery by service providers to families. Alternate delivery systems, such as Internet or computer-based deliveries and television or video-based approaches (eg, Triple P's "Driving Mum and Dad Mad" television series) need to be evaluated for their effectiveness at child maltreatment prevention.[29] Sanders and colleagues reported online and workbook approaches for delivering Triple P produced comparable clinically significant improvements in parent-reported child behavior problems and dysfunctional parenting outcomes, with effect sizes similar to programs with similar delivery intensity.[64] Comparing alternative approaches to the existing evidence-based child maltreatment prevention programs or examining child maltreatment outcomes would provide information about the approaches' effectiveness for preventing child maltreatment. Additional research should also address the conditions under which these various dissemination strategies may be effective, for whom and for how long. Some of the research questions to answer include:

— "What are the best formats and channels for delivering interventions?"

— "How do these formats influence parent and family engagement?"

— "Do alternative delivery systems produce comparable child maltreatment outcomes?"

Conclusion

Child maltreatment remains a significant public health problem. Despite the progress research has made in describing this issue, identifying important risk factors, developing promising interventions, and promoting evidence-based programs, much work remains to be done before these programs are widely adopted and used effectively. Public health impact depends on large numbers of health care professionals, service providers, and families adopting the best child maltreatment prevention practices over time. By articulating the key activities embedded within Stage 4 of the public health model—translation, capacity building, adoption and implementation, and dissemination—we highlighted the critical research needs that, if addressed, can help close the gap between research and practice in child maltreatment prevention.

REFERENCES

1. US Department of Health and Human Services; Administration for Children and Families; Administration on Children, Youth and Families; Children's Bureau. *Child Maltreatment 2012.* Washington, DC: US Department of Health and Human Services; Administration for Children and Families; Administration on Children, Youth and Families; Children's Bureau; 2013. Administration for Children and Families Web site. http://www.acf.hhs.gov/programs/cb/research-data-technology/statistics-research/child-maltreatment. Accessed September 30, 2016.

2. Fang X, Brown DS, Florence C, Mercy J. The economic burden of child maltreatment in the United States and implications for prevention. *Child Abuse Negl.* 2012;36(2):156-165.

3. Hammond WR. Public health and child maltreatment prevention: The role of the Centers for Disease Control and Prevention. *Child Maltreat.* 2003;8(2):81-83.

4. Chambless DL, Hollon SD. Defining empirically supported treatments. *J Clin Consult Psychol.* 1998;66(1):7-18.

5. Chaffin M, Friedrich B. Evidence-based treatments in child abuse and neglect. *Child Youth Serv Rev.* 2004;26(11):1097-1113.

6. Chaffin M, Schmidt S. An evidence-based perspective on interventions to stop or prevent child abuse. In: Lutzker JR, ed. *Preventing Violence: Research and Evidence-based Intervention Strategies.* Washington, DC: American Psychological Association; 2006:49-68.

7. MacMillan HL, Wathen CN, Barlow J, Fergusson DM, Leventhal JM, Taussig HN. Interventions to prevent child maltreatment and associated impairment. *Lancet.* 2009;373:250-266.

8. Olds DL, Eckenrode J, Henderson CR Jr, et al. Long-term effects of home visitation on maternal life course and child abuse and neglect: fifteen-year follow-up of a randomized trial. *JAMA.* 1997;278(8):637-643.

9. Dias MS, Smith K, deGuehery K, Mazur P, Li V, Shaffer ML. Preventing abusive head trauma among infants and young children: a hospital-based parent education program. *Pediatrics.* 2005;115(4):e470-e477.

10. Dubowitz H, Feigelman S, Lane W, Kim J. Pediatric primary care to help prevent child maltreatment: the Safe Environment for Every Kid (SEEK) Model. *Pediatrics.* 2009;123(3):858-864.

11. Mersky JP, Topitzes JD, Reynolds AJ. Maltreatment prevention through early childhood intervention: a confirmatory evaluation of the Chicago Child-Parent Center preschool program. *Child Youth Serv Rev.* 2011;33(8):1454-1463.

12. Chaffin M, Silovsky J, Funderburk B, et al. Parent-child interaction therapy with physically abusive parents: efficacy for reducing future abuse reports. *J Consult Clin Psychol.* 2004;72(3):491-499.

13. Chaffin M, Funderburk B, Bard D, Valle LA, Gurwitch R. A combined motivation and Parent-Child Interaction Therapy package reduces child welfare recidivism in a randomized dismantling field trial. *J Consult Clin Psychol.* 2011;79(1):84-95.

14. Prinz RJ, Sanders MR, Shapiro CJ, Whitaker DJ, Lutzker JR. Population-based prevention of child maltreatment: the U.S. Triple P System population trial. *Prev Sci.* 2009;10(1):1-12.

15. Chaffin M, Hecht D, Bard D, Silovsky JF, Beasley WH. A statewide trial of the SafeCare home-based services model with parents in child protective services. *Pediatrics*. 2012;129(3):509-516.

16. Proctor E. Implementaton science and child maltreatment: methodological advances. *Child Maltreat*. 2012;17(1):107-112.

17. Self-Brown S, Whitaker D, Berliner L, Kolko D. Disseminating child maltreatment interventions: Research on implementing evidence-based programs. *Child Maltreat*. 2012;17(1):5-10.

18. Bronson DE. Evidence-based practice: identifying and removing barriers to implementation. *The APSAC Advisor*. 2006;18(1):2-6.

19. Buckley H, Tonmyr L, Lewig K, Jack S. Factors influencing the uptake of research evidence in child welfare: a synthesis of findings from Australia, Canada, and Ireland. *Child Abuse Rev*. 2014;23(1):5-16.

20. Hurlburt M, Aarons GA, Fettes D, Willging C, Gunderson L, Chaffin MJ. Interagency Collaborative Team Model for Capacity Building to Scale-Up Evidence-Based Practice. *Child Youth Serv Rev*. 2014;30:160-168.

21. Shapiro CJ, Prinz RJ, Sanders MR. Population-based provider engagement in delivery of evidence-based parenting interventions: challenges and solutions. *J Prim Prev*. 2010;31(4):223-234.

22. Shapiro CJ, Prinz RJ, Sanders MR. Facilitators and barriers to implementation of an evidence-based parenting intervention to prevent child maltreatment: The Triple P-Positive Parenting Program. *Child Maltreat*. 2012;17(1):86-95.

23. Thomas R, Zimmer-Gembeck MJ, Chaffin M. Practitioners' views and use of evidence-based treatment: Positive attitudes but missed opportunities in children's services. *Adm Policy Ment Health*. 2014;41(3):368-378.

24. Chen EK, Reid MC, Parker SJ, Pillemer K. Tailoring evidence-based interventions for new populations: A method for program adaptation through community engagement. *Eval Health Prof.* 2012;36(1):73-92.

25. Tseng V. The uses of research in policy and practice. *Soc Poly Rep*. 2012;26(2):1-19.

26. Goldhaber-Fiebert JD, Snowden LR, Wulczyn R, Landsverk J, Horwitz SM. Economic evaluation research in the context of child welfare policy: a structured literature review and recommendations. *Child Abuse Negl.* 2011;35(9):722-740.

27. Foster EM, Prinz RJ, Sanders MR, Shapiro CJ. The costs of a public health infrastructure for delivering parenting and family support. *Child Youth Serv Rev*. 2008;30:493-501.

28. Saldana L, Chamberlain P, Bradford WD, Campbell M, Landsverk J. The cost of implementing new strategies (COINS): a method for mapping implementation resources using the stages of implementation completion. *Child Youth Serv Rev*. 2014;39:177-182.

29. Sanders MR. Triple P: a population approach to parenting and family support. Paper presented at: Centers for Disease Control and Prevention; November, 2012; Atlanta, GA.

30. Aarons GA, Palinkas LA. Implementation of evidence-based practice in child welfare: service provider perspectives. *Adm Policy Ment Health*. 2007;34(4):411-419.

31. Mazzucchelli TG, Sanders MR. Facilitating practitioner flexibility within an empirically supported intervention: Lessons from a system of parenting support. *Clin Psychol Sci Pract.* 2010;17(3):238-252.

32. Bauman BL, Kolko DJ, Collins K, Herschell AD. Understanding practitioners' characteristics and perspectives prior to the dissemination of an evidence-based intervention. *Child Abuse Negl.* 2006;30(7):771-787.

33. Kohl PL. Engaging fathers in Triple P. Paper presented at: Society for Social Work and Research Conference; January, 2013; San Diego, CA.

34. Metzler CW, Sanders MR, Rusby JC, Crowley RN. Using consumer preference information to increase the reach and impact of media-based parenting interventions in a public health approach to parenting support. *Behav Ther.* 2012;43(2):257-270.

35. Ingoldsby EM, Baca P, McClatchey MW, et al. Quasi-experimental pilot study of intervention to increase participant retention and completed home visits in the Nurse-Family Partnership. *Prev Sci.* 2013;14(6):525-534.

36. Chaffin M, Valle LA, Funderburk B, et al. A motivational intervention can improve retention in PCIT for low-motivation child welfare clients. *Child Maltreat.* 2009;14(4):356-368.

37. Shera W, Dill K. Promoting evidence-informed practice in child welfare in Ontario: Progress, challenges, and future directions. *Res Soc Work Pract.* 2012;22(2):204-213.

38. Palinkas LA, Fuentes D, Finno M, Garcia AR, Holloway IW, Chamberlain P. Inter-organizational collaboration in the implementation of evidence-based practices among public agencies serving abused and neglected youth. *Adm Policy Ment Health.* 2014;41(1):74-85.

39. McHugh RK, Barlow DH. The dissemination and implementation of evidence-based psychological treatments. *Am Psychol.* 2010;65(2):73-84.

40. Oxman AD, Thompson MA, Davis DA, Haynes RB. No magic bullets: a systematic review of 102 trials of interventions to improve professional practice. *CMAJ.* 1995;153(10):1423-1431.

41. Funderburk B, Chaffin M, Bard E, Shanley J, Bard D, Berliner L. Comparing client outcomes for two evidence-based treatment consultation strategies. *J Clin Child Adolesc Psychol.* 2015;44(5):730-41.

42. Whitaker DJ, Ryan KA, Wild RC, Self-Brown S, Lutzker RJ, Shanley JR, Hodges AE. Initial implementation indicators from a statewide rollout of SafeCare within a child welfare systems. *Child Maltreat.* 2012;17(1):96-101.

43. Nelson MM, Shanley JR, Funderburk BW, Bard E. Therapists' attitudes toward evidence-based practices and implementation of Parent-Child Interaction Therapy. *Child Maltreat.* 2012;17(1):47-55.

44. Aarons GA, Fettes DL, Sommerfeld DH, Palinkas LA. Mixed methods for implementation research: Application to evidence-based practice implementation and staff turnover in community-based organizations providing child welfare services. *Child Maltreat.* 2012;17(1):67-79.

45. Aarons GQ, Sommerfeld DH, Hecht DB, Silovsky JF, Chaffin MJ. The impact of evidence-based practice implementation and fidelity monitoring on staff turnover: evidence for a protective effect. *J Consult Clin Psychol.* 2009;77(2):270-280.

46. Fixsen DL, Naoom SF, Blase KA, Friedman RM, Wallace F. *Implementation Research: A Synthesis of the Literature*. Tampa, FL: University of South Florida, Louis de la Parte Florida Mental Health Institute, The National Implementation Research Network; 2005.

47. Aarons GA, Sawitzky AC. Organizational culture and climate and mental health provider attitudes toward evidence-based practice. *Psychol Serv*. 2006;3(1):61-72.

48. Klein KJ, Sorra JS. The challenge of innovation implementation. *Acad Manage Rev*. 1996;21(4):1055-1080.

49. Saul J, Duffy J, Noonan R, et al. Bridging science and practice in violence prevention: Addressing ten key challenges. *Am J Community Psychol*. 2008;41(3-4):197-205.

50. Romney S. Triple P in San Francisco: implementation variation and outcomes. Paper presented at: Centers for Disease Control and Prevention; November, 2012; Atlanta, GA.

51. Self-Brown S, Frederick K, Binder S, Whitaker D, Lutzker J, Edwards A, Blankenship J. Examining the need for cultural adaptations to an evidence-based parent training program targeting the prevention of child maltreatment. *Children Youth Serv Rev*. 2011;(33):1166-1172.

52. Smith TB, Rodriquez MD, Bernal G. Culture. *J Clin Psychol*. 2011;67(2):166-175.

53. Lau AS. Making the case for selective and directed cultural adaptations of evidence-based treatments: Examples from parent training. *Clin Psychol Sci Pract*. 2006;13(4):295-310.

54. Damashek A, Bard D, Hecht D. Provider cultural competency, client satisfaction, and engagement in home-based programs to treat child abuse and neglect. *Child Maltreat*. 2012;17(1):56-66.

55. Chaffin M, Bard D, Bigfoot DS, Maher EJ. Is a structured, manualized, evidence-based treatment protocol culturally competent and equivalently effective among American Indian parents in Child Welfare? *Child Maltreat*. 2012;17(3):242-252.

56. McCabe K, Yeh M. Parent-child interaction therapy for Mexican Americans: a randomized clinical trial. *J Clin Child Adolesc Psychol*. 2009;38(5):753-759.

57. McCabe K, Yeh M, Lau A, Argote CB. Parent-child interaction therapy for Mexican Americans: results of a pilot randomized clinical trial at follow-up. *Behav Ther*. 2012;43(3):606-618.

58. Sanders MR, Pidgeon AM, Gravestock F, Connors MD, Brown S, Young RW. Does parental attributional retraining and anger management enhance the effects of the Triple P-Positive Parenting Program with parents at risk of child maltreatment? *Behav Ther*. 2004;35:513-535.

59. Silovsky JR, Bard D, Chaffin M, Hecht D, Burris L, Owora A, Lutzker J. Prevention of child maltreatment in high-risk rural families: A randomized clinical trial with child welfare outcomes. *Child Youth Serv Rev*. 2011;33:1435-1444.

60. Aarons GA, Miller EA, Green AE, Perrott JA, Bradway R. Adaptation happens: a qualitative case study of implementation of The Incredible Years evidence-based parent training programme in a residential substance abuse treatment programme. *J Child Serv*. 2012;7:233-244.

61. Aarons GA, Green AE, Palinkas LA, et al. Dynamic adaptation process to implement an evidence-based child maltreatment intervention. *Implement Sci.* 2012;7:32.

62. Lee SJ, Altschul I, Mowbray CT. Using planned adaptation to implement evidence-based programs with new populations. *Am J Community Psychol.* 2008;41(3-4):290-303.

63. McCabe KM, Yeh M, Garland AF, Lau AS, Chavez G. The GANA Program: a tailoring approach to adapting parent child interaction therapy for Mexican Americans. *Educ Treat Children.* 2005;28:111-129.

64. Sanders MR, Dittman CK, Farruggia SP, Keown LJ. A comparison of online versus workbook delivery of a self-help positive parenting program. *J Prim Prev.* 2014;35:125-133.

The findings and conclusions in this chapter are those of the authors and do not necessarily represent the official position of the Centers for Disease Control and Prevention.

Section III

Preventing Different Types of Abuse

Chapter 10

Promising Approaches for Preventing Child Neglect

Diane DePanfilis, PhD, MSW
Howard Dubowitz, MD, MS

Introduction

Child neglect is the type of child maltreatment most frequently reported to Child Protective Services (CPS) agencies and the most frequently identified type of maltreatment in national incidence studies.[1,2] Child neglect is also more likely than other forms of maltreatment to reoccur, and the consequences of neglect are equally damaging as, if not more damaging than, other forms of maltreatment.[3-9] Of the 1593 children estimated to have died due to maltreatment in 2012, 69.9% suffered neglect either exclusively or in combination with other types of maltreatment.[2]

Given the extent and effects of child neglect, one might assume that the attention to the problem would be commensurate to the serious nature and extent of the problem; however, most experts would agree that this is not the case. Despite the fact that the field has been calling attention to the "neglect of neglect" for over 2 decades, the field continues to spend less attention on understanding what interventions may be most effective to prevent it, compared to physical and sexual abuse.[10-13] The purpose of this chapter is to briefly define the neglect of children, consider a conceptual framework for designing and implementing preventive interventions designed to reduce risk factors for neglect, and to review programs and practices that may have promise for preventing the neglect of children.

Defining Child Neglect

Child neglect is usually defined as omissions in care resulting in significant harm or the risk of significant harm.[14] The uniform definition of neglect suggests that child neglect is failure to provide for a child's basic physical, emotional, or educational needs or failure to protect a child from harm or potential harm.[15] Neglect by omission relates to failure to provide physical neglect, emotional neglect, medical/dental neglect, and educational neglect and failure to supervise related to inadequate supervision and exposure to violent environments.

Despite having evolved to a uniform definition, historically there has been debate about whether neglect should be defined based on measurable harm to a child or the actions or omissions of caregivers regardless of whether a child is harmed.[16,17] A second conceptual debate centers on whether neglect should be viewed as occurring when a child's basic needs (eg, adequate food, shelter, protection/supervision, clothing, health care) are not met or whether neglect should be viewed as occurring based on the conventional focus on parental omissions in care.[18,19]

From a prevention perspective, it is important to arrive at a definition to clarify a conceptual understanding of child neglect and in order to tailor preventive interventions for child neglect. For the purposes of this chapter, we choose to use the broader definition assuming that child neglect occurs when a child's basic needs go unmet.[18] Most preventive interventions are focused on the role of parents or other caregivers to meet those basic needs; thus, this uniform definition is appropriately matched to the preventive interventions included in this chapter. Fewer focus on the inattention to children's basic needs that may be related to broader societal conditions such as poverty. Further complicating this picture is that there are many ways in which a child's basic needs may be unmet. For example, lack of supervision, inadequate food and nutrition, and the lack of adequate health care are different experiences for children. And because many forms of child neglect occur at the same time, developing interventions to prevent it must clearly focus on these differences and clarify exactly which behaviors and conditions the preventive intervention is designed to address. While it is beyond the scope of this chapter to tease out these differences, this chapter will address promising preventive interventions that purport to prevent all forms of neglect.

Consequences of Child Neglect

Because of the heterogeneity of neglect (ie, because the consequences of a single instance of neglect is different than chronic inattention), preventive interventions need not only to focus on preventing child neglect but also on the consequences of neglectful conditions if they are apparent in children at the time of identification and assessment. And because the consequences of neglect will vary, understanding these differences influences the conceptual framework for prevention in families with children of different ages.[8]

A review of the research on the effects of child neglect on children has confirmed that child neglect can have severe, deleterious short- and long-term effects on children's cognitive, socioemotional, and behavioral development.[8] Moreover, this same review suggests that relative to physically abused children, neglected children have more severe cognitive and academic deficits, social withdrawal and problematic peer interactions, and internalizing (as opposed to externalizing) problems.

In what ways does neglect affect children over time? The effect of neglect on children appears to be impacted by a combination of factors, including the age of the child, type and severity of neglect, whether neglect has occurred in combination with other types of maltreatment, and related risks that may impact specific families in their environments.[20] As children age, research indicates that children who experience parental neglect, with or without parental alcohol or drug abuse, are at high risk for substance use disorder.[21]

Overview of Conceptual Framework

It is generally recognized that a prevention science framework works best to guide the development, implementation, and testing of preventive interventions. Prevention science is built on the premise that there are precursors to health and social problems, and thus, the goals of prevention science are to decrease risk factors (ie, precursors to child neglect) and increase protective factors (ie, by utilizing strengths, developing resources).[22-26] This framework is consistent with a public health approach and an ecological-developmental model.[27,28] Consistent with a public health model, child neglect preventive interventions may be classified at 3 levels: (1) universal strategies designed for entire populations (eg, an entire community) and not based on individual risks, (2) selective strategies designed for families with significant risk factors commonly associated with child neglect (eg, poverty, multiple children, parental alcohol or drug problems), and (3) indicated strategies targeting families with children who have already experienced neglect.[29] Indicated strategies are synonymous to treatment, aimed at preventing continued neglect as well as its negative outcomes. However, most preventive interventions do not fit perfectly into only one category, as the same intervention (eg, a parent group) may serve different levels of risk.

Prevention Programs

This chapter describes 8 prevention programs, all of which have demonstrated some evidence for preventing neglect, reducing risk factors associated with neglect, and/or promoting protective factors that may reduce the likelihood of neglect: Family Connections (FC), Healthy Families America (HFA), The Incredible Years (TIY), Nurse-Family Partnership (NFP), Nurturing Parenting Program (NPP), Safe Environment for Every Kid (SEEK), SafeCare (SC), and Triple P – Positive Parenting Program (TP). Each preventive intervention is briefly described, followed by a summary of the conceptual/theoretical basis, goals, program services, and a synthesis of research evaluating the program.

Family Connections

Family Connections (FC), originally developed in Baltimore through a federal demonstration project, is a multifaceted community-based program that works with families in their homes, in the context of their neighborhoods, to help them meet the basic needs of their children and prevent child neglect.[30] FC has been formally replicated in 8 sites through federal funding and in additional sites through a combination of federal, state, foundation, and local funding. Families with children age newborn to 18 years may be enrolled for services if they meet eligibility criteria (ie, risk factors related to child neglect) and are provided services for 3, 6, 9, or 12 months, depending on the target population. FC has been implemented as a selective strategy (ie, targeting families identified with significant risk but not involved with child protective services) and as an indicated strategy for families reported for maltreatment, determined to be safe from immediate harm, but assessed to be at risk for child neglect or physical abuse.

Goals

The goals of FC are geared to increase protective factors (eg, parenting attitudes, parenting skills, parenting competence, family functioning, social support), to decrease risk factors (eg, parental depressive symptoms and substance abuse, every day stress, parenting stress), and ultimately, to increase the safety (prevention of child neglect) and well-being of children.

Conceptual/Theoretical Basis

FC operates from an ecological developmental framework that views neglect within a system of risk and protective factors interacting across 4 levels: (1) the individual or ontogenic level, (2) the family microsystems, (3) the exosystem, and (4) the social macro system.[31] Developed primarily to prevent child neglect, the program conceptualizes the problem evolving when risk factors related to the child, caregivers, family system, and the environment challenge the capacity of caregivers and broader systems to meet the basic needs of children. This view was first formulated in Bronfenbrenner's theory of social ecology.[27] FC was designed based on a prevention science framework and uses 10 practice principles to guide FC interventions: community outreach, individualized family assessment, tailored interventions, helping alliance, empowerment approaches, strengths perspective, cultural competence, developmental appropriateness, outcome-driven service plans, and competence of the helping professional.[32]

Program Description

FC uses a home-based, family centered model of practice consistent with other home-based approaches.[33,34] Individualized intervention targeting families with children at all ages, outlined in an intervention manual, is designed to increase protective factors (ie, social support) and decrease risk factors (eg, parental depressive symptoms) associated with maltreatment. The core components of FC include (1) intake and screening for eligibility, (2) outreach and engagement, (3) concrete and/or emergency assistance, (4) comprehensive family assessment with the use of standardized assessment instruments, (5) outcome-driven family plans with SMART goals, (6) change-focused intervention including direct in-home counseling as well as facilitation of targeted service referrals provided by community agencies when indicated, (7) progress assessment at least every 90 days (ie, to measure change with the standardized assessment instruments and achievement of SMART goals and outcomes), and (8) case closure.

The original FC program and some replicating sites also supplement the core intervention with multi-family supportive and recreational activities. FC uses screening criteria as clear inclusion criteria for targeting and screening program clients. FC initiates the therapeutic relationship through prompt face-to-face contact with the family.[35] An FC worker (usually a BSW or MSW trained social worker) is assigned to work with the qualified family and provides weekly individual and group supervision. Workers deliver tailored and direct therapeutic services to help families reduce risks, maximize protective factors, and achieve service outcomes and goals. Workers provide at least one hour of face-to-face services to families at least once per week for at least 3 months following the comprehensive assessment period (30 days).

Evaluations

FC has been recognized by the Children's Bureau as an effective program for preventing neglect and by the California Evidence-Based Clearinghouse for Child Welfare as a program with promising research evidence and high relevance to child welfare in 2 categories: child neglect and prevention.[36]

FC was developed in 1996 through a demonstration project supported by the Children's Bureau. Families were randomly assigned to receive shorter versus longer services. Findings from the initial study indicated positive change over time in risk factors (eg, parental depressive symptoms, life stress, parenting stress), protective factors (eg, parenting attitudes, parenting competence, social support), child safety (ie, physical and psychological care of children), and child behavior problems (eg, internalizing, externalizing) between the beginning, end, and 6 months after a case closure follow-up period for families served for 3 and 9 months.[30,37]

A separate study of cost effectiveness determined that the 3-month intervention was more cost effective than the 9-month intervention in relation to positive changes in risk and protective factors and child safety.[38] However, cost effectiveness analysis indicated that the 9-month intervention was more cost effective (CE ration=$276) than the 3-month intervention (CE ratio=$337) in relation to improvements in the child's behavior between baseline and 6 months after service closure. Results from a cross-site evaluation by James Bell Associates (JBA) of 8 programs replicating FC found similar positive changes in risk and protective factors and demonstrated consistent and significant improvement from baseline to post-test and follow-up for 9 out of 11 outcomes.[39-43] Interestingly, analysis also suggests that families served by workers who implement FC with greater fidelity also achieve greater improvement in family and child level outcomes. Agencies replicating FC have collected cost data using a standard template and cost analysis illustrated significant differences in costs per unit family between programs replicating FC in different formats with different target populations.[41,44,45] Evidence from qualitative research indicate that FC is easily adapted to cultural groups, is successful in engaging families to increase safety for their children, and that caregivers report the benefit of the program for building support and services, skill building, and helping to improve affect and behavior.[46-48]

Conclusions

FC has demonstrated success for reducing risk factors, enhancing protective factors, and increasing child safety and child behavioral outcomes in the original demonstration as well as in a cross-site evaluation of programs replicating FC with varied target populations. Further evaluations should examine variations in program fidelity for programs replicating FC and evaluate the degree to which these promising results will be achieved by other programs replicating this intervention.

Healthy Families America

Healthy Families America (HFA), a home visitation model based on the Healthy Start Program (HSP) developed in Hawaii, was designed to work with overburdened families who are at risk for child abuse and neglect and other adverse childhood experiences. HFA exists in over 440 communities across the United States and Canada. It is designed to enroll families during pregnancy or immediately after birth and provides services for 3 to 5 years after enrollment. Thus, Healthy Families America is an example of a universal preventive program.

Goals

HFA aims to promote positive parenting, enhance child health and development, and prevent child maltreatment. These goals are to be achieved via a variety of approaches, including crisis intervention, parental support and education to enhance their skills, and identifying a medical home for the baby (ie, a consistent setting for providing comprehensive health care).[50] HFA program goals include: (1) to systematically reach out to parents to offer resources and support; (2) to cultivate the growth of nurturing, responsive, parent-child relationships; (3) to promote healthy childhood growth and development; and (4) to build the foundations for strong family functioning.

Conceptual/Theoretical Basis

HFA operatives from a set of core philosophical principles for program development and implementation: emphasis on infant mental health, strength-based practice, family-centered intervention, culturally sensitive services, use of a nurturing parallel process between the home visitor and family members, and use of a reflective continuous process that involves attention to all relationships, including the relationships between the infant and the parent, the parent and the home visitor, and the home visitor and the supervisor.[49]

Program Description

Mothers eligible for home visitation are assessed by staff prenatally or shortly after the birth of their baby using Kempe's Family Stress Checklist to identify those most in need of services and considered to be at risk for child maltreatment.[51] The screen includes risk factors such as substance abuse, intimate partner violence, being a single parent, social isolation, and low income. HFA programs aim to provide families with weekly home visits for the first 6 to 9 months of the child's life; subsequently, the frequency is determined by family functioning and needs. Services are continued for 3 to 5 years after the child's birth.

The staff of paraprofessionals receives basic training to identify and address risk factors that impair family functioning and contribute to child maltreatment. They provide parenting education, link families to a medical professional, and try to promote positive parenting by focusing on strengths and building trust as well as linking families to community resources. There is ongoing supervision by professional staff (eg, nurses, social workers) to enhance the home visitors' services and help prevent burnout.

Evaluations

While there have been at least 35 evaluations of HFA programs, a review by Harding et al is useful to synthesize findings across studies.[50] This review focuses on the 4 rigorous randomized controlled trials conducted in Hawaii, New York, San Diego, and Alaska. Results from all 4 have indicated no program effects concerning childhood injuries or other objective measures of maltreatment, although some outcomes such as those pertaining to parenting are promising.

Compared to controls, Healthy Families New York (HFNY) parents reported one-quarter as many seriously abusive acts when the children were aged 2 years.[52] Findings were especially encouraging in 2 subgroups. Young, first-time mothers who joined the program when 30 weeks pregnant reported less minor physical aggression in the past year than did controls (51% versus 70%). Among women who were "psychologically vulnerable," HFNY mothers were one-quarter as likely to report engaging in serious abuse and neglect as did control mothers (5% versus 19%) at age 2. The term, "psychologically vulnerable" in this study was a measure of mothers with depressive symptoms and low coping resources. A follow-up study found that HFNY effectively increased positive parenting, such as maternal responsivity and cognitive engagement.[53] In addition, young HFNY, first-time mothers who were recruited during pregnancy were less likely than controls to use harsh parenting.

Healthy Families Alaska (HFAK) mothers reported less use of milder physical and psychological discipline; severe forms of discipline did not differ.[54] HFAK also found improved home environments for children to learn, less parental stress, and children's improved cognitive development and behavior at age 2. These outcomes were attributed partially to the program improving maternal self-efficacy and the learning environment in the home. The follow-up of HFAK found a 42% decrease in referrals for physical abuse among program participants, but a similar decline occurred among comparison families.[55] HFAK did not improve children's health, maternal life course and household functioning, or psychosocial problems, such as maternal depression and partner violence.

In the evaluation of the Hawaiian Healthy Start Program (HSP), there were no effects regarding most measures of maltreatment including substantiated CPS reports.[56] HSP mothers, however, reported less frequent corporal and verbal punishment as well as less neglectful behavior. Of note, home visitors seldom observed or identified maltreatment. Of note, HSP did appear to reduce rates of intimate partner violence during participation in the program; HSP mothers reported lower rates of victimization as well as perpetration.[57] During follow-up, rates of IPV victimization and perpetration decreased, with insignificant intergroup differences.

A randomized control trial (RCT) of an HFA program in San Diego found favorable effect of the intervention on mental development and child behavior but no effect on other measured outcomes. Although the program was well implemented, Landsverk and colleagues did not find significant impact on child maltreatment, intimate partner violence, substance abuse, or maternal mental health.[58]

Most recently, an evaluation of Healthy Families Florida (HFF) has yielded encouraging findings.[59] HFF followed the HFA model as a voluntary long-term home visiting program serving families assessed as high-risk for child abuse and neglect. Home visiting services began prenatally or within 3 months after the birth of a baby or target child and lasted from 3 to 5 years, depending on the needs of the family, with the intensity and frequency of services decreasing over time. Home visiting services were delivered by trained paraprofessionals.

The evaluation employed a post-test-only, quasi-experimental design with multiple treatment and comparison groups. Instead of the more rigorous "intention to treat" approach, the researchers evaluated those who completed the program to those who had not been recruited. They also compared those with high and low fidelity (eg, participation less than 3 months) to the program. In general, greater participation in HFF was associated with fewer maltreatment reports (effect sizes ranging from -0.22 to -0.85). Findings remained significant after controlling for potential confounding.

Conclusions

There have been a mix of findings from evaluations of HFA, some that may be interpreted as favorable related to some outcomes with other studies indicating no effect related to the same outcomes. Those from New York and Florida are most promising. The variability in findings is not that surprising given the variation across programs, populations served, and research methodologies. Such differences make it difficult to compare programs. Researchers have offered various explanations for the inconsistent effectiveness of some HFA programs. One is that the programs were not well implemented. For example, in Hawaii, workers may have been overly enthused with a strengths-based approach, while not attending to substantial problems such as substance abuse. In addition, they were unable to involve fathers, and they were not successful in linking families to community resources. Inadequate training and supervision were thought to be responsible.[56] Another issue is that the benefits may be primarily in specific high risk groups, as was found in New York. Targeting such groups seems important for future efforts. There have also been problems in implementing the model. For example, in HFAK, 38% of families active at one year had no individual family service plans. While most visits included content on child development and parent-child interaction, developmental screens were completed for about only half the children whose families were active in HFAK.[54] Only half the families had any visits that included discussion of health services.

Attrition from some HFA programs has been another major problem. In the Alaskan study, services were intended for 3 to 5 years, but the highest site-specific retention rate was 46% at 2 years. Addressing this is critical to improving engagement in the program. The relatively low base rate of identified and reported abuse and neglect—even in high-risk populations—presents a formidable challenge to programs and researchers: large samples are needed to show a statistically significant difference. Home visitors, privy to what is happening in the home, may need to report maltreatment, resulting in higher rates due to surveillance bias. A new generation of innovative HFA programs, built on lessons learned, is being evaluated, which will hopefully find greater effectiveness.

The Incredible Years

The Incredible Years (TIY) is a parenting and child behavior management skills training program with curricula for parents, teachers, and children. TIY has been delivered as treatment for child behavior disorders as well as a school-based behavior problem prevention program for high-risk populations. It offers an example of a well-evaluated parenting program, and while the TIY is concerned with parenting behaviors and discipline, it has not specifically focused on child maltreatment. It was selected for inclusion in this chapter because even though the program was not specifically designed to prevent child neglect, the focus on promotion of positive parent and teacher interactions and relationships with children as well as promotion of children's emotional literacy and self-regulation, social competence and problem solving skills, and reduction of behavior problems suggest it would be relevant for families who struggle to meet the basic needs of their children. Since it has been used in both prevention and clinic populations, it may be appropriate as a universal or selective child neglect prevention program.

Goals

The primary goal of TIY is to support parents and enhance their skills in managing difficult child behaviors.

Program Description

The program is delivered in 12 weekly 2-hour group sessions with a trained facilitator leading discussions about parenting and child behavior management. Materials include video vignettes that cover a range of parenting challenges, such as use of praise and rewards, effective limit setting, handling noncompliance, and problem solving, and they feature real parents modeling effective parenting techniques. Group discussions follow the viewing of vignettes and role playing to build skills is encouraged. Parents are given weekly homework assignments to generalize and apply new skills.[60,61] It has been provided to parents with children at various ages (eg, day care, elementary school).

The intervention teaches positive discipline strategies, effective parenting skills, strategies for coping with stress, and ways to strengthen children's social skills. The group leaders' discussion with parents encourages problem-solving and self-management.

Evaluations

Several randomized controlled trials have shown TIY to be effective for child behavior problems and parenting outcomes, outside of a child welfare context. TIY has been found to reduce harsh, critical, and ineffective parenting and to increase supportive, consistent, and positive parenting in samples of mothers in Head Start.[61,62] A trial of the program in low-income urban communities found that the parents demonstrated higher self-efficacy (ES = .40), less coercive discipline (ES = .42 at baseline, ES = .34 at 1 year follow-up), and more positive parenting (ES = .30) than controls.[60] In a child welfare context, TIY has been evaluated in one RCT with biological and foster parents, compared to "usual" services. Parents randomized to TIY showed greater improvement in areas of positive parenting with 3-month follow-up effect sizes as high as .59.[63]

Conclusions

There is considerable evidence supporting TIY for improving and preventing child behavior problems. Trials have included high risk samples. To date, maltreatment outcomes have not been directly measured in a TIY trial, but other outcomes pertaining to disciplinary approaches may be related to physical and psychological abuse. TIY offers a group delivery format, videotaped vignettes for modeling parenting skills, an established training and dissemination infrastructure, and materials in multiple languages.

Nurse-Family Partnership (NFP)

The NFP program was started in Elmira, New York in 1977 as a randomized, controlled trial of home intervention by nurses for low-income, mostly white, first-time mothers. NFP is a maternal and early childhood health program that aims to foster long term success for first-time mothers and their babies. It's an example of a selected intervention, focused on a subgroup considered at risk for maltreatment.

Goals

NFP's goals are to: (1) improve outcomes of pregnancy, (2) improve children's health and development, including preventing maltreatment, and (3) improve families' economic self-sufficiency. Another goal has been to help mothers to space subsequent births and diminish the stress of caring for multiple young children.

Conceptual/Theoretical Basis

It was thought that optimizing fetal development by, for example, limiting exposure to alcohol, would lead to babies being easier to parent.[64] Enabling parents to provide responsive care should enhance children's development. Women pregnant for the first time are thought to offer "a window of opportunity" for engaging them in supportive services. Nurses are selected for intervention based on their ability to address health issues during pregnancy and of the infant. It is also felt that nurses have greater credibility with parents than paraprofessionals.

Program Description

NFP has aimed to recruit first time pregnant, low-income women, many of whom were unmarried and adolescents. Home visits were offered every 2 weeks, although there was flexibility to tailor these to women's needs. NFP is a universal preventive intervention.

Evaluations

The first study in Elmira, New York included 400 women who were randomized into one of 4 treatment groups.[65] One group received the nurse visits during pregnancy, until the child was aged 2 years, as well as referrals for health and developmental services. One group, serving as controls, received standard health care as well as transportation for routine prenatal care, infant developmental screening, and referrals for evaluation and treatment. Two groups received intermediate levels of home visiting support. The second study conducted in Memphis used a similar approach but with primarily African American women.[66] The third study was conducted in Denver and included many Latinos and a group that received services from paraprofessionals rather than nurses.[67]

In the first study, low-income, unmarried teenage mothers had fewer reports for maltreatment than did controls during the first 2 years (1 (4%) versus 8 (19%), although this was not statistically significant).[68] There was also a 32% reduction in emergency department visits, partly due to fewer injuries and ingestions. This finding continued during the 2 years after the program ended; however, the rate of maltreatment was still not significant in the ensuing 2 years. Other related findings were encouraging: fewer women smoked during pregnancy, mothers identified more social support, nurse-visited smokers had 75% fewer preterm babies and very young adolescents had higher birth weight babies than did controls. In the first 4 years of the child's life, the nurse-visited group demonstrated less punishment, more appropriate play, and provided safer and more nurturing home environments. Child development outcomes were improved. Finally, nurse-visited mothers had fewer subsequent pregnancies, longer delays until subsequent births, and were more likely to be employed.[65]

In a 15-year follow-up, nurse-visited participants had an average of 0.29 substantiated reports for maltreatment; the control group had 0.54.[69] This was especially evident among those who at the outset were unmarried and poor. This difference was not evident if intimate partner violence was also a problem.

In Memphis, the overall low rate of child maltreatment (3% to 4%) precluded examining this as an outcome. During the children's first 2 years, nurse-visited children had 23% fewer health care encounters for injuries and ingestions than controls.[66] This was especially evident in children of "psychologically vulnerable" mothers. By age 9, there was a trend with more children in the control group having died.[70] Of the 10 deaths among controls, 3 related to prematurity, 3 to sudden infant death syndrome, and 3 were due to injuries. One death was related to congenital anomalies. The one death in the nurse-visited group was due to a chromosomal problem.

In Denver, the low rate of CPS reports precluded using this as an outcome.[67] Lacking access to health data, the researchers could not examine injuries and ingestions. Nurse-visited children and mothers interacted more positively and the children had better language and mental development in the first few years; this was again most evident among children of psychologically vulnerable mothers. Nurse-visited mothers were less likely to have subsequent births, had longer delays until subsequent births, and experienced less intimate partner violence compared to controls. Of note, those served by paraprofessionals had effects roughly half the size of those visited by nurses. During the subsequent follow-up period, more benefits to families served by paraprofessionals became apparent, such as mothers and children showing greater sensitivity to each other.[71]

A Canadian study examined whether nurse home visitation (similar to the Nurse-Family Partnership program) could reduce recurrent physical abuse and neglect among preteens identified as having been abused or neglected within the prior 3 months and living with their biological family.[72] Those randomized to the intervention group received home visits for 2 years, beginning weekly and tapering to monthly during the second year. The goals were (1) to meet families' needs and reduce stress, (2) educate parents about child development, and (3) connect families to community health and social services. "Standard care" involved routine follow-up by caseworkers, parent education, and referrals for further parent education. After 3 years, there were no differences between the groups in CPS reports, and the intervention group had higher rates of maltreatment documented in hospital records.

Conclusions

Nurse home visitation appears promising, although the findings in terms of preventing child maltreatment are more mixed than commonly recognized.[73] Of note, the main findings in the Elmira study pertained to the highest risk group of low income, single, teenage first-time mothers receiving the most comprehensive and extensive version of the intervention.

Nurturing Parenting Programs

The Nurturing Parenting Programs (NPP) are family-based programs used for the prevention and treatment of child abuse and neglect. Programs are intended to target: emotional abuse, exposure to domestic violence, physical abuse, and physical neglect. NPP has been used as selective and indicated preventive intervention.

Goals

The goals of the curriculum are to (1) teach age-appropriate expectations and neurological development of children; (2) develop empathy and self-worth in parents and children; (3) utilize nurturing, nonviolent strategies and techniques in establishing family discipline; (4) empower parents and children to utilize their personal power to make healthy choices; and (5) to increase awareness of self and others in developing positive patterns of communication while establishing healthy, caring relationships.

Conceptual/Theoretical Basis

Underpinning the NPP is the belief that human behavior is multidimensional and that the positive and negative impact of life's past events shape our cognitive and emotional responses to current events.[74] As a result of this basic principle, Nurturing Parenting Programs employ psychoeducational and cognitive-behavioral approaches to learning. The program embraces the theory of re-parenting. By helping parents become more self-aware of their personal histories, the focus is on teaching parents to learn new skills and helping families learn new and healthier ways to live together.

Program Description

Nurturing Parenting Programs are designed for the prevention and treatment of child abuse and neglect. Programs are offered in home-based, group-based, and combination home-based/group-based models. There are different programs that are designed to meet the varied needs of families. Program length and number of sessions (dose) vary according to individual programs:

1. Nurturing Program Prenatal Families: Nine group-based sessions, each session lasting 2.5 hours. Can also be offered as in-home sessions.
2. Nurturing Program for Parents and their Infants, Toddlers and Preschoolers: Group-based program contains 24 sessions, each lasting 2.5 hours. Home-base program contains 48 sessions, each 90 minutes in length.
3. Nurturing Program for Parents and School-Aged Children: Fifteen group-based sessions, each lasting 2.5 hours.
4. Nurturing Program for Parents and Adolescents: Twelve group-based sessions, each lasting 3 hours.
5. Nurturing Program for Teen Parents: Twenty-six group-based sessions, each lasting 2.5 hours. Home-based program contains 49 sessions, each lasting 1.5 hours.
6. Nurturing Skills Programs: Programs have variable session lengths, based on the assessed needs of the family. Intervention programs are generally 12 to 16 sessions in length and can be offered in home settings, group settings, and combination home/group settings.
7. ABC's School-Based Program: Nine sessions in length, each session lasting 2.5 hours. This program is designed for parents and kindergarten-aged children preparing for school entry.
8. Cultural Programs include group- and home-based programs for Hispanic families, Hmong families, Haitian families, Arabic families, and a supplemental instructional booklet for African American families.
9. Additional programs for families in substance abuse recovery/special needs families, parents, and children with health challenges.
10. Community-Based Education Program: Ten 90-minute sessions. Unlike in the treatment programs, families in the community-based programs can attend any of the 10 classes, which are typically offered in community settings such as a library, school, hospital, or church.

Evaluations

Since the original validation in 1983 of the first Nurturing Program funded by the National Institute of Mental Health (NIMH), 23 additional field-based research studies have been conducted over the past 25 years. No studies have included random assignment to treatment and control groups. Study designs have included traditional pre-posttests (without follow-up), pre-posttests with longitudinal follow-up, and comparison studies that compare outcomes of families completing NPP versus families completing other programs. Most evaluations of the NPP have used the Adult Adolescent Parenting Inventory (AAPI) to measure change over time in 5 dimensions of parenting: (1) inappropriate developmental expectations of children, (2) lack of empathy toward children's needs, (3) strong belief in the value and use of physical punishment, (4) parents reversing family roles expecting children to take on adult responsibilities, and (5) oppressing parenting behavior that limits/reduces children's power and independence.[75]

The initial study funded by NIMH offered some support for the original NPP designed as a 15-week classroom-based model. A pre-post design suggested changes over time in self-reported parenting attitudes and practices. In addition, only 7% of program participants were known by Child Protective Services (CPS) to have future reports of child abuse or neglect within 2 years following intervention.[76]

Most evaluations of the NPP have not been published. Two studies that were published are selected to represent the range of evaluations that have been conducted on the efficacy of this program. In one study, 154 primarily white parents in Iowa demonstrated statistically significant improvements in 4 dimensions of parenting over time: inappropriate expectations, low empathy, strong belief in the value of punishment, and role reversal.[77] In another study, 323 ethnically diverse parents in New Mexico demonstrated improvements in the following domains: inappropriate expectations, empathy, belief in corporal punishment, and role reversal.[78]

Conclusions

Nurturing parenting programs have been classified in the promising research evidence category, as defined by the California Evidence-Based Clearinghouse for Child Welfare. The particular focus of the program on building empathy in high-risk parents makes the program relevant to families at risk of neglect. The varied program formats makes it possible to select the program type that best matches the particular risks identified in families.

A Safe Environment for Every Kid (SEEK)

SEEK is a model of enhanced pediatric primary care that includes a systematic approach to identifying and addressing major psychosocial risk factors that have been associated with child maltreatment: maternal depression, substance abuse, major stress, and intimate partner violence.[79]

Goals

By helping address risk factors for child maltreatment, SEEK aims to strengthen families; support parents; enhance children's health, development, and safety; and prevent child maltreatment. SEEK has 2 levels of intervention both universal and selective, with different interventions based on the target of the intervention component.

Conceptual/Theoretical Basis

It is thought that certain problems impair parents' abilities to adequately protect and nurture their children, contributing to abuse and neglect. Pediatric primary care usually involves a trusting relationship with a health professional. Routine checkups, especially in the first few years of a child's life, are rather frequent and include concerns with parents and the child's critical home environment, thus providing an excellent opportunity to help address prevalent problems.

Program Description

The SEEK model begins with training child health care professionals to briefly assess and initially manage the targeted psychosocial problems. Parents bringing in preschoolers for checkups are given the parent screening questionnaire (PSQ) to complete while waiting for their appointment. The PSQ has a brief introduction that strikes an empathic tone, conveying a concern that all children be in a safe, healthy environment. The screening questions have been tested to briefly identify families with possible problems (eg, substance abuse).[80-83] Parents then give the PSQ to their child's health professional at the start of the visit.

Health professionals, trained to briefly assess and initially manage identified problems, can choose to do so alone with the parent(s), or they may involve the SEEK social worker. The social worker may not be present on site, but is available by phone to both health professionals and parents. Health professionals and/or the social worker help facilitate necessary referrals to community agencies for evaluation and possible intervention. SEEK includes parent handouts for the targeted problems; these are user-friendly and customized to each local area.

Evaluations

The first randomized controlled trial was conducted in a university-based primary care clinic for pediatric trainees. Two days of the week were randomized to SEEK and 2 to controls. Controls received standard pediatric care. Five hundred and fifty-eight parents, mostly mothers, were recruited for the evaluation. Child maltreatment was assessed in 3 ways[79]:

— Parents self-reported less use of severe physical punishment than did controls.

— Review of the children's medical records approximately 2 years after SEEK had been implemented revealed fewer instances of nonadherence (or noncompliance) to medical care and delays in immunizations.

— There were fewer CPS reports in the SEEK families over the 2 years compared to controls (12% versus 19%).

The second RCT was conducted in 18 private pediatric practices in central Maryland with a mostly middle class white sample. Practices were randomized to SEEK or control and 1119 mothers were recruited for the evaluation. Again, SEEK mothers reported using less psychological aggression and minor physical violence than controls, both initially and 12 months later.[84] It should be noted that most of the behaviors included here would not generally cross the threshold for legal definitions of abuse. Nevertheless, it is clear that they may be quite damaging to children.[85-89] Concerns with maltreatment should not be limited to legal definitions. The finding with regard to physical violence was even stronger in an at-risk subgroup with demographic or psychosocial risk factors.

Conclusions

SEEK appears to be a promising strategy for helping address prevalent psychosocial problems via enhanced pediatric primary care. By potentially strengthening families and supporting parents, children's health, development, and safety may be enhanced and child maltreatment prevented. There is a need to further evaluate the SEEK model in other settings.

SafeCare

SafeCare is a structured behavioral training protocol with a primary goal of preventing or reducing physical abuse and neglect of children.[90] SafeCare is an in-home parenting model program that provides direct skill training to parents in child behavior management and planned activities training, home safety training, and child health care skills to prevent child maltreatment. It has been used as a selective and indicated prevention program.

Goals

The goal of SafeCare is to prevent child maltreatment by facilitating change of parenting behavior in the following areas: difficulty managing behavior, inability to prevent challenging behavior, and child health and safety concerns. All areas are relevant to families who are at risk for neglect. Child health and safety domains are specific dimensions where omissions in care may be defined as child neglect. The focus on child behavior is particularly relevant to families with neglect problems due to the effect of neglect on child behavior.

Conceptual/Theoretical Basis

SafeCare is based on the ecobehavioral model, which posits that maltreatment arises from a combination of factors, including individual parent factors, parent-child interactions, family factors, and broader cultural and societal factors.[91] Furthermore, the ecobehavioral model suggests that family social ecology must be considered in any examination of parent-child relationships and in developing effective behavioral intervention treatment strategies.[92]

Program Description

SafeCare intervention is provided in the home for approximately 1.5 hours weekly over 18 to 20 weeks. The primary focus is on building parenting skills related to child behavior management, home safety, and child health care. Staff must have a college education and be trained to performance criteria.

Evaluations

SafeCare is a parenting program with established research via single case and quasi-experimental studies. The original program, known as Project 12-Ways, was established 30 years ago in Illinois.[93,94] Randomized clinical trials are currently in progress. A quasi-experimental study in California established that 41 families who participated in SafeCare were significantly less likely to have a recurrence of child maltreatment (15% over 3 years) compared to families who received services as usual (44% over 3 years).[95] In the same study, the effectiveness of individual training components was evaluated as the change in the parents' scores in roleplay situations for child health problems, hazards present in the home, and the frequency and quality of parent-child interactions during activities of daily living. Statistically significant improvements were seen in health, safety, and parenting over baseline measures. However, the authors note that there was a high level of attrition from the program [decrease in using program components] among those who were referred, with only 10% completing all of the training components.[96]

SafeCare has been classified in the promising research evidence category, defined by the California Evidence-Based Clearinghouse for Child Welfare. It has been implemented in multiple jurisdictions across the country and the tightly controlled methods of implementing the program with fidelity suggest that current studies may further demonstrate the efficacy of this intervention when compared to services as usual.[97]

The particular focus of the program on building empathy in high-risk parents makes the program relevant for families identified at risk of neglect. The varied program formats makes it possible to select the program type that best matches the particular risks identified in families.

Triple P – Positive Parenting Program

The Triple P - Positive Parenting Program is a multi-level system of parenting and family support. The program is intended for the prevention of social, emotional, and behavioral problems in childhood, the prevention of child maltreatment, and the strengthening of parenting and parental confidence, although its original focus was to address behavioral problems in children. The programs are tailored to family needs through flexible formats and delivery. Its levels of intervention are used as both a universal and selective preventive intervention.

Goals

Triple P aims to prevent severe behavioral, emotional, and developmental problems in children by enhancing the knowledge, skills, and confidence of parents.

Conceptual/Theoretical Basis

Triple P draws on social learning, cognitive-behavioral and developmental theory, as well as research into risk and protective factors associated with the development of social and behavioral problems in children.

Program Description

Triple P targets 5 different developmental periods from infancy to adolescence. Within each developmental period, the reach of the intervention can vary from being very broad (targeting an entire population) to quite narrow (targeting only high-risk children). The program can be provided individually, in a group, or a self-directed format. Level 1 – Universal Triple P is a coordinated information campaign using print and electronic media and other health promotion strategies to promote awareness of parenting issues. Level 2 – Selected Triple P and Selected Teen Triple P targets parents with specific concerns about their child's development or behavior. Services involve provision of specific advice on how to solve common child development issues and minor child behavior problems. These programs may involve face-to-face or telephone contact with a practitioner (about 20 minutes over 2 sessions) or seminars (about 90 minutes). Level 3 – Primary Care Triple P or Primary Care Teen Triple P targets parents with specific concerns who require consultations or active skills training. A brief program (about 80 minutes over 4 sessions) combining advice with rehearsal and self-evaluation as required to teach parents to manage a discrete child problem behavior. This intervention may involve face-to-face or telephone contact with a practitioner. It is offered for parents of children aged birth to 12 years and parents of adolescents. Level 4 – Standard Triple P, Group Triple P, Group Teen Triple P, Self-Directed Triple P targets parents wanting intensive training in positive parenting skills. Typically, these parents have children with more severe behavior problems, such as aggressive or oppositional behavior. The services involve about 10 hours of services over 8-10 sessions and may be provided in individual, group, or self-directed (with or without telephone assistance) options. Level 5 – Enhanced Triple P is an enhanced family intervention that targets parents of children with concurrent child behavior problems and family dysfunction, such as parental depression or stress or conflict between partners. This intensive individually tailored program is provided in up to 11 sessions and includes practice sessions to enhance parenting skills, mood management strategies, stress coping skills, partner support skills, attribution retraining, and anger management. Other specialist programs are also available for parents of children with a disability and Pathways Triple P – a level 5 program that targets parents at risk of child maltreatment. Pathways Triple P is provided in 4 sessions as an adjunctive intervention used in combination with either group or standard Triple P. This intervention addresses parental anger and explanations for their children's behavior.

Evaluations

The program has been developed over 30 years and has had extensive research, particularly related to the effectiveness of the Level 4 Triple P interventions for children with disruptive behavior problems. A complete review of this research is beyond the scope of this chapter, but a recent meta-analysis of randomized controlled trials of this version of Triple P is available on the Triple P Web site.[98] The results indicated that Level 4 of Triple P interventions reduced disruptive behaviors in children and these improvements were sustained with further improvements in long-term follow-up.

An evaluation of Level 1 Triple P – related to a population level trial found that counties receiving Triple P showed significantly lower levels of maltreatment related outcomes than the control counties that did not receive the Level 1 intervention.[99]

Conclusions

The multi-level nature of Triple P interventions suggests that this intervention may be beneficial to prevent child neglect, but most of the research has focused on addressing child behavior problems or prevention of child maltreatment broadly at a system level.

Triple P has received the highest scientific rating by the California Evidence-Based Clearinghouse for Child Welfare. However, it has achieved only a medium relevance to child welfare rating (ie, the program was designed, or is commonly used, to serve children, youth, young adults, and/or families who are similar to child welfare populations).

Summary, Conclusions, and Recommendations

This chapter has summarized what is known about key programs and approaches relevant to the prevention of child neglect. Programs are typically applied in varied ways. Most of those described in this chapter focus on families considered at risk for neglect (or maltreatment). Alternatively, they may be used as treatment interventions for families after maltreatment has been identified. A few programs are applied broadly at a community level without regard to risk or maltreatment status. Finally, some programs target related problems, such as children's behavior problems, and their ability to prevent maltreatment remains untested. To the extent that they support and strengthen parenting, they might well enhance children's development, health, and safety and help prevent neglect. Conceptually, this makes sense.

The quest for evidence on prevention programs has been hampered by limited funding and the pressing priority to deliver much needed services. However, it remains important that prevention efforts be carefully evaluated. Most of the programs described in this chapter need further replication and evaluation before broad implementation. In some instances, valuable lessons have been learned, which can be incorporated into innovative improvements of existing models. But, in this era of accountability, the "need to do something" is not enough—we need to learn what works and what does not. "Promising" is just a good start.

Finally, the ecology of child neglect attests to the broad, underlying systemic problems that contribute to this prevalent phenomenon. Effective programs are needed, but that will not be enough. Broader social supports are also necessary to help ensure children's and families' basic needs are adequately met and to help prevent neglect.

The Level 1 – Universal Triple P preventive intervention has been designed and tested to reach all families in a community.[99] NFP and HFA have both targeted pregnant women and their first-born children. FC, SEEK, and SafeCare have been designed targeting specific risk factors that may increase risk for child neglect and/or child maltreatment more broadly. NPP has multiple formats and has been implemented most widely for parents whose children have already been identified as maltreated; however, other parents have received services because someone in the community believes they may be at risk for neglect or abuse. Triple P and TIY have many years of design and testing although most of the research has documented the relevance of these preventive interventions in enhancing parenting competencies in relation to problematic child behaviors. However, the focus of these programs on strengthening parenting behaviors suggests that these interventions may be useful for work with families at risk for neglect.

Given the variations of the theories that guide these various preventive interventions, along with differences in conceptual frameworks, preventive intervention formats, and target populations, programs considering program replication should carefully review these variations in an effort to match the program with the goals or purposes of the replicating site. Furthermore, it is important to continue to study the fidelity of implementation as well as the outcomes of these preventive interventions and to specifically examine the relevance for families at risk for neglect (versus other forms of child maltreatment or related social problems).

References

1. Sedlak AJ, Mettenburg J, Basena M, et al. *Fourth National Incidence Study of Child Abuse and Neglect (NIS-4): Report to Congress.* Washington, DC: US Department of Health and Human Services, Administration of Children and Families; 2010.

2. US Department of Health and Human Services; Administration for Children and Families, Administration on Children, Youth and Families; Children's Bureau. Child Maltreatment 2012. Washington, DC: US Department of Health and Human Services; Administration for Children and Families; Administration on Children, Youth and Families; Children's Bureau; 2013. Children's Bureau Web site. http://www.acf.hhs.gov/programs/cb/research-data-technology/statistics-research/child-maltreatment. Accessed October 19, 2016.

3. DePanfilis D, Zuravin SJ. Rates, patterns, and frequency of child maltreatment recurrences among families known to CPS. *Child Maltreat.* 1998;3(1):27-42.

4. DePanfilis D, Zuravin SJ. Epidemiology of child maltreatment recurrences. *Social Services Review.* 1999;73(2):218-239.

5. Erickson MF, Egeland B. Child neglect. In: Myers JB, Berliner L, Briere J, Hendrix CT, Jenny C, Reid TA, eds. *The APSAC Handbook on Child Maltreatment.* 2nd ed. Thousand Oaks, CA: Sage Publications; 2002:3-20.

6. Fluke JD. Child protective services reporting and recurrence: context and considerations regarding research. *Child Abuse Negl.* 2008;(32):749-751.

7. Fluke JD, Yuan YY, Edwards M. Recurrence of maltreatment: an application of the National Child Abuse and Neglect Data System (NCANDS). *Child Abuse Negl.* 1999;23(7):633-650.

8. Hildyard KL, Wolfe DA. Child neglect: developmental issues and outcomes. *Child Abuse Negl.* 2002;26(6-7):679-695.

9. Trickett PK, McBride-Chang C. The developmental impact of different forms of child abuse and neglect. *Dev Rev.* 1995;15(3):311-337.

10. Dubowitz H. Understanding and addressing the "neglect of neglect": digging into the molehill. *Child Abuse Negl.* 2007;31(6):603-606.

11. Kaplan SJ, Pelcovitz D, Labruna V. Child and adolescent abuse and neglect research: a review of the past 10 years. part 1: physical and emotional abuse and neglect. *J Am Acad Child Adolesc Psychiatry.* 1999;38(10):1214-1222.

12. McSherry D. Understanding and addressing the neglect of neglect: why are we making a mole-hill out of a mountain? *Child Abuse Negl.* 2007;31(6):607-614.

13. Wolock I, Horowitz B. Child maltreatment as a social problem: the neglect of neglect. *Am J Orthopsychiat.* 1984;54(4):530-543.

14. Dubowitz H. What is child neglect? In: Dubowitz H, DePanfilis D, eds. *Handbook for Child Protection Practice.* Thousand Oaks, CA: Sage Publications; 2000:10-14.

15. Leeb RT, Paulozzi L, Meanson C, Simon T, Arias I. *Child Maltreatment Surveillance: Uniform Definitions for Public Health and Recommended Data Elements, Version 1.0.* Atlanta, GA: Centers for Disease Control and Prevention, National Center for Injury Prevention and Control; 2008.

16. Straus MA, Kantor GK. Definition and measurement of neglectful behavior: some principles and guidelines. *Child Abuse Negl.* 2005;29(1):19-29.

17. Zuravin SJ. Child neglect: a review of definitions and measurement research. In: H. Dubowitz, ed. *Neglected Children: Research, Practice and Policy.* Thousand Oaks, CA: Sage Publications; 1999:24-46.

18. Dubowitz H, Black M, Starr R, Zuravin S. A conceptual definition of child neglect. *Crim Justice Behav.* 1993;(20):8-26.

19. Dubowitz H, Pitts SC, Litrownik AJ, Cox CE, Runyan D, Black MM. Defining child neglect based on child protective services data. *Child Abuse Negl.* 2005;29(5):493-511.

20. English DJ, Upadhyaya MP, Litrownik AJ, et al. Maltreatment's wake: the relationship of child maltreatment dimensions to child outcomes. *Child Abuse Negl.* 2005;29(5):597-619.

21. Dunn MG, Tarter RE, Mezzich AC, Vanyukov M, Kirisci L, Kirillova G. Origins and consequences of child neglect in substance abuse families. *Clin Psychol Rev.* 2002;22(7):1063-1090.

22. Cole JD, Watt NF, West SG, et al. The science of prevention: a conceptual framework and some directions for a national research program. *Am Psychol.* 1993;48(10):1013-1022.

23. Hawkins JD, Horn MLV, Arthur MW. Community variation in risk and protective factors and substance use outcomes. *Prev Sci.* 2004;5(4):213-220.

24. Kellam SG, Koretz D, Mościcki EK. Core elements of developmental epidemiologically based prevention research. *Am J Community Psychol.* 1999;27(4):463-482.

25. Institute of Medicine. *Reducing Risks for Mental Disorders: Frontiers for Preventive Intervention Research.* Washington, DC: National Academy Press; 1994.

26. Weissberg RP, Greenberg MT. Prevention science and collaborative community action research: combining the best from both perspectives. *J Ment Health.* 1998;7(5):479-492.

27. Bronfenbrenner U. *The Ecology of Human Development: Experiments by Design and Nature.* Cambridge, MA: Harvard University Press; 1979.

28. Institute of Medicine. *Future of the Publics' Health in the 21st Century.* Washington, DC: Institute of Medicine; 2002.

29. Mrazek PJ, Haggerty RJ. *Reducing Risks for Mental Disorders: Frontiers for Preventive Intervention Research.* Washington, DC: National Academy Press; 1994.

30. DePanfilis D, Dubowitz H. Family Connections: a program for preventing child neglect. *Child Maltreat.* 2005;10(2):108-123.

31. Belsky J. Child maltreatment: an ecological integration. *Am Psychol.* 1980;35(4):320-335.

32. DePanfilis D. Using prevention science to reduce the risk of child neglect. *Children Australia.* 2009;34(1):40-44.

33. Dunst CJ, Trivette CM, Deal AG. *Enabling and Empowering Families: Principles and Guidelines for Practice.* Cambridge, MA. Brookline Books; 1988.

34. Kinney J, Strand K, Hagerup M, Bruner C. *Beyond the Buzzwords: Key Principles in Effective Frontline Practice*. Falls Church, VA: National Center for Safety Initiatives Information Clearinghouse; 1994.

35. De Panfilis D, Glazer-Semmell E, Farr M, Ferretto G. *Family Connections Intervention Manual*. Baltimore, MD: University of Maryland, Baltimore; 1999.

36. US Department of Health and Human Services. *Emerging Practices in the Prevention of Child Abuse and Neglect*. Washington, DC: Office on Child Abuse and Neglect; 2003.

37. Girvin H, DePanfilis D, Daining C. Predicting program completion among families enrolled in a child neglect preventive intervention. *Res Soc Work Pract*. 2007;17(6):674-685.

38. DePanfilis D, Dubowitz H, Kunz J. Assessing the cost-effectiveness of family connections. *Child Abuse Negl*. 2008;32(3):335-351.

39. DePanfilis D, Filene JH, Brodowski ML. Introduction to family connections and the national replication effort. *Prot Child*. 2009;24(3):4-14.

40. DePanfilis D, Smith EG, Filene JH, Rice K. Assessing final outcomes: predicting time to CPS report. Paper presented at: Society for Social Work & Research 14th Annual Conference: Social Work Research: A World of Possibilities; January 14-17, 2010; San Francisco, CA.

41. James Bell Associates, Inc. *National Cross-Site Evaluation of the Replication of Family Connections: Final Evaluation Report*. Arlington, VA: James Bell Associates, Inc; 2011.

42. Smith EG, Filene JH, DePanfilis D. Assessing intermediate outcomes: increasing protective factors and decreasing risk factors. Society for Social Work & Research 14th Annual Conference, Social Work Research: A World of Possibilities; January 14-17, 2010; San Francisco, CA.

43. Theriott MT, O'Day KR, Hatfield K. Client and service use predictors of successfully completing a child maltreatment prevention program. *Prot Child*. 2009;24(3):38-49.

44. Brodowski ML, Filene JH. Engaging program staff in economic evaluation: lessons learned and recommendations for practice. *Prot Child*. 2009;24(3):69-76.

45. Corso P, Filene JH. Cost analysis of the Family Connections program. *Prot Child*. 2009;24(3):77-87.

46. Sharpe T, DePanfilis D, Strieder F, Gregory G. Replication of Family Connections: lessons learned from grandparents. *Prot Child*. 2009;24(3):58-68.

47. Stephens K, Mills C, Williams C, Bridge T, Massie E. Maximizing the therapeutic helping alliance with high-risk families. *Prot Child*. 2009;24(3):27-37.

48. Wu ST, Mimura-Lazare A, Petrucci C, Kageyama N, Suh C. Culturally competent practice with Cambodian and Korean families in Los Angeles: results from a 5 year replication of Family Connections. *Prot Child*. 2009;24(3):15-26.

49. Healthy Families America. Healthy Families America philosophy. Healthy Families America Web site. http://www.healthyfamiliesamerica.org/about_us/philosophy.shtml. Accessed February 13, 2014.

50. Harding K, Galano J, Martin J, Huntington L, Schellenbach CJ. Healthy Families America effectiveness: a comprehensive review of outcomes. *J Prev Interv Community*. 2007;34(1-2):149-179.

51. Korfmacher J. The Kempe Family Stress Inventory: a review. *Child Abuse Negl.* 2000;24(1):129-140.

52. DuMont K, Mitchell-Herzfeld S, Greene R, et al. Healthy Families New York (HFNY) randomized trial: effects on child abuse and neglect. *Child Abuse Negl.* 2008;32(3):295-315.

53. Rodriguez M, Dumont K, Mitchell-Herzfeld SD, Walden NJ, Green R. Effects of Healthy Families New York on the promotion of maternal parenting competencies and the prevention of harsh parenting. *Child Abuse Negl.* 2010;34(10):711-723.

54. Duggan AK, Caldera DL, Rodriguez K, Burrell L, Rohde C, Crowne SS. Impact of a statewide home visiting program to prevent child abuse. *Child Abuse Negl.* 2007;31:829-852.

55. Gessner BD. The effect of Alaska's home visitation program for high-risk families on trends in abuse and neglect. *Child Abuse Negl.* 2008;32(3):317-333.

56. Duggan AK, McFarlane E, Fuddy L, et al. Randomized trial of a statewide home visiting program to prevent child abuse: impact preventing child abuse and neglect. *Child Abuse Negl.* 2004;28(6):597-622.

57. Bair-Merritt M, Jennings J, Chen R, et al. Reducing maternal intimate partner violence after the birth of a child: a randomized controlled trial of the Hawaii Healthy Start home visitation program. *Arch Pediatr Adolesc Med.* 2010;164(1):16-23.

58. Landsverk J, Carrilio T, Connelly C, et al. *Healthy Families San Diego Clinical Trial: Technical Report.* San Diego, CA: Child and Adolescent Services Research Center and San Diego Children's Hospital and Health Center; 2002.

59. Falconer MK, Clark MH, Parris D. Validity in an evaluation of Healthy Families Florida—a program to prevent child abuse and neglect. *Child Youth Serv Rev.* 2001;33(1):66-77.

60. Gross D, Fogg L, Webster-Stratton C, Garvey C, Julion W. Parent training of toddlers in day care in low-income urban communities. *J Consult Clin Psychol.* 2003;71(2):261-278.

61. Reid MJ, Webster-Stratton C, Beauchaine TP. Parent training in Head Start: a comparison of program response among African American, Asian American, Caucasian, and Hispanic mothers. *Prev Sci.* 2001;2(4):209-227.

62. Baydar N, Reid MJ, Webster-Stratton C. The role of mental health factors and program engagement in the effectiveness of a preventive parenting program for Head Start mothers. *Child Development.* 2003;74(5):1433-1453.

63. Linares LO, Montalto D, Li M, Oza VS. A promising parenting intervention in foster care. *J Consult Clin Psychol.* 2006;74(1):32–41.

64. Olds DL, Kitzman H, Cole R, Robinson J. Theoretical foundations of a program of home visitation for pregnant women and parents of young children. *Journal of Community Psychology.* 1997;25(1):9-25.

65. Olds DL, Henderson CR, Tatelbaum R, Chamberlin R. Improving the life-course development of socially disadvantaged mothers: a randomized trial of nurse home visitation. *Am J Public Health.* 1988;78(11):1436-1445.

66. Kitzman H, Olds DL, Henderson CR, et al. Effect of prenatal and infancy home visitation by nurses on pregnancy outcomes, childhood injuries, and repeated childbearing: a randomized controlled trial. *JAMA.* 1997;278(8):644-652.

67. Olds DL, Robinson J, O'Brien R, et al. Home visiting by paraprofessionals and by nurses: a randomized, controlled trial. *Pediatrics.* 2002;110(3):486-496.

68. Olds DL, Henderson CR, Chamberlin R, Tatelbaum C. Preventing child abuse and neglect: A randomized trial of nurse home visitation. *Pediatrics.* 1986;78(1):65-78.

69. Olds DL, Eckenrode J, Henderson CR, et al. Long-term effects of home visitation on maternal life course and child abuse and neglect: fifteen-year follow-up of a randomized trial. *JAMA.* 1997;278(8):637-643.

70. Olds DL, Kitzman H, Hanks C, et al. Effects of nurse home visiting on maternal and child functioning: age 9 follow-up of a randomized trial. *Pediatrics.* 2007;120(4):832-845.

71. Olds DL, Robinson J, Pettitt LM, et al. Effects of home visits by paraprofessionals and by nurses: age 4 follow-up results of a randomized trial. *Pediatrics.* 2004;114(6):1560-1568.

72. MacMillan HL, Thomas BH, Jamieson E, et al. Effectiveness of home visitation by public-health nurses in prevention of the recurrence of child physical abuse and neglect: a randomized controlled trial. *Lancet.* 2005;365(9473):1786-1793.

73. Gomby DS. The promise and limitations of home visiting: implementing effective programs. *Child Abuse Negl.* 2007;31(8):793-799.

74. Bavolek SJ. Successful implementation of the Nurturing Parenting Programs. Nurturing Parenting Web site. http://www.nurturingtrainisng.com/pp5.html. Accessed February 13, 2014.

75. Bavolek S, Keene R. *Adult-Adolescent Parenting Inventory.* Park City, UT: Family Development Resources; 1999.

76. Bavolek SJ, Comstock CM, McLaughlin JW. The Nurturing Program: a validated approach for reducing dysfunctional family interactions. Nurturing Parenting Web site. http://www.nurturingparenting.com/research_validation/The%20Nurturing%20Program%20NIMH%20Study%20-%20.pdf. Accessed February 13, 2014.

77. Cowen PS. Effectiveness of a parent education intervention for at-risk families. *J Soc Pediatr Nurs.* 2001;6(2):73-82.

78. Devall EL. Positive parenting for high-risk families. *J Fam Consum Sci.* 2004;96(4):22-28.

79. Dubowitz H, Feigelman S, Lane W, Kim JW. Pediatric primary care to help prevent child maltreatment: the Safe Environment for Every Kid (SEEK) Model. *Pediatrics.* 2009;123(3):858-864.

80. Dubowitz H, Feigelman S, Lane W, et al. Screening for depression in an urban pediatric primary care clinic. *Pediatrics.* 2007;119(3):435-443.

81. Dubowitz H, Prescott L, Feigelman S, Lane W, Kim J. Screening for intimate partner violence in an urban pediatric primary care clinic. *Pediatrics.* 2008;121(1):85-91.

82. Feigelman S, Dubowitz H, Lane W, Kim J. Screening for harsh punishment in a pediatric primary care clinic. *Child Abuse Negl.* 2009;33(5):269-277.

83. Lane W, Dubowitz H, Feigelman S, et al. Screening for parental substance abuse in an urban pediatric primary care clinic. *Ambul Pediatr.* 2007;7(6):458-462.

84. Dubowitz H, Lane WG, Semiatin JN, Magder LS, Venepally M, Jans M. The safe environment for every kid model: impact on pediatric primary care professionals. *Pediatrics.* 2011;127(4):e962-e970.

85. Knox M. On hitting children: a review of corporal punishment in the United States. *J Pediatr Health Care.* 2010;24(2):103-107.

86. Miller-Perrin C, Perrin R, Kocur J. Parental physical and psychological aggression: Psychological symptoms in young adults. *Child Abuse Negl.* 2009;33(1):1-11.

87. Straus M, Sugarman D, Giles-Sims J. Spanking by parents and subsequent antisocial behavior of children. *Arch Pediatr Adolesc Med.* 1997;151(8):761-767.

88. Taylor C, Manganello J, Lee S, Rice J. Mothers' spanking of 3-year-old children and subsequent risk of children's aggressive behavior. *Pediatrics.* 2010;125(5):e1057-e1065.

89. Zolotor A, Theodore A, Chang J, Berkoff M, Runyan D. Speak softly—and forget the stick: corporal punishment and child physical abuse. *Am J Prev Med.* 20058;35(4):364-369.

90. Whittaker DJ, Crimmins D, Edwards AE, Lutzker JR. Safety training and violence prevention using the SafeCare training model. In: O'Donohue W, Fisher JE, eds. *Cognitive Behavior Therapy: Applying Empirical Supported Techniques in Your Practice.* New York, NY: John Wiley; 2009:473-477.

91. Edwards A, Lutzker JR. Iterations of the SafeCare model, an evidence based child maltreatment prevention program. *Behav Modif.* 2008;32(5):736-756.

92. Lutzker JR, Bigelow KM, Doctor RM, Gershater RM, Greene BF. An ecobehavioral model for the prevention and treatment of child abuse and neglect. In: Lutzker JR, ed. *Handbook of Child Abuse Research and Treatment.* New York, NY: Plenum Press; 1998:239-266.

93. Lutzker JR, Rice JM. Project 12-ways: measuring outcome of a large in-home service for treatment and prevention of child abuse and neglect. *Child Abuse Negl.* 1984;8(4):519-524.

94. Tertinger DA, Greene BF, Lutzker JR. Home safety: development and validation of one component of an ecobehavioral treatment program for abused and neglected children. *J Appl Behav Anal.* 1984;17(2):159-174.

95. Gershater-Molko RM, Lutzker JR, Wesch D. Using recidivism data to evaluate Project SafeCare: teaching bonding, safety, and health care skills to parents. *Child Maltreat.* 2002;7(3):277-285.

96. Gershater-Molko RM, Lutzker JR, Wesch D. Project Safe Care: improving health, safety, and parenting skills in families reported for, and at-risk for child maltreatment. *J Fam Violence.* 2003;18(6):377-386.

97. Hecht DB, Silvosky JF, Chaffin M, Lutzker JR. Project SafeCare: an evidence-based approach to prevent child neglect. *APSAC Advisor.* 2008;20(1):14-17.

98. de Graaf I, Speetjens P, Smit F, de Wolff M, Travecchio L. Effectiveness of the Triple P Positive Parenting Program on behavioral problems in children: a meta-analysis. *Behav Modif.* 2008;32(5):714-735.

99. Prinz RJ, Saunders MR, Shapiro CJ, Whitaker DJ, Lutzker JR. Population-based prevention of child maltreatment: the U.S. Triple P system population trial. *Prev Sci.* 2009;10(1):1-12.

Chapter 11

Corporal Punishment and Child Abuse: Policy and Prevention Programs

Adam J. Zolotor, MD, MPH

Overview of Corporal Punishment

Corporal punishment (CP) includes use of any physical punishment against a child in response to a specific misbehavior. In the United States, this most often takes the form of spanking, but many other forms of CP are widely practiced in the United States and abroad. There can be a fine line between CP and child physical abuse. In the United States, spanking and hitting with an object (eg, a belt, switch) in the home are legal, if no significant injury occurs. For practical purposes, many child protective services agencies and consulting physicians use a 24-hour rule; that is, if a mark from CP lasts greater than 24 hours, injury is said to have occurred and the fine line between CP and physical abuse has been crossed.[1] CP should be considered in the context of discussions of child abuse because (1) it is associated with numerous harms to the well-being of the child, (2) it is closely associated with child physical abuse, and (3) it is considered by some child rights advocates to be a form of physical abuse. This chapter will consider the harms associated with CP, trends and international variations in CP, and the prevention of CP through policies and programs.

Many experts and advocates recommend CP as an option for discipline or even a necessary part of good parenting.[2-4] It is clear that CP can be effectively used to alter immediate compliance.[5] However, it is also clear that CP has many unintended consequences. A systematic review of over 300 original articles on CP by Gershoff demonstrated that CP has adverse associations in childhood, including moral internalization, aggression, delinquent and antisocial behavior, decreased quality of parent-child relationship, and behavioral symptoms. In addition, CP during childhood is associated with adult consequences: aggression, criminal and antisocial behavior, worse mental health, and abuse of one's own child and spouse.[5]

Spanking is associated with an increased risk of physical abuse. Previous research has shown that protective service substantiated abuse often results from escalated spanking[6] and is usually in response to child misbehavior.[7] Other studies have shown that abusive parents are 3 to 5 times more likely to spank than nonabusive parents.[8-9] If a child is spanked often, spanking will become less effective at modifying behavior. If spanking is ineffective, a parent may spank more, harder, or use an object.[6,10-11] A recent study reported that spanking frequency and intensity (use of an object) are associated with increasing probability of self-reported abuse.[12]

CP is widespread in the United States. Population-based data on spanking is often difficult to compare based on differences in methodology and sampling. The most systematically comparable data on CP over time comes from the 1975 and 1985 National Family Violence Surveys and the 1995 Gallup survey on discipline.[13-14] A recent report compared the results from those studies over 3 decades to 2002 data from North and South Carolina, demonstrating a decline of 18% in spanking over nearly 4 decades. This study accounted for the potential of higher rates of spanking in the Southeast by restricting previous samples to the Southeast and the results were nearly identical. Analysis was restricted to children between ages 3 and 11 because spanking very young and older children is less common. Overall rates of spanking have declined 18%—from 765/1000 (1975 national sample) to 623/1000 (2002, Carolinas) among children 3 to 11. Spanking peaks among 3 to 5 year olds, with a rate of 788/1000 in 2002, down 4% from 822/1000 in 1975. Hitting with an object is reported less often, with a rate of 332/1000 in 2002. This type of punishment peaks somewhat later, with nearly 50% of 7 to 9 year olds receiving this type of punishment in the past year.[15] It should be noted that this data comes from self-report. Therefore, the decline might be a real decline in the use of spanking, but it also may reflect a decline in the social acceptability of spanking with greater impact of social desirability bias in more recent surveys.

Spanking in very early childhood may represent a special problem for a number of reasons. Numerous studies have shown that earlier abuse and neglect has a greater impact on development than later abuse and neglect.[16-18] Less is known about the consequences of early spanking relative to later spanking regarding differential developmental consequences. One longitudinal study of discipline at age 3 found that among girls, physical discipline was associated with a lower IQ of the physically disciplined child.[19] A subsequent study with a much larger sample and more effective control of confounding variables reported that spanking at 1 year of age was associated with aggressive behavior at 2 years of age and lower developmental scores at 3 compared to children who were not spanked.[20] A recent prospective cohort study reported that spanking at 3 was associated with increased aggressive behavior at 5, further reinforcing that the groundwork for adverse developmental and behavioral consequences of spanking may be laid at a young age.[21] A survey of nearly 3000 mothers in North Carolina reported that spanking starts early. Thirty percent of children under 2 have been spanked by their mother in the last year. At 3 months, 6% of children have been spanked, and at 24 months, 75% of children have been spanked.[22]

International Variation in Corporal Punishment

Since 1979, 50 countries have enacted legislation to ban CP in the home.[23] CP around the world most commonly takes the form of spanking (also known as smacking, whupping, popping, etc), but may also include slapping, pinching, pulling hair, twisting ears, or hitting with an object such as a rod or stick. There are few multinational comparative studies by which to judge various rates of CP. One exception to this is the WorldSAFE study, including 6 national or multi-city representative samples. Spanking by a mother or her partner on a specific child in the last year varied from 16% of children in non-slum New Delhi to 76% of children in the Philippines. Of the common types of CP, spanking on the buttocks is most common in the United States (44%), Philippines (76%), Chile (53%), and Brazil (55%). Different forms of punishment were common in Egypt (slapping on the face 42%, shaking 68%, pinching 45%, ear twisting 29%).[24]

Programmatic Approaches to Corporal Punishment

There are 2 primary approaches toward a reduction or elimination of CP against children: parents can either be taught other effective approaches to discipline, or laws that ban the use of CP can be passed. Educational approaches have the primary advantage of voluntary behavior change and demonstrated effectiveness. However, the most effective approaches are costly and often only available to serve high-risk families.

In considering educational approaches to CP, it is useful to consider appropriate service delivery settings and developmentally appropriate timing for messages. As previously discussed, CP is common even in the first 6 months of life. There are 2 approaches to universal education: primary care and mass media. Rigorous evaluations of standalone media campaigns to decrease CP are lacking. Media campaigns often introduce and reinforce legislative bans on CP. Furthermore, media campaigns have been part of other evidence-based, community-wide interventions such as Triple P. In this context, media campaigns may play a role in decreasing CP.[25]

Primary care medical visits are nearly universal in the United States and most high-income countries, and are an appropriate setting for education about discipline. A typical well child schedule in the United States includes 6 visits through the first birthday. The American Academy of Pediatrics states unequivocally that children under 2 should not be spanked and that parents should be encouraged to develop and use alternative behavior management strategies for children of all ages.[26] Pediatric health care professionals, public health programs, and child development programs should assist parents of very young children in developing a discipline skill set including positive and negative reinforcement without physical punishment as well as setting appropriate behavioral expectations for children. Well child visits are crowded with dozens of suggested topics for screening and anticipatory guidance, and primary care clinicians are limited by time and reimbursement schemes to the number of topics they can address reasonably well.[27-28] However, primary care clinicians have been reported to be expert sources for parenting and safety advice.[29] One approach is the use of supplementary educational materials. One study randomized parents attending a primary care clinic to use an interactive DVD to view 4 behavior conflicts and parenting strategies out of 16 available versus usual care. In this study, parents reported immediately after the intervention that they planned to spank less and were more likely to feel like clinic visits had helped them to develop discipline strategies.[30] Other models that use primary care offices for parenting education have potential or demonstrated success in reducing CP but require relatively more resources.[31-33] One additional approach that has involved primary care clinics is Triple P, in which some nurses were trained in Triple P approaches as part of countywide interventions which have been shown to reduce CP.[25] Second to primary care, the next most common service for young children is daycare. Triple P has included daycare workers for training in parenting techniques as well, though many studies have evaluated daycare centers as places to disseminate parenting advice, no studies to date have evaluated CP rates as a result of parent education in daycare.[25]

Parents who are at high risk of abusing their children due to risk factors such as young age, depression, substance abuse, partner violence, and poverty may have more intensive services available. These types of services often focus on child-rearing strategies in the context of health and development and parent wellness. Several programs have been shown in rigorous evaluation or experimental design to reduce CP or improve positive discipline. Healthy Families America and Healthy Start have shown a reduction in harsh parenting.[34-35] The Nurse-Family Partnership has shown more positive discipline. Incredible Years has reported less harsh discipline (verbal and physical), less physical punishment, more positive discipline, and improved child behavior.[36] A particular therapeutic model, Parent-Child Interaction Therapy has been shown to improve positive parental responses to appropriate behavior.[37]

Policy Approaches to Corporal Punishment

One approach to curtailing CP globally is the enactment of legislative bans on CP. As of November 2016, there are 50 countries (53 by another count) with such bans.

Arguments for banning CP can be advanced on several fronts. First, CP can cause numerous scientifically demonstrated harms to the developing child, including being an important risk factor for child physical abuse. Furthermore, bans on CP are often advanced as a human rights issue. Briefly stated, in most civil societies, it is illegal to strike an adult. Such use of force is considered a violation of human rights. The United Nations has argued that the state of childhood should confer, if anything, special rights, not the abdication of rights.[38-39] The Convention on the Rights of the Child (CRC) supports the human rights argument to prohibit CP. There are 195 countries which have ratified the UN Convention on the Rights of the Child, including all recognized member states, with the exception of the United States.[40] The original language of the CRC was not explicit regarding CP, but it generally advocated to protect children from "all forms of physical and mental violence, injury or abuse."[41] CRC committee opinions have clarified this position. "Addressing widespread acceptance of CP and eliminating it is an obligation of States and a key strategy in reducing all forms of violence."[42] Legal prohibitions against CP are in effect in only 26% of countries.

Thirty-two European countries, 10 Central and South American countries, 2 Middle Eastern countries, 6 African countries, and 1 country in Oceania have legislative bans on CP. All Scandinavian and near Scandinavian countries (Sweden, Norway, Denmark, Iceland, Greenland, and Finland) have CP bans and were among the first countries to adopt such legislation. Over four-fifths of all bans have been enacted since 2000.[43] (See the **Table 11-1** for more details about some of the first countries that have enacted such bans.)

There are many common threads in the laws and penalties related to CP. Most laws mention prison as a possible consequence of CP. Most cite short maximum terms, but usually incarceration is an option presented among other punishments, including fines and community service. There are 6 countries which list prison terms as the only available punishment for CP; however, all but 2 of these include language that allows no prosecution or sentencing for minor or inconsequential CP. Only 2 countries make reference in the law to limitations in parental authority (Greece and Latvia). Only one country (Croatia) states that cases shall be referred to social services for examination. Bans on CP are based on new laws in 11 instances, amendments to existing laws in 16 instances, a new constitutional bill of rights in one instance, and judicial interpretation in one instance.

Legislative bans on CP may be associated with changes in attitudes and behaviors around CP. Sweden has been systematically collecting data on support for CP since the 1960s. According to national opinion polls, public support for CP has been declining in Sweden for some time. In 1965, 53% of Swedish adults indicated that they supported the use of CP. This number declined in years following and was only 11% in 1994.[44-45] Results from a 1981 study suggest that Swedish attitudes condoning CP have decreased dramatically following the legislative ban.[46] Changing attitudes toward CP started years before 1979 and there is no evidence of causality.[47]

There is some evidence of decreasing public support for CP in the Netherlands that predates the ban on CP of 2007, according to an analysis of judicial case reports on child abuse. Before the ban, parents talked candidly about severe physical punishments used for discipline. Recent cases showed perpetrators noticeably less forthcoming about severe abuses and more aware of public attitudes of disapproval toward CP.[48]

There is some evidence of declines in the prevalence of beliefs that physical discipline benefits children. In 2001, 3 pre-ban studies were replicated concerning attitudes toward and prevalence of CP. Interviews conducted with 3000 parents of children under the age of 18 revealed small decreases in attitudinal measures of acceptance of CP compared to identical interviews (n=2000) conducted in 1996.[49]

Table 11-1. Summaries of National Legislative Bans on Corporal Punishment

Country	Year	Penalty	Legislation	Type of Government
Austria	1989	Up to 1 year imprisonment or fine.	Amendment of civil code: "use of force... inadmissible."	Federal parliamentary republic
Bulgaria	2000	Up to 3 years for light bodily harm.	New law, child protection act: "Every child has a right to protection...against physical...violence."	Parliamentary democracy
Costa Rica	2008	May include imprisonment.	New article to code on children. Amendment to family code.	Democratic republic
Croatia	1999	Notice of such cases shall be examined by the Center for Social Welfare.	Amendment to family code: "May not subject the child to ...physical violence."	Parliamentary republic
Cyprus	1994	Imprisonment, fine, or probation.	New law with amendment declares unlawful "any act of violence (between family members) which results in physical, sexual, or psychological injury."	Parliamentary republic
Denmark	1997	Prison up to 2 years, in extenuating circumstances: simple detention or fine.	Amendment to the parental custody and care act: "Children... must not be exposed to corporal punishment."	Parliamentary democracy and constitutional monarchy
Finland	1983	Fine or prison (up to 2 years).	New law: Child Custody and Right of Access Act: "He (the child) shall not be corporally punished."	Semi-presidential republic
Germany	2000	Fine or up to 1 year in prison. Only prosecuted upon complaint.	Amendment to civil code: Physical punishments are inadmissible.	Federal parliamentary republic
Greece	2006	May order any appropriate measure, including restricting (wholly or partially) parental care.	New law prohibits "physical violence against a minor ...in the context of upbringing."	Parliamentary republic

(continued)

Table 11-1. Summaries of National Legislative Bans on Corporal Punishment *(continued)*

Country	Year	Penalty	Legislation	Type of Government
Hungary	2005	Felony imprisonment up to 3 years.	Amendment to act on the children: "The child cannot be subject to ... corporal punishment."	Parliamentary republic
Iceland	2003	Fines or imprisonment up to 3 years.	The child may not be subject to physical punishment.	Parliamentary republic
Israel	2000	Particular test case, 3 years in prison.	Supreme court ruling: "Corporal punishment is ...entirely impermissible."	Republic under parliamentary democracy
Kenya	2010	Civil code	New constitutional bill of rights	Semi-presidential republic
Latvia	1998	*Civil law:* Limitation of parental wishes. In the case of violence, provision of extra-familial care. *Criminal law:* Intentional slight bodily injury, up to 3 years in prison, custodial arrest, community service, or fine.	New law, protection of the rights of the child: "Shall not be...physically punished."	Parliamentary republic
Liechtenstein	2008	Civil code.	Children and Youth Act.	Parliamentary democracy
Luxembourg	2008	Penal code. Punishment includes imprisonment and fines.	Law on Children and Families	Parliamentary democracy
Netherlands	2007	Up to 3 years in prison or fine.	Amendment to civil code: "Parents will not use violence."	Parliamentary democracy and constitutional monarchy
New Zealand	2007	Imprisonment up to 2 years, exclusion for 'inconsequential' force.	Amendment to the crimes act: Nothing "justifies the use of force for the purposes of correction."	Parliamentary democracy and constitutional monarchy
Norway	1987	Civil penal code, fine or prison up to 6 months.	Amendment to the children act: "The child must not be subjected to violence."	Parliamentary democracy under constitutional monarchy

(continued)

Table 11-1. Summaries of National Legislative Bans on Corporal Punishment *(continued)*

Country	Year	Penalty	Legislation	Type of Government
Poland	2010	Amendment to the Family Code		Parliamentary republic
Portugal	2007	Confinement of 1-5 years.	Amendment to penal code, includes corporal punishment as physical maltreatment.	Parliamentary republic
Spain	2007	6 to 12 months in prison or 31-80 days of service.	Amendment to civil code.	Constitutional monarchy
Sweden	1979	Petty crime, fine, or up to 6 months in prison. Not prosecuted unless the crime is serious in nature.	Amendment to the children and parents code: "Children…may not be subjected to corporal punishment." Constitution: "All citizens shall be protected against corporal punishment."	Parliamentary democracy and constitutional monarchy
Republic of Moldova	2009	Requires bodily harm, may range from small fine to 6-12 years in prison.	Amendment to family code.	Parliamentary democracy
Romania	2004	6-12 months in prison or fine.	New law: "Child….may not be subject to physical punishments."	Unitary semi-presidential republic
Tunisia	2010	Amendment to penal code		Presidential republic
Uruguay	2007	3-12 months in prison (requires injury).	Incorporated into code of childhood a prohibition of physical punishment.	Democratic republic
Venezuela	2007	3-12 months in prison.	New article to Law for the protection of children.	Federal republic
Ukraine	2004	Fine, community service, or correctional labor.	Amendment to the family code: "Physical punishment….[is] prohibited."	Unitary semi-presidential republic

Adapted from Zolotor AJ, Puzia ME.[43]

One cross-cultural study of young children comparing 102 Swedish and 107 Canadian mothers' attitudes toward CP found that whereas the majority of mothers in either country disapprove of physical punishment, a greater percentage of Swedish mothers reported holding views that condemn its use.[50]

Associations between the prohibition of CP and more general views on child-rearing are not as consistently supported by research. In 2005-2006 a study of adults in 7 countries in Europe was conducted. Three countries (Bulgaria, Latvia, and Ukraine) had, at the time of the study, laws prohibiting CP. Two countries (Moldova and Poland) did not have a legal prohibition of CP at the time but have since passed such laws. Two countries (Lithuania and Macedonia) do not have laws prohibiting the CP of children in the home. This study suggests that the legality of CP in a country did not influence the frequency with which respondents indicated agreement with the beliefs that "Children should be afraid of their parents, because fear fosters obedience," "Tough treatment by parents strengthens the child and, ultimately, is of benefit to him or her," or "A child is his/her parents' property, so the parents should be the only ones to make decisions about his/her fate." Respondents from countries with a legal ban on CP did not seem to differ from respondents from countries with no such ban in their reported beliefs about what situations would warrant third-party intervention (eg, parents "punishing their child with a spanking," parents "beating a child with a belt or another object"). Respondents also did not differ in their indications of situations where they would consider CP to be justifiable.[51]

One study compared how an act that a parent considers to be "violent" changed over time. In 2001, 61.9% of German parents indicated that they considered a child being slapped across the face by a teacher to be an act of violence, whereas only 30.7% indicated that they considered a child being slapped across the face for disobedience by his or her parent to be an act of violence.[49] CP in the school has been illegal in Germany since the 1970s, while at the time of the study, CP in the home had only been recently been banned.[52] Results of a pre-post law study show that most parents have more sensitive perceptions of what is "violent," especially regarding more severe forms of CP. In 1996, 37.2% of German parents reported that they considered "thrashing" to be an act of violence; in 2001, 48.2% of parents indicated this belief. In 1996, 12.5% of parents reported that they considered a forceful smack on the bottom to be an act of violence, and in 2001 this number had increased to 18.2%.[49]

Adult participants from the multinational study in Europe were asked about their beliefs regarding the appropriateness of parental use of CP. Respondents from countries where CP was or is now legal did differ from respondents in countries where CP of children was legal in their reported beliefs.[51] Respondents from the professional populations in the same countries (primary school teachers working in the capital cities) were asked similar questions regarding their opinions of the appropriateness of CP as a disciplinary measure. Respondents from countries where CP was illegal and respondents from countries where CP is legal did not differ in response to the question "Should the way parents treat their children be regulated by law?" It is important to note that respondents from countries where CP was illegal at the time of the study more frequently supported a ban on CP than respondents in countries where CP was legal.[51]

Perceptions of social norms regarding CP may affect endorsement of physical discipline and beliefs about CP. The study in Central and Eastern Europe addressed this, asking about perceived CP prevalence. Responses did not vary by legality of CP; however, when the same question was asked to professionals working with children respondents in countries where CP was prohibited indicated a lower estimated prevalence of spanking but not of more severe CP.[51]

One important policy question is whether or not legal prohibitions on CP change rates of physical punishment or child abuse. In 2002, interviews with 2000 adolescents between the ages of 12 and 18 were conducted in Germany, replicating a 1992 study (n= 2400) of the prevalence of physical punishment after the passage of a legislative ban in 2000. In 1992, 81.2% of adolescents reported ever being lightly slapped across the face by parents; in 2002, this number had fallen to 68.9%. In 1992, 43.6% of adolescents reported ever having received severe slaps, and in 2002 this was reported by only 13.9% of adolescents.[49]

The Swedish response to the UN's survey of violence against children referenced 2 studies that aimed to determine the prevalence of CP in Sweden. In 1980, a sample of Swedish children was asked whether a parent had ever used some form of physical punishment in the last year; 51% report that they had. In 2000, a similar study found that only 14% of children indicated that they had ever experienced CP. The available data on CP of children in Sweden indicated that in the 1960s, use of CP was widespread. In the 1970s, about 50% of children were subject to CP. By the 1980s, the number had fallen to about one-third and then further declined to about 20% in the 1990s.[53]

The study in Central and Eastern European countries asked teachers, "Have you encountered cases of child victims of family violence in your professional practice in the past year?" Respondents from countries where CP is illegal seemed to indicate that they had seen such cases less frequently than those in countries where CP was legal at the time of the study.[51]

In 2002, only 4.8% of German adolescents reported ever having been beaten on the bottom with a rod, compared to 41.3% 10 years earlier. Additionally, in 2002, only 3.2% of adolescents in Germany reported ever having been beaten to the point of bruising, compared to 30.6% in 1992. This study of CP experienced by German adolescents looked separately at the results found in families that reported frequently using CP compared to other, nonviolent disciplinary measures. Even in these "violence-prone" families, adolescent surveys indicated decreases in the severity of the punishments. In 1992, 54.2% of adolescents in "violence-prone" families reported having been beaten on the bottom with a rod; in 2002 this number had decreased to 29.7%. Almost all of adolescents in "violence-prone" families in the 1992 study reported being beaten to the point of bruising (98.9%), compared with only 20.1% in 2002.[49]

Police reports on physical child abuse in Sweden indicate a significant increase in the number of reported cases between 1981 and 1996; however, this may reflect an increase in Swedes' tendency to report suspected cases of abuse rather than in the true prevalence of abuse in Sweden.[44,54] According to an analysis of 182 case files dealing with child physical abuse between the 1960s and the 1990s in the district of Dordrecht, a provincial town in the Netherlands, decreases in severe child abuse rates could be detected before the legislative reform in 2007.[48] Although there is insufficient information to determine a trend in child homicides resulting from abuse, child deaths as a result of physical abuse did not decrease between 1971 and 1998 in Sweden.[44] This may reflect a type of family violence that is most severe and intractable and, therefore, not as susceptible to legislative or educational efforts.

Finally, it is important that data obtained from social service agencies on reports of child abuse is considered carefully. In Croatia, New Zealand, Norway, Romania, Bulgaria, Greece, and Portugal, official reports of child abuse, neglect, and maltreatment indicate higher rates of reporting abuse and/or higher conviction rates after CP has been legally prohibited.[55-62] These findings, however, do not necessarily reveal an increase in the prevalence of abuse. They may reflect a change in reporting bias commensurate with legislative change.

Corporal Punishment in Schools

Most countries (112) have enacted federal legislation to ban CP in the schools.[63] The United States and Australia are the only developed countries without such federal bans on CP.[63] United States federal law does not specifically prohibit CP in the schools.[63] However, 31 United States states and the District of Columbia prohibit CP in schools. In North Carolina, a state which allows CP in the schools, 55 of 115 local school districts forbid CP of students as a matter of policy.[64] The United States is the only developed country to allow CP in schools.[63] One study estimates that over 220 000 students in the United States are subject to CP in schools each year, with African American and disabled children disproportionately subjected to CP.[65] Among countries with a national ban on CP, legislation banning CP in the schools often precedes a more global ban.[63] It may reflect a societal context in which the relative place of children has improved or the relative embracing of violence as a means to control behavior has decreased. Thus, continued efforts on a state-by-state or federal basis to ban CP in schools may be a key ingredient to banning or diminishing the use of CP in the United States.[66]

Conclusion

CP is common worldwide.[67-68] It is most common among preschool-aged children.[15] A long list of potential negative consequences has been associated with CP during childhood, including child and adult mental health problems, child abuse victimization, future drug use, aggressive behavior, and criminality.[5] These consequences represent one argument for decreasing the use of CP as a tool of child-rearing. The other important argument against CP considers a child's right to be free from violence. Children are the only members of American society that are legal to hit. The UN Convention on the Rights of the Child advances a child rights–based approach to limiting or banning CP. Legislative policy against CP will always be difficult in a country or society where CP is so common and support for a parent's right to spank so widely supported. Representative governments which have successfully limited parent's right to spank have done so in the context of declining support for spanking. There may be potential to limit more severe types of spanking (eg, the use of a belt or switch) or spanking under certain circumstances (eg, very young children). In addition to policy considerations, it is critical to advance education in parenting. Parents need information about behavior modification techniques that work without violence. Parents also need to learn a variety of techniques to be most effective. Parenting programs that teach such techniques have been shown to lead to less CP, less violent discipline, and more positive discipline. Parents need such education early in child-rearing, as CP begins to emerge around 3 months of age. They need repetitive information in an accessible and developmentally appropriate format. Parent education could ultimately lead to and support productive dialogue around legislative bans on CP that would reinforce changing popular sentiment.[43]

References

1. Committee on Child Abuse and Neglect. When inflicted skin injuries constitute child abuse. *Pediatrics*. 2002;110(3):644-645.

2. Baumrind D, Larzelere RE, Cowan PA. Ordinary physical punishment: is it harmful? comment on Gershoff. *Psychol Bull.* 2002;128(4):580-589; discussion 602-511.

3. Larzelere RE, Baumrind D, Polite K. Two emerging perspectives of parental spanking from two 1996 conferences. *Arch Pediatr Adolesc Med.* 1998;152(3):303-305; author reply 306-307.

4. Focus on the Family. Discipline: wisdom for raising children in today's culture. Focus on the Family Web site. http://www.family.org/parenting/Discipline/. Accessed November 7, 2007.

5. Gershoff ET. Corporal punishment by parents and associated child behaviors and experiences: a meta-analytic and theoretical review. *Psychol Bull.* 2002;128(4):539-579.

6. Kadushin A, Martin JA. *Child Abuse: An Interactional Event.* New York, NY: Columbia Univeristy Press; 1981.

7. Gil DG. *Violence Against Children.* Cambridge, MA: Harvard University Press; 1973.

8. Smyth SM. *The Battered Child Syndrome.* London, England: Thomas Butterworth; 1975.

9. Oates RK, Davis AA, Ryan MG, Stewart LF. Risk factors associated with child abuse. *Child Abuse Negl.* 1979;3(2):547-553.

10. Straus MA, Gelles RJ. *Physical Violence in American Families: Risk Factors and Adaptations to Violence in 8145 Families.* New Brunswick, NJ: Transaction Publishers; 1999.

11. Kempe RS, Kempe CH. *Child Abuse.* London, England: Fontana/Open Books; 1978.

12. Zolotor AJ, Theodore AD, Chang JJ, Berkoff MC, Runyan DK. Speak softly--and forget the stick. corporal punishment and child physical abuse. *Am J Prev Med.* 2008;35(4):364-369.

13. Straus MA, Donnelly DA. *Beating the Devil Out of Them: Corporal Punishment in American Families and Its Effects on Children.* New Brunswick, NJ: Transaction Publishers; 2005.

14. Straus MA, Hamby SL, Finkelhor D, Moore DW, Runyan D. Identification of child maltreatment with the Parent-Child Conflict Tactics Scales: development and psychometric data for a national sample of American parents. *Child Abuse Negl.* 1998;22(4):249-270.

15. Zolotor AJ, Theodore AD, Runyan DK, Chang JJ, Laskey AL. Corporal punishment and physical abuse: population-based trends for three-to-11-year-old children in the United States. *Child Abuse Rev.* 2011;20(1):57-66.

16. Kaplow JB, Widom CS. Age of onset of child maltreatment predicts long-term mental health outcomes. *J Abnorm Psychol.* 2005;116:176-187.

17. Keiley MK, Howe TR, Dodge KA, Bates JE, Pettit GS. The timing of child physial maltreatment: a cross-domain gwoth analysis of impact on adolescent externalizing and internalizing symptoms. *Dev Psychopathol.* 2001;13(4):891-892.

18. Kotch JB, Lewis T, Hussey JM, et al. Importance of early neglect for childhood aggression. *Pediatrics.* 2008;121(4):725-731.

19. Smith JR, Brooks-Gunn J. Correlates and consequences of harsh discipline for young children. *Arch Pediatr Adolesc Med.* 1997;151(8):777-786.

20. Berlin LJ, Ispa JM, Fine MA, et al. Correlates and consequences of spanking and verbal punishment for low-income white, African American, and Mexican American toddlers. *Child Dev.* 2009;80(5):1403-1420.

21. Taylor CA, Manganello JA, Lee SJ, Rice JC. Mothers' spanking of 3-year-old children and subsequent risk of children's aggressive behavior. *Pediatrics.* 2010;125(5):e1057-e1065.

22. Zolotor AJ, Robinson TW, Runyan DK, Barr RG, Murphy RA. The emergence of spanking among a representative sample of children under two years of age in North Carolina. *Front Psychiatry.* 2011;2:36.

23. Center for Effective Discipline. Discipline and the law. Center for Effective Discipline Web site. http://www.stophitting.com/index.php?page=laws-main. Updated December 21, 2011. Accessed March 10, 2013.

24. Runyan DK, Shankar V, Hassan F, et al. International variations in harsh child discipline. *Pediatrics.* 2010;126(3):e701-e711.

25. Prinz RJ, Sanders MR, Shapiro CJ, Whitaker DJ, Lutzker JR. Population-based prevention of child maltreatment: the U.S. Triple P system population trial. *Prev Sci.* 2009;10(1):1-12.

26. Stein MT, Perrin EL. Guidance for effective discipline. *Pediatrics.* 1998;101(4 pt 1):723-728.

27. Norlin C, Crawford MA, Bell CT, Sheng X, Stein MT. Delivery of well-child care: a look inside the door. *Acad Pediatr.* 2011;11(1):18-26.

28. Rourke L, Leduc D, Constantin E, Carsley S, Rourke J. Update on well-baby and well-child care from 0 to 5 years: what's new in the Rourke Baby Record? *Can Fam Physician.* 2010;56(12):1285-1290.

29. Zolotor AJ, Burchinal M, Skinner D, Rosenthal M; Key Family Life Project Investigators. Maternal psychological adjustment and knowledge of infant development as predictors of home safety practices in rural low-income communities. *Pediatrics.* 2008;121(6):e1668-e1675.

30. Scholer SJ, Hudnut-Beumler J, Dietrich MS. A brief primary care intervention helps parents develop plans to discipline. *Pediatrics.* 2010;125(2):e242-e249.

31. Dubowitz H, Lane WG, Semiatin JN, Magder LS, Venepally M, Jans M. The safe environment for every kid model: impact on pediatric primary care professionals. *Pediatrics.* 2011;127(4):e962-e970.

32. Minkovitz CS, Hughart N, Strobino D, et al. A practice-based intervention to enhance quality of care in the first 3 years of life: the Healthy Steps for Young Children Program. *JAMA.* 2003;290(23):3081-3091.

33. Dubowitz H, Lane WG, Semiatin JN, Magder LS. The SEEK model of pediatric primary care: can child maltreatment be prevented in a low-risk population? *Acad Pediatr.* 2012;12(4):259-268.

34. DuMont K, Mitchell-Herzfeld S, Greene R, et al. Healthy Families New York (HFNY) randomized trial: effects on early child abuse and neglect. *Child Abuse Negl.* 2008;32(3):295-315.

35. Duggan A, Fuddy L, Burrell L, et al. Randomized trial of a statewide home visiting program to prevent child abuse: impact in reducing parental risk factors. *Child Abuse Negl.* 2004;28(6):623-643.

36. Letarte MJ, Normandeau S, Allard J. Effectiveness of a parent training program "Incredible Years" in a child protection service. *Child Abuse Negl.* 2010;34(4):253-261.

37. Thomas R, Zimmer-Gembeck MJ. Accumulating evidence for parent-child interaction therapy in the prevention of child maltreatment. *Child Dev.* 2011;82(1):177-192.

38. UN Committee on the Rights of the Child. General comment no. 1: the aims of education. http://www.unhcr.org/refworld/docid/4538834d2.html. Published April 17, 2001. Accessed March 10, 2013.

39. Fiji Court of Appeal. *Naushad Ali v State.* Cited in: General comment no. 8. The right of the child to protection from corporal punishment and other cruel and degrading forms of punishment. http://www.unhchr.ch/tbs/doc.nsf/898586b1dc7b4043c1256a450044f331/6545c032cb57bff5c12571fc002e834d/$FILE/G0740771.pdf. Published March 2, 2007. Accessed March 10, 2013.

40. Convention on the Rights of the Child: frequently asked questions. UNICEF Web site. http://www.unicef.org/crc/index_30229.html. Updated November 30, 2005. Accessed October 19, 2009.

41. Hodgkin R, Newell P; United Nations Children's Fund, eds. *Implementation Handbook for the Convention on the Rights of the Child.* 2nd ed. Geneva, Switzerland: United Nations Children's Fund; 2002.

42. General comment no. 8. the right of the child to protection from corporal punishment and other cruel and degrading forms of punishment. http://www.unhchr.ch/tbs/doc.nsf/898586b1dc7b4043c1256a450044f331/6545c032cb57bff5c12571fc002e834d/$FILE/G0740771.pdf. Published March 2, 2007. Accessed March 10, 2013.

43. Zolotor AJ, Puzia ME. Bans against corporal punishment: a systematic review of the laws, changes in attitudes, and behaviours. *Chil Abuse Rev.* 2010;19(4):229-247.

44. Durrant JE. Evaluating the success of Sweden's corporal punishment ban. *Child Abuse Negl.* 1999;23(5):435-448.

45. Ministry for for Affairs, Sweden. Response to the United Nation's study on violence against children. http://www2.ohchr.org/english/bodies/CRC/docs/study/responses/Sweden.pdf. Published September 17, 2004. Accessed October, 2009.

46. Ziegert K. The Swedish prohibition of corporal punishment: a preliminary report. *J Marriage Fam.* 1983;45(4):917-926.

47. Roberts JV. Changing public attitudes towards corporal punishment: the effects of statutory reform in Sweden. *Child Abuse Negl.* 2000;24(8):1027-1035.

48. Komen M. Physical child abuse and social change: judicial intervention in families in the Netherlands, 1960-1995. *Child Abuse Negl.* 2003;27(8):951-965.

49. Bussmann K. Evaluating the subtle impact of a ban on corporal punishment of children in Germany. *Child Abuse Rev.* 2004;13(5):292-311.

50. Durrant JE, Rose-Krasnor L, Broberg AG. Physical punishment and maternal beliefs in Sweden and Canada. *J Comp Fam Stud.* 2003;34(4):585-604.

51. Sajkowska M. *The Problem of Child Abuse: Attitudes and Experiences in Seven Countries of Central and Eastern Europe.* Warsaw, Poland: Warsaw University; 2007.

52. Global Initiative to End Corporal Punishment of Children. Germany: full country report. Global Initiative to End Corporal Punishment of Children Web site. http://www.endcorporalpunishment.org/pages/frame.html. Accessed October 19, 2009.

53. Janson S. *Children and Abuse: Corporal Punishments and Other Forms of Child Abuse in Sweden at the End of the Second Millenium.* Stockholm, Sweden: Ministry of Health and Social Affairs; 2003.

54. Lindell C, Svedin CG. Physical child abuse in Sweden: a study of police reports between 1986 and 1996. *Soc Psychiatry Psychiatr Epidemiol.* 2001;36(3):150-157.

55. National Statistical Institute. Punished criminality and persons convicted in 2003. National Statistical Institute Web site. http://www.nsi.bg/Stat_e/SearchFrame.htm?query=child+abuse&stpos=0&Submit=Search&stype=AND. Accessed October 19, 2009.

56. United Nations, Human Rights, Office of the High Commissioner. Response to the United Nation's study on violence against children. United Nations, Human Rights, Office of the High Commissioner Web site. http://www2.ohchr.org/english/bodies/CRC/docs/study/responses/Croatia.pdf. Published September 14, 2004. Accessed October 19, 2009.

57. United Nations, Human Rights, Office of the High Commissioner. Response of the government of New Zealand to the questionnaire from United Nation's Independent Expert on Violence Against Children. United Nations, Human Rights, Office of the High Commissioner Web site. http://www2.ohchr.org/english/bodies/CRC/docs/study/responses/NewZealand.pdf. Published 2005. Accessed October 19, 2009.

58. United Nations, Human Rights, Office of the High Commissioner. United Nations Secretary-General's Study on violence against children: questionnaire to governments: Portugal. United Nations, Human Rights, Office of the High Commissioner Web site. http://www2.ohchr.org/english/bodies/CRC/docs/study/responses/Portugal.pdf. Published 2005. Accessed October 19, 2009.

59. United Nations, Human Rights, Office of the High Commissioner. United Nations Study on Violence Against Children: response to the questionnaire received from the Government of Republic of Bulgaria. United Nations, Human Rights, Office of the High Commissioner Web site. http://www2.ohchr.org/english/bodies/CRC/docs/study/responses/Bulgaria.pdf. Published 2005. Accessed October 19, 2009.

60. United Nations, Human Rights, Office of the High Commissioner. United Nations Study on Violence Against Children: response to the questionnaire received from the Government of Republic of Finland. United Nations, Human Rights, Office of the High Commissioner Web site. http://www2.ohchr.org/english/bodies/CRC/docs/study/responses/Finland.pdf. Published 2005. Accessed October 19, 2009.

61. United Nations, Human Rights, Office of the High Commissioner. United Nations Secretary-General's Study on violence against children: questionnaire to governments. United Nations, Human Rights, Office of the High Commissioner Web site. http://www2.ohchr.org/english/bodies/CRC/docs/study/responses/Romania.pdf. Published 2005. Accessed October 19, 2009.

62. United Nations, Human Rights, Office of the High Commissioner. United Nations Study on Violence Against Children: response to the questionnaire received from the Government of the Kingdom of Denmark. United Nations, Human Rights, Office of the High Commissioner Web site. http://www2.ohchr.org/english/bodies/CRC/docs/study/responses/Denmark.pdf. Published Agust 2004. Accessed October 19, 2009.

63. Global Initiative to End Corporal Punishment of Children. Homepage. Global Initiative to End Corporal Punishment of Children Web site. http://www.endcorporalpunishment.org. Accessed June 12, 2011.

64. North Carolina Child. Fact or fiction: corporal punishment in North Carolina public schools. North Carolina Child Web site. http://www.ncchild.org/sites/default/files/Corporal_Punishment_Issue_Brief_final.pdf. Published April 2008. Accessed March 10, 2013.

65. Human Rights Watch, American Civil Liberties Union. A violent education: corporal punishment of children in the US Public Schools. http://www.aclu.org/pdfs/humanrights/aviolenteducation_execsumm.pdf. Published February 2009. Accessed March 10, 2013.

66. Corra AJ, Stephan SH. *Corporal Punishment in Schools*. Baltimore, MD: Center for School Mental Health, Department of Psychiatry, University of Maryland School of Medicine; 2009. http://csmh.umaryland.edu/Resources/Briefs/CorporalPunishmentBrief.pdf. Published March 2009. Accessed March 10, 2013.

67. Lansford JE, Deater-Deckard K. Childrearing discipline and violence in developing countries. *Child Dev*. 2012;83(1):62-75.

68. Runyan DK, Shankar V, Hassan F, et al. International variations in harsh child discipline. *Pediatrics*. 2010;126(3):e701-e711.

Chapter 12

Physical Abuse Prevention

Randell Alexander, MD, PhD
Debra Esernio-Jenssen, MD

Introduction

Physical abuse was the first form of child abuse that received substantial attention.[1] Likewise physical abuse prevention is perhaps the oldest category of child abuse prevention. Physical abuse prevention may be targeted to a specific type of physical abuse (eg, shaken baby syndrome, burns), broader aspects of physical abuse (eg, coping with crying), or linked with other forms of abuse (eg, general child abuse prevention, positive parenting programs).

Physical abuse is the commission of physical harm to a child by a caregiver through an intentional action. The caregiver may not intend to cause harm. Many caregivers who report that they spank their child and subsequently note bruising probably did not intend to leave marks. Nevertheless they employ forces serious enough to cause injury. When shaking children, caregivers are angry and probably are not thinking about the specific brain consequences of their actions. However, the range of forces they employ includes the possibility of injury or severe injury. Except perhaps for torture, this failure of caregivers not to think through the consequences of their actions is one potential opportunity for prevention intervention.

Physical abuse prevention has taken a variety of forms but may be summarized as falling into several main categories:

1. ***Awareness***: Programs aimed at shaken baby syndrome have for several decades promoted the message not to shake babies. Awareness is perhaps a cornerstone to prevention. While it is not clear that awareness alone changes behavior, it may be an important first step to gain acceptance by legislators, other potential funders, and the public. Awareness may prompt social change, which ultimately is a sustainable means for prevention. Five decades ago shaken baby syndrome was virtually unrecognized. Now it is common knowledge. While shaking violently enough to cause serious or fatal injuries would have been known by any observer as being potentially dangerous even years ago,[2] the overt awareness of this form of abuse was not. Now, prevention programs that incorporate the terminology of "shaken baby syndrome" create some familiarity and images in the mind of the general public: that shaking is bad in general and that children should not be handled this way. This awareness is very useful when tailoring a prevention approach.
2. ***General media efforts***: Similar to awareness, media through news articles (often about a tragic child abuse case) or entertainment serve to increase recognition and, to some degree, perhaps motivation about child abuse prevention. Media can both tell a story and be educational. Some burn prevention efforts have used media to promote the benefits of lowering the temperature of water heaters. It is also possible that the many stories about physical abuse cases have an inhibitory prevention effect on some individuals.

abuse, dependent adult abuse, animal cruelty, or other forms of violence/mistreatment exist. While violence can be assigned different categories by professionals, the reality of many situations is that multiple forms of overlapping violence occur. Child physical abuse prevention may be only one facet of the overall situation and primary or tertiary prevention needs to take this into account when measuring effectiveness or even considering the likelihood of effectiveness.

4. ***The caregiver often has been using video games, watching television, or using the computer immediately prior to the abuse.*** Young children in particular require frequent attention and supervision. While a caregiver distracted by video games/TV/computers may significantly increase the risk for child neglect, a caregiver may also become angered when interrupted. This is usually not in isolation, but may be coupled with a caregiver who is sleep deprived (eg, parent of an infant) or has other coexisting risk factors (eg, substance abuse). Prevention efforts should highlight that adults are likely to engage in such activities and thus steer them away from simultaneous child care and video usage, or to find ways to train caregivers how to shift from one activity to the other seamlessly. For example, having a "pause" function on a game system might allow interruption without as much adult distress.

5. ***Abusive caregivers often have inappropriate developmental expectations.*** The specific type of physical abuse may be provoked by the developmental activities of the child and possible mismatches with caregiver expectations. The specific type of abuse may also follow the age/size of the child. Examples include:

   a. Infants: Crying is part of normal development, perhaps an evolutionary adaptation to "prime" the mother's lactation. However in a modern setting with enclosed spaces, sleep deprived parents, and cultural expectations that crying babies might reflect upon the parent's capability, crying may not be seen as normal. The combination of frustrations can lead to harsh behaviors or to physical abuse. Thus a caregiver who is angry or frustrated with a crying infant would likely act impulsively wherever the infant is at the time. Abuse might consist of hitting, putting a hand over the mouth to suffocate, or shaking.

   b. Toddlers: As part of normal development, toddlers explore their environment. They test their physical skills and test boundaries set by their parents. With incomplete brain myelination, toddlers are not good at inhibiting (stopping an undesirable behavior). Redirection is a better response by a caregiver in many situations. Independent toilet training occurs at approximately 3 to 3 ½ years of age for many children. A caregiver who expects toilet training without accidents at an earlier age is at variance with actual development. Should the caregiver be angry with the pace of a toddler's toilet training, they might be in a bathroom cleaning the child and near hot water at the same time. Thus it is no coincidence that unlike impulsive hitting at the location where the irritation occurs, many bathtub burns occur during toddlerhood when the angry caregiver is adjacent to hot water.

   c. Older children: It is difficult to shake or immerse an older child. However, older children may be hit with hands or objects such as belts. Often caregivers would not hit an infant because of a cultural expectation that they are too little. Perceived infractions such as talking back, disobedience, and poor grades may elicit beatings. The abuser will often explain that this is to help the child learn.

By being aware of the spectrum of development and common inappropriate expectations by some caregivers, prevention can be better focused on development-specific education and behavior management training.

ABUSIVE HEAD TRAUMA/SHAKEN BABY SYNDROME

SCOPE OF THE PROBLEM

Shaken Baby Syndrome (SBS), a form of abusive head trauma, is caused by violently shaking an infant with or without impacting the head and leading to brain injury.[2] SBS can cause permanent neurological, developmental, and/or behavioral sequelae or death.[5] Estimates of the annual incidence of SBS range from 1200 to 1600 in the United States. Rates of SBS most typically range from 24.6 per 100 000 children under one year of age in Scotland[6] to 30 per 100 000 children under 1 year of age in one United States study.[7] The actual incidence of SBS is likely higher due to misdiagnosis and underreporting.[8,9] **Table 12-1** shows a variety of estimates for SBS from around the world. Interestingly, one argument against those who deny SBS exists is the similarity of frequencies in a wide range of studies from different countries. Epidemiologic studies have shown that premature infants, male infants, male caretakers, and having a nonbiological male living in the home are some of the risk factors for abusive head trauma.[7,10-14]

Abusive head trauma victims also have longer hospital stays and incur more direct costs than children with nonabusive serious head injuries.[15] Therefore, preventing SBS is cost effective. Friedman and colleagues found that the cost of abusive head trauma cases in New Zealand was about $836 019 (US) per child, but the projected lifetime care for disabled survivors was $26 877 950 (US).[16] Estimates in the United States for lifelong care of a brain injured infant is $14 million per child.[17] In another study, the estimated total medical cost alone attributable to abusive head trauma in the 4 years after diagnosis was $47 952.[18]

Table 12-1. Incidence of Abusive Head Trauma/Shaken Baby Syndrome in Infancy

LOCATION	WHAT IS MEASURED	RATE	CITATION
Southwest England and Wales	SDH (under 1 year of age)	21 per 100 000	Jayawant et al (1998)
Scotland	SDH (under 1 year of age [retrospective])	11.2 per 100 000	Barlow et al (1998)
Scotland	SDH (under 1 year of age [prospective])	24.6 per 100 000	Barlow et al (2000)
North Carolina	Hospital surveillance (prospective)	29.7 per 100 000	Keenan et al (2003)
Canada	Hospital surveillance (retrospective)	40 cases per year	King et al (2003)
New Zealand		14.7 to 19.6 per 100 000	Kelly et al (2008)
Estonia	Hospital surveillance (retrospective)	13.5 per 100 000	Talvik et al (2006)
Estonia	Hospital surveillance (prospective)	40.5 per 100 000	Talvik et al (2006)

Intervention Approaches

According to the American Academy of Pediatrics, "the act of shaking leading to shaken baby syndrome is so violent that individuals observing it would recognize it as dangerous and likely to kill the child."[2,19] Thus the problem is not one of knowledge (it should not be necessary to teach that stabbing a child is dangerous either), but of motivation. Compounding this is that a frequent purpose of shaking (to get the infant to quit crying) is actually accomplished by the activity (the infant is dazed, has a concussion or worse – but quiets nevertheless).[20] Programs that create awareness that shaking is dangerous have been in existence for 30 years or more, but the rate of SBS appears to be unchanged. More recently in the last decade or two there has been an increased emphasis on the point of stress/decision making versus the medical outcome of shaking per se. Rather than emphasizing that SBS is dangerous and can cause brain damage, the approaches are to train the caregiver that at the point of frustration to redirect their own activity. At the moment when the adult might shake the child, by being well trained that crying is normal, the adult can be taught to leave the room for a short period to calm down instead (ie, reduce their adrenaline level). This may be a more useful tactic.

Intervention Descriptions

Initial prevention efforts focused on public awareness of the dangers of SBS.[21] One radio campaign seemed to have promising results. On August 14, 2001, The Shaken Baby Syndrome Association of Milwaukee convinced 18 stations covering 95% of the listening audience to play the same public service announcement simultaneously. The PSA began with the incessant crying of an infant, and then followed with, "No matter how long she cries, or how frustrated you get, never, ever, shake a baby." In the 7 months prior to this PSA "radio roadblock" 26 cases of SBS were reported by local hospitals. During the ensuing 4½ months, only one child was reported to have been shaken. However the effectiveness of this campaign appears to have been time limited. The number of SBS cases at Milwaukee Children's Hospital almost doubled from 17 in 2007 to 30 in 2008.[22] (See *Volume 1, Chapter 14, "Nonprogrammatic Approaches to Child Maltreatment."*)

Another public awareness campaign was implemented during Child Abuse Prevention Month in April 2009. SBS prevention messages and images were displayed on the 11 NASDAQ and Reuters screens in Times Square New York for 2 minutes, hourly, for 3 weeks. "If you are stressed or frustrated by a crying baby. Put the baby down in a safe place. Walk away. Crying does not harm a baby. But SHAKING a baby can cause brain damage or death." And "REAL MEN have a soft touch? NEVER SHAKE A BABY!" 1.5 million people viewed these screens daily.[23] The effectiveness of this campaign in reducing SBS is difficult to ascertain.

Television is another avenue for public awareness. SBS has found its way into entertainment pop culture. In the animated television sitcom Family Guy, the star tries to comfort his wife at their infant son's grave by saying, "I thought if I shook him enough he'd stop crying…I was kinda right…" Although perverse, the message that shaking can kill is clearly dramatized.[24]

In addition to public awareness, prevention efforts included educating parents of newborns and having them commit to not shaking their baby. In 2005, the results of a hospital-based parent education program concerning violent infant shaking were published. This comprehensive program in western New York State involved maternity unit nurses distributing SBS prevention leaflets to parents of all newborns, encouraging viewing the video "Portrait of a Promise: Preventing Shaken Baby Syndrome," and asking parents to sign a commitment statement confirming the receipt and understanding of the materials. As a result of this program, there was a 47% reduction in the annual incidence of abusive head injuries in Western New York State.[25]

This study spearheaded the passage of SBS prevention education laws in New York State. As of 2012, 22 states, the Virgin Islands, and Puerto Rico had some form of SBS prevention laws.[26] Eighteen states and Puerto Rico had enacted legislation for hospitals/birthing centers to provide SBS educational materials for parents of newborns, 8 states had enacted SBS education for childcare providers, 11 states and the Virgin Islands enacted creation of a statewide public awareness campaign, 2 states require incorporating SBS curriculum in school health classes, and New York State law requires inclusion of SBS instructional materials in the education program at correctional facilities. The efficacy of these legislative efforts has not yet been determined.

The Hudson Valley Shaken Baby Prevention Initiative (HVSBPI) was modeled after the program in Western New York. The HVSBPI includes 22 hospitals in the lower Hudson Valley Region in New York State and 58 hospitals in New York City and Long Island. The initiative also utilizes a video, brochure, and commitment statement and nurse educators to remind parents about the dangers of shaking. The nurses provided this prevention message to nearly 40 000 individuals during the past 3 years. The program evaluated methods by which cases of SBS were tracked across New York State and demonstrated a downward trend in SBS cases since initiation (Jennifer Canter, MD, personal communication 2009).

Evidence supports that infant crying may be the final trigger that sets off many cases of SBS. In one study in the Netherlands, 5.6% of parents with infants aged 1 to 6 months reported they smothered, slapped, or shook their baby at least once because of its crying.[27] Another study assessed "soothing" techniques for crying infants by surveying mothers in Amsterdam. Of all respondents, 3% reported slapping the infant, 5% reported shaking the infant, and 2% reported smothering the infant to quiet it. Of the mothers who reported their infant "cries a lot," reports of shaking, slapping, or smothering increased by 2 to 3 fold.[28] A more recent American study found that 2.6% of mothers self-reported shaking their children under 2 years of age as a means of discipline.[29] Further support that frustration with trying to calm a crying infant could lead to shaking has been shown by several studies showing a temporal relationship between the peak of normal infant crying and SBS.[30-34] **Figure 12-1** shows that the 3 studies looking at the peak of SBS show an approximate 2 week "phase shift" from the peak of crying, suggesting that often SBS is the result of repeated frustrations as described in a study looking at perpetrator confessions.[20]

An indication that shaking is perceived as a means to stop an infant from crying was the release in April 2009 of an iPhone application called "Baby Shaker." The object of the game was to stop the incessant crying of a baby pictured on the screen by violently shaking the phone until 2 red "x" marks appeared over the baby's eyes. Although Apple removed this application within 2 days amid outcries from child abuse prevention and SBS victim groups, a video demonstrating this application has been viewed more than 600 000 times on YouTube.[35]

Since stress or frustration when trying to calm a crying infant may lead to shaking, prevention efforts have more recently focused on educating new parents about infant crying and alternative coping strategies. For example, Prevent Child Abuse Georgia and the Georgia Chapter of the American Academy of Pediatrics piloted a program that focused on coping with infant crying. At the 2-week, 2-month, and 4-month well child visits at the pediatricians' offices, parents are presented with the education materials and asked to sign a "crying pledge." Success of this statewide program, however, was not adequately evaluated.[36] Parents signing the crying pledge would make the following promises to their child:

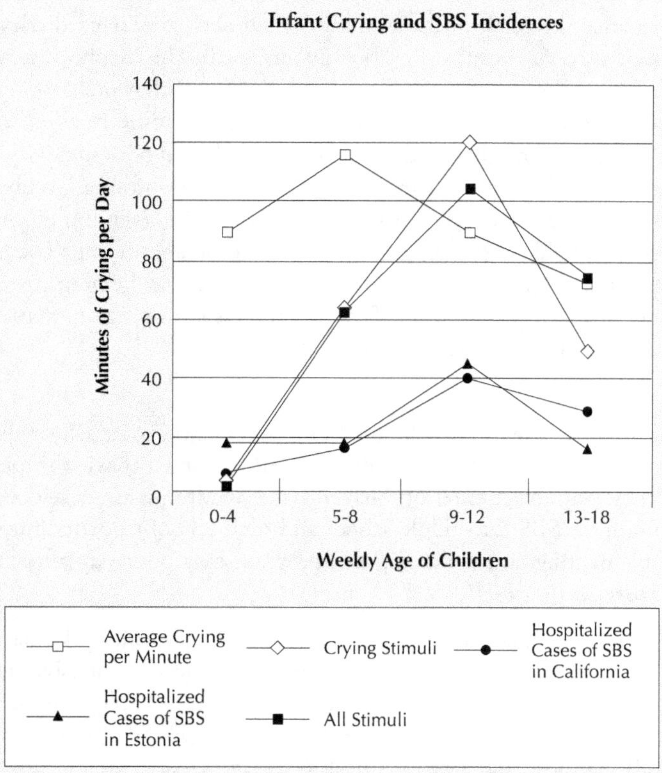

Figure 12-1

Figure 12-1. Infant crying incidence and incidence of shaken baby syndrome in 3 studies.

1. To always check to see if their baby is crying for a reason.
2. To understand that sometimes, babies cry for no reason.
3. To be calm if their baby is simply crying, even if it lasts for hours.
4. To be proud that their baby is healthy and strong.
5. To get help if they feel frustrated.
6. To teach their baby's caregivers about crying and that no one should yell at, hit, or shake their baby.
7. To sign their pledge and have all of their baby's other caregivers sign it and keep it.

Another universal approach that focuses on parent education is The Period of PURPLE Crying (PURPLE). PURPLE, developed by Dr. Ronald Barr and the National Center on Shaken Baby Syndrome, educates caregivers about normal infant crying behaviors, provides strategies to cope with crying infants, alerts them to the possibility that their infant may be shaken, and encourages them to share this information with other caregivers of their infant (www.dontshake.org). Two randomized, controlled trials used PURPLE materials to evaluate maternal knowledge and behavior regarding infant shaking.[37,38] In Washington State, mothers were recruited from prenatal classes, maternity units, and pediatric offices during a 2-year period. In Vancouver, mothers were recruited from hospitals during a 6-month period. Eighty-five percent of mothers had some college or postgraduate education. Nurses gave mothers from maternity units from both sites the PURPLE materials or control materials on infant safety during a home visit 2 weeks after the birth of their child. All mothers completed diaries at 5 weeks and a telephone survey 2 months after their infants' birth. The telephone survey included knowledge scales about crying, the dangers of shaking, behavioral responses to usual and inconsolable crying, and questions regarding sharing of information with others. Intervention and control mothers had similar demographics at both sites. Crying knowledge was higher in all intervention mothers as was sharing information about walking away if frustrated and the dangers of shaking an infant. Intervention mothers in Vancouver were also more likely to walk away during inconsolable crying. The fact that these parameters attained statistical significance is important as helping stressed caregivers cope with crying may prevent SBS. This parent education program may not generalize to male caregivers or less educated mothers.

Bottom Line

It has not been consistently shown that these existing interventions actually reduce SBS.[39] It may be more effective to broadly influence culture and behavior through educating children. The National Center on Shaken Baby Syndrome has developed a school-based curriculum on SBS for middle school and high school students (http://dontshake.org/). Implementing and evaluating this program may positively affect the future generation of parents.

Such a program was developed and implemented in Gainesville, Florida in 2010. An educational intervention for ninth and twelfth graders on abusive head trauma and safe sleep environment, the number-one cause of physical abuse deaths and the second leading cause of neglect deaths in Florida, respectively, was initiated. A 20-question test was administered prior to two 45-minute power point presentations and 4 months later on completion of both lectures. One hundred and eighty-five pretests were compared to 165 posttests. Fourteen questions elicited statistically significant differences between pre-post deployments ($p < 0.01$). Specifically, students were better able to understand that even healthy infants can cry for 5 or more hours per day. Thus, this program was effective in improving knowledge. Changing attitudes and behaviors in conjunction with other prevention efforts may reduce AHT deaths (Poster Presentation; Pediatric Academic Societies Annual Meeting; May 4-7, 2013; Washington, DC).

The Centers for Disease Control and Prevention have additional resources to assist with SBS prevention efforts (www.cdc.gov/injury). A booklet titled *Preventing Shaken Baby Syndrome—A Guide for Health Departments and Community-Based Organizations* outlines steps to: implement evidence-based intervention strategies; integrate specific education strategies into existing programs for new parents, caregivers, professionals, and the general public; engage in activities that impact policy development that is effective in preventing SBS. (See *A Journalist's Guide to Shaken Baby Syndrome: A Preventable Tragedy*.[40]) This provides background and resources to help journalists cover SBS and give their audiences a better understanding of causes and how to help with tips for coping with a crying baby, how parents and caregivers can calm themselves, how others can support parents, and additional resources.

Additional research might include:

1. How to reach the highest risk populations (eg, males—especially boyfriends, babysitters)
2. Considering how to educate about the evolutionary advantage of crying and whether such education mediates a caregiver's frustration/anger
3. Technology adjuvants such as:

a. Screening applications that might simulate crying and provide scoring for a person involved in a complex task

b. Reminders on videogames that ask for input if a child is present in the house and periodically pause or inquire

c. Crying recognition on mobile devices that can cue in on prolonged crying and attempt interventions

4. Determining how sleep deprivation and other coexisting risk factors play a role and how to ameliorate these effects.

Impact Injuries

Scope of the Problem

Impact can include hitting with hands or objects, punching, kicking, or stomping. Skin injuries constitute the most frequent form of physical abuse, with bruising being most common.[41] Bruising can occur by biting or pinching, but most commonly, it results from some form of impact.[42]

Intervention Approaches

Hitting another individual is not unique to humans but is common in all mammals. This often reflects displays of dominance, helping to define a hierarchy of power. Because forms of communication with the young are limited by the nonvocal behavioral repertoire of a parent, physical force may be employed to teach and accomplish the desired goal (eg, a mother lion snapping/gently biting her young). A key difference with humans is that they have greatly expanded behavioral choices when dealing with preverbal children and also the ability to verbally mediate with older children.

Probably the most powerful predictor of whether parents will hit a child (and possibly how hard) is how the parents themselves were raised. Thus, prevention must target this generational cycle. Prevention strategies may not be effective if parents do not wish to change their parenting style or state that their use of even harsher punishment is helpful or worthwhile for them. This may overcome their latent emotional distress in knowing that hitting and hurting a child is contrary to how adults expect to be treated by other adults.

Prevention opportunities can capitalize on how inappropriate it is to hit someone smaller and younger. Relabeling may be important. When a parent hits a child and leaves bruising and calls it "corporal punishment," the American Academy of Pediatrics distinguishes it as "abuse."[43] Thus the phrase "excessive corporal punishment" is a misnomer—it is physical abuse. By relabeling semi–socially acceptable terms such as "swat," "whupping," "whipping," "whooping," and "pop" into terms such as "hitting" or, when bruising occurs, as "abuse," some caregivers may feel less likely to engage in such actions.

Experimental psychologists have long understood the efficacy of positive reinforcement versus negative reinforcement as a means of inducing various desired behaviors. The American Academy of Pediatrics endorses alternate forms of behavior management of children instead of punishment.[44] Avoidance of physical punishment has also been endorsed by the Canadian Paediatric Society, which "recommends that physicians strongly discourage disciplinary spanking and all other forms of physical punishment. The physician's role is to take an anticipatory approach to discipline, which involves asking questions about techniques used in the home. Physicians should actively counsel parents about discipline and specifically discourage all forms of physical punishment, including the use of spanking."[45]

One approach to prevention of impact abuse would be to provide repetitive training and repetitive practice on how to implement such alternatives for caregivers, because many adults were not exposed to such methods in their own childhood. Eventually a caregiver's behavior management approach needs to be so well learned that it is instinctive and will be used even in times of stress or anger. The CDC has a program, "Essentials for Childhood," that gives advice about how to optimize behavior management.[46]

Changing the culture would be an important way to reduce such behaviors and injuries. Part of this involves increasing empathy for children's behaviors and often understanding them in the context of normal development. Observers of a parent hitting children in public can express how difficult a child can be when exhibiting certain behaviors and sometimes help to diffuse the situation. Because this is awkward and may be perceived as eliciting some caregiver hostility toward the observer or the child, many people feel helpless as to what to do. If there was extensive media demonstration of scenarios in which an observer successfully mediated with a parent hitting a child, this intervention could be expected and conventional in public.

In 1979, Sweden became the first of 50 countries to ban corporal punishment in any setting by law as of November 2016.[47] While support for corporal punishment has greatly decreased in Sweden, physical abuse statistics are not clear enough at this time to identify the magnitude of any possible decrease. A total of 117 countries have banned corporal punishment in schools (sometimes public schools only). The impact of this worldwide social change is yet to be determined. However, recent studies have demonstrated that physical punishment has significant consequences for children. Harsh physical punishment has been associated with psychiatric disorders, and maternal spanking has been correlated with externalizing behaviors in children.[48,49]

Intervention Descriptions

Modeling of positive behaviors is the focus of many physical abuse prevention programs and many programs that do not explicitly have child abuse prevention as a goal. Programs such as Healthy Families America, Healthy Start, many state early development programs, Head Start, and others attempt to help parents by didactic instruction and by modeling desired parental behaviors. Some programs are universal, but more often, they are targeted at high-risk or high-need populations. Sometimes they include tertiary prevention (prevention after the abuse has occurred), but the efficacy is uncertain when problems are of this magnitude.

Bright Futures (formerly VIPP) is a set of programs begun by the Maternal and Child Health Bureau in 1990 and focused at the American Academy of Pediatrics. It is a collaborative of other federally funded and state-funded Bright Futures projects. A broad range of health issues are addressed throughout childhood, including effective behavior management and developmental milestones.

Connected Kids is another initiative of the American Academy of Pediatrics. "Connected Kids includes a Clinical Guide and 21 handouts for parents and teens topics such as bullying, discipline, interpersonal skills, parenting, suicide, and television violence."[50]

More indirectly, programs that foster optimal child development include Reach Out & Read (http://www.reachoutandread.org/), which encourages positive interactions between parent and child in the context of improving literacy. The Medical-Legal Partnership for Children also has tips on parenting (www.mlpforchildren.org).

Bottom Line

Positive parenting programs can be shown to have educational benefits but have not been widely adopted in the population. The multitude of efforts may reflect a change in the culture (eg, versus the parenting practices of the 1800s). Whether the projects or the long-term cultural change is responsible for changed practices is uncertain. Currently, over half the states have laws that ban corporal punishment in schools. Yet all states allow corporal punishment at home in the United States. Research as to whether countries that ban corporal punishment have less physical abuse is yet to be extensively demonstrated.

A key concern is what to do? Parents who hit children often express the need to change behavior and may refer to such practices as a last resort. They may feel that they do not have any realistic options that would work or that they are comfortable using. Other parents have different beliefs and usually incorporate nonpunitive practices in a way that does not feel awkward. More research might elucidate these factors and suggest opportunities to aid parents.

For physical abuse that is more anger-driven, societal change is perhaps most likely to influence those who are otherwise difficult to reach. Special attention might be given to babysitters and to mothers' paramours as they are overrepresented in physical abuse statistics in general.

Burns

Scope of the Problem

Burns are a significant cause of pediatric morbidity and mortality and consequently, a drain on national health care resources. Fire and burns are the fifth leading cause of injury-related deaths to children in the United States. There were 128 500 children less than 19 years of age injured due to a fire or burn in 2010. Three hundred and sixty-five children died, of which 47% were less than 4 years of age.[51]

Children 2 years of age or younger who are nonwhite and male children under 18 years have the highest rates of burn-associated hospitalizations. The total cost for pediatric burn-associated hospitalizations in the United States for children less than 18 years old was greater than 2 billion dollars in 2000.[52]

Although burns are a well-recognized form of child abuse, the incidence of inflicted burns varies, ranging from 1% to 25% of burn center admissions.[53-56] Abuse victims tend to be younger, have more significant burns, and are more likely to have been scalded. Abusive burns are more common among families of lower socioeconomic status.[52]

Children whose injuries are suspicious for abuse compared to accidental burn victims of similar demographic and injury profiles also have longer intensive care stays, total hospital days, and are at greater risk of death.[57] Intentional scalds are frequently immersion injuries that are caused by hot tap water.[55,57] Burns may also occur as a result of neglect. In one center, neglect accounted for 9.3% of hospitalized pediatric burn patients. Single-parent households, parental drug use, lack of treatment for their injuries, and delay in seeking medical care was statistically more prevalent in these neglected children. Neglected children were also more likely to have deeper burns and require skin grafting.[58]

Intervention Approaches

Aside from general approaches to physical abuse prevention or promoting positive parental behaviors, there is little prevention that is specific to abusive burns. There are approaches that are targeted to the prevention of all burns—abusive or accidental.

Intervention Descriptions

Over the past several decades, many preventive interventions have been implemented to reduce pediatric burn-associated injury and decrease national health care expenditure.

As scalds caused by hot tap water are the leading cause of burns and hospital admissions, universal prevention strategies were targeted to reduce water heater temperatures to 120 degrees Fahrenheit, where it would take 10 minutes to cause a full thickness burn in adult skin. In the 1980s, Florida and Washington enacted legislation requiring water heaters to be pre-set at the factory or at installation to these lower, safer temperatures. In addition, both the American Academy of Pediatrics and American Public Health Association issued policy statements recommending that water heaters be set to less than 130 degrees Fahrenheit.[59,60] One study demonstrated that implementation of the state law was very effective as 84% of homes with water heaters installed after the law went into effect remained set at less than 130 degrees Fahrenheit. More importantly, there was a 56% reduction in scald burn admission rates.[61] Legislation in at least one major urban setting was shown to be inadequate, as many existing dwellings were not covered under the law. Tap water scald rates increased from 170 per year to 182 per year with 19 deaths and a cost of $100 million to the city after passage of the law. More than 90% of injuries occurred in residential settings, many within older constructed or renovated dwellings and thus were exempt from the existing law.[62]

Selective prevention interventions targeting high-risk groups have had some success. Smoke alarm promotion initiatives were developed to reduce residential fires, another significant cause of thermal injury and death in children. The Safe Block Project in Philadelphia targeted poor minorities in an urban setting. One component of the project involved home inspection and distribution of materials, including smoke detectors and batteries. The prevalence of smoke alarms was 19% higher in intervention areas.[63] In Oklahoma City, free smoke alarms were distributed door-to-door in an area where there were high rates of severe and fatal burns from residential fires. Serious fire-related injuries had declined by 80% in the target region 4 years later.[64] As these studies were not randomized controlled trials, systematic bias between study groups may have influenced the results.

Several studies focused on the effectiveness of community-based prevention programs designed to reduce burns and scalds in children. MacKay evaluated Project Burn Prevention, a school curriculum, community outreach intervention for adults, and mass media education campaign, in 2 communities within the Boston Standard Metropolitan Statistical Area (SMSA) from October 1977 to May 1978.[65] Two control groups were used: 2 communities also within Boston SMSA that received the mass media component of the education only, and 2 communities 100 miles away that received no intervention. Educational content included prevention of scalds, flame and smoke injuries, electrical and contact burns, and first aid for burns. To evaluate the effectiveness of the intervention, burn incidence rates and severity of injuries 4 years before, during the 8 months of the program, and for 12 months after the program were measured in the 6 communities. The school curricula did not reduce the incidence or severity of burn injuries. The community-initiated intervention may have caused a moderate and temporary reduction in burn injuries during the program as compared to before the program. Surprisingly, there was an increase in the rate of burn injuries for the communities in the intervention and control group residing within Boston SMSA that received the broadcast educational messages. The authors felt this reflected random variation in burn incidence.

Guyer and colleagues evaluated the effectiveness of the Statewide Childhood Injury Prevention Program (SCIPP) between September 1980 and June 1982.[66] Five injury prevention projects created to reduce the incidence of burns, falls in the home, motor vehicle occupant injuries, and poisonings and suffocations among children ages 0 to 5 were implemented in 9 Massachusetts cities. Included in the intervention was Project Burn Prevention. Control communities were matched on demographics including socioeconomic status, education level, ethnicity, hospital usage pattern, and characteristics of local pediatricians, school districts, and boards of health. During the 22-month study period, 42% of households participated in the SCIPP prevention projects whereas only 10% participated in Project Burn Prevention. Safety knowledge and practices increased in both intervention and control communities. However, participating households had higher safety knowledge and behavior scores over baseline via telephone survey after completion of the intervention. Burn-related injury in children 5 years and younger actually increased in both intervention and control communities, compared to baseline. This may reflect difficulties in implementing the program as well as the short evaluation time period.

Unlike the previous 2 studies, Ytterstad and Sogaard reported a decrease in childhood injury rates due to burns and scalds.[67] A community-based injury prevention program was initiated in Harstad, a city of 22 000 inhabitants in Norway in 1987 and evaluated by data received from a hospital-based injury recording system. The study was divided into a 19.5-month baseline period of no intervention and a 7-year period of education with both passive and active prevention strategies. Education was focused on both prevention including reducing hot tap water thermostat settings and cooker safeguards and immediate medical treatment of burns and scald injuries. This was accomplished through several means, one-on-one parent counseling sessions by public health nurses at the mandatory home visit 2 weeks postpartum, health fairs and shopping malls, and local media. The control city of Trondheim, although larger, had similar demographics in terms of child population, income levels, employment base and other socioeconomic factors. The mean burn injury rate decreased 52.9% after the intervention, from 52.4 to 24.7 per 10 000 person years ($P<0.05$) in Harstad. In the control city, the rates increased from 61.9 to 68.0 per 10 000 person years.

Since the mid-1990s the Internet has expanded into popular use and has become an integral component of everyday life. Capitalizing on this innovation, prevention programs could be inexpensively implemented for a larger number of individuals or communities. A study in Seattle, Washington created a Web-based intervention, "My Healthy Child" that provided information on prevention topics before a scheduled well-child visit.[68] Thirteen topics were selected for which there was a reasonable evidence base and clear prevention recommendation. Included among the topics were hot water heater temperature and smoke detectors. Eight hundred and eighty-seven children from 0 to 11 years of age were randomly assigned to 4 groups: (1) usual care (in which parents had no access to the Web site); (2) content only (in which) parents could select and access relevant topics; (3) content and notification (in which the parent selected and read about the topics, and providers had access to what the parents selected); and (4) notification only (in which parents could select topics but not access them, and providers had access to the selected topics). Outcomes were determined by telephone surveys 2 to 4 weeks after their child's visit. The results showed that an Internet-based intervention increased discussion and implementation overall. Parents in the notification/content group and in the notification-only group reported discussing more prevention topics with their providers and parents in the content/notification and in the content-alone groups reported implementing more prevention topic suggestions, such as use of a safety device. More than 80% of the study families had home Internet access. Thus, universal use of this Web site may not be feasible for other pediatric practices.

Bottom Line

Prevention efforts targeted at reducing the possibility of burns show that burns can be prevented. If the water is not too hot, it is difficult to sustain an abusive or accidental burn. If a smoke detector works, then fire burns may be decreased. Both can be set up as passive prevention—an advantage in that no decisions have to be made in a moment of anger or in a neglectful situation. They both can and should be assessed by any child protective services worker or public health nurse visiting the home.

However, a more specific opportunity to prevent at least immersion burns might be warranted. Would educational messages on disposable diapers help reduce anger when a child has a toileting mishap? Could media affect how toileting is perceived by teaching more realistic milestones? A similar opportunity also presents itself for irons and curling iron burns caused by neglect and occasionally by physical abuse.

Measurements

While neglect and sexual abuse are likely considerably under reported, serious physical abuse that results in hospitalization (or death) can be better documented and can serve as a bellwether for the larger problem of physical abuse (ie, rates of serious physical abuse likely co-vary with all physical abuse). However, for a condition as uncommon as shaken baby syndrome, it may be better to measure all serious physical abuse. For example, suppose a catchment area has 5 SBS cases per year. If next year there is a reduction to 3 cases, is this a statistically significant number? In contrast, if in the same area serious physical abuse (including SBS) averages 50 cases per year and then decreases to 30, a better statistical argument could be made that a prevention intervention made a difference.

The criteria for hospital admission for a burned child likely have not varied significantly for years. Thus the incidence of significant abusive burns could be determined largely through hospitalization data. The limitation is that abuse cases would have to be accurately identified from among all burn cases.

Undoubtedly there are many instances of physical abuse caused by hands, belts, and other objects that never get reported. Thus the proxies of known physical abuse should be understood as underestimates of the total problem.

General Approaches to Physical Abuse Prevention

Home Visiting

The incidence of premature birth, infant mortality, and child abuse was very high in Elmira, New York in the 1970s. To address these issues, David Olds, PhD developed a nurse home visitation program targeted to help high-risk mothers and their first-born infants in 1977. His program was effective in reducing child abuse and neglect.[69] Subsequently, with the support of the Robert Wood Johnson Foundation, this Nurse-Family Partnership (NFP) was expanded to include more than 20 000 mothers in 20 states across the United States.[70]

However, in the United States, for children living in poorer communities and for African Americans, there are still disproportionally higher rates of death due to sudden infant death syndrome, unintentional injuries, and homicides.[71] In Memphis Tennessee, primarily African American pregnant women with no previous live births and at least 2 of the following risk characteristics—unmarried, less than 12 years education, and unemployed—were enrolled and randomized to participate in the NFP in 1990-1991. During the 2-decade period from 1990-2011, children of mothers who were visited from pregnancy until their child's second year, were less likely to have died from preventable causes (SIDS, unintentional injuries, homicides) compared to controls. Although the numbers were small "0" versus "9", reducing child death is certainly a desirable outcome for maltreatment prevention.[72]

Intimate Partner Violence (IPV)

Nearly 1 in 5 women in the United States and 1 in 3 women globally will experience physical or sexual violence from an intimate partner during their lifetime.[73,74] Children who witness violence in their homes are much more likely to be abused and neglected. Therefore, preventing IPV would also prevent child maltreatment. SASA! is a community-based violence prevention program that may help reduce IPV in low-income settings. The acronym—Start, Awareness, Support, and Action—details how communities can identify both male and female "activists" who can educate, support, and help change behaviors associated with victims of IPV.[75]

Parental Attitudes

The use of corporal punishment is widespread in the United States as it is deeply rooted in religious, cultural, and familial beliefs.

Intergenerational transmission of corporal punishment stems from the belief that this method of discipline is appropriate, effective, and sometimes necessary.[76] Results from the longitudinal Child Development Project in Tennessee revealed that 74% of adolescents studied had experienced physical punishment, and 19% had a history of suspected physical maltreatment. Adolescents from lower socioeconomic households, African American adolescents, and adolescents who had experienced physical punishment were more likely to endorse physical punishment. Adolescents without a history of suspected physical maltreatment were less likely to endorse this discipline strategy except if they were chronic victims of physical punishment.[77]

According to a prospective study of mostly black, low-income women in Philadelphia, mothers who were physically abused as children were 1.5 times more likely to use infant spanking when compared to nonabused mothers.[78] Among an urban community sample of parents, the strongest predictors of positive attitudes toward the use of corporal punishment were perceived support by the professional from whom they sought discipline advice. Forty-eight percent of these parents selected their pediatricians, 21% their religious leaders, and 18% their mental health professionals.[79] Parents who sought advice from religious leaders compared to pediatricians had nearly 4 times the odds of reporting use of corporal punishment. Parents who were white, college educated, financially well off, had a younger index child, or were Catholic or low in religiosity were more likely to seek advice from their pediatrician, whereas previously married black parents, who were less than college educated, less financially well off, who had lower "knowledge of child development" scores, and were non-Catholic Christians or high in religiosity sought advice from religious leaders.[80]

The Multiple Indicator Cluster Survey is an international household survey developed by the United Nations Children Fund. Data from MICS3 from nationally representative samples in 25 low- and middle-income countries, conducted in 2005-2010, revealed that women who condone the notion that husbands are entitled to hit their wives were more likely to endorse that corporal punishment is fundamental to rearing children. Children in countries with high rates of domestic violence and corporal punishment are more likely to be psychologically and physically victimized. As such, harsh behaviors toward children likely result from embracing prevailing social practices rather than individual practices.[81]

Does the media highlighting celebrity child abuse, delineating the detrimental effects of corporal punishment, influence parents' child rearing? Altering attitudes and behaviors would be necessary to effect real change. And parental education may be the most helpful and healthful means. In a recent study involving children aged 2 to 8 years, their parents were randomized to a group to read either very brief research summaries on the problems associated with corporal punishment or a comparison group that read research on the relationship of daycare to child behaviors. A significant decrease in positive attitudes toward spanking was observed in the intervention group.[82]

Other

A recent study evaluated the effectiveness of 11 state policies on preventing child maltreatment. Only 2 were significantly associated with decreased child maltreatment rates: lack of waitlists to access subsidized child care and policies that facilitate continuity of child health care.[83]

Summary

Physical abuse can be prevented but not easily. Whether a project targeted to a specific physical abuse is more efficacious than a more general approach to positive parenting is not clear. What a community can do may reflect available resources, as well. Only when significant cultural change occurs in how children are treated will there be major improvement in an all-too-common aspect of childhood.

References

1. Kempe CH, Silverman FN, Steele BF, Droegemueller W, Silver HK. The battered-child syndrome. *JAMA*. 1962;181(1):17-24.

2. American Academy of Pediatrics: Committee on Child Abuse and Neglect. Shaken baby syndrome: rotational cranial injuries-technical report. *Pediatrics*. 2001;108(1):206-210.

3. Felitti VJ, Anda RF, Nordenberg D, et al. Relationship of childhood abuse and household dysfunction to many of the leading causes of death in adults. the Adverse Childhood Experiences (ACE) Study. *Am J Prev Med*. 1998;14(4):245-258.

4. Florida Child Abuse and Death Review Committee. *Child Abuse and Neglect Deaths in Florida*. Tallahassee, Florida: Florida Child Abuse and Death Review Committee; 2012. http://www.flcadr.com/reports/_documents/2012-annual-report.pdf. Accessed November 4, 2016.

5. Christian CW, Block R; Committee on Child Abuse and Neglect; American Academy of Pediatrics. Abusive head trauma in infants and children. *Pediatrics*. 2009;123(5):1409-1411.

6. Barlow KM, Minns RA. Annual incidence of shaken impact syndrome in young infants. *Lancet*. 2000;356(9241):1571-1572.

7. Keenan HT, Runyan DK, Marshall SW, Nocera MA, Merten DF, Sinal SH. A population-based study of inflicted traumatic brain injury in young children. *JAMA*. 2003;290(5):621-626.

8. Jenny C, Hymel KP, Ritzen A, Reinert SE, Hay TC. Analysis of missed cases of abusive head trauma. *JAMA*. 1999;281(7):621-626.

9. Jones R, Flaherty EG, Binns HJ, et al. Clinician's description of factors influencing their reporting of suspected child abuse: report of the Child Abuse Reporting Experience Study Research Group. *Pediatrics*. 2008;122(2):259-256.

10. Hunter RS, Kilstron N, Kraybill EN, Loda F. Antecedents of child abuse and neglect in premature infants: a prospective study in a newborn intensive care unit. *Pediatrics*. 1978;61(4):629-635.

11. Schnitzer PG, Ewigman BG. Child deaths resulting from inflicted injuries: household risk factors and perpetrator characteristics. *Pediatrics*. 2005;116(5):e687-e693.

12. Starling SP, Holden JR, Jenny C. Abusive head trauma: the relationship of perpetrators to their victims. *Pediatrics*. 1995;95(2):259-262.

13. Starling SP, Holden JR. Perpetrators of abusive head trauma: a comparison of two geographic populations. *South Med J*. 2000;93(5):463-465.

14. Starling SP, Patel S, Burke BL, Sirotnak AP, Stronks S, Rosquist P. Analysis of perpetrator admissions to inflicted traumatic brain injury in children. *Arch Pediatr Adolesc Med*. 2004;158(5):454-458.

15. Libby AM, Sills MR, Thurston NK, Orton HD. Costs of childhood physical abuse: comparing inflicted and unintentional traumatic brain injuries. *Pediatrics*. 2003;112:58-65.

16. Friedman J, Reed P, Sharplin, Kelly P. Primary prevention of pediatric abusive head trauma: a cost audit and cost-utility analysis. *Child Abuse Negl*. 2012;36(11-12):760-770.

17. Ornstein A, Dipenta JC. Abusive head trauma in infants and why we can afford to prevent it. *Paediatr Child Health*. 2011;16(2):e9-e10.

18. Peterson C, Xu L, Florence C, et al. The medical cost of abusive head trauma in the United States. *Pediatrics*. 2014;134(1):91-99.

19. American Academy of Pediatrics Committee on Child Abuse and Neglect: shaken infant syndrome: inflicted cerebral trauma. *Pediatrics*. 1993;92(6):872-875.

20. Adamsbaum C, Grabar S, Mejean N, Rey-Salmon C. Abusive head trauma: judicial admissions highlight violent and repetitive shaking. *Pediatrics*. 2010;126(3):546-555.

21. Showers J. "Don't shake the baby": the effectiveness of a prevention program. *Child Abuse Negl*. 1992;16(1):11-18.

22. Stephenson C. Radio spot to raise awareness of shaken baby syndrome. *Journal Sentinel*. May 13, 2009. Journal Sentinel Web site. http://www.jsonline.com/news/milwaukee/44891012.html. Accessed October 21, 2016.

23. Shaken babies. http://www.timessquare2.com/clientlist/shaken_babies/. Accessed May 22, 2015.

24. Juice is loose [transcript]. *Family Guy*. Fox Broadcasting Company. March 15, 2009.

25. Dias MS, Smith K, DeGuehery K, Mazur P, Li V, Shaffer ML. Preventing abusive head trauma among infants and young children: a hospital-based, parent education program. *Pediatrics*. 2005;115(4):e470-e477.

26. Shaken baby syndrome prevention legislation. National Conference of State Legislatures Web site. http://www.ncsl.org/research/human-services/shaken-baby-syndrome-prevention-legislation.aspx. Updated January 2014. Accessed October 21, 2016.

27. Reijneveld SA, van der Wal MF, Brugman E, Sing RA, Verloove-Vanhorick SP. Infant crying and abuse. *Lancet*. 2004;364(9442):1340-1342.

28. van der Wal MF, van den Boom DC, Pauw-Plomp, de Jonge GA. Mother' reports of infant crying and soothing in a multicultural population. *Arch Dis Child*. 1998;79(4):312-317.

29. Theodore AD, Chang JJ, Runyan DK, Hunter WM, Bangdiwala SI, Agans R. Epidemiologic features of the physical and sexual maltreatment of children in the Carolinas. *Pediatrics.* 2005;115(3):e331-e337.

30. Brazelton TB. Crying in infancy. *Pediatrics.* 1962;29:579-588.

31. Barr RG. The normal crying curve: what do we really know? *Dev Med Child Neurol.* 1990;32(4):356–362.

32. Barr RG, Trent RB, Cross J. Age-related incidence curve of hospitalized shaken baby syndrome cases: convergent evidence for crying as a trigger to shaking. *Child Abuse Negl.* 2006;30(1):7-16.

33. Lee C, Barr R, Catherine N, Wicks A. Age-related incidence of publicly reported shaken baby syndrome cases: is crying a trigger for shaking? *J Dev Behav Pediatr.* 2007;28(4):288-293.

34. Talvik I, Alexander RC, Talvik T. Shaken baby syndrome and a baby's cry. *Acta Paediatr.* 2008;97(6):782-785.

35. Siegler MG. YouTube Web site. https://www.youtube.com/watch?v=CAM9VFM6HzY; %20accessed%209/5/09. Published April 22, 2009. Accessed October 21, 2016.

36. Alexander R. Prevention of inflicted childhood neurotrauma-response. *Inflicted Childhood Neurotrauma: Proceedings of a Multi-disciplinary, Modified, Evidence-based Conference.* Elkgrove Village, IL: American Academy of Pediatrics; 2003:282.

37. Barr RG, Rivera FP, Barr M, et al. Effectiveness of educational materials designed to change knowledge and behaviors regarding crying and shaken-baby syndrome in mothers of newborns: a randomized, controlled trial. *Pediatrics.* 2009;123(3):972-980.

38. Barr RG, Barr M, Fujiwara T, Conway J, Catherine N, Brant R. Do educational materials change knowledge and behaviour about crying and shaken baby syndrome? a randomized controlled trial. *CMAJ.* 2009;180(7):727-733.

39. Mikton C, Butchart A. Child maltreatment prevention: a systemic review of reviews. *Bull World Health Organ.* 2009;87(5):353-361.

40. Centers for Disease Control and Prevention. *A Journalist's Guide to Shaken Baby Syndrome: A Preventable Tragedy.* Atlanta, GA: Centers for Disease Control and Prevention; 2010. https://stacks.cdc.gov/view/cdc/5865. Accessed November 4, 2016.

41. Kemp AM, Maguire SA, Nuttall D, Collins P, Dunstan F. Bruising in children who are assessed for suspected physical abuse. *Arch Dis Child.* 2014;99(2):108-113.

42. Kaczor K, Pierce MC, Makoroff, K, Corey TS. Bruising and physical child abuse. *Clin Ped Emerg Med.* 2006;7:153-160.

43. American Academy of Pediatrics Committee on Child Abuse and Neglect. When inflicted skin injuries constitute child abuse. *Pediatrics.* 2002;110(3):644-645.

44. Guidance for effective discipline. American Academy of Pediatrics. Committee on Psychosocial Aspects of Child and Family Health. *Pediatrics.* 1998;101(4 pt 1):723-728.

45. Nieman P, Shea S; Canadian Paediatric Society, Community Paediatrics Committee. Effective discipline for children. *Paediatr Child Health.* 2004;9(1):37-41.

46. Centers for Disease Control and Prevention. Essentials for childhood framework: steps to create safe, stable, nurturing relationships and environments for all children. http://www.cdc.gov/violenceprevention/childmaltreatment/essentials.html. Accessed November 4, 2016.

47. States which have prohibited all corporal punishment. http://www.endcorporalpunishment.org/progress/prohibiting-states/. Accessed November 4, 2016.

48. Afifi TO, Mota NP, Dasiewicz P, MacMillan HL, Sareen J. Physical punishment and mental disorders: results from a nationally representative US sample. *Pediatrics.* 2012;130(2):184-192.

49. Mackenzie MJ, Nicklas E, Waldfogel J, Brooks-Gunn J. Spanking and child development across the first decade of life. *J Pediatrics.* 2013;132(5):e1118-e1125.

50. Connected Kids: Safe, Strong, Secure.™ https://www2.aap.org/connectedkids/. Accessed November 4, 2016.

51. National Safe Kids Campaign. *Burn Injury Fact Sheet.* Washington, DC: National Safe Kids Campaign; 2013

52. Shields BJ, Comstock RD, Fernandez SA, Xiang H, Smith GA. Healthcare resource utilization and epidemiology of pediatric burn-associated hospitalizations, United States, 2000. *J Burn Care Res.* 2007;28(6):811-826.

53. Hight DW, Bakalar HR, Lloyd JR. Inflicted burns in children. recognition and treatment. *JAMA.* 1979;242(6):517-520.

54. Stone NH, Rinaldo L, Humphrey CR, Brown RH. Child abuse by burning. *Surg Clin North Am.* 1970;50(6):1419-1424.

55. Purdue GF, Hunt JL, Prescott PR. Child abuse by burning--an index of suspicion. *J Trauma.* 1988;28(2):221-224.

56. Thombs BD. Patient and injury characteristics, mortality risk, and length of stay related to child abuse by burning: evidence from a national sample of 15,802 pediatric admissions. *Annals of Surgery.* 2008;247(3):519-523.

57. Maguire S, Moynihan S, Mann M, Potokar T, Kempe AM. A systematic review of the features that indicate intentional scalds in children. *Burns.* 2008;34(8):1072-1081.

58. Chester DL, Jose RM, Aldlyami E, King H, Moiemen NS. Non-accidental burns in children - are we neglecting neglect? *Burns.* 2006;32:222-228.

59. American Academy of Pediatrics. Office-based counseling for injury prevention. *Pediatrics.* 1994;94(4):566-567.

60. American Public Health Association. Tap water scald injuries. *Am J Public Health.* 1979.

61. Erdmann TC, Feldman KW, Rivera FP, Heimbach DM, Wall HA. Tap water burn prevention: the effect of legislation. *Pediatrics.* 1991;88(3):572-577.

62. Leahy NE, Hyden PJ, Bessey PQ, Rabbitts A, Freudenberg N, Yurt RW. The impact of a legislative intervention to reduce tap water scald burns in an urban community. *J Burn Care Res.* 2007;28:805-810.

63. Schwarz DF, Grisso JA, Miles C, Holmes JH, Sutton RL. An injury prevention program in an urban African-American Community. *Am J Public Health.* 1993;83:675-680.

64. Mallonee S, Istre GR, Rosenberg M, et al. Surveillance and prevention of residential-fire injuries. *N Engl J Med.* 1996;335(1):27-31.

65. MacKay AM, and Rothman KJ. The incidence and severity of burn injuries following Project Burn Prevention. *Am J Public Health.* 1982;72(3):248-252.

66. Guyer B, Gallagher, SS, Chang BH, Azzara CV, Cupples LA, Colton T. Prevention of childhood injuries: evaluation of the state-wide childhood injury prevention programme (SCIPP). *Am J Pub Health.* 1989;79:1521-1527.

67. Ytterstad B, Sogaard AJ. The Harstad Injury Prevention Study; prevention of burns in small children by a community-based intervention. *Burns.* 1995;21(4):259-266.

68. Christakis DA, Zimmerman FJ, Rivera FP, Ebel B. Improving pediatric prevention via the internet: a randomized, controlled trial. *Pediatrics.* 2006;118(3):1157-1166.

69. Olds DL, Echenrode J, Henderson CR Jr, et al. Long-term effects of home visitation on maternal life course and child abuse and neglect. fifteen-year follow-up of a randomized trial. *JAMA.* 1997;278(8):637-643.

70. Goodman A. The story of David Olds and the nurse home visiting program. *Grants Results Special Report.* July 25, 2006.

71. Singh GK, Kogan MD. Widening socioeconomic disparities in US childhood mortality, 1969-2000. *Am J Public Health.* 2007;97(9):1658-1665.

72. Olds DL, Kitzman H, Knudson MD, Anson E, Smith JA, Cole R. Effect of home visiting by nurses on maternal and child mortality: results of a 2-decade follow-up of a randomized clinical trial. *JAMA Pediatr.* 2014;168(9):800-806.

73. Breiding MJ, Smith SG, Basile KC, Walters ML, Chen J, Merrick MT. Prevalence and characteristics of sexual violence, stalking, and intimate partner violence victimization – national intimate partner and sexual violence survey, United States, 2011. *MMWR.* 2014;63(SS08):1-18.

74. Devries KM, Mak JY, Garcia Moreno C, et al. Global health. the global prevalence of intimate partner violence against women. *Science.* 2013;340(6140):1527-1528.

75. Kyegombe N, Starmann E, Devries KM, et al. 'SASA! is the medicine that treats violence'. qualitative findings on how a community mobilization intervention to prevent violence against women created change in Kampala, Uganda. *Glob Health Action.* 2014;7:25082. doi: 10.3402/gha.v7.25082.

76. Holden GW, Miller PC, Harris SD. The instrumental side of corporal punishment: parent's reported practices and outcome expectancies. *J Marriage Fam.* 1991;61:908-919.

77. Deater-Deckard K, Lansford JE, Dodge KA, Pettit GS, Bates JE. The development of attitudes about physical punishment: an 8-year longitudinal study. *J Fam Psychol.* 2003;17(3):351-360.

78. Chung EK, Leny M, Rothkopf AC, Elo IT, Coyne JC, Culhane JF. Parenting attitudes and infant spanking: the influence of childhood experiences. *Pediatrics.* 2009;124(2):e278-e286.

79. Taylor CA, Hamvas L, Rice J, Newman DL, DeJong W. Perceived social norms, expectations, and attitudes toward corporal punishment among an urban community sample of parents. *J Urban Health.* 2011;88(2):254-269.

80. Taylor CA, Moeller W, Hamvas L, Rice JC. Parents' professional sources of advice regarding child discipline and their use of corporal punishment. *Clinical Pediatrics.* 2013;52(2):147-155.

81. Lansford JE, Deater-Deckard K, Bornstein MH, Putnick DL, Bradley RH. Attitudes justifying domestic violence predict endorsement of corporal punishment and physical and psychological aggression towards children: a study in 25 low- and middle-income countries. *J Peds.* 2014;164(5):1208-1213.

82. Holden GW, Brown AS, Baldwin AS, Croft Caderao K. Research findings can change attitudes about corporal punishment. *Child Abuse Negl.* 2014;38(5):902-908.

83. Klevens J, Barnett SB, Florence C, Moore D. Exploring policies for the reduction of child physical abuse and neglect. *Child Abuse Negl.* 2015;40:1-11.

Chapter 13

Primary Prevention of Childhood Sexual Abuse

Cindy Miller-Perrin, PhD
Sandy K. Wurtele, PhD

Introduction

Childhood sexual abuse (CSA) is a type of child maltreatment that refers to the "involvement of the child in sexual activity to provide sexual gratification or financial benefit to the perpetrator."[1] When perpetrated by adults, sexual abuse involves the exploitation of children's naiveté, trust, and obedience. CSA can include physical contact between a perpetrator and victim (eg, fondling, intercourse) and also "interactions" where there is no physical contact (eg, showing a child pornography, photographing or videotaping a child for pornographic purposes).

Although incidence and prevalence estimates vary depending on the participant sample and definition of sexual abuse used, it is clear that CSA is a significant public health problem in the United States as well as globally.[2,3] The results of the most recent National Incidence Study (NIS-4) revealed an estimated 180 500 children were victims of CSA in the United States during the study year.[4] In their US National Survey of Children's Exposure to Violence, Finkelhor, Vanderminden, et al[5] examined the incidence of CSA and found that 2.2% of youth experienced sexual assault or sexual abuse during 2011. In terms of childhood prevalence of CSA, 2 recent meta-analyses demonstrated that the prevalence of CSA is alarmingly high all over the world, with 18% to 20% of women and 8% of men reporting sexual abuse during their childhood.[6,7] Another meta-analysis of 55 studies from 24 countries conducted with children and adolescents found that about 9% of girls and 3% of boys are victims of forced intercourse.[8]

Sexual victimization can result in a broad range of negative short- and long-term outcomes. Compared to non–sexually abused individuals, CSA victims have been found to experience more emotional disorders (eg, depression, anxiety), cognitive disturbances (eg, poor concentration, dissociation), physical problems (eg, sexually transmitted diseases, teenage birth and pregnancy, substance abuse, coronary attacks in men), problem behaviors (eg, running away from home, violence, unsafe sexual behaviors, self-injurious behaviors), and interpersonal difficulties, including relationship distress, partner violence, sexual and nonsexual revictimization, and sexual offending in males.[9-32] CSA victims account for more than half of all individuals in the United States who receive mental health counseling or therapy, at an estimated cost of between $8.3 billion and $9.7 billion (in 1991 figures).[33] The costs of child sexual victimization to society are high, as it affects families, communities, and the entire nation.

Based on the magnitude of the problem and its association with a range of both mental and physical health outcomes, CSA has been identified as a significant public health challenge by both the US Centers for Disease Control and Prevention (CDC) and the World Health Organization.[34,35] In the public health field, consensus has emerged that the

Social-Ecological Model of the Effects of Child Abuse

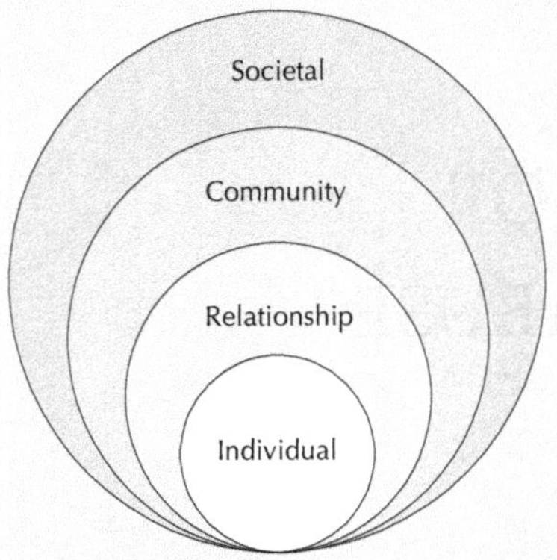

Figure 13-1

***Figure 13-1.** The Social-Ecological Model. Reprinted from Centers for Disease Control and Prevention.*[41]

etiology of many health problems (including CSA) arise from multiple levels of the ecology and that interventions focused on a single level of influence are limited.[36] The social-ecological model emphasizes that behaviors happen within a context and examines the bidirectional transactions between human beings and the systems in which they interact.[37] This process is affected by relations both between settings and by the larger contexts in which the settings are embedded. Increasingly, health-related prevention efforts are moving from a sole focus on individual-level activities to changing macrosystem characteristics, like legislation and social norms. As can be seen in **Figure 13-1**, these efforts target risk and protective factors at the individual, relationship, community, and societal levels.[38-40]

With the identification of CSA as a public health issue, there has been a subsequent call for the development of a public health approach to the primary prevention of CSA. The goal of primary prevention is to keep abuse from ever happening in the first place and provide services to everyone, regardless of risk status (ie, universal prevention). Several experts have recommended a public health approach to CSA prevention that promotes the social-ecological model.[2,3,42-49] Taking a comprehensive, ecological approach is particularly important with CSA prevention, as this form of victimization is very different from other forms of child maltreatment. Compared to physical abuse and neglect, which is more common during a child's first 6 years of life, children of all ages (especially adolescents) are at risk of sexual abuse.[50,51] In CSA, perpetrators include not only family members but adult acquaintances, including nonfamily adults serving in positions of trust (eg, teachers, mentors, religious leaders, coaches). Again, in contrast to neglect and physical abuse, sexual abuse happens in the home and often in nonfamily settings, such as youth-serving organizations (eg, sports, schools, faith-based institutions). Risk factors for CSA vary across children's developmental stages and the settings in which they develop, including institutions where youth have opportunities to form close relationships with adults outside of the home.

This chapter will describe CSA prevention strategies using an ecological framework by focusing on individual, relationship, community, and societal level targets of prevention, including children, parents/caretakers, youth-serving organizations, and society. For each of these target groups, the need for prevention efforts will be demonstrated, empirical findings about effectiveness will be presented, and suggestions for expanding these interventions will be offered.

Child-Focused Approaches: Child Education

The first ecological level focuses on the individual and identifies factors that increase the likelihood of becoming a victim; therefore, prevention strategies at this level often include education and training designed to prevent abuse.[43,52] Many child-focused prevention education programs were developed in the United States during the late 1970s and were widely disseminated in the early to mid-1980s. Unlike efforts to prevent the physical abuse or neglect of children (which focus on modifying caregiver behavior and providing family support and home visitation services), the primary focus of CSA prevention efforts has been to educate children about how to protect themselves. Most of the education has been offered to groups of children, usually conducted in educational settings. School systems became the obvious choice for teaching children about personal safety, given that their primary function is to inform and educate and also because of their ability to reach large numbers of diverse children in a relatively cost-efficient fashion. A universal primary prevention approach of this nature also eliminates the stigma of identifying specific children or families as being at risk for sexual abuse and, thus, avoids costly and intrusive interventions into family privacy.

One of the earliest programs designed for children was the Child Assault Prevention Program developed by Women Against Rape in Columbus, Ohio. Shortly thereafter, the "good touch, bad touch, confusing touch" continuum was developed by Cordelia Anderson of the Hennepin County Attorney's Office in Minnesota. Stimulated by federal funding allocated in 1980 by the National Center on Child Abuse and Neglect, several books, films, plays, and structured prevention education curricula started to appear. Many children participated in these programs; in fact, in 1990 over 85% of US school districts surveyed offered CSA prevention programs.[53] A 1993 telephone survey of 2000 young people between the ages of 10 and 16 found that 67% of respondents reported having participated in a school-based CSA prevention program at some point in their educational careers.[54] Current rates of school-based program implementation are unknown.

Most child-focused personal safety programs share common goals, including (a) helping children recognize potentially abusive situations or potential abusers; (b) encouraging children to refuse the request by saying "No," (c) teaching children to resist by getting away from the potential perpetrator, (d) encouraging children to report previous or ongoing abuse to a trusted authority figure, and (e) explaining that secret or inappropriate touching is never the child's responsibility.[55] Thus, classroom-based curricula emphasize understanding these "5 Rs": recognize, refuse, resist, report, and responsibility. Programs typically cover various concepts to help children better recognize the abusive context (eg, victims can be both boys and girls, perpetrators can be both strangers and people they know). Some programs also teach children the correct terminology for the genitals so they can effectively communicate experiences of inappropriate touching.

Need for Child-Focused Prevention Education

In general, children report minimal knowledge of sexual abuse and self-protection skills.[56] In one study of 406 children ages 3.5 years to 5.5 years, only 38% correctly recognized inappropriate touch requests; the majority regarded sexual touching as acceptable.[57] Furthermore, half of the children in this sample believed that abuse was the child's fault, and few participants thought that children should report secret touching. Few children were willing to tell anyone about the abusive incident, and even fewer knew how to report. Other research has found that although almost all preschool children know the correct terminology for nongenital body parts, very few know the correct names for genitals.[58-60] Knowing the correct terminology for genitals facilitates helpful communication regarding children's disclosures of abuse. In contrast, children who make disclosures using incorrect and idiosyncratic terminology (eg, "She touched my snake.") may not be understood and, consequently, may not receive a positive, supportive response. As a result, adults may be less likely to report abuse and child protection agencies may be reluctant to investigate reports perceived as difficult to substantiate.

Empirical Findings of Child-Focused Education

Widespread implementation of child-focused prevention programs was followed closely by efforts to evaluate program effectiveness. A sizeable number of evaluation studies have been published examining this type of programming, along with several meta-analyses. These evaluations document that both school- and preschool-aged children demonstrate enhanced knowledge about CSA prevention concepts following program participation. For example, in their meta-analysis of CSA prevention evaluation studies, reported large effect sizes for both preschool-aged children (d = .86) and elementary school-aged children (d = .98).[61] Furthermore, knowledge gains have been shown to be maintained for up to 1 year.[62] Research also shows that preschool- and school-aged children can learn certain preventive skills. In their meta-analysis, Rispens et al found a significant and considerable mean post-intervention effect size for skill gains (d = .71), and concluded that victimization prevention programs are successful in teaching children sexual abuse concepts and self-protection skills.[63] Reviews have generally concluded that school-based educational programs have a positive impact on child knowledge and self-protection skills.[63-67] After participating in personal safety classes, children have demonstrated increased ability to (a) recognize potentially abusive situations; (b) resist potential lures; (c) report abusive situations; (d) blame the perpetrator, not the child; and (e) report positive feelings about their bodies and genitals.[57]

Only 1 study has determined whether participation in personal safety programs might prevent sexual victimization. In 2000, Gibson and Leitenberg asked 825 undergraduate women to report both their past histories of CSA and participation in school-based prevention programs during childhood.[68] Young women who had not participated in a prevention program in childhood were about twice as likely to have experienced CSA as those who had participated in a program. This study provides preliminary support for the assertion that, at least for women, child-focused CSA prevention programs are associated with a decreased occurrence of sexual abuse. In his review of child-focused educational programs, childhood victimization expert Finkelhor concluded that "the weight of currently available evidence shows that it is worth providing children with high-quality prevention-education programs."[69]

What constitutes a "high-quality" program? Ample research concludes that programs incorporating modeling (eg, demonstrating the skill to be learned) and rehearsal (eg, role plays) are more effective than programs that primarily rely on individual study or passive exposure. For example, the US General Accounting Office's summary of CSA educational programs concluded that concepts and skills are better grasped when taught with active participation (eg, modeling, roleplaying, or behavioral rehearsal techniques) than with more passive methods (eg, films or lectures).[70] A similar conclusion was reached by Finkelhor and Dziuba-Leatherman who asked 2000 youth about their experiences and responses regarding actual or threatened sexual assaults.[54] Children were more likely to use self-protection strategies if they had received comprehensive prevention instruction, which included opportunities to practice the skills in class.[71] Likewise, Roberts and Miltenberger concluded that "a behavioral skills training approach to prevention results in the greatest improvement in sexual abuse knowledge and prevention skills relative to approaches involving plays, films, lecture/discussion, and written materials."[72] In their meta-analysis, Rispens et al found that resistance skill scores were higher when children participated in active-learning programs that provided multiple opportunities for children to practice the skills during the program.[63] Davis and Gidycz also concluded that "programs that allowed physically active participation and made use of behavioral skills training such as modeling, rehearsal, and reinforcement produced the largest changes in performance level."[64] Likewise, Topping and Barron concluded that effective school-based abuse prevention programs need to incorporate modeling, discussion, and skills rehearsal and be at least 4 to 5 sessions long.[65]

Expanding Child-Focused Prevention Efforts

In summary, ample empirical evidence exists attesting to the importance of behavioral skills training for teaching children self-protection skills.[73-76] Behavioral techniques that include instructions; teacher modeling of desired behavior, practice, corrective feedback, and social reinforcement produce changes in children's behavior. Such findings are significant because they justify expending the time and effort necessary to provide active practice in CSA prevention programs. Indeed, these research findings have been translated into practice guidelines. The National Center for Missing and Exploited Children (NCMEC) has published guidelines for CSA prevention programs.[77] These guidelines suggest that prevention programs (a) use developmentally appropriate language, content, and teaching methods; (b) use behavior rehearsal, roleplaying, and feedback to teach skills; (c) occur on multiple occasions over several years and include periodic reviews and supplemental sessions to reinforce skills; and (d) include homework and active parental involvement.

Despite empirical evidence and NCMEC recommendations to employ behavioral approaches to teach personal safety skills, a survey of 87 select CSA prevention programs found that only 37% of programs used roleplay activities for the children to practice the skills.[78] Instead, children were much more likely to be shown movies or videos (74%) and the majority (63%) of programs used one-time sessions to educate youth. Inadequate programming may be due to limited resources, a problem reported by over 70% of the programs surveyed. It may also be driven by the pressures on schools for accountability, perhaps accelerated in the United States by the No Child Left Behind Act of 2001, which has forced educators to focus on improving test scores in reading and mathematics, leaving less time for implementation of "social-emotional programs."[79] CSA prevention programs also compete for limited time during the school day with prevention programs targeting other social problems (eg, bullying, dating violence, sexual harassment). Letourneau and colleagues have also suggested that failure to implement CSA prevention programming may be due to policy resistance resulting from not only the complex and poorly understood nature of CSA, but because it engenders strong emotional and defensive responses that limit objective discussion of its prevention, causes, and consequences.[2]

Child-focused prevention programs have been criticized for expecting children to be solely responsible for their own protection and for overemphasizing secondary prevention (ie, disclosing abuse) while underemphasizing primary prevention (ie, stopping the development of perpetrating behaviors). Stopping the development of sexual offending behaviors among youth must be emphasized by helping children and youth develop healthy relationship skills, promoting healthy sexuality and acceptance of sexual diversity, and helping youth understand the moral and legal consequences of sexually disrespectful and exploitative behaviors.

More work is needed to develop and evaluate educational materials for prepubescent youth (ie, "tweens") and teenagers. As adolescence is a key developmental risk period for the onset of CSA offending, educational approaches should prepare youth as they begin to experience sexual thoughts, feelings, and attractions to others (starting around age 10); help them adjust to the biological and physical changes of puberty (generally starting between ages 10 and 14); and assist adolescents with the transition to establishing sexual partnerships.[80-83] Given that adolescents are the perpetrators in a significant minority of CSA cases (between 20% and 50%), youth (ie, preteen, early adolescents) need to be taught that it is morally and legally wrong to sexually experiment with or exploit children.[84] In addition to targeting this age group, innovative ways to educate teens about sexuality and prevention of exploitation are needed (eg, using the Internet or online interactive games). Evaluations of Web-based training to prevent CSA are appearing and showing promise.[85]

Another criticism of child-focused prevention programs has been the lack of attention and sensitivity to diverse populations and specific cultural values of participants. Some programs shown to be effective for building knowledge and skills among children in an average socioeconomic environment have been less effective in a multiethnic and underprivileged urban environment.[86,87] Plummer's review of 87 child-focused CSA prevention programs found that just 17% of programs addressed diversity, while only about one-third addressed special needs populations (ie, deaf, developmentally or physically disabled).[78] Children who are deaf or hard of hearing (DHH) are at increased risk of sexual abuse, particularly DHH youth who attend residential schools for the deaf.[88] Encouragingly, guidelines and research are beginning to fill this void. McEachern provides much-needed guidance for adapting prevention information for children with disabilities.[89] In another study, researchers examined changes in children's knowledge of sexual abuse prevention concepts using a culturally tailored school-based curriculum that was implemented in diverse communities across Hawaii.[90] Students attending intervention schools significantly increased their knowledge of appropriate and inappropriate touch and what to do if they experienced sexual abuse, as compared to nonintervention schools.

Another study attempted to target ethnic diversity by administering a personal safety educational program designed for Latino families attending preschools in a large metropolis.[91] Compared to a control group, Latino children who completed the program showed significant improvements in all measures of CSA-related skills and knowledge, with essentially no negative side effects. Although these initial findings are promising, more efforts to meet the unique needs of diverse populations (eg, sexual minority youth, special needs children, immigrant children) and specific cultural values are needed.

Parent-Focused Approaches: Education and Support

A logical partnership to enhance the efficacy of child-focused prevention strategies is with children's parents, who play key roles in the sexual socialization of their children.[92] Forming a prevention partnership with parents has long been recommended and has many advantages.[93-97] One role parents can play in prevention efforts is to support their child's participation in a school-based program. Parents who have concerns about these programs or believe they may endanger or harm their children may refuse to allow them to participate. By consenting to have their children participate in school-based programs, parents indirectly support prevention efforts. Parents can also be enlisted to provide more direct support as adjunct teachers of personal safety.

When parents are trained to be prevention educators, their children receive repeated exposure to prevention information in their natural environment, thus providing booster sessions to supplement classroom presentations. Involving the family in the educational process may help reduce the secrecy surrounding the topic of CSA and can stimulate parent-child discussions about sexuality in general.[98,99] Encouraging parents of preschool-aged children to discuss this topic at home may help prevent abuse at early ages, before the children have an opportunity to participate in a school-based program. Educated parents would also be better able to identify child victims and respond appropriately to victim disclosures.

Another reason for targeting parents is that the home is the most proximal level of the child's ecology. Parents can do much to make the home environment safer for their children. Many of the factors that heighten a child's risk for sexual exploitation relate to the home environment (ie, lack of supervision or privacy, presence of unrelated males, restricted parent-child communication about sexuality, high-frequency use of substitute caregivers, etc). Parent-directed educational programs have the potential to build assets in the home and reduce the child's risk for being sexually abused.[100] Parents can also be provided with suggestions about how to limit access of potential perpetrators to their children. For example, parents could be trained to "safety-screen" potential babysitter candidates, romantic partners, households in which their children play, and youth-serving community programs.[101-104] By following the tenets of the situational prevention model for CSA, parents can be informed about ways to modify their home environments to reduce the risk of sexual abuse, eliminate interactions between potential perpetrators and their children, and to increase the supervision and guardianship of their children.[80]

Need for Parent-Focused Prevention Efforts

Preliminary research provides support for parental involvement in personal safety education. Several surveys of parents have shown that the majority of parents strongly support the education of children on this topic and that parents are receptive to learning more about CSA.[94,93,105-108] Results from these surveys also show that parents have much to learn about CSA. There are many myths about CSA held by the public in general and parents in particular—myths which may affect a parent's willingness to allow his or her child to participate in a personal safety program. For example, parents who believe that their children are at low risk for sexual exploitationor are too young to understand the topic[106] may not support their children's personal safety education.[109,110]

Despite alarming rates of CSA, along with adults' fears of child sex offenders, few parents discuss CSA with their children, although parent-child communication about CSA is increasing.[107,108,111-115] Furthermore, some of what parents tell their children is inaccurate. For example, parents have described child molesters as "dirty old men" or, most frequently, as "strangers."[105,108,113,116-120] Rarely do parents include family members, relatives, substitute caregivers, teenagers, or trusted authority figures in the list of potential perpetrators, despite the fact that these are the most likely perpetrators of sexual abuse.[121] Parents are also more likely to warn children about being lured into a car by strangers than they are to discuss the types of ploys perpetrators use to engage children in inappropriate sexual interactions, including emotional coercion, bribes, and threats.[122] Parents need to be informed about how to identify potential offenders, the types of ploys and manipulations molesters use to gain the trust and acceptance of the child (and often the child's parent), and how to talk to their children about this threat. Given the potential for children to be abused via cyberspace through online sexual solicitation and access to pornography, it is critical that parents also be informed about safe Internet use and how to talk to their children about online safety.[123,124]

Empirical Findings of Parent-Focused Efforts

One way parents have been involved in the education of children about CSA is when schools inform parents about personal safety programs being implemented in the classroom. Typically, parents are invited to view the materials before program implementation. According to Kolko et al, parents who attended the informational meetings demonstrated greater improvements in knowledge and reported enhanced communication in the home about CSA 6 months after the meeting.[125] Likewise, MacIntyre and Carr reported significant increases in knowledge scores and attitudes toward prevention programs among the parents attending an informational meeting about the Stay Safe program in Ireland.[126] Unfortunately, attendance at these informational meetings has been quite low (eg, 21% of parents in a study by Tutty, 20% in a study by Hébert et al), and fathers rarely attend.[86,94,107,109,120]

Other programs send handouts home to parents describing the skills and concepts their children are learning in the classroom. In 1995, Finkelhor and Dziuba-Leatherman[54] reported 11% of programs sent materials home to parents. In Plummer's review of 87 child-focused programs, only half provided take-home educational materials.[78] The depth and effectiveness of these parent-focused efforts are unknown.

There have been a limited number of studies evaluating standalone parent educational workshops. Campis et al recruited 165 mothers of elementary school-aged children to read educational materials about CSA and then complete a questionnaire asking about their intentions to present the information to their children.[127] The strongest intentions to inform their children about sexual abuse came from parents who had read material designed to enhance their self-efficacy beliefs. In a subsequent investigation of parental self-efficacy beliefs, Burgess and Wurtele randomly assigned 45 parents of preschool-aged children to participate in either a CSA prevention workshop or a home safety presentation.[128] Parents who participated in the CSA workshop reported significantly greater intentions to talk to their children about CSA, as compared to the control group. At follow-up, the workshop parents also reported having had significantly more discussions about CSA with their children compared with the control parents. As predicted, parents' self-efficacy beliefs were significantly related to intentions, and intentions predicted parent-child communications. In 2008, Wurtele et al evaluated a 3-hour educational workshop designed to inform parents about CSA, promote parent-child communication about the topic of CSA, and help parents create safer environments for their children.[129] Subsequent to the workshop, parents significantly increased their knowledge about the characteristics of perpetrators and reported increased parent-child communication about CSA. Findings were limited by the small and select sample, and the effects of the parent workshop on children's knowledge and skill levels were not determined.

Parents can also be recruited to educate their own children about CSA. With a few exceptions, extant research suggests that parents can effectively teach their children to recognize, resist, and report CSA.[98,99,130-132] Studies have also demonstrated that preschoolers retain more knowledge about correct genital terminology when taught by parents as compared to teachers.[60,133]

Expanding Parent-Focused Prevention Efforts

Although there are many advantages of having parents talk to their children about CSA, there are several challenges to developing a full partnership with parents. Home-based educational approaches would be difficult to implement with families experiencing abuse and/or dysfunction. Children in these homes not only need personal safety education at school, but finding a way to intervene with the parent(s) should be a priority. Additionally, school-sponsored workshops for parents tend to be poorly attended. More research is needed to identify predisposing factors for parent participation in CSA prevention programs.[109,110,134] Research is also needed to determine more effective ways of reaching parents. Possible venues include offering brown-bag lunches at the parents' worksites or having employer- or health care–sponsored workshops. Other potential sites for groups of parents include their own homes, parenting centers, medical establishments, faith-based institutions, libraries, or other community agencies. Early childhood home visitation programs, showing promise in preventing child physical abuse and neglect, could incorporate personal safety and children's sexual development into materials given to parents.[51] Internet-based interventions (IBIs) may be especially useful for youth and their parents, yet few existing IBIs are aimed at children, adolescents, or parent-child dyads.[135] Web-based interventions can reach a large population at relatively low cost and can be accessed privately and conveniently from the household—a plus for parents who may be reluctant or unable to attend school-based workshops. Future research also needs to develop and evaluate in-home educational materials, particularly materials describing how parents can eliminate potentially risky situations and create safer environments for their children.[102,104,122] In addition, Wurtele has suggested that routine well-child examinations afford excellent opportunities to (a) educate children and their parents about normal sexual development and inappropriate sexual behavior, (b) facilitate parent-child communication about sexual issues, (c) provide guidance to parents on handling young children's sexual behavior (eg, masturbation, peer sex play), (d) encourage parents to provide developmentally appropriate personal safety education, and (e) strengthen parents' awareness and vigilance of situations that might increase their child's risk for CSA.[136]

Community-Focused Approaches: Youth-Serving Organizations

The third ecological level focuses on settings (eg, schools, workplaces, neighborhoods) where social relationships occur. Prevention strategies at this level should theoretically impact the climate, processes, and policies in such systems.[43,137] Youth-serving organizations (YSOs) are an example of such systems and include establishments, organizations, and clubs that serve children for various purposes. They include schools, youth groups, youth correctional and residential treatment facilities, faith-based institutions, and recreational or sporting clubs. As noted by Trocmé and Schumaker, "participation in these activities provide children with important protective factors against sexual abuse, including increased self-esteem and skills development, relationships with adults outside the home who may act as role models and confidants, and relationships with peers."[138] Many of these organizations promote close and caring relationships between youth and adults outside the family, but this same closeness and trust can provide opportunities for CSA to occur.

Sexual abuse in YSOs can be approached through the lens of situational prevention theory that shifts attention from an exclusively individual-level focus to the context in which the potential offender and potential victim interact.[139] Situational prevention of CSA depends on a thorough understanding of abusers' characteristics; how they select and groom their victims, and the characteristics of the settings that might contribute to abuse. The concept of institutional betrayal (ie, institutional action and inaction that exacerbate the impact of sexual trauma) is another useful heuristic to guide empirical examination into these systemic factors within YSOs.[140]

In the vast majority of accounts of CSA occurring in YSOs, perpetrators obtain a trusted role or position where they have access to and power and authority over vulnerable children. Some sex offenders purposefully choose their work for the opportunity it presents for targeting and sexually abusing children. Sullivan and Beech refer to these offenders as "professional perpetrators."[141] Perpetrators are often trusted by other adults (ie, staff members, parents) and set up or take advantage of opportunities to be alone with and sexually exploit children. As noted by Moulden, Firestone, and Wexler, professional perpetrators are difficult to detect due to their "unsupervised access to victims and the trust that is bestowed upon them."[142] Along with privacy, power and authority are the most important ingredients that enable a person to coerce a child into sexual compliance.[104]

Need for Community-Focused Prevention Efforts

Although the exact prevalence of CSA in YSOs is unknown, news reports clearly demonstrate that CSA in institutional settings is a serious problem. Research reports are beginning to appear that confirm these observations. Research in the United States has revealed widespread sexual abuse of children by Catholic priests, teachers or other school employees, employees of youth detention and treatment facilities, and staff in youth groups such as the Boy Scouts of America.[143-151] CSA in formal and informal daycare facilities has also been reported.[152] CSA has been documented in several competitive sports, including hockey, swimming, gymnastics, basketball, wrestling, and football.[153-163] Although few researchers have conducted surveys of youth in YSOs about sexually abusive experiences, initial studies suggest that approximately 10% of youth report incidents of staff sexual misconduct.[146,149]

In addition to the magnitude of CSA in YSOs, there is also evidence that employees in YSOs lack awareness of and knowledge about the problem of CSA. In 1 study that examined the perceptions of youth sport administrators relating to child maltreatment in general, the administrators tended to view child abuse as a problem within society, but they did not always believe it was a significant issue within their own organizations.[164] In the same study, one third of administrators were not confident in their ability to detect child sexual abuse. In addition, nearly one third of respondents were unsure or did not believe they should be mandated reporters. Studies evaluating teachers' knowledge and understanding of child maltreatment find that many teachers report a lack of knowledge, and the majority of teachers report receiving inadequate training in child abuse signs, symptoms, and reporting procedures.[53,165,166]

CSA prevention experts also note the existence of several characteristics of organizations that might increase the risks of sexual abuse, including physical and cultural characteristics.[80,103,167] Physical characteristics of facilities that might increase risk of victimization include offices and classrooms with no windows or lack of security cameras in high-risk areas. There are also several conditions related to agency culture that can contribute to CSA in YSOs. One example of the influence of agency culture was illustrated in the Freeh Report, produced by a law firm that investigated the facts and circumstances surrounding the Penn State Sandusky scandal.[168] The report concluded that the "culture of reverence for the football program" contributed to the most influential leaders at the university placing the interests and image of the football program before the safety of children. Other agency cultural barriers that threaten the safety of children include leadership that lacks awareness about issues related to child abuse, transparency in decision-making, and open discussion and dissent.[103,168,169] In addition, agencies that instill an environment not conducive to reporting and acting on incidents of abuse, such as concerns over the agency's image, also put children at risk.[103,168,170] Many YSO cultures also adhere to a "code of silence," whereby individuals do not act or report abuse incidents because they fear repercussions (eg, being branded as a traitor, reprisal from supervisors).[168,171,172]

Empirical Findings of Community-Focused Efforts

One potential prevention strategy for YSOs is to screen out potential perpetrators from obtaining positions in these institutions.[103,164,173] Most YSOs conduct criminal background checks on all employees and volunteers working with children; applicants' names can also be checked against the state's Sex Offender Registry. However, criminal history record checks and sex offender registries will not identify most sexual offenders, because the majority of people who commit sex offenses do not get caught, let alone convicted. For example, Smallbone and Wortley found that more than three-quarters of their sample of CSA offenders did not have previous sexual offense convictions.[174] As suggested by Kendrick and Taylor, although criminal checks are not the sole answer, they can act as a deterrent.[175] Wurtele and Kenny recommend additional methods for thoroughly screening staff, including administering personality tests or instruments assessing potential for abusing children, conducting informal Internet searches, in-depth personal interviews (eg, asking applicants about their motives for wanting to work with children, substance abuse problems, and past rule-breaking or nonsexual criminal activities), and reference checks.[37] In the guidebook, *Preventing Child Sexual Abuse Within Youth-Serving Organizations*, Saul and Audage suggest that interviewers describe possible scenarios that involve personal boundary issues or youth protection policy violations in order to gauge the applicant's response.[173] These authors also recommend informing applicants about an organization's policies and procedures relevant to CSA prevention. Likewise, Finkelhor urges organizations to do "foreground checks," meaning that the topic of child protection be brought to the "fore" in recruitment and hiring.[121] Saul et al also recommend requiring an applicant to sign a document that describes the agency's commitment to protecting children and its expectation that employees will abide by this policy.[49] By emphasizing child protection, it sends a very clear message: children in this organization are "off limits" to sexual abusers.[104]

In addition to implementing stringent screening procedures, organizations can also establish policies to reduce high-risk situations.[37,103,164,173,176] One strategy to prevent CSA in institutions is to minimize opportunities for staff to be alone with children. Some organizations have a policy limiting one-on-one interactions between youth and adults. For example, Boy Scouts of America (BSA) has a "two-deep leadership" policy, which requires that at least 2 adults be present on all trips and outings.[177] BSA also prohibits youth workers from transporting children alone in a vehicle. Another high-risk situation is when staff has contact with youth outside the context of the program. Organizations can set a policy limiting contact between staff and youth to organization-sanctioned activities.[37] Other YSOs have developed codes of conduct providing clear guidance to staff on standards of behavior. Several standards of practice for preventing the sexual abuse of children in sports are also available.[178-181]

Once selected for positions, it is critical that in-service training programs be offered to all employees and volunteers to raise their awareness of CSA in YSOs.[103,173] Trainees need opportunities to discuss ethical principles underlying their care of youth, particularly the need to maintain professional boundaries, knowing what constitutes sexual misconduct, and acknowledging the potential for exploiting their greater status and power. Training should also be provided to staff on how to recognize and respond to questionable behaviors exhibited by fellow staff members (ie, when a coworker has a special relationship with a particular child, is seen touching the child in questionable or inappropriate ways, or communicates with a child via cell phone, e-mail, text messages, letters about personal or intimate issues. Education in the identification and reporting of CSA is available at both the pre-professional and in-service levels for early childhood educators, teachers, school counselors, and medical professionals.[182-189]

Evaluations of these training programs are scarce. One adult-focused CSA prevention program is offered by Darkness to Light (D2L), whose mission is to empower adults to prevent CSA. Darkness to Light's[192] Stewards of Children program teaches adults in YSOs (ie, staff, volunteers, parents) how to prevent, recognize, and react responsibly to CSA. The program is available both in-person and online (at a cost of $10 per person).

Topics include:

1. Prevalence rates, risks, and consequences of CSA
2. Ways to minimize opportunities for CSA to occur
3. Talking about CSA with adults and children
4. Recognizing signs and symptoms of CSA
5. Responding to a child's disclosure
6. Acting on suspicions and using intuition
7. Getting others involved in preventing CSA

Rheingold and colleagues have conducted studies showing the program's promise for efficacy and have also compared different formats, both in-person and Web-based.[191,192]

YSOs also need to develop monitoring and supervision protocols.[103,164,173,193] All employees and volunteers should be informed about the monitoring protocol and clear about their roles and responsibilities regarding reporting inappropriate or harmful behavior. A well-designed supervisory plan can reduce the risks of sexual misconduct. Organizations must also have policies for dealing appropriately with allegations of staff-child and youth-on-youth sexual abuse. It is also essential that there are easily accessible ways for children to disclose abuse. Saul et al[48] recommend empowering youth as partners in the prevention process by encouraging them to intervene or tell someone when they see inappropriate interactions between adults and youth or between youth (ie, encouraging bystander intervention). Similarly, Finkelhor recommended that a bystander mobilization strategy be incorporated into both adult- and child-focused CSA education.[194]

Expanding Community-Focused Efforts

Encouragingly, several YSOs have adopted many of the above strategies in an effort to stop the exploitation of youth in their care (eg, Boy Scouts of America, Catholic Dioceses of Wilmington, USOC's "Safe Sport" program). Although the various strategies described previously may be potentially promising ways to prevent CSA from occurring in YSOs, the research available to confirm their effectiveness is very limited.[195] As Saul et al caution, "without a solid evidence-base, it is impossible to know if the current prevention strategies employed by youth-serving organizations are making the difference they set out to make."[49] More evaluation research examining the effectiveness of prevention policies in YSOs is needed.

Another issue worthy of consideration in expanding community-focused prevention efforts is the number of potential problems that have been identified in implementing prevention policy and other measures designed to protect children in institutions. Lack of personnel and resources to implement mandatory educational programs for staff is a frequently mentioned problem.[103,176,195,196]

Wurtele recommends several suggestions to help agencies defray costs, including partnering with other organizations to develop and implement in-service training and using more informal training approaches (eg, roundtable discussions, accessing resources on the Web or in handbooks, brown-bag lunch discussions).[103]

Another potential problem to implementing CSA prevention is reticence on the part of employees about addressing the subject. Agency administrators are sometimes concerned that pushing prevention may arouse fear within the organization, possibly leading members to worry that measures are being implemented because sexual abuse exists in their organization.[195] Staff members might also become fearful of false allegations due to heightened sensitivity and monitoring by parents, coworkers, and supervisors about engaging in various forms of nonsexual physical contact (eg, e-communication, social media with students).[197-199] There may be denial among employees and administrators that CSA abuse exists within their organization, with many refusing to believe that their colleagues are capable of such behavior.[103,200] Believing that sexual boundary violations are committed by "professional perpetrators" can result in an "us versus them" attitude and lead to a denial of the inherent vulnerability to commit this type of transgression.[103] Letourneau et al argue that such polarization is the result of media coverage about CSA that promotes angry or fearful responses to the problem, resulting in the perception of "CSA perpetrators as monsters who are nothing like ourselves."[2] To break through this denial, Celenza and Gabbard suggest asking trainees to explain why sexual misconduct does not occur in most staff–youth relationships.[201] Trainees can then brainstorm answers to the question: "What are the safeguards other staff employ to prevent crossing those boundaries?"

Administrative difficulties have also been cited as a potential problem to implementing CSA prevention policies.[166,176,195,202] Noble and Vermillion observe that while administrators of sports programs may be well-versed about their child protection policies, they may encounter problems in carrying them out, such as delays in criminal background checks or reluctance to share information about offending coaches.[164] Similarly, Hartill and Lang describe some of the challenges faced by those charged with implementing child protection and safeguarding policies in sport, including lack of support from senior management.[204] In her comprehensive exposé of USA Swimming's sordid history of handling sexual abuse cases, writer Rachel Sturtz points out the significant limitations of having a sporting organization adjudicate sex crimes in its own ranks.[161] Several experts have called for an independent national body or center to oversee the safety of children in YSOs In addition, materials for youth explaining their rights to learn, play, and socialize in abuse-free environments are sorely needed.[2,44,47,136,203,204]

Society-Focused Efforts: Public Awareness and Statewide Programming and Policy

In addition to focusing on individual, relationship, and community levels, a public health approach to preventing the sexual abuse of children necessarily focuses on macro-level factors that exist within society and culture. This fourth ecological level emphasizes the broad societal factors that impact the cultural climate around CSA, such as social and cultural norms and social policies.[43,52] Unfortunately, very little research has addressed societal-level risk factors for CSA, despite the calls for prevention efforts targeting adults and systems within the broader society.[205]

It is important to identify and consider social norms, shared beliefs and attitudes, and statewide programming and policy around the issue of CSA and its prevention. Norms and policies that support abuse (or fail to condemn it) can be used to justify abusive behavior and practices, excuse perpetrators' actions, and blame victims for events while trivializing or minimizing their suffering. Attitudes, programs, and policies toward CSA are indicators of the level of the status afforded to children within a given society, the level of knowledge commonly held about the issue, and the public's willingness and motivation to confront it.[205]

Need for Society-Focused Prevention Efforts

Social attitudes in the United States about CSA have varied over time, and even today, there is no consensus that sexual interactions between an adult and child is an abusive and harmful problem. Although there is no doubt that CSA is recognized by many today as a significant social problem, both the media as well as researchers have often used neutral terms to describe CSA. They refer to it as "childhood sexual experiences" or "adult-child sexual contact," suggesting that such interactions are neither abusive nor harmful.[206,207] Empirical research has also formally examined attitudes of the general public toward CSA, and suggests that many American attitudes reflect a lack of knowledge about the problem. A study by the advocacy organization Stop It Now! found that only 44% of a large sample (N = 5241) reported that CSA was a major problem in their community.[208]

One key societal factor in shaping attitudes and norms related to CSA, and in shaping public policy, is the media. Given that mass media shapes the way we think about social problems, media campaigns could be used to transform CSA from a shameful individual secret to a more public issue, to encourage more bystander intervention, and to shift from an exclusive focus on "stranger danger" to help the general public recognize more common perpetrators of CSA. In the past, the news media has perpetuated the "stranger danger" misconception.[209-211] In addition, media accounts have often served to inappropriately "frame" the problem of CSA by either promoting "angry and fearful reactions" (eg, by presenting rare and extreme cases as if they were commonplace and by replacing predictability with randomness) or by promoting "victim blaming" (eg, by introducing skepticism about a victim's report or shifting blame to the victim). These reactions result in either unduly vilifying perpetrators or ignoring and minimizing the seriousness of CSA, respectively.[129,130] Indeed, in a recent review of media coverage, Mejia et al found that CSA remains largely absent from the news, unless there is a high-profile case to report.[212]

Other reviews of news coverage of CSA cases suggest that the news tends to report on criminal justice responses rather than contextual information about causes of and solutions to CSA. In a review examining news coverage appearing between 2007 and 2009, Dorfman et al found that stories about CSA typically focused on the criminal justice details of specific incidents, thereby making CSA crimes appear as though they occur in a vacuum and are not the product of broader social conditions.[213] In addition, prevention-oriented solutions rarely appeared. Only 18% of articles described some type of preventive measure, and half of these suggested prevention education for children and their parents. By contrast, only 7 articles (4% of total) suggested policy changes or other broader scale prevention activities focused on either potential victims or potential perpetrators. Only 2% of the articles advocated for broad changes in the media as a preventive measure, such as reducing the amount of sex shown on television. Other reviews of news coverage have found similar voids and biases in news coverage.[212,214] Clearly there is a need to move attitudes about CSA beyond a criminalization perspective to include a view of CSA as a public health threat warranting primary prevention efforts.

Empirical Findings of Society-Focused Efforts

One approach to addressing macro-level societal factors is through public education, which has primarily been delivered through various media campaigns. Although a range of technologies (eg, television, Web sites) have been employed to reduce child (physical) maltreatment, few media campaigns targeting CSA have been mounted in the United States.[215] One exception is the Stop it Now! campaign developed by a nonprofit advocacy organization in Vermont which is one of the best known examples of this type of prevention programming.[208] The program operates through public education and media campaigns aimed at the public at large, as well as adult offenders, those at risk of offending, parents of youth with sexual behavior problems, and families and close friends of these individuals. Prevention messages are delivered through newspaper advertisements, television and radio ads, talk shows, articles, billboards, posters, and news features. The general public is encouraged to call a toll-free helpline for information and referrals.

Evaluations of such society-level media campaigns in the United States have shown promise.[216,217] An evaluation of the Stop It Now! program, for example, was shown to effectively change public awareness and knowledge over a 2-year period.[134] Other evaluations of media campaigns on the issue in other US cities, as well as other countries, show similar positive outcomes (eg, increased knowledge, awareness, disclosures).[218] Despite the methodological limitations of these evaluations, such public awareness initiatives hold great promise for focusing on the most appropriate targets: potential offenders and bystanders.

Another prevention approach targeting the societal ecological level is statewide CSA prevention programs. In Massachusetts, the Enough Abuse Campaign is a statewide education and community mobilization effort whose mission is "to prevent people from sexually abusing children now and to prevent children from developing sexually abusive behaviors in the future."[219] The Enough Abuse Campaign provides information about conditions and social norms associated with the occurrence of CSA and offers training for parents and child care professionals to identify and respond to sexual behaviors of children. Along with media coverage, community presentations, and workshops, the campaign also provides a variety of CSA prevention materials and resources on their Web site. The Enough Abuse Campaign also works to strengthen the capacity of YSOs to reduce the risks of sexual abuse occurring in these settings. In addition to facilitating changes in organizational settings, the Campaign also supports efforts to affect public policies related to CSA (eg, reforming the state's statute of limitations).[220]

Evaluation of the Enough Abuse Campaign supports this approach as a promising avenue for CSA prevention. Following the campaign, it was demonstrated that more Massachusetts residents were likely to endorse the belief that adults, rather than children, should take responsibility for preventing CSA (an increase from 69% in 2003 to 93% in 2007).[220] As another potential indicator of program impact, substantiated reports of CSA in Massachusetts declined 69% from 1990 to 2007. Similar effects were observed in Georgia, as substantiated reports of CSA decreased 4 of the 5 years of the implementation period.[221] These findings suggest that a statewide effort can impact rates of CSA and promote community responsibility for preventing CSA.

The CDC recently provided funding for 3 additional public health projects including Prevent Child Abuse Georgia, Project Pathfinder, Inc. (Minnesota), and Massachusetts Citizens for Children.[137] These are statewide prevention collaboratives designed to build capacity at the state and local level to implement CSA prevention programming and strategies that focus on adult and community responsibility for CSA. Each program is conducting a statewide inventory of child sexual abuse prevention programs, creating a collaborative to guide prevention programming and selecting, implementing, and evaluating pilot programs. The organizations will focus on adult or community responsibility and response in preventing the perpetration of CSA. Strategies include use of media campaigns (eg, billboard, radio, and print ads), Internet-based resources, training for parents and professionals, general workshops and presentations, and efforts to change policies at various levels. The impact of these new efforts on CSA has yet to be empirically determined.

Other examples of societal-level prevention efforts are criminal justice system responses that target CSA offenders. All US states have laws criminalizing CSA.[222] Criminal laws, however, vary widely by state in terms of the minimum age at which a person is considered to be legally competent to consent to sexual activity, with the most common age of consent in the United States being 16 years of age. This means that under certain circumstances, it is not technically illegal for an adult to have sex with a 16 year old, which has implications for legal responses pertaining to CSA by staff in YSOs. Sex is legal in Massachusetts, for example, between a student and teacher as long as the student is at least 16.[223] However, states are beginning to raise the age of consent if the abuser is in a position of authority over the young person, such as being a teacher, manager, or parent, with over 30 US states implementing statutes criminalizing sexual relations between minors and adults serving in positions of authority.[103,224]

In addition to criminal charges and incarceration, criminal justice responses also include community protection policies such as lifetime offender registries, lifetime online community notification, indefinite postincarceration civil commitment, and expansive sex offender residency restrictions.[194,225] These approaches are most often considered to be tertiary rather than primary prevention strategies since they apply after abuse has already occurred. However, because of the potential deterrent effect on future acts of abuse, they might also be considered primary prevention. Unfortunately, most legislative initiatives have not been adequately evaluated, and what research is available suggests that sex offender policies (including notification, registration, and residency restrictions) do not prevent sex offenders from repeating their crimes.[225-227] Thus, the impact of these legislative initiatives on primary prevention of CSA perpetration is unknown. Letourneau et al argue that strong emotional reactions engendered by CSA often lead to reactionary legislation that may actually be counterproductive to CSA prevention efforts because such legislation leaves the impression that "legislators are doing everything that can be done," which results in complacency.[2] Such reactive legislation is often quickly implemented in response to a dramatic case of CSA (eg, legislation that includes the name of the child victim in its title) in order to protect children. There are recent signs, however, that the tide of reactive legislation may be subsiding, as several US states have not complied with all of the requirements of the Adam Walsh Child Protection and Safety Act of 2006, potentially signaling greater willingness on the part of legislators to consider alternative prevention policies.[2]

Expanding Society-Focused Efforts

Prevention efforts targeting societal-level efforts are in their infancy and need further development and evaluation, but several current approaches do show promise. This is seen particularly in media campaigns and statewide prevention programs. Several challenges to such efforts exist, including the fact that CSA represents a very complex human phenomenon that elicits strong emotional reactions.[2,228] These challenges make disseminating knowledge and understanding about the topic difficult. In addition, such programs are financially costly and, unfortunately CSA does not receive the same funding as other public health problems. In 2009, the CDC conducted a review of public health agencies and found that 71% offered programs targeting intimate partner violence, whereas only 20% offered CSA prevention programs.[231] Other research suggests that whereas $2 is spent on research for every $100 in cost for cancer, only 5 cents is spent for every $100 in cost for child maltreatment.[230] These findings suggest that CSA prevention receives lower priority relative to other public health concerns. Increased federal, state, and foundational funding for CSA-related research and prevention implementation is definitely needed. When weighed against the psychological, medical, and economic costs of CSA, investing in its prevention is clearly a worthwhile endeavor.

Although research has shown that news coverage of CSA is often limited, sensationalistic, and biased or uninformed, no prevention efforts directly focus on this group of professionals. Education for media professionals about the empirical realities of CSA is greatly needed.[2,212] Public media campaigns likely impact some media professionals, but the development of comprehensive toolkits to help the media disseminate information free of bias and sensationalism would be helpful.[231] More research on the nature and impact of media coverage of CSA would also be important to help influence routine coverage in a way that links CSA to preventive policies.[212] In addition, rigorous experimental studies are needed to assist advocates and media researchers in learning about the impact of routine news coverage on opinion leaders and their policy decisions.[212] Greater efforts to provide education and proper training on CSA and trauma to all persons who may work with children and adolescents (including daycare workers, teachers, and practitioners) are needed and could be presented early in the academic training of such individuals.[231,232]

Future CSA prevention efforts could benefit from following the lead of policy and prevention initiatives developed to end sexual violence against women and need to shift the primary focus of CSA prevention efforts from preventing child sexual victimization to stopping child sexual perpetration.[233] Toward this end, more research and efforts are needed to target at-risk populations of adolescents and adults. Research and efforts are also needed to increase early detection of problems associated with sexual offending such as sexual behavior problems, along with family concerns of offender-like behavior (eg, viewing of child pornographic material).

Finally, continued efforts are needed to enhance broad-based efforts to change the social norms that support and condone the sexual abuse of children. These efforts should include addressing the sexualization of women and especially young children, as well as problematic gender norms that can lead to justification of offending. The American Psychological Association Task Force on the Sexualization of Girls concluded that "virtually every media form studied provides ample evidence of the sexualization of women, including television, music videos, music lyrics, movies, magazines, sports media, video games, the internet, and advertising."[234] Likewise, the American Academy of Pediatrics alerts pediatricians and parents about how sexual messages and images in music and videos can impact sexual behaviors of young viewers.[235] Levin and Kilbourne describe how the fashion industry and mainstream advertisers are pushing youth down the "slippery slope of sexualized childhood."[236] Embedded in these sexualized images is the dangerous message that it is socially acceptable to view children as sexual objects and to use them sexually for personal or financial gain. Efforts are needed to ban ads that sexually objectify children, messages that sexually degrade or violate children, and "sex sells" messages involving children. Parents can be encouraged to take a stand against the commercial sexualization of children and to help children and teens become critical consumers of what they see and hear.[103,236] Rather than promoting perceptions that children are objects for sexual use or economic gain, mass media could instead be used to recognize the worth and value of all children.

Conclusions and Implications

Since CSA has been recognized as a social and public health problem, prevention advocates have devoted considerable effort to the development, implementation, and evaluation of primary prevention programs. Public health's broad view emphasizes population health—not just the health of individuals. Youth are directly harmed by sexual exploitation, but its consequences also affect society in general. Thus, the long-term goal of public health is to achieve lasting change in the factors and conditions that place people at risk by making changes at the individual, relationship, community, and societal levels. Most of the programs reviewed in this chapter are universal, and most have been directed at the micro level rather than the macro level of the child's ecology. The bulk of primary prevention efforts to date have targeted young children via child-focused, classroom-based educational programs. To a lesser extent, parents have been provided with information about CSA and encouraged to instruct and practice personal safety knowledge and skills with their children. Fewer comprehensive attempts have focused on preventing CSA in youth-serving organizations, and there has been minimal involvement in prevention at the societal level, although several recent developments appear to be promising.

Encouragingly, substantiated cases of sexual abuse have significantly decreased over the past 2 decades. Although this decline cannot be definitively attributed to the sexual abuse prevention movement, prevention efforts have most likely played a role. (See Finkelhor and Jones for other explanations.[237]) Because the sexual exploitation of minors is a complex public health problem, the eradication of CSA calls for complex and comprehensive solutions, necessitates that we extend the focus outward from individual to systemic factors, and requires that we all "share the responsibility" for preventing CSA.[97]

References

1. US Department of Health & Human Services. *Child Maltreatment 2005: Reports From the States to the National Child Abuse and Neglect Data System*. Washington, DC: US Government Printing Office; 2007.

2. Letourneau EJ, Eaton WW, Bass J, Berlin FS, Moore SG. The need for a comprehensive public health approach to preventing child sexual abuse. *Public Health Reports*. 2014;129:222-228.

3. Wurtele SK, Miller-Perrin CL. Global efforts to prevent sexual exploitation of minors. In: Dubowitz H, ed. *World Perspectives on Child Abuse*. 10th ed. Denver, CO: International Society for Prevention of Child Abuse and Neglect; 2012:82-88.

4. Sedlak AJ, Mettenburg J, Basena M, et al. *Fourth National Incidence Study of Child Abuse and Neglect (NIS-4): Report to Congress*. Washington, DC: US Department of Health and Human Services, Administration for Children and Families; 2010.

5. Finkelhor D, Vanderminden J, Turner HA, Hamby SL, Shattuck A. Child maltreatment rates assessed in a national household survey of caregivers and youth. *Child Abuse Negl*. 2014;38(9):1421-1435.

6. Pereda N, Guilera G, Forns M, Gomez-Benito J. The prevalence of child sexual abuse in community and student samples: a meta-analysis. *Clin Psychol Rev*. 2009;29(4):328-338.

7. Stoltenborgh M, van Ijzendoorn MH, Euser EM, Bakermans-Kranenburg MJ. A global perspective on child sexual abuse: meta-analysis of prevalence around the world. *Child Maltreatment*. 2011;16(2):79-101.

8. Barth J, Bermetz L, Heim E, Trelle S, Tonia T. The current prevalence of child sexual abuse worldwide: a systematic review and meta-analysis. *Int J Public Health*. 2013;58(3):469-483.

9. Arata CM. From child victim to adult victim: a model for predicting sexual revictimization. *Child Maltreatment*. 2000;5(1):28-38.

10. Barnes JE, Noll JG, Putnam FW, Trickett PK. Sexual and physical revictimization among victims of severe childhood sexual abuse. *Child Abuse Negl.* 2009;33(7):412-420.

11. Berliner L, Elliott DM. Sexual abuse of children. In: Myers JEB, Berliner L, Briere J, Hendrix CT, Jenny C, Reid TA, eds. *The APSAC Handbook on Child Maltreatment.* 2nd ed. Thousand Oaks, CA: Sage Publications; 2002:55-78.

12. Chen LP, Murad MH, Paras ML, et al. Sexual abuse and lifetime diagnosis of psychiatric disorders: Systematic review and meta-analysis. *Mayo Clinic Proceedings.* 2010;85(7):618-629.

13. Classen CC, Palesh O, Aggarwal R. Sexual revictimization: a review of the empirical literature. *Trauma Violence Abuse.* 2005;6(2):103-129.

14. Dube SR, Anda RF, Whitfield CL, et al. Long-term consequences of childhood sexual abuse by gender of the victim. *American J Prev Med.* 2005;28(5):430-438.

15. Fuller-Thomson E, Bejan R, Hunter JT, Grundland T, Brennenstuhl S. The link between childhood sexual abuse and myocardial infarction in a population-based study. *Child Abuse Negl.* 2012;36:656-665.

16. Gilbert R, Widom CS, Browne K, Fergusson D, Webb E, Janson S. Burden and consequences of child maltreatment in high-income countries. *The Lancet.* 2009;373(9657):68-81.

17. Kilpatrick DG, Ruggerio KJ, Acierno R, Saunders BE, Resnick HS, Best CL. Violence and risk of PTSD, major depression, substance abuse/dependence, and comorbidity: results from the national survey of adolescents. *J Consult Clin Psychol.* 2003;71(3):692-700.

18. Lacelle C, Herbert M, Lavoie F, Vitaro F, Tremblay RE. Sexual health in women reporting a history of child sexual abuse. *Child Abuse Negl.* 2012;36:247-259.

19. Maniglio R. The impact of child sexual abuse on health: a systematic review of reviews. *Clin Psyhcol Rev.* 2009;29:647-657.

20. Noll JG, Haralson KJ, Butler EM, Shenk CE. Childhood maltreatment, psychological dysregulation, and risky sexual behaviors in female adolescents. *J Pediatr Psychol.* 2011;3:1-10.

21. Noll JG, Shenk CE. Teen birth rates in sexually abused and neglected females. *Pediatrics.* 2013;131(4):e1181-e1187.

22. Noll JG, Trickett PK, Putnam FW. A prospective investigation of the impact of childhood sexual abuse on the development of sexuality. *J Consult Clin Psychol.* 2003;71:575-586.

23. Ogloff JRP, Cutajar MC, Mann E, Mullen P. Child sexual abuse and subsequent offending and victimisation: a 45 year follow-up study. *Trends and Issues in Criminal Justice.* 2012;440:1-6.

24. Paolucci EO, Genuis ML, Violato C. A meta-analysis of the published research on the effects of child sexual abuse. *J Psychol.* 2001;135:17-36.

25. Perez-Fuentes G, Olfson M, Villegas L, Morcillo C, Wang S, Blanco C. Prevalence and correlates of child sexual abuse: a national study. *Compr Psychiatry.* 2013;54:16-27.

26. Pollio E, Deblinger E, Runyan MK. Mental health treatment for the effects of child sexual abuse. In: Myers JEB, ed. *The APSAC Handbook on Child Maltreatment.* 3rd ed. Los Angeles, CA: Sage; 2011:253-256.

27. Putnam FW. Ten-year research update review: child sexual abuse. *J Am Acad Child Adolesc Psychiatry.* 2003;42(3):269-278.

28. Raghavan R, Bogart LM, Elliott MN, Vestal KD, Schuster MA. Sexual victimization among a national probability sample of adolescent women. *Perspect Sex Reprod Health.* 2004;36(6):225-232.

29. Roberts R, O'Connor T, Dunn J, Golding J; ALSPAC Study Team. The effects of child sexual abuse in later family life; mental health, parenting and adjustment of offspring. *Child Abuse Negl.* 2004;28:525-545.

30. Suris A, Lind L. Military sexual trauma: a review of prevalence and associated health consequences in veterans. *Trauma Violence Abuse.* 2008;9(4):250-269.

31. Tyler KA. Social and emotional outcomes of childhood sexual abuse: a review of recent research. *Aggress Violent Behav.* 2002;7:567-589.

32. van Roode T, Dickson N, Herbison P, Paul C. Child sexual abuse and persistence of risky sexual behavior and negative sexual outcomes over adulthood: findings from a birth cohort. *Child Abuse Negl.* 2009;33:161-172.

33. Cohen M, Miller T. The cost of mental health care for victims of crime. *J Interpers Violence.* 1988;13(1):93-110.

34. Whitaker DJ, Lutzker JR, Shelley GA. Child maltreatment prevention priorities at the Centers for Disease Control and Prevention. *Child Maltreatment.* 2005;10(3):245-259.

35. Butchart A, Harvey AP, Mian M, Furniss T. *Preventing Child Maltreatment: A Guide to Taking Action and Generating Evidence.* Geneva, Switzerland: WHO; 2006.

36. Wandersman A, Florin P. Community interventions and effective prevention. *Am Psychol.* 2003;58:441-448.

37. Wurtele SK, Kenny MC. Preventing child sexual abuse: an ecological approach. In: Goodyear-Brown P, ed. *Handbook of Child Sexual Abuse: Identification, Assessment, and Treatment.* Hoboken, NJ: Wiley Press; 2012:531-565.

38. Belsky J. Etiology of child maltreatment: a developmental-ecological analysis. *Psychological Bulletin.* 1993;114:413-434.

39. Bronfenbrenner U. *The Ecology of Human Development.* Cambridge, MA: Harvard University Press; 1979.

40. Zielinski D, Bradshaw C. Ecological influences on the sequelae of child maltreatment: a review of the literature. *Child Maltreatment.* 2006;11:49-62.

41. Centers for Disease Control and Prevention. The social-ecological model: a framework for prevention. http://www.cdc.gov/violenceprevention/overview/social-ecologicalmodel.html. Accessed November 3, 2016.

42. Anderson JF, Mangels NJ, Langsam A. Child sexual abuse: a public health issue. *Crim Justice Stud.* 2004;17:107-126.

43. Dahlberg LL, Krug EG. Violence-a global public health problem. In: Krug E, Dahlberg LL, Mercy JA, Zwi AB, Lozano R, eds. *World Report on Violence and Health.* Geneva, Switzerland: World Health Organization; 2002:1-56.

44. Kaufman KL. Future directions for the prevention of sexual violence. In: Kaufman KL, ed. *The Prevention of Sexual Violence: A Practitioner's Sourcebook.* Holyoke, MA: NEARI Press; 2010:489-501.

45. Kenny MC, Wurtele SK. Preventing childhood sexual abuse: an ecological approach. *J Child Sex Abuse.* 2012;21:361-367.

46. Krugman RD. It's time to broaden the agenda. *Child Abuse Negl.* 1998;22:475-479.

47. McMahon PM, Puett RC. Child sexual abuse as a public health issue: recommendations of an expert panel. *Sex Abuse.* 1999;11:257-266.

48. Mercy JA. Having new eyes: viewing child sexual abuse as a public health problem. *Sex Abuse.* 1999;11:317-321.

49. Saul J, Patterson J, Audage N. Preventing sexual maltreatment in youth-serving community organizations. In: Kaufman KL, ed. *The Prevention of Sexual Violence: A Practitioner's Sourcebook.* Holyoke, MA: NEARI Press; 2010:449-463.

50. Flaherty EG, Thompson R, Dubowitz H, et al. Adverse childhood experiences and child health in early adolescence. *JAMA Pediatrics.* 2013;167(7):622-629.

51. Nelson G, Caplan R. The prevention of child physical abuse and neglect: an update. *J Appl Res Child.* 2014;5(1):3.

52. Centers for Disease Control and Prevention. The social-ecological model: a framework for prevention. Centers for Disease Control and Prevention Web site. http://www.cdc.gov/violenceprevention/overview/social-ecologicalmodel.html. Accessed November 2, 2016.

53. Abrahams N, Casey K, Daro D. Teachers' knowledge, attitudes, and beliefs about child abuse and its prevention. *Child Abuse Negl.* 1992;16:229-238.

54. Finkelhor D, Dziuba-Leatherman J. Victimization prevention programs: a national survey of children's exposure and reactions. *Child Abuse Negl.* 1995;19:129-139.

55. Wurtele SK. Behavioral approaches to educating young children and their parents about child sexual abuse prevention. *The Journal of Behavior Analysis of Offender and Victim Treatment and Prevention.* 2008;1(1):52-64.

56. Wurtele SK. School-based child sexual abuse prevention: questions, answers, and more questions. In: Lutzker JR, ed. *Child Abuse Research and Treatment.* New York, NY: Plenum Press; 1998:501-516.

57. Wurtele SK, Owens JS. Teaching personal safety skills to young children: an investigation of age and gender across five studies. *Child Abuse Negl.* 1997;21:805-814.

58. Kenny MC, Wurtele SK. Preschoolers' knowledge of genital terminology: a comparison of English and Spanish speakers. *Am J Sex Ed.* 2008;3(4):345-354.

59. Wurtele SK. Enhancing children's sexual development through child sexual abuse prevention programs. *J Sex Ed Ther.* 1993;19(1):37-46.

60. Wurtele SK, Melzer A, Kast L. Preschoolers' knowledge of and ability to learn genital terminology. *J Sex Ed Ther.* 1992;18:115-122.

61. Berrrick JD, Barth RP. Child sexual abuse prevention: research review and recommendations. *Soc Work Res Abstr.* 1992;28:6-15.

62. Briggs F, Hawkins RMF. Follow-up data on the effectiveness of New Zealand's national school based child protection program. *Child Abuse Negl.* 1994;18:635-643.

63. Rispens J, Aleman A, Goudena PP. Prevention of child sexual abuse victimization: a meta-analysis of school programs. *Child Abuse Negl.* 1997;21:975-987.

64. Davis MK, Gidycz CA. Child sexual abuse prevention programs: a meta-analysis. *J Clin Child Psychol.* 2000;29:257-265.

65. Mikton C, Butchart A. Child maltreatment prevention: a systematic review of reviews. *Bull World Health Org.* 2009;87:353-361.

66. Topping KJ, Barron IG. School-based child sexual abuse prevention programs: a review of effectiveness. *Rev Educ Res.* 2009;79(1):431-463.

67. Zwi KJ, Woolfenden SR, Wheeler DM, O'Brien TA, Tait P, Williams KW. School-based education programmes for the prevention of child sexual abuse. *Cochrane Database Syst Rev.* 2007;18(3):CD004380.

68. Gibson LE, Leitenberg H. Child sexual abuse prevention programs: do they decrease the occurrence of child sexual abuse? *Child Abuse Negl.* 2000;24:1115-1125.

69. Finkelhor D. Prevention of sexual abuse through educational programs directed toward children. *Pediatrics.* 2007;120(3):640-645.

70. US General Accounting Office. *Preventing Child Sexual Abuse: Research Inconclusive About Effectiveness of Child Education Programs.* Washington, DC: US Government Printing Office; 1996.

71. Finkelhor D, Asdigian N, Dziuba-Leatherman J. The effectiveness of victimization prevention instruction: an evaluation of children's responses to actual threats and assaults. *Child Abuse Negl.* 1995;19:141-153.

72. Roberts JA, Miltenberger RG. Emerging issues in the research on child sexual abuse prevention. *Education & Treatment of Children.* 1999;22(1):84-102.

73. Hazzard A, Webb C, Kleemeier C, Angert L, Pohl J. Child sexual abuse prevention: evaluation and one year follow up. *Child Abuse Negl.* 1991;15:123-138.

74. Poche C, Yoder P, Miltenberger R. Teaching self-protection to children using television techniques. *J Appl Behav Anal.* 1988;21:253-261.

75. Wurtele SK. Teaching personal safety skills to four-year-old children: a behavioral approach. *Behavior Therapy.* 1990;21:25-32.

76. Zhang W, Chen J, Feng Y, Li J, Liu C, Zhao X. Evaluation of a sexual abuse prevention education for Chinese preschoolers. *Res Soc Work Pract.* 2014;24(4):428-436.

77. National Center for Missing and Exploited Children. *Guidelines for Programs to Reduce Child Victimization: A Resource For Communities when Choosing a Program to Teach Personal Safety to Children.* Lake Park, FL: National Center for Missing and Exploited Children; 1999.

78. Plummer CA. Prevention of child sexual abuse: a survey of 87 programs. *Violence Vict.* 2001;16:575-588.

79. Zins JE, Weissberg RP, Wang MC, Walberg HJ, eds. *Building Academic Success on Social and Emotional Learning: What Does the Research Say?* New York, NY: Teachers College Press; 2004.

80. Smallbone S, Marshall WL, Wortley R. *PPreventing Child Sexual Abuse: Evidence, Policy and Practice.* Portland, OR: Willan Publishing; 2008.

81. Herdt G, McClintock M. The magical age of 10. *Arch Sex Behav.* 2000;29(6):587-606.

82. DeLamater J, Friedrich WN. Human sexual development. *J Sex Res.* 2002;39(1):10-14.

83. Wurtele SK, Kenny MC. Normative sexuality development in childhood: implications for developmental guidance and prevention of childhood sexual abuse. *Counseling and Human Development.* 2011;43(9):1-24.

84. Barbaree HE, Marshall WL, eds. *The Juvenile Sex Offender.* 2nd ed. New York, NY: Guilford; 2006.

85. Muller AR, Roder M, Fingerle M. Child sexual abuse prevention goes online: introducing "Cool and Safe" and its effects. *Comput Educ.* 2014;78:60-65.

86. Hébert M, Lavoie F, Piché C, Poitras M. Proximate effects of child sexual abuse prevention program in elementary school children. *Child Abuse Negl.* 2001;25:505-522.

87. Daigneault I, Hébert M, McDuff P, Frappier JY. Evaluation of a sexual abuse prevention workshop in a multicultural, impoverished urban area. *J Child Sex Abus.* 2012;21:521-542.

88. Schenkel LS, Rothman-Marshall G, Schlehofer DA, Towne TL, Burnash DL, Priddy BM. Child maltreatment and trauma exposure among deaf and hard of hearing young adults. *Child Abuse Negl.* 2014;38:1581-1589.

89. McEachern AG. Sexual abuse of individuals with disabilities: prevention strategies for clinical practice. *J Child Sex Abus.* 2012;21:386-398.

90. Baker CK, Gleason K, Naai R, Mitchell J, Trecker C. Increasing knowledge of sexual abuse: a study with elementary school children in Hawaii. *Res Soc Work Pract.* 2012;23:167-178.

91. Kenny MC, Wurtele SK, Alonso L. Evaluation of a personal safety program with Latino preschoolers. *J Child Sex Abus.* 2012;21(4):368-385.

92. Martin KA, Luke K. Gender differences in the ABC's of the birds and bees: what mothers teach young children about sexuality and reproduction. *Sex Roles.* 2010;62:278-291.

93. Babatsikos G. Parents' knowledge, attitudes and practices about preventing child sexual abuse: a literature review. *Child Abuse Rev.* 2010;19:107-129.

94. Elrod JM, Rubin RH. Parental involvement in sexual abuse prevention education. *Child Abuse Negl.* 1993;17:527-538.

95. Reppucci ND, Jones LM, Cook SL. Involving parents in child sexual abuse prevention programs. *J Child Fam Stud.* 1994;3:137-142.

96. Wurtele SK, Kenny MC. Partnering with parents to prevent childhood sexual abuse. *Child Abuse Rev.* 2010;19:130-152.

97. Wurtele SK, Miller-Perrin CL. *Preventing Child Sexual Abuse: Sharing the Responsibility.* Lincoln, NE: University of Nebraska Press; 1992.

98. Wurtele SK, Gillispie EI, Currier LL, Franklin CF. A comparison of teachers vs. parents as instructors of a personal safety program for preschoolers. *Child Abuse Negl.* 1992;16:127-137.

99. Wurtele SK, Kast L, Melzer A. Sexual abuse prevention education for young children: a comparison of teachers and parents as instructors. *Child Abuse Negl.* 1992;16:865-876.

100. Fieldman JP, Crespi TD. Child sexual abuse: offenders, disclosure, and school-based initiatives. *Adolescence.* 2002;37:151-160.

101. Kaufman KL, Mosher H, Carter M, Estes L. An empirically based situational prevention model for child sexual abuse. In: Smallbone S, Wortley R, eds. *Situational Prevention of Child Sexual Abuse.* Monsey, NY: Criminal Justice Press; 2006. *Crime Prevention Studies*; vol 19.

102. Wurtele SK. *Out of Harm's Way: A Parent's Guide to Protecting Young Children From Sexual Abuse.* Seattle, WA: Parenting Press; 2010.

103. Wurtele SK. Preventing the sexual exploitation of minors in youth-serving organizations. *Child Youth Serv Rev.* 2012;34:2442-2453.

104. Wurtele SK, Berkower F. *Off Limits: A Parent's Guide to Keeping Kids Safe from Sexual Abuse.* Brandon, VT: Safer Society Press; 2010.

105. Chen JQ, Chen DG. Awareness of child sexual abuse prevention education among parents of grade 3 elementary school pupils in Fuxin City, China. *Health Education Research.* 2005;20(5):540-547.

106. Olsen ME, Kalbfleisch JH. A survey of pregnant women's knowledge about sexual abuse. *J Pediatr Adolesc Gynecol.* 1999;12:219-222.

107. Tutty LM. Parent's perceptions of their child's knowledge of sexual abuse prevention concepts. *J Child Sex Abus.* 1993;2:83-103.

108. Wurtele SK, Kvaternick M, Franklin CF. Sexual abuse prevention for preschoolers: a survey of parents' behaviors, attitudes, and beliefs. *J Child Sex Abus.* 1992;1:113-128.

109. Tang CS, Yan EC. Intention to participate in child sexual abuse prevention programs: a study of Chinese adults in Hong Kong. *Child Abuse Negl.* 2004;28:1187-1197.

110. Collins ME. Parents' perceptions of the risk of CSA and their protective behavior: findings from a qualitative study. *Child Maltreatment.* 1996;1:53-64.

111. Kernsmith PD, Craun SR, Foster J. Public attitudes toward sexual offenders and sex offender registration. *J Child Sex Abus.* 2009;18:290-301.

112. Levenson JS, Brannon YN, Fortney T, Baker J. Public perceptions about sex offenders and community protection policies. *Anal Soc Issues Public Policy.* 2007;7(1):1-25.

113. Deblinger E, Thakkar-Kolar RR, Berry EJ, Schroeder CM. Caregivers' efforts to educate their children about child sexual abuse: a replication study. *Child Maltreatment.* 2010;15(1):91-100.

114. Finkelhor D. *Child Sexual Abuse: New Theory and Research.* New York, NY: The Free Press; 1984.

115. Walsh K, Brandon L, Chirio L. Mother-child communication about sexual abuse prevention. *J Child Sex Abus.* 2012;21(4):399-421.

116. Morison S, Greene E. Juror and expert knowledge of child sexual abuse. *Child Abuse Negl.* 1992;16:595-613.

117. Berrick JD. Parental involvement in child abuse prevention training: what do they learn? *Child Abuse Negl.* 1988;12:543-553.

118. Calvert JF Jr, Munsie-Benson M. Public opinion and knowledge about childhood sexual abuse in a rural community. *Child Abuse Negl.* 1999;23:671-682.

119. Chen JQ, Dunne MP, Han P. Prevention of child sexual abuse in China: knowledge, attitudes, and communication practices of parents of elementary school children. *Child Abuse Negl.* 2007;31:747-755.

120. Tutty LM. Child sexual abuse prevention programs: evaluating who do you tell. *Child Abuse Negl.* 1997;21:869-881.

121. Finkelhor D. *Child Victimization: Violence, Crime, and Abuse in the Lives of Young People.* New York, NY: Oxford University Press; 2008.

122. Dombrowski SC, Gischlar KL, Durst T. Safeguarding young people from cyber pornography and cyber sexual predation: a major dilemma of the Internet. *Child Abuse Rev.* 2007;16:153-170.

123. Wurtele SK. *Safe Connections: A Parent's Guide to Protecting Young Teens from Sexual Exploitation.* Seattle, WA: Parenting Press; 2012.

124. Wurtele SK, Miller-Perrin C. Preventing technology-initiated sexual victimization of youth: a developmental perspective. In: Kenny MC, ed. *Sex Education: Attitude of Adolescents, Cultural Differences and Schools' Challenges.* New York, NY: Nova; 2014:147-175.

125. Kolko D, Moser J, Litz J, Hughes J. Promoting awareness and prevention of child sexual victimization using the Red Flag/Green Flag program: an evaluation with follow-up. *J Fam Violence.* 1987;2:11-35.

126. MacIntyre D, Carr A. Evaluation of the effectiveness of the Stay Safe primary prevention program for child sexual abuse. *Child Abuse Negl.* 1999;23:1307-1325.

127. Campis LK, Prentice-Dunn S, Lyman RD. Coping appraisal and parents' intentions to inform their children about sexual abuse:aA protection motivation theory analysis. *J Soc Clin Psychol.* 1989;8:304-316.

128. Burgess ES, Wurtele SK. Enhancing parent-child communication about sexual abuse: a pilot study. *Child Abuse Negl.* 1998;22:1167-1175.

129. Wurtele SK, Moreno T, Kenny M. Evaluation of a sexual abuse prevention workshop for parents of young children. *Journal of Child and Adolescent Trauma.* 2008;1:1-10.

130. Miltenberger RG, Thiesse-Duffy E. Evaluation of home-based programs for teaching personal safety skills to children. *J Appl Beha Anal.* 1988;21:81-87.

131. Miltenberger RG, Thiesse-Duffy E, Suda KT, Kozak C, Bruellman J. Teaching prevention skills to children: the use of multiple measures to evaluate parent versus expert instruction. *Child & Family Behavior Therapy.* 1990;12:65-87.

132. Wurtele SK, Currier LO, Gillispie EI, Franklin CF. The efficacy of a parent-implemented program for teaching preschoolers personal safety skills. *Behavior Therapy*. 1991;21:25-32.

133. Deblinger E, Stauffer L, Steer R. Comparative efficacies of supportive and cognitive behavioral group therapies for children who were sexually abused and their nonoffending mothers. *Child Maltreatment*. 2001;6(4):332-343.

134. Chasen-Taber L, Tabachnick J. Evaluation of a child sexual abuse prevention program. *Sex Abuse*. 1999;11:279-292.

135. Amstadter AB, Broman-Fulks J, Zinzow H, Ruggiero KJ, Cercone J. Internet-based interventions for traumatic stress-related mental health problems: a review and suggestions for future research. *Clin Psychol Rev*. 2009;29:410-420.

136. Wurtele SK. Preventing sexual abuse of children in the twenty-first century: preparing for challenges and opportunities. *J Child Sex Abus*. 2009;18:1-18.

137. Centers for Disease Control and Prevention. Preventing child maltreatment: program activities guide. Centers for Disease Control and Prevention Web site. http://www.cdc.gov/violenceprevention/pub/preventingcm.html. Accessed November 2, 2016.

138. Trocmé N, Schumaker K. Reported child sexual abuse in Canadian schools and recreational facilities: implications for developing effective prevention strategies. *Child Youth Serv Red*. 1999;21(8):621-642.

139. Tonry M, Farrington D. *Building a Safer Society: Strategic Approaches to Crime Prevention*. Chicago, IL: Chicago University Press; 1995.

140. Smith CP, Freyd JJ. Dangerous safe havens: institutional betrayal exacerbates sexual trauma. *J Trauma Stress*. 2013;26(1):119-124.

141. Sullivan J, Beech A. Professional perpetrators: sex offenders who use their employment to target and sexually abuse the children with whom they work. *Child Abus Rev*. 2002;11:153-167.

142. Moulden HM, Firestone P, Wexler AF. Child care providers who commit sexual offenses: a description of offenders, offense and victim characteristics. *Int J Offender Ther Comp Criminol*. 2007;51(4):384-406.

143. John Jay College of Criminal Justice. *The Causes and Context of the Problem of Sexual Abuse of Minors by Catholic Priests and Deacons in the United States*. New York, NY: City University of New York; 2011.

144. Terry KJ, Ackerman A. Child sexual abuse in the Catholic Church: how situational crime prevention strategies can help create safe environments. *Crim Justice Behav*. 2008;35(5):643-657.

145. Terry KJ, Freilich JD. Understanding child sexual abuse by Catholic priests from a situational perspective. *J Child Sex Abus*. 2012;21:437-455.

146. Shakeshaft C. *Educator Sexual Misconduct: A Synthesis of Existing Literature*. Washington, DC: US Department of Education; 2004.

147. Shoop R. *Sexual Exploitation in Schools: How to Spot It and Stop It*. Thousand Oaks, CA: Corwin Press; 2003.

148. Teichroeb R. Abuse and silence: examining America's schools for the deaf. *Seattle Post Intelligencer*. November 27, 2001.

149. Beck AJ, Harrison PM, Guerino P. *Sexual Victimization in Juvenile Facilities Reported by Youth, 2008-09*. Washington, DC: US Department of Justice, Office of Justice Programs, Bureau of Justice Statistics; 2010.

150. Twill SE, Green DM, Traylor A. A descriptive study on sexually exploited children in residential treatment. *Child Youth Care Forum*. 2010;39:187-199.

151. Yardley W. $18.5 million in liability for scouts in abuse case. *New York Times*. April 23, 2010. http://www.nytimes.com/2010/04/24/us/24scouts.html?_r=1.

152. Finkelhor D, Williams L. *Nursery Crimes: Sexual Abuse in Day Care*. Newbury Park, CA: Sage; 1988.

153. Adelson E. Why sports and sex abuse too often mix. http://www.thepostgame.com/features/201111/how-widespreadsex-abuse-sports. Accessed March 25, 2013.

154. Brackenridge CH, Bishopp D, Moussalli S, Tapp J. The characteristics of sexual abuse in sport: a multidimensional scaling analysis of events described in media reports. *Int J Sport Exerc Psychol*. 2008;6:385-406.

155. Brackenridge CH, Rhind D. Child protection in sport: reflections on thirty years of science and activism. *Social Sciences*. 2014;3:326-340.

156. Chuchmach M, Patel A. ABC News investigation: USA swimming coaches molested, secretly taped dozens of teen swimmers. http://abcnews.go.com/Blotter/abc-news-investigation-usa-swimming-coaches-raped-molested/story?id=10322469#.UAf9. Published April 9, 2010. Accessed November 2, 2016.

157. Fibkins WL. *Innocence Denied: A Guide to Preventing Sexual Misconduct by Teachers and Coaches*. Lanham, MD: Rowman & Littlefield Education; 2006.

158. Nack W, Yaeger D. Every parent's nightmare: the child molester has found a home in the world of youth sports, where as a coach he can gain the trust and loyalty of kids—and then prey on them. *Sports Illustrated*. September 13, 1999. http://www.si.com/vault/1999/09/13/266260/every-parents-nightmare-the-child-molester-has-found-a-home-in-the-world-of-youth-sports-where-as-a-coach-he-can-gain-the-trust-and-loyalty-of-kids--and-then-prey-on-them. Accessed November 2, 2016.

159. Willmsen C, O'Hagan M. Coaches who prey: the abuse of girls and the system that allows it. *Seattle Times*. December 14-17, 2003. http://old.seattletimes.com/news/local/coaches/about.html. Accessed November 2, 2016.

160. O'Keeffe M. End zone: sexual predators prowling the sidelines. *New York Dialy News*. April 9, 2011. http://www.nydailynews.com/sports/i-team/sexual-predators-prowling-sidelines-parents-trust-article-1.110165. Accessed November 2, 2016.

161. Sturtz R. Unprotected. *Outside*. December 2014. http://www.outsideonline.com/outdoor-adventure/water-activities/swimming/The-Sex-Abuse-Scandal-Plaguing-USA-Swimming.html. Accessed November 2, 2016.

162. United Nations Children's Fund. *Protecting Children From Violence in Sport: A Review With a Focus on Industrialized Countries*. Florence, Italy: United Nations Children's Fund; 2010.

163. Zinser L. Coaching gives abusers opportunity and trust. *New York Times*. December 10, 2011. http://www.nytimes.com/2011/12/11/sports/culture-of-sports-works-against-children-especially-boys-reporting-abuse. Accessed November 2, 2016.

164. Noble J, Vermillion M. Youth sport administrators' perceptions and knowledge of organizational policies on child maltreatment. *Child Youth Serv Rev.* 2014;38:52-57.

165. Kenny M. Child abuse reporting: teachers' perceived deterrents. *Child Abuse Negl.* 2001;25(1):81-92.

166. Kenny MC. Teachers' attitudes toward and knowledge of child maltreatment. *Child Abuse Negl.* 2004;28(12):1311-1319.

167. Smith CP, Freyd JJ. Institutional betrayal. *Am Psychol.* 2014;69(6):575-587.

168. Freeh Report. http://www.TheFreehReportonPSU.com. Published on July 12, 2012. Accessed November 26, 2014.

169. Robinson GJ. Changing the culture. In: Plante TG, McChesney KL, eds. *Sexual Abuse in the Catholic Church: A Decade of Crisis, 2002-2012.* Santa Barbara, CA: Praeger; 2011:91-102.

170. Plante TG. Keeping kids safe from institutional child sexual abuse. http://www.psychologytoday.com/node/97726. Published June 11, 2012. Accessed November 2, 2016.

171. English K, Heil P, Dumond R. *Sexual Assault in Jail and Juvenile Facilities: Promising Practices for Prevention and Response: Final Report.* Denver, CO: Colorado Division of Criminal Justice; 2010.

172. Smith BV, Yarussi JM. Addressing sexual violence against youth in custody: youth workers' handbook on identifying and addressing sexual violence in juvenile justice settings. http://www.wcl.american.edu/endsilence/documents/JuvenileHandbook-WHITEPAPER.pdf. Accessed November 2, 2016.

173. Saul J, Audage N. *Preventing Child Sexual Abuse Within Youth-Serving Organizations: Getting Started on Policies and Procedures.* Atlanta, GA: Centers for Disease Control and Prevention; 2007.

174. Wortley R, Smallbone S. Emotional arousal and child sex offending: a situational perspective. In: Van Gelder JL, Elffers H, Nagin D, Reynald D, eds. *Affect and Cognition in Offender Decision Making.* New York, NY: Routledge; 2013.

175. Kendrick A, Taylor J. Hidden on the ward: the abuse of children in hospitals. *J Adv Nurs.* 2000;31(3):565-573.

176. Read D. It takes a team. *Athletic Management.* 2013;25(2):31-35.

177. Boy Scouts of America. Youth protection. http://www.scouting.org/Training/YouthProtection.aspx. Accessed November 2, 2016.

178. Child Protection in Sport Unit. *Standards for Safeguarding and Protecting Children in Sport.* Leister, UK: Child Protection in Sport Unit; 2003.

179. Irish Sports Council. Code of ethics and good practice for children's sport. http://www.irishsportscouncil.ie/Participation/Code_of_Ethics/Code_of_Ethics_Manual/Content_PDF_/. Published 2000. Accessed November 2, 2016.

180. Play by the Rules. Maintaining appropriate boundaries. http://www.playbytherules.net.au. Published 2011. Accessed November 2, 2016.

181. USA Gymnastics. Participant welfare policy. http://www.californiatnt.com/USA%20Welfare.pdf. Published 2009. Accessed November 2, 2016.

182. Bryant JK. School counselors and child abuse reporting: a national survey. *Sch Couns.* 2009;12(5):333-342.

183. Bryant J, Baldwin PA. School counselors' perceptions of mandatory reporter training and mandatory reporting experiences. *Child Abuse Rev.* 2010;19:172-186.

184. Cavanagh M, Read J, New B. Sexual abuse inquiry and response: a New Zealand training program. *NZ J Psychol.* 2004;33(3):137-144.

185. Hinkelman L, Bruno M. Identification and reporting of child sexual abuse: The role of elementary school professionals. *Elm Sch J.* 2008;108(5):376-391.

186. Kenny MC. Web-based training in child maltreatment for future mandated reporters. *Child Abuse Negl.* 2007;31(6):671-678.

187. McKee BE, Dillenburger K. Child abuse and neglect: training needs of student teachers. *Int J Educ Res.* 2009;48(5):320-330.

188. Smith MC. Early childhood educators: perspectives on maltreatment and mandated reporting. *Child Youth Serv Rev.* 2010;32(1):20-27.

189. Walsh KM, Bridgstock RS, Farrell AM, Rassafiani M, Schweitzer R. Case, teacher and school characteristics influencing teachers' detection and reporting of child physical abuse and neglect: results from an Australian survey. *Child Abuse Negl.* 2008;32(10):983-993.

190. Darkness To Light. *Stewards of Children.* Charleston, SC: Darkness To Light; 2004.

191. Rheingold AA, Zajac K, Chapman JE, et al. Child sexual abuse prevention training for childcare professionals: an independent multi-site randomized controlled trial of Stewards of Children. *Prev Sic.* 2015;16(3):374-385.

192. Rheingold AA, Zajac K, Patton M. Feasibility and acceptability of a child sexual abuse prevention program for childcare professionals: comparison of a Web-based and in-person training. *J Child Sex Abus.* 2012;21(4):422-436.

193. Gula RM. *Just Ministry: Professional Ethics for Pastoral Ministers.* Mahwah, NJ: Paulist Press; 2010.

194. Finkelhor D. The prevention of childhood sexual abuse. *Future Child.* 2009;19(2):53-78.

195. Parent S, Demers G. Sexual abuse in sport: a model to prevent and protect athletes. *Child Abuse Rev.* 2011;20:120-133.

196. Wiersma LD, Sherman CP. Volunteer youth sport coaches' perspectives of coaching education/certification and parental codes of conduct. *Res Q Exerc Sport.* 2005;76(3):324-338.

197. Andrzejewski CE, Davis HA. Human contact in the classroom: exploring how teachers talk about and negotiate touching students. *Teaching and Teacher Education.* 2008;24:779-794.

198. Preston J. Rules to stop pupil and teacher from getting too social online. New York Times. December 17, 2016. http://www.nytimes.com/2011/12/18/business/media/rules-to-limit-how-teachers-and-students-interact-online.html. Accessed November 2, 2016.

199. Vamos M. The concept of appropriate professional boundaries in psychiatric practice: a pilot training course. *Aust N Z J Psychiatry*. 2001;35:613-618.

200. Malkin K, Johnston L, Brackenridge C. A critical evaluation of training needs for child protection in UK sport. *Managing Leisure*. 2000;5(3):151-160.

201. Celenza A, Gabbard GO. Analysts who commit sexual boundary violations: a lost cause? *FOCUS: The Journal of Lifelong Learning in Psychiatry*. 2007;4:483-492.

202. Hartill M, Lang M. "I know people think I'm a complete pain in the neck": an examination of the introduction of child protection and "safeguarding" in English sport from the perspective of National Governing Body Safeguarding Lead Officers. *Soc Sci*. 2014;3:606-627.

203. Freyd JJ, Putnam FW, Lyon TD, et al. Psychology. the science of child sexual abuse. *Science*. 2005;308(5721):501.

204. Muchnick I. Outside magazine's USA Swimming sex abuse article: is this just a 2010 media hit reset - or is real accountability at hand? http://concussioninc.net/?p=9666. Published November 12, 2014. Accessed November 2, 2016.

205. United Nations Children's Fund. *Hidden in Plain Sight: A Statistical Analysis of Violence Against Children*. New York, NY: United Nations Children's Fund; 2014.

206. Hunter SV. *Childhood Sexual Experiences: Narratives of Resilience*. Oxon, OX: Radcliffe Publishing LTD; 2010.

207. Rind B, Tromovitch P, Bauserman R. A meta-analytic examination of assumed properties of child sexual abuse using college samples. *Pscyhol Bull*. 1998;124(1):22.

208. Stop It Now! what do U.S. adults think about child sexual abuse? measures of knowledge and attitudes among six states. http://www.stopitnow.org/sites/default/files/documents/files/RDD_Survey_Report_Briefing_Sheet1.pdf. Accessed November 2, 2016.

209. Cheit RE, Shavit Y, Reiss-Davis Z. Magazine coverage of child sexual abuse, 1992-2004. *J Child Abuse*. 2010;19(1):99-117.

210. Doan C. 'Subversive stories and hegemonic tales' of child sexual abuse: from expert legal testimony to television talk shows. *Int J Law Context*. 2005;1(3):295-309.

211. Kitzinger J. *Framing Abuse: Media Influences and Public Understanding of Sexual Violence Against Children*. London, England: Pluto Press; 2004.

212. Mejia P, Cheyne A, Dorfman L. News coverage of child sexual abuse and prevention, 2007-2009. *J Child Sex Abus*. 2012;21(4):470-487.

213. Dorfman L, Mejia P, Cheyne A, Gonzalez P. *Case by Case: News Coverage of Child Sexual Abuse*. Berkeley, CA: Berkeley Media Studies Group; 2011.

214. Dorfman L, Mejia P, Gonzalez P, Cheyne A. *Breaking News on Child Sexual Abuse: Early Coverage of Penn State*. Berkeley, CA: Berkeley Media Studies Group; 2012.

215. Barlow J, Calam R. A public health approach to safeguarding in the 21st Century. *Child Abuse Rev*. 2011;20:238-255.

216. Rheingold AA, Campbell C, Self-Brown S, de Arellano M, Resnick H, Kilpatrick D. Prevention of child sexual abuse: evaluation of a community media campaign. *Child Maltreatment*. 2007;12(4):352-363.

217. Self-Brown S, Rheingold AA, Campbell C, de Arellano MA. A media campaign prevention program for child sexual abuse: community members' perspectives. *J Interpers Violence*. 2008;23(6):728-743.

218. Lalor K, McElvaney R. Child sexual abuse, links to later sexual exploitation/high risk sexual behavior, and prevention/treatment programs. *Trauma Violence Abuse*. 2010;11(4):159-177.

219. Enough Abuse Campaign. Home page. http://www.enoughabuse.org. Accessed November 2, 2016.

220. Schober DJ, Fawcett SB, Bernier J. The Enough Abuse Campaign: building the movement to prevent child sexual abuse in Massachusetts. *J Child Sex Abus*. 2012;21(4):456-469.

221. Schober DJ, Fawcett SB, Thigpen S, Curtis A, Wright R. An empirical case study of a child sexual abuse prevention initiative in Georgia. *Health Education Journal*. 2012;71(3):291-298.

222. Myers JEB. Criminal prosecution of child maltreatment. In: Myers JEB, ed. *The APSAC Handbook on Child Maltreatment*. 3rd ed. Thousand Oaks, CA: Sage Publications; 2011:87-99.

223. Most D. No more pencils, no more books, no more teachers' dirty looks. Boston Magazine. October 2003. http://www.bostonmagazine.com/2006/05/no-more-pencils-no-more-books-no-more-teachers-dirty-looks/. Accessed November 2, 2016.

224. Weiss K. Authority as coercion: when authority figures abuse their positions to perpetrate child sexual abuse. *J Child Sex Abuse*. 2002;11(1):27-51.

225. Letourneau EJ, Levenson JS. Preventing sexual abuse: community protection policies and practice. In: Myers JEB, ed. *The APSAC Handbook on Child Maltreatment*. 3rd ed. Thousand Oaks, CA: Sage; 2011:307-321.

226. Letourneau EJ, Levenson JS, Bandyopadhyay D, Sinha D, Armstrong K. Effects of South Carolina's sex offender registration and notification policy on adult recidivism. *Crim Justice Policy Rev*. 2010;21(4):435-458.

227. Zandbergen PA, Levenson JS, Hart T. Residential proximity to schools and daycares: an empirical analysis of sex offense recidivism. *Crim Justice Behav*. In press. 2010;37(5):482-502.

228. Zollner H, Fuchs KA, Fegert JM. Prevention of sexual abuse: improved information is crucial. *Child Adolesc Psychiatry Ment Health*. 2014;8(5):1-9.

229. Centers for Disease Control and Prevention. *Findings From the 2009 Child Maltreatment Prevention Environmental Scan of State Public Health Agencies*. Atlanta, GA: Centers for Disease Control and Prevention; 2009.

230. Putnam FW. Why is it so difficult for the epidemic of child abuse to be taken seriously? In: Franey K, Geffner R, Falconer R, eds. *The Cost of Child Maltreatment: Who Pays?* San Diego, CA: Family Violence and Sexual Assault Institute; 2001:185-198.

231. Collin-Vézina D, Daigneault I, Hebert M. Lessons learned from child sexual abuse: research, prevalence, outcomes, and preventive strategies. *Child Adolesc Psychiatry Ment Health*. 2013;7(22):1-9.

232. Kissee JL, Miller-Perrin CL, Isaacson LJ. An analysis of child maltreatment content in introductory psychology textbooks. *J Aggress Maltreat Trauma*. 2014;23(3):215-228.

233. DeGue S, Simon TR, Basile KC, Yee SL, Lang K, Spivak H. Moving forward by looking back: reflecting on a decade of CDC's work in sexual violence prevention, 2000-2010. *Journal of Women's Health*. 2012;21(12):1211-1218.

234. American Psychological Association. *Report of the APA Task Force on the Sexualization of Girls*. Washington, DC: American Psychological Association; 2007

235. American Academy of Pediatrics. Policy statement: impact of music, music lyrics, and music videos on children and youth. *Pediatrics*. 2009;124(5):1488-1494.

236. Levin DE, Kilbourne J. *So Sexy so Soon: The New Sexualized Childhood and What Parents Can Do to Protect Their Kids*. New York, NY: Ballantine Books; 2008.

237. Finkelhor D, Jones L. Why have child maltreatment and child victimization declined? *Journal of Social Issues*. 2006;62(4):685-716.

Chapter 14

Nonprogrammatic Approaches to Child Maltreatment Prevention

Randell Alexander, MD, PhD
Sandra Alexander, MEd
Debra Esernio-Jenssen, MD
Lynn Sheets, MD, FAAP

Introduction

Child abuse prevention efforts often follow a certain process. A particular group within a community (ie, local, state, national) identifies an area of concern, reviews research on the problem to see what others have done, develops an idea for intervention, and implements an intervention. Increasingly, this intervention is being developed with some sort of structured feedback or even formal research on various aspects of effectiveness.

The intervention is often a program. The term "program" is not a rigid concept but usually would be understood to include a plan of action with a series of activities and procedures. For child abuse prevention, this usually means that a core group of people will initiate a type of time-limited process to reach individual people with the intention of modifying behavior. Examples include: face to face work with at-risk populations (eg, those who screen for being at risk in the newborn unit, as with many home visitation programs), programs for related problems (eg, drug or alcohol treatment), and interventions to reduce risk for abuse (eg, respite care, parenting classes).

Many child abuse prevention programs are individual to individual. There may be excellent reasons for this. Modeling is the key means by which humans and other species have learned. Lion cubs learn to hunt by observing their mothers. Chimpanzees learn some use of tools from adults in their troop. Humans have parents and other adults who teach folklore and techniques, as well as model how things should be done. Didactic learning (eg, reading) is a recent historical invention and has not been the primary way that humans have learned throughout history. If new parents learn how to be a parent, it has historically been by the modeling they observed while growing up and with the help of parents and others once they have a child. Thus, interventions that use this form of learning could be said to be capitalizing on millennia of tested methodology.

When confronted with wanting to do something to help prevent child abuse, professionals and others are also the product of what they have been taught, what they have seen, and orientations to the problem that reflect their own horizons. It is no surprise that social workers are often the group in a community that begin many of the child abuse programs. Not only do they care about children as much as anyone personally, but professionally they usually perceive an obligation to improve children's lives. Yet when approaching what to do, social work orientations tend to lead down certain pathways. Exposed to programs in their professional training and work life, it is natural to approach child abuse prevention similarly. Such approaches have created successes and constitute much of the effort to date. But how would a banker approach the subject? Or an engineer? And especially a health care professional?

Even if programs have had a certain amount of success, are they the structure to prevent child abuse (or at least take it to the next level of significant reduction)? Since no single approach to child abuse prevention will cover its many different types and populations, is the response to develop a program to address a problem the right approach most of the time?

Problems With Programs

An argument that decades of programs have yet to actually prevent child abuse is too simplistic an argument against this approach. However, programs may have some limitations that lessen the likelihood that they will achieve widespread child abuse reduction. There are multiple potential problems with the concept of "programs" to have a major impact on child abuse. Their very structure virtually ensures they will have limited impact.

Programs often involve individual or group contact. With estimates of child abuse ranging over 30% of the population,[1] direct encounter programmatic approaches would require the mobilization of millions to provide the interventions—an exceptionally unlikely proposition.

There also can be problems reaching the desired population:

1. A prenatal program might address women who actually get prenatal care, but often, it is the women who don't get such care that are considered at risk. Men/fathers are rarely seen in this setting, yet they are responsible for more physical abuse than women.

2. Birth of a child is another opportunity, since most babies in the United States are born in hospitals. Absent complications, most women and infants are discharged home in 48 hours. During that 48 hours, the new mother begins to learn about her baby, feed it, deal with her own physical health, get some sleep, receives visitors, often makes phone calls, texts, and is on social media. She is taught to bathe the baby, sees several physicians and multiple nurses, and has other activities. Child abuse prevention messages have to compete with all of this, with someone who probably would not be identified as an ideal student in these circumstances.

3. For many children under 5 years of age, the only professional that they see is their pediatrician/family practitioner. Well-child visits have many messages that need to be conveyed within a limited time. However, some messages can be conveyed by others in the practice (eg, nurse, receptionist) or by handouts or media in the waiting room. Some children see dentists, and some are enrolled in child care or preschool. All of these settings often do not have a large proportion of men attending.

4. Public or private school is relatively universal, except for primarily home schooling, and is a sustained opportunity to reach out to and affect children, teenagers, and their families.

5. Many adults do not attend college. Newspaper popularity has declined, but social media has increased. If a program wishes to access adults, it may be difficult to identify how to do so. What do 20 year olds watch or listen to? How could they be reached? How does this vary by socioeconomics, race, ethnicity, education, and life circumstances? Organizations such as the military might make an intervention mandatory for their entire population, but this does not apply to the general population.

Programs almost always depend on continual financing:

1. Programs depend on money and will likely die when the money ends unless new sources of funding can be found. They usually are not structured to be fully sustainable or to achieve a goal and be done.
2. They rely on funding that is likely to disappear. Foundations and communities often give for a limited period and then move on to another area of interest. Government and health are 2 funding sources that are most likely to be able to sustain long-term financing, but there are limits to these resources as well.

Even if they have an impact, it does not get translated to larger populations:

1. Some programs begin as pilot programs. Plans to increase such programs are often more nebulous than the original program idea itself. What works with the original group of people involved in the project may not be able to be extended financially or with program fidelity. Typically, the notion is to prove that it can be done first before thinking of how to expand to much larger populations.
2. Some programs serve an entire population that is small. A community that is granted funds to provide respite care, even if they were to achieve full funding, probably is not planning to expand outside the population in question. If the program is part of some larger network (eg, a large social service agency) then the issue is how to move the program to other communities with the same enthusiasm and community support.
3. Local programs often suffer because they do not have the researchers necessary for rigorous evaluation. Without this, other communities may have less incentive to adopt a program based on what appears to be only anecdotal success. Continued financing may suffer in the absence of data about effectiveness.

Even if they somehow got translated to larger populations, they may not be sustainable:

1. Core people eventually retire or leave. If a program was successful because of a charismatic leader, subsequent leadership may not be able to maintain or advance the effort.
2. Financial underwriting for small programs may not be adequate for growth. For example, some foundations provide funding for only limited geographical areas and efforts to widen the scope are beyond their charter.

Even if all this works, programs eventually die for lack of proof. At some point, child abuse programs face the challenge to prove that they actually reduced child abuse. This is difficult if the research component is not strong. Even if the program shows some success by operational measures, child abuse can be difficult to measure. Because most child abuse is not reported compared to its incidence,[1-4] a program that reduces child abuse by 50% but increases child abuse reporting by the same amount will appear to be ineffective. For example, if child abuse in a given area is reduced by 1000 cases, it would be offset if programs encouraged reporting and caused 1000 previously unknown cases to be identified. Teaching child safety in a school might encourage a child to tell about abuse that is happening to them now. More sophisticated research designs can help demonstrate a specific effect, but it has been difficult to date to show that an entire state's child abuse rate, for example, has been significantly reduced.

Programs also need to be adaptable. During the course of a child abuse prevention program better ideas might emerge. Continued work on the original program may become irrelevant. For this reason it is important, but not often done, that programs integrate a rapid cycle of quality improvement in response to outcomes and new evidenced-based practices.

Programs can Work Despite These Limitations

An example of a program that has sustained core leadership over time, kept program fidelity, and has a strong research component is the nurse home visitation program by David Olds and colleagues.[5] In this study from Memphis TN, one long-term study showed that long-term survival was better with the program. The intervention groups had home visitation that began prenatally and continued regularly for the first 2 years of life. Contrasted to nonvisiting comparison groups, the visitation sample of both mothers and children were significantly more likely to be alive 20 years later. That a program intervention would matter nearly 20 years later is impressive and gives hope for many other types of child abuse prevention efforts. However, the same difficulties remain if this program were to be taken to scale: development of the next generation of program leadership, finances to sustain and grow the effort, and the limits on finding enough nurses for large populations of infants and their families.

Another program that has shown long-term success for health outcomes decades later is the Carolina Abecedarian Project (ABC).[6] This has been an early childhood stimulation program near Chapel Hill, NC. "Disadvantaged" (ie, low-income) children were enrolled between 1972 and 1977. There were 57 "treatment" children and 54 well-matched children in the comparison group. The treatment consisted of 2 phases: birth to 5 years, and 6 to 8 years of age. In the first phase, there was an emphasis on enhancing language skills, emotional regulation, and cognitive skills of the children by an 8-hour day of periods of cognitive and social stimulation interspersed with caregiving and supervised play. This continued for 5 years. In the second phase, there was an emphasis on improving early math and reading skills with home school resource teachers. The researchers found that the second phase had no effect on health outcomes several decades later. More importantly, the first phase for those in the treatment group resulted in a lower prevalence of risk factors for cardiovascular and metabolic disease for when the original children were in their mid-30s. Treated males had healthier BMI in their childhood years extending into adulthood. The mean systolic blood pressure in the males in the comparison group was 143 mm Hg, but only 126 mm Hg for those who decades earlier had phase 1 intervention. Metabolic syndrome consists of increased blood pressure, high blood sugar level, excess body fat around the waist, and abnormal cholesterol levels. These symptoms occurred together, increasing risk of heart disease, stroke, and diabetes. For males in the control group, 1 in 4 had evidence of developing metabolic syndrome in their mid-30s. In contrast, none of those in the intervention group had metabolic syndrome. The cost of the program includes 5 years and $67 000 (in 2002 dollars) per child. But the outcome was sustained and substantial health benefits. Like the Memphis nurse home visitation program,[5] there was a strong benefit years later and long after the program itself ended. But this is an intensive program that might be difficult to take to a larger scale.

Nonprogrammatic Approaches

Nonprogrammatic approaches, as used here, are interventions that affect more people than a 1-to-1 program might. While there is a spectrum of intervention, key areas that are addressed include novel public awareness, systematic approaches for individuals, approaches to reduce fatalities, social norms, and policy and systems approaches. Clearly these programs overlap and have an interrelatedness that may be more than the name itself might imply. For example, public awareness may be part of some of the other nonprogrammatic approaches beyond those examples named in the following text. Thus the following examples are grouped in a fashion that should not be inferred to necessarily be exclusive of one another.

Public Awareness

Public awareness may not directly reduce child abuse, but it is often a springboard for individuals, communities, organizations, and government to do more. Public awareness can reach many people, often more than 1-to-1 programs can. Even if behavior is not substantially changed overall, it may make a difference to an individual. Messages can have lasting power; ads on TV can be remembered decades later. Indeed, companies would not spend their money on advertising if it did not generally work. Adults may know the words and tunes of TV shows from their distant childhood; older adults might remember the tunes and many of the words to such American TV shows such as Gilligan's Island or the Brady Bunch more than algebra formulas. Child abuse messages have not yet achieved such penetration and staying power. Four examples of public awareness follow, in which novel strategies have been used to capture attention and strengthen the messages.

Milwaukee Radio Roadblock

For difficult-to-reach populations, one way might be to use a media saturation strategy. In Milwaukee, Wisconsin, a "radio roadblock" helped to ensure that a large portion of the general population heard abusive head trauma prevention messages.

Abusive head trauma is a leading cause of abusive fatality and disability in young children. Prevention efforts primarily have been focused on parental support and caregiver education about coping with crying, yet the effectiveness of these approaches is not yet known. Given the serious consequences of abusive head trauma, novel approaches to prevention should be considered. If a caregiver's violence toward an infant can be mediated by education, then a novel and reasonable approach might include a public media campaign.

In August of 2001, and again in May of 2009, times when abusive head trauma cases admitted to Children's Hospital of Wisconsin were dramatically increased, public media campaigns including a "radio roadblock" were implemented. The radio roadblock consisted of a radio broadcast of the sound of a crying infant on all radio stations simultaneously in the Milwaukee market for 50 seconds followed by a short public service announcement. No matter what radio station a person might change to, the same message was heard. It could not be easily escaped. The notion was that 50 seconds would seem very long and create feelings and discussions, even though such crying does not compare to the daily experiences of a parent with an infant.

The results were impressive. On average the Children's Hospital of Wisconsin admits 20 infants and young children with abusive head trauma each year, and rarely is there a month without a new case. By early August 2001, 25 cases had already been admitted that year. A radio roadblock was developed and launched; what followed was more than 3 months without a new case. The radio roadblock intervention was used again 8 years later. In the economic recession of 2008, a record-breaking 30 cases were admitted. In May 2009, another 11 cases already had been seen. A comprehensive media campaign that included another radio roadblock was launched on May 15, 2009. Afterward, nearly 4 months passed without a new case. Media campaigns without a radio roadblock were used in 2003 and 2006 without a significant effect on the abusive head trauma-free intervals. In fact, in the last 10 years, the only abusive head trauma–free intervals longer than 2 months occurred after a public media campaign that included a radio roadblock. The results when compared to media campaigns without a roadblock were significant at $p < .001$ (Lynn Sheets MD, presentation to the Helfer Society, 2011).

Based upon both successes, a radio roadblock is a potentially effective strategy in the prevention of abusive head trauma. However, it has a certain novelty effect. Were this done twice a year, would the effect be the same? Would there be adaptation to the intervention and less effect on reducing abusive head trauma? For the children who were not injured in these time periods, there were clear benefits.

Times Square Media Saturation

A novel public awareness campaign was implemented in April 2009 during Child Abuse Prevention Month in New York City. For 3 weeks, messages about shaken baby prevention were displayed on the 11 NASDAQ and Reuters screens in Times Square. (See Volume 1, Chapter 12, "Physical Abuse Prevention.") The messages were shown for 2 minutes each hour for 3 weeks. The messages included content such as: "If you are stressed or frustrated by a crying baby. Put the baby down in a safe place. Walk away. Crying does not harm a baby. But SHAKING a baby can cause brain damage or death." And "REAL MEN have a soft touch? NEVER SHAKE A BABY!"

Approximately 1.5 million people viewed these screens daily. Although there was no means to assess the effect directly on the incidence of shaken baby syndrome thereafter; like the Milwaukee radio blockade, this intervention utilized the novelty effect and media saturation in communicating child abuse prevention.

Buddy Day

A novel approach to raising awareness about children and child abuse is Buddy Day in New Zealand. Begun in November 2011, this annual event is held each year in multiple cities in New Zealand. Buddies are cardboard cutouts that are shaped by school children into child facsimiles with a name, face, clothing, and other decorations (**Figure 14-1**). A story is created by schoolchildren for each Buddy in an accompanying booklet with extra pages for comments (**Figure 14-2**). On the front, the Buddy Day booklet states: "I understand that it takes a community to look after a child and I will be a 'buddy' by looking out and speaking up for children to keep them safe."

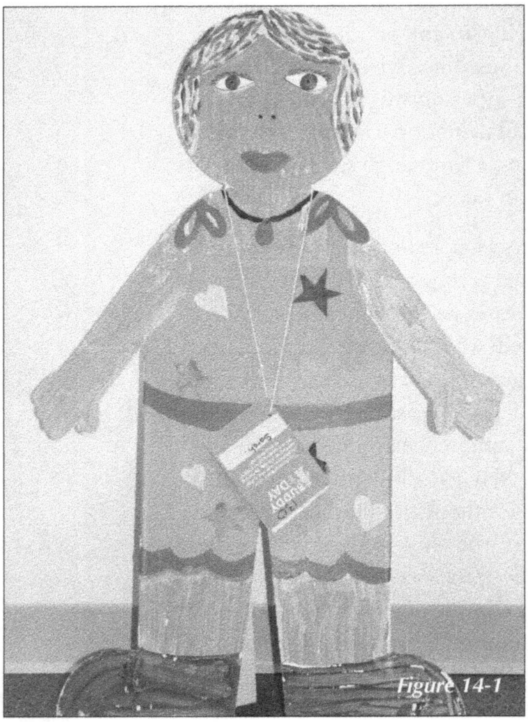

Figure 14-1. An example of a Buddy. "Sarah" was decorated by school children.

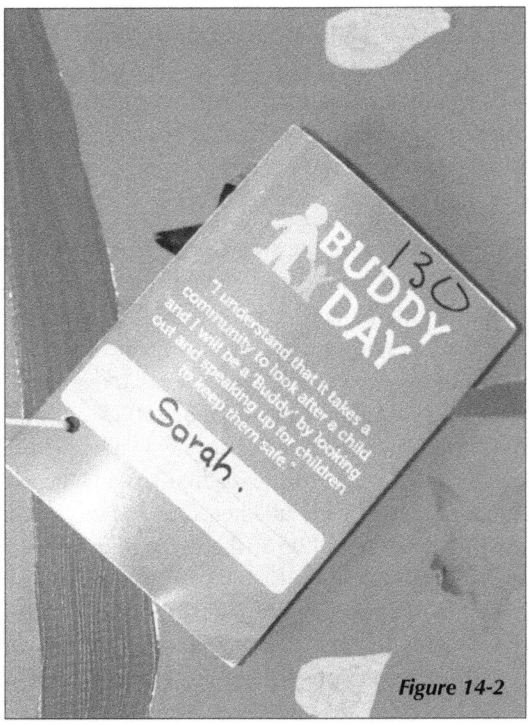

Figure 14-2. The booklet accompanying Sarah.

On Buddy Day, special breakfasts are held to distribute the Buddies to adults in all walks of life. Buddies are carried around during the day for everything the "carer" does. This creates conversations and sharing of messages. One example of a Buddy is the story of Sarah:

This is Sarah. Sarah's mum has left her in the care of her dad with 2 brothers and 1 sister. Sarah says, "All I need is a warm house, cozy bed, and a little soft teddy bear." She also needs to have a shower/bath every day. She loves to drink milk and eat vegetables. Most of all she enjoys coming to school every day. Sarah is very quiet and well mannered.

Some of the handwritten comments for Sarah by children and adults who saw her include:

— "Hi, Sarah! Every child needs to be loved and encouraged. Enjoy your day with Marie."

— "Kia ora, Sarah! I hope you have a super rad day with Marie."

— "Lovely to meet Sarah—made a difference after reading another sad tale of child abuse in today's paper."

— "A great reminder of children's simple needs. Lovely to meet you, Sarah."

Buddy Day is the creation of Child Matters, a nongovernmental organization dedicated to training about child abuse and its prevention. There are a variety of sponsors of Buddy Day, with the major sponsor being Sovereign, the largest insurance company in New Zealand. Sovereign has a business rationale for child abuse prevention[7]:

Sovereign is proud to be the principal partner of Child Matters Buddy Day. Buddy Day is New Zealand's only community event aimed at raising awareness of child abuse and the role every adult can play in keeping our children safe.

Sovereign partners with intervention programs because the health and wellbeing of New Zealanders has a direct impact on our business and the communities in which we all live.

Thousands of New Zealanders participate in Buddy Day; taking their Buddy to work, school, and other activities of the day. Top government officials and legislators take their Buddy to work, as well.

In addition to raising media and community awareness about children in general, Buddies generate discussions about protecting children, nurturing, and ways to increase their general well-being. Each year more thousands of Buddies are created and cities added to this effort.

Figure 14-3. *Sign upon entering the city limits of Morrinsville, New Zealand.*

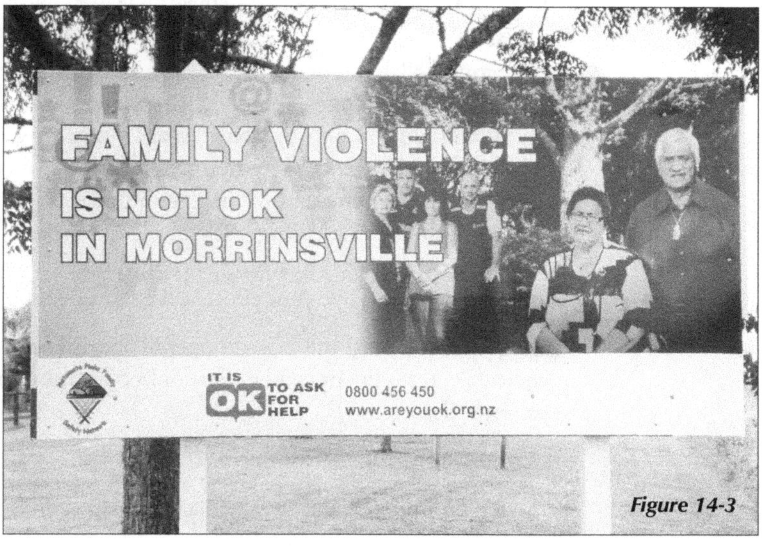
FAMILY VIOLENCE
IS NOT OK
IN MORRINSVILLE
IT IS OK TO ASK FOR HELP
0800 456 450
www.areyouok.org.nz
Figure 14-3

Family Violence is Not OK

The New Zealand Ministry of Social Development has developed a multimedia strategy of saying that "Family violence is not okay." **Figure 14-3** shows a billboard at the entrance to one small town. The Ministry measured the impact of television public service advertisements with 3 surveys between December 2007 and September 2008.

The Ministry described the results of their television interventions[8]:

— Overall, 68% of the people who recalled one of the ads surveyed in September 2008 agreed that the ads helped them to understand more about behaviors that should not be tolerated.

— The ads created the expectation that a violence-free life is possible. Of the people who recalled one of the ads, 88% agreed that the ads made them see change is possible.

— Of the people who recalled one of the ads, 57% agreed that the advertisements made them feel that they could help to influence someone to change their violent behavior. This feeling was particularly strong for Pacific peoples.

— The TV ads generated discussion among viewers. Overall, 68% of the people who recalled one of the ads reported having discussed them. This rose from 56% in survey 2.

— Of the people who recalled one of the ads, 22% (over 1 in 5) reported taking at least one action as a result of seeing them. This number of people reporting action is consistent across the 3 surveys.

— The people surveyed who took some action were most likely to talk to family and friends (14%) and to try and stop violence they were worried about (12%).

This governmental intervention helps to set an expectation and climate of a violence-free society. These messages are relatively ubiquitous within the country and may help with physical abuse reduction at various ages. This effort is one way in which the government and organizations are trying to improve the life of children. The Agenda for Children is one of the strategies in this regard.[9]

While the public may become accustomed to any message and, therefore, it might lose its impact, when such messages are being regularly adapted and there is saturation of public consciousness the opportunity exists to make a substantial difference. However, the net effect might be to raise child abuse reporting rates, and documentation of any positive effect could be swamped by such numbers.

Systematic Approaches Designed for Individual Education and Behavior Change

Text4Baby

In a unique collaboration between the mobile telephone industry and government and child advocacy groups, a mobile information service was developed that promotes maternal and child health by text messages (https://www.text4baby.org/). **Table 14-1** shows the founding partners, government partners, media partners, and some health nonprofit partners. In addition, there are numerous other organizations involved with this project. The idea is that over 80% of the American population with cell phones send and receive text messages. Reaching the population of expectant and new parents without requiring more than a one-time effort is, therefore, feasible and a relatively passive strategy.

Signing up for the text messaging hopefully begins prenatally, but can be done at birth or thereafter. Enrollment can be done online or by phone. For the latter, the following steps are undertaken:

1. Text BABY (or BEBE for Spanish) to 511411
2. When prompted, enter the due date and zip code

Table 14-1. Text4Baby Partners

Founding Partners:
— National Healthy Mothers, Healthy Babies Coalition
— Founding Sponsor: Johnson & Johnson
— Voxiva, Inc.
— The Wireless Foundation
— Grey Healthcare Group

Government Partners:
— US Department of Health and Human Services (HHS)
— White House Office of Science and Technology Policy
— US Department of Defense Military Health System
— US Department of Agriculture
— US Consumer Product Safety Commission
— Social Security Administration

Media Partners:
— MTV
— VME
— Discovery Fit & Healthy

Health Outreach Partners:
— American Academy of Pediatrics
— American Academy of Pediatric Dentistry
— American Association of Poison Control Centers
— American College of Nurse-Midwives
— American College of Obstetricians and Gynecologists
— America's Health Insurance Plans (AHIP)
— American Public Health Association
— The AOA Foundation, InfantSEE program
— Association of Community Affiliated Plans

That is all that has to be done. All information is kept private and not sold. Once someone has signed up, text messages will be sent that contain health-related issues timed to when the baby is born. For example, a mother might receive 3 messages per week reminding her about getting her baby shots, other health messages, injury and violence prevention, car seats, expected development, and other information. Among many others, the Centers for Disease Control and Prevention (CDC) was instrumental in message development. The text messages are free and do not count against the quota of minutes on nearly all telephone plans. Messages can be sent in English or Spanish. While it is necessary to sign up only once, if the due date changes, then texting "UPDATE" to 511411 will allow for adjustments.

Text4Baby lists sample messages that would be sent for a new baby[10]:

— Free msg: It's time for baby's 1-month Dr.'s visit. Your baby had blood tests right after she was born. At this visit, ask your Dr. for the results.

— Free msg: Not sure if your car seat is installed right? Get it inspected. Department of Transportation can help. Call for locations near you.

— Free msg: Your baby's mouth needs cleaning now—even before the first tooth! Wipe your baby's gums each day with a wet washcloth or use a soft baby toothbrush.

— Free msg: Worried about keeping baby warm at night? Infant pajamas & infant sleep sacks are safe for baby to wear to sleep. But no loose blankets in the crib.

— Free msg: Babies can get very sick from the flu. You & everyone who cares for your baby should get the flu shot during flu season. Call for info.

— Free msg: Have you gone back to work? It can be tough. Take it one day at a time & know you're not alone in this balancing act.

Hundreds of thousands of women have signed up to use this service in the United States. According to Text4Baby, over 39% of participants enrolled during the first trimester. Women in high-poverty areas enroll at a higher rate than the overall population. In one study, nearly half of enrolled women reported their household income as $16 000 or less.[11] In another study from Emory University, 99% of WIC participants had no concerns about enrolling with Text4Baby; 95% found the process to be easy, 92% read the messages regularly, and 88% planned to continue.[12] Ratings of the program are high.[11,13] Improvements include health knowledge and comfort in being a new parent,[11,14] appointment attendance and behavior change,[15] and improved access to health services.[11]

Text4Baby is a project that can extend into other countries, where cell phone use is likely to be relatively common as well. While a person can decide to delete an unread message, the attention of getting a message might increase the likelihood that some of the content will be delivered.

Anticipatory Guidance

Anticipatory guidance refers to recommendations given by physicians at the end of the medical encounter. Typical recommendations might include advice on feeding, developmental milestones, safety, and community resources. Pediatricians are often the only professional to see a child (and family) prior to kindergarten. These moments of opportunity enable delivery of child abuse prevention messages. These can take the form of asking about violence in the home, encouraging positive parenting, and explaining child development so it is not misunderstood. The success of the Back to Sleep campaign by the American Academy of Pediatrics is an example. Teaching parents to put their baby to sleep on their backs instead of their stomachs has saturated culture beyond that of 1-to-1 teaching. To the extent that the message has changed the culture, the effects may be long-term and self-perpetuating.

The difficulties for pediatricians (and family practitioners) are the numerous teaching points vs. the amount of time available for a well-child visit. Holding group teaching sessions can partially alleviate this, but media in the waiting room and use of other personnel are necessary in the delivery of such information. One example is the Coping with Crying program developed by Prevent Child Abuse Georgia and the Georgia Chapter of the American Academy of Pediatrics in 2003 and 2004. (See Volume 1, Chapter 12, "Physical Abuse Prevention.") In addition to education of the physician, this program involved all office staff, including receptionists, in an attempt to provide information saturation with all possible encounters a parent might have within the office.

Bystander Approach

Bystander programs to help prevent sexual mistreatment at college have been developed and increasingly used.[16] They are designed to help students develop the motivation and methods to intervene. The same dilemma exists for witnessing child mistreatment. People often express uncertainty about what to do when they observe a child being treated badly in public. In some cases, they mall call child protective services, but often, they do not. In many instances of public physical mistreatment of children there would be no physical injury if examined.

Such situations raise concerns about what to do. What is the right thing to say? Is someone being "nosey" for something that is "none of their business"? What rights do parents have to punish in their own way? Another concern is personal safety. Would intervening actually increase the risk to the child? What if intervening caused verbal or physical hostility to the person trying to help? There is little to no modeling in the media as to what can be done. There is no social saturation such that the person who is being overly aggressive/abusive would recognize what the bystander is doing and respond in a nonhostile fashion. However, a widespread educational campaign about intervening in a nonthreatening and supportive fashion could be very helpful for the many people frustrated about what to do.

Safety Checklists

Neglect is the most common form of child abuse, and kills more children than physical abuse. One of the most common forms of neglect is environmental neglect. Many people may have messy or cluttered homes, but the real risk is for those that are major safety hazards. Filthy homes reflect the chaos of the caregiver. This may be because of mental health problems, drug abuse, or other situational factors that impinge on some modicum of cleanliness. The challenge when working with families in such situations is not merely to get the house cleaned, but to address the underlying problem.

Often such environments take the form not of just dirty households, but actually unsafe and unsanitary homes. While there is a risk of disease with filthy living conditions, the actual number of diseases or hospital admissions for diseases is not very common. But the risk of injuries can be significant. In homes that are not as filthy, there can also be a safety concern with unanticipated risks by the caregiver.

While such lists can be used to document multiple ways in which a caregiver has created a dangerous house, these can also be used proactively to prevent injuries before they occur. Given to families with newborns, distributed with any agency home visit, passed out with pediatric visits, and available at stores that cater to young parents (eg, Toys "R" Us stores),–such information could be helpful to families willing to childproof their homes and seek assistance if that proves difficult.

Adverse Childhood Experiences Screening

Considerable research has shown that adverse childhood experiences (ACEs) have a strong effect on later adult health and functioning.[17] ACEs have such a strong effect on neurohormonal development, stress-related diseases, and overall health that they are perhaps the most preventable challenges to the nation's health.[1]

Yet using ACE screening with adults might help to identify and intervene to prevent additional abuses, or recognize those at risk for abusing others. Multiple groups exist and much research is exploring this important health domain. Aces Connection maintains a newsletter helping to share information about several such interventions, including prevention programs (http://www.acesconnection.com/).

Viewed in a different direction, it may be of help to educate parents and prevention partners about the consequences for abused children. For example, if a parent knew that their child's telomeres might shorten with abuse,[18] thereby possibly shortening lifespan and/or causing chronic diseases to appear at an earlier age, would that modify their behavior? The tremendous advances in understanding the biological harm of abuse might form a basis for education of the public as to what is at risk, why it is too costly to just respond after the fact, and why it is too costly not to prevent abuse and neglect.

Some Approaches to Reduce Fatalities

Of the estimated 2000 or more child abuse-related deaths each year in the United States, most are from neglect.[19] These numbers have remained relatively constant over the years. The major causes of child abuse and neglect deaths are unsafe sleep and drownings, followed in many states by physical abuse.[20] Prevention efforts for these neglect deaths include a number of specific teaching interventions such as education of the mother after birth of her child, in the pediatrician's office, the media, and others.

Unsafe Sleep

Bed sharing with a child has been discouraged by the American Academy of Pediatrics and others.[21] Sleeping on a sofa is especially dangerous.[22] Co-sleeping with an infant in a bed or sofa is more dangerous when the adult uses drugs or alcohol. However, sleeping in the same room early in infancy is often encouraged. As typically conceived, bed sharing means the infant is in bed with an adult without any protection. However, several countries have a more systematic method to allow both bed sharing and safety through the use of sleep boxes.

Since 1938, Finland expectant mothers have been given a box by the government that is both a sleeping environment for their newborn and contains clothes, blankets, diapers, and other items for their baby.[23] Starting first with low-income populations, in 1949 this service was extended to all expectant mothers. Mothers can choose between the box or a cash payment, but about 95% opt for the box. The sturdy box is lined with a close-fitting mattress which later can be used as a bed. The boxes have different colors and styles for different years. Thus, it becomes a social discussion as to what color box a person had. Boxes often become a keepsake from infancy.

The impetus for this was the high infant mortality rate in 1938, coupled with a generally poor population. In 1938 the infant mortality rate was 65 deaths per 1000 children, but in 2013 had dropped to 2 per 1000.[24] Some of this drop has been credited to the safer sleep environment.

In response to earthquakes in Christchurch, New Zealand in 2011, a safe sleep program was begun that uses boxes for infants. Called Pepi-Pod™, they have become a public health intervention for vulnerable or high-risk infants. After a decade of relatively stable infant mortality rates (already low because New Zealand initiated the concept of "back to sleep"), since 2010-2011 the infant mortality rates have fallen; especially in the native Maori population.[25,26] This is a statistical association and it cannot be causally proven, but (as in Finland) the program continues in part on the belief it might be making a difference (Anthea Simcock, Child Matters, personal communication).

Drowning

When a young child dies from drowning, it can be difficult for authorities to label it as neglect in the face of intense family grief. However, if a toddler were to wander outside and fall into a pool, it was the failure of the caregiver to have layers of protection to avoid this preventable situation. Another scenario when drowning occurs is when a toddler or infant is in a tub (sometimes with another child) and the parent goes away for a period of time to attend to another task. This too is predictable and preventable. The numbers of cases of drowning recognized as neglect likely is an underestimate because of the sympathy for the parents mourning the nonintentional loss of their child.

Education about pool safety and bath time safety may be of value, but consideration should also be given to more passive methods of prevention.[27] Zoning laws about pool safety, requiring 4 sided fencing for example, can help to reach people that might not be reachable by educational means alone. Door and pool alarms should not be relied upon alone, but can be one of the multiple means of protection. In part, these can be implemented by regulation of new and existing housing and do not require individual effort.

Policy and Systems Approaches

Policy and systems approaches have a benefit in that they might not require much individual effort, but have a preventive effect nonetheless. The goal is to change a way of acting or encourage desired behaviors through custom, media, or legislation.

Center-Based Day Care

Research suggests that well-run center-based day care can provide a safe alternative to other caregiving situations with less controlled environments. Child deaths were reviewed that occurred at day care facilities from Cook County, Illinois; Fulton County, Georgia; San Diego County, California; and the State of New Mexico from 1986 to 1990.[28] These jurisdictions have a combined population of 37 million people. Records included investigation, autopsy, and toxicology. After excluding deaths that occurred in the care of a babysitter, there were 9 deaths that were found to have occurred at a day care facility: "natural" in 6 cases and "unintentional" in 3 cases. The natural deaths consisted of sudden infant death or infections. Two deaths were from accidental asphyxiation and one from a motor vehicle/pedestrian accident. There were no deaths from falls or abuse. In a review of this study, Chadwick and Phillips[29] noted that the child population would have been about 700 000. Based upon California data of incidence, they estimated that the predicted number of deaths in the general population would have been 10, not 0. They concluded that center-based day care was substantially safer.

Chadwick and Salerno conducted a record review of children from birth to 6 years of age between 1984 to 1992 who were brought to a trauma center for serious head injury resulting from accidental trauma or physical abuse.[30] Motor vehicle accidents were excluded. At total of 338 records were examined and separated into: large, licensed child care centers and all other sites. The San Diego County referral base had a population of 232 084 children aged birth to 6 years, and the population of children attending part- or full-time center-based care was about 35 000. Of the 338 patients, 41 died and 191 had an Abbreviated Injury Scale (AIS) of 4 or 5. Only one child was from a day care, and that child had an AIS of 3 (stayed overnight in the hospital for observation from a nonabusive fall). Based upon a calculation of hours spent in day care, the risk of serious head injury was 19 children per million per year in day care versus 227 children per million per year in the general population. The conclusion was that child care centers are highly protective against life-threatening head injury.[29,30]

In a national survey that examined center-based care versus homes and family child care homes, the incidence of sexual abuse was considerably less in center-based care.[31] When corrected for numbers of children in an individual setting, the estimate of sexual abuse in centers was 5.5 per 10 000 children versus 8.9 per 10 000 children cared for in a home or family child care. Most of the sexual abuse in the centers centered on toilet training and consisted of fondling and touching.

Reasons for the relative safety of center-based care vs. home or family daycare settings include[29,32]:

1. Such centers have dedicated premises that are subject to inspection and therefore have less opportunity for neglect injuries, such as falling from a great height because of improper zoning regulation.
2. The presence of more than one caregiver most of the time. Since most physical abuse of children is hidden from other adults, the mere presence of another person may have a protective effect.
3. In addition, a center-based employee only has to handle any stress due to a child for a defined work period and can use other employees for respite.
4. Centers are typically open and subject to a person walking in at any time. This potential scrutiny may also be protective.
5. Caregivers in licensed centers receive some screening, which might reduce the possibility of known criminals or child abusers from being employed.

Implications for child abuse prevention could include:

1. More extensive screening of potential caregivers.
2. Increase in surveillance. Some centers and schools have cameras that allow parents to watch their children online at their convenience. This provides reassurance and is a message that someone might be watching at any time. (This can also be done in a home setting.) Centers could substantially increase the use of such cameras, often providing reassurance to parents about their child, not just as a child abuse prevention measure.
3. Increased access to center-based child care. Data suggest that center-based day care as a child abuse prevention strategy might be considerably more effective than virtually any existing child abuse prevention program. Compared to the costs of child abuse, this strategy might prove strongly cost effective.

TrustLine

An example of a system to help prevent abuse by in-home child care providers, tutors, in-home counselors, and child care staff is the TrustLine established in California in 1987. The concept arose from an effort to help parents find out whether their child's provider might be known to have child abuse concerns. While most states have some sort of screening of day care providers, TrustLine is a means for parents to find out if their provider has passed a screen successfully. TrustLine is a voluntary system in which a potential provider pays a one-time fee of approximately $124 to the Department of Social Services. A search is then made for 3 databases to include the fingerprint records from the California Department of Justice's California Criminal History System, the Child Abuse Central Index of California, and fingerprint records of the FBI Criminal History System (http://trustline.org/).

If the potential provider passes the background check they are listed on the TrustLine database. Parents can then call a phone number to check on the status of an applicant or receive information on how to apply. Sometimes the parent may pay the fee for a potential caregiver, but only the applicant can authorize the background check. If a provider refuses the background check, the parent may elect not to hire him/her. What the parent can learn for those who agree, is whether the potential provider has any disqualifying criminal convictions or substantiated child abuse reports in California (a pass/fail report). Details are not given. TrustLine is endorsed by the California Chapter of the American Academy of Pediatrics and administered by the California Department of Social Services and the nonprofit California Child Care Resource and Referral Network.

While there is a somewhat high price for this, the reassurance for parents can be substantial. The program pays for itself, therefore requiring no taxpayer subsidy. The information obtained is based on by a certain date the potential provider has passed the screens or not. Just because a person's record may be clear at the time the TrustLine is queried is not a guarantee that future abuse may not occur. But it is hoped that it reduces the chances, at least by potentially eliminating known risky caregivers. Since its inception, thousands of applicants have been screened out for failing the background checks. Some of these potential providers might be at increased risk of abusing children.

Laws About Spanking

As of November 2016, there are 50 countries that have banned corporal punishment in their society. Even if the laws were not strictly followed, these laws create a legal expression of what behaviors are desired. There is some evidence that these bans reduce physical abuse and perhaps some emotional abuse as well. (See Volume 1, Chapter 11, "Corporal Punishment and Child Abuse: Policy and Prevention Programs.") Building a cultural expectation that children (and adults) should not be hit might be an evolutionary step towards changing societal norms more fundamentally.

Business and Infrastructures

Prevention should involve a greater community than child abuse professionals if it is to succeed. The business community has an investment in safe and healthy employees, and that begins during their childhood.

Adverse childhood experiences (ACEs) were examined for 9633 currently employed adult members of Kaiser Foundation Health Plan in San Diego.[33] The authors found a strong graded relationship between a person's ACE score and each measure of impaired worker performance. Each of the ACE categories was associated with an increased likelihood of job problems, financial problems, and absenteeism. A strong dose response relationship was also found between the ACE score and the annual probability of a work-related injury. Findings such as these help the business community appreciate that having a childhood that avoids major adversities, such as various forms of child abuse, is in their economic interest. Helping the communities prevent child abuse then becomes part of the long-range business plan.

For example, Sovereign is the largest insurance company in New Zealand. Its former CEO, Symon Brewis-Weston, points out that his company has to think in 90 year spans. An insurance policy written today with a newborn might be relevant for a lifetime. Child abuse prevention and avoidance of many of the associated short- and long-term health problems make Sovereign financially stronger as well as serving the moral needs of the community.

With its scale and financial resources, the business community can be a powerful agent for prevention. Approaches to changing the business environment to consider long-term interests corresponds to changing the social norms of society as a whole.

Changing Social Norms

Ultimately, much of child abuse prevention depends upon changing the way society sees children, teaches how to interact with them, and helps parents to understand the exciting potential of children. As seen in Volume 1, Chapter 1, "Preventing Child Maltreatment Through the Positive Community Norms Framework," social norm change can be approached systematically, with some expectation of changing how people view themselves and others.

The Center for Health & Safety Culture in the Montana Institute has helped several states and the CDC develop approaches to reinforce positive behaviors that hope to reduce the risk of child abuse.[34]

Two examples of social norms change projects follow:

1. ***Positive Community Norms Project to Reduce Child Maltreatment in Wisconsin***: The Center for Health and Safety Culture is working in partnership with the Wisconsin Children's Trust Fund and Child Abuse Prevention Fund to reduce child maltreatment in Wisconsin through the utilization of the Positive Community Norms (PCN) framework. Specifically, the group is working to develop context and system linkages at the community and state levels that increase safe, stable, nurturing environments in which children are healthy, thrive, and develop free of maltreatment.
2. ***Reducing and Preventing Child Maltreatment in West Virginia***: TEAM for West Virginia Children and the Center for Health and Safety Culture are engaged in a multiyear project supporting efforts to reduce and prevent child maltreatment and promote positive outcomes for children in West Virginia. They are doing this by growing positive parenting norms supporting safe, stable, nurturing relationships; creating safe sleeping environments and behaviors; and reducing shaken baby syndrome. The Center will provide training on the PCN framework and develop and implement baseline surveys to measure existing positive norms, perceived norms, and critical gaps regarding safe infant sleeping practices and shaken baby syndrome. The Center will develop communications strategies to hear and steer public conversations on these critical issues.

By explicitly targeting strategies to highlight and change social norms, projects may help alter the general tenor of the community about child maltreatment and teach expectations to adults and children.

Essentials for Childhood

As a contrast to a sole focus on child abuse and its outcomes, the Division of Violence Prevention at the CDC has developed a framework of actions that can increase prevention effectiveness and a vision for what a positive childhood would look like. Their goals include:

— Raise awareness and commitment to promote safe, stable, nurturing relationships and environments and prevent child maltreatment.

— Use data to inform actions.

— Create context for healthy children and families through norms change and programs.

— Create context for healthy children and families through policies.

The Essentials for Childhood approach envisions the key building blocks of safe, stable, and nurturing relationships and environments as necessary for optimum development and as a way to avoid child maltreatment:

— ***Safety***: The extent to which a child is free from fear and secure from physical or psychological harm within their social and physical environment

— ***Stability***: The degree of predictability and consistency in a child's social, emotional, and physical environment

— ***Nurturing***: The extent to which a parent or caregiver is available and able to sensitively respond to and meet the needs of their child

Note that nurturing should include a strong component of stimulation as well. It is not enough to just be safe and stable, but all organisms grow best when stimulation and learning help to mold brain development and overall health.

Safe, stable, nurturing relationships can also be established in social environments that children encounter outside of the home and extended to relationships with caregivers other than the parents of the child. Providing safe, stable, nurturing relationships and environments outside the home (eg, high-quality child care) might have the potential for buffering their absence in the home. And safe, stable, nurturing relationships are important for adults as well, not only for their own well-being but to make them better parents for their children.

In response to this initiative, the CDC asked state health departments to join in using a Collective Impact approach in developing a plan of implementation. Key components of this initiative include[35]:

— Coordinate and manage existing and new partnerships with other child maltreatment prevention organizations and nontraditional partners

— Work with partners to identify strategies across sectors

— Identify, coordinate, monitor, and report on the strategies implemented by multisector partners

— Coordinate improvement processes (eg, continuous quality improvement) for multisector partners to refine strategies

— Document state-level impact of these efforts

Funding was only available for 5 states: California, Colorado, Massachusetts, North Carolina, and Washington. Yet the interest level was so high, that over 30 states continue to work with CDC without federal funding on this project. The states are applying the collective impact approach to work on the 4 Essentials goal areas. Collective impact approaches begin with communities working first to understand each other's points of view, conducting a landscape assessment of current strategies and services. Next, common goals are identified and then problem solving occurs, including identifying and implementing common strategies and common measures. A cycle of feedback and revision is continuous throughout the process.

Balancing Programmatic and Nonprogrammatic Approaches

Programs that address individuals directly are a mainstay of traditional approaches to child abuse prevention. They have become increasingly sophisticated and have scientific support in some instances. Their popularity speaks in part to the conceptual attractiveness, funding, and resources available and, perhaps, to the philosophical leanings of those who conduct them.

In the future, nonprogrammatic approaches may become more common in an effort to apply multiple means to substantially reduce child maltreatment. Increasing innovative, nonprogrammatic thinking can be difficult almost by definition. Familiarity with novel approaches may make new ideas easier to imagine. Child abuse has proven stubborn to prevent and will only likely be seriously diminished when the culture of caregiving changes.

References

1. Felitti VJ, Anda RF, Nordenberg D, et al. The relationship of adult health status to childhood abuse and household dysfunction. *Am J Prev Med.* 1998;14:245-258.

2. Gilbert L, Breiding M, Merrick M, et al. Childhood adversity and adult chronic disease: an update from ten states and the District of Columbia, 2010. *Am J Prev Med.* 2014;48(3):345-349.

3. Berger R, Fromkin J, Stutz H, et al. Abusive head trauma during a time of increased unemployment: a multicenter analysis. *Pediatrics.* 2011;128:637-643.

4. Finkelhor D, Jones L. *Have Sexual Abuse and Physical Abuse Declined Since the 1990s?* Durham, NH: Crimes Against Children Research Center; 2012:CV267.

5. Olds D, Kitzman H, Knudtson M, Anson E, Smith J, Cole R. Effect of home visiting by nurses on maternal and child mortality: results of a 2-decade follow-up of a randomized clinical trial. *JAMA Pediatr.* 2014;168:800-806.

6. Campbell F, Conti G, Heckman J, et al. Early childhood investments substantially boost adult health. *Science.* 2014;343:1478-1485.

7. Buddy Day. Thank you to our 2015 sponsors. http://buddyday.org.nz/47/supporters/sponsors. Accessed November 2, 2016.

8. Ministry of Social Development. Campaign for action on family violence: impact of the 'It's not ok' television advertisements. http://www.msd.govt.nz/about-msd-and-our-work/publications-resources/research/campaign-action-violence-tv/. Accessed November 3, 2016.

9. Agenda for Children. *Making Life Better for Children.* Wellington, New Zealand: Ministry of Social Development; 2001.

10. text4baby. Message content. https://www.text4baby.org/about/message-content. Accessed November 3, 2016.

11. Martinez K, Uekusa S. National survey of text4baby participants. http://www.csusm.edu/anthropology/docsandfiles/Text4baby.pdf. Published 2013. Accessed November 3, 2016.

12. Gazmararian JA, Elon L, Yang B, Graham M, Parker R. Text4baby program: an opportunity to reach underserved pregnant and postpartum women? *Matern Child Health J.* 2014;18(1):223-232.

13. Kaleka A, Olsen R, Sweet M. Utilization of text4baby to improve maternal and infant outcomes with an interdisciplinary team. Paper presented at: STFM Annual Conference; Seattle, Washington; April 26, 2012.

14. Evans WD, Wallace JL, Snider J. Pilot evaluation of the text4baby mobile health program. *BMC Public Health.* 2012;12:1031.

15. Grabosch S, Gavard J, Mostello D. Text4baby improves glycemic control in pregnant women with diabetes. American Journal of Obstetrics and Gynecology Web site. http://www.ajog.org/article/S0002-9378(13)01249-0/pdf. Accessed November 3, 2016.

16. Potter S, Stapleton J, Moynihan M. Designing, implementing, and evaluating a media campaign illustrating the bystander role. *J Prev Interv Community.* 2008;36:39-55.

17. Centers for Disease Control and Prevention. Adverse childhood experiences (ACEs). http://www.cdc.gov/violenceprevention/acestudy/. Accessed November 3, 2016.

18. Shalev I, Moffitt TE, Sugden K, et al. Exposure to violence during childhood is associated with telomere erosion from 5 to 10 years of age: a longitudinal study. *Mol Psychiatry*. 2012;18(5):576-581.

19. US Advisory Board on Child Abuse and Neglect. *A Nation's Shame: Fatal Child Abuse and Neglect in the United States*. Washington, DC: US Department of Health and Human Services; 1995.

20. Florida Child Abuse Death Review Committee. *Death Review: Annual Report December 2010*. Tallahassee, FL: Florida Child Abuse Death Review Committee; 2011.

21. American Academy of Pediatrics, Task Force on Sudden Infant Death Syndrome. SIDS and other sleep-related infant deaths: expansion of recommendations for a safe infant sleeping environment. *Pediatrics*. 2011;128:e1341-e1367.

22. Rechtman L, Colvin J, Blair P, Moon R. Sofas and infant mortality. *Pediatrics*. 2014;134:e1293-e1300.

23. Lee H. Why Finnish babies sleep in cardboard boxes. http://www.bbc.com/news/magazine-22751415. Published June 4, 2013. Accessed November 3, 2016.

24. World Bank. Mortality rate, infant (per 1,000 live births). http://data.worldbank.org/indicator/SP.DYN.IMRT.IN. Accessed November 3, 2016.

25. Statistics New Zealand. Births. http://www.stats.govt.nz/browse_for_stats/population/births?BirthsAndDeaths_MRYeDec12.asp. Accessed November 3, 2016.

26. Ihaka J. Sudden infant death rate drops. *New Zealand Herald*. December 9, 2013. http://www.nzherald.co.nz/nz/news/article.cfm?c_id=1&objectid=11169518. Accessed November 3, 2016.

27. Feldman K. Drowning in child fatality review. In: Alexander R, ed. *Child Fatality Review: An Interdisciplinary Guide and Photographic Reference*. Saint Louis, MO: GW Medical Publishing; 2007:319-330.

28. Good S, Parrish G, Ing R. Children's deaths at day-care facilities. *Pediatrics*. 1994;94:1039-1041.

29. Chadwick D, Phillips M. Safety in numbers: protection of children from death and serious injuries by licensed childcare centers. In: Alexander R, ed. *Child Fatality Review: An Interdisciplinary Guide and Photographic Reference*. Saint Louis, MO: GW Medical; 2007:709-718.

30. Chadwick D, Salerno C. Likelihood of the death of an infant or young child in a short fall of less than 6 vertical feet. *J Trauma*. 1993;35:968.

31. Finkelhor D, Moore D, Hamby S, Straus M. Sexually abused children in a national survey of parents: methodological issues. *Child Abuse Negl*. 1997;21:1-9.

32. Alexander R. Child abuse and protective child care. In: Murph J, ed. *Health in Child Care: A Manual for Health Professionals*. Chicago, IL: American Academy of Pediatrics; 2005.

33. Anda RF, Fleisher VI, Felitti VJ, et al. Childhood abuse, household dysfunction, and indicators of impaired adult worker performance. *Perm J*. 2004;8(1):30-38.

34. Center for Health & Safety Culture. The Montana model of social norms. http://chsculture.org/montana-model-of-social-norms/. Accessed November 3, 2016.

35. Centers for Disease Control and Prevention. Essentials for Childhood Framework: steps to create safe, stable, nurturing relationships and environments for children. http://www.cdc.gov/violenceprevention/childmaltreatment/essentials.html. Accessed November 3, 2016.

The findings and conclusions in this chapter are those of the authors and do not necessarily represent the official position of the Centers for Disease Control and Prevention.

Chapter 15

Prevention of the Commercial Sexual Exploitation of Children

Jordan Greenbaum, MD

Introduction

Commercial sexual exploitation of children (CSEC) is a particularly egregious form of child maltreatment that involves multiple violations of human rights and warrants major global efforts for primary prevention. This chapter will begin with a definition and overview of CSEC, describe challenges to primary prevention, and finish by focusing on current prevention efforts and highlights of interesting programs.

CSEC involves the sexual abuse of a child by another person in return for remuneration, in cash or kind, paid to the child or paid to a third person or persons.[1] CSEC includes child prostitution, child pornography, trafficking in children for sexual purposes, child sex tourism, and child marriage for the purposes of sexual abuse or sexual exploitation. Essential to this definition is the commercial transaction that occurs in exchange for the sex act. The remuneration may not be in the form of money but instead involve exchange of sex acts for food, shelter, or other valued commodity. Thus, it includes "survival sex" that occurs commonly among runaway and thrownaway youth.[2]

The exact number of children and youth CSEC victims is unknown because the databases and research necessary to calculate prevalence and annual incidence are lacking. Estimates vary substantially given varied measurement strategies, populations studied, terminology used, and the inherent difficulty in identifying victims of illegal activities. In one study, 1078 American-born youth in Ohio were thought to have been victims of trafficking during the course of a year.[3] Estes and Weiner estimated that over 244 000 United States youth were at risk of CSEC during the year 2000, although it should be noted that there have been criticisms of the methodology leading to this estimate.[4,5] As it stands, any figures offered for total numbers of CSEC victims should be considered only estimates.

Children at risk for CSEC include those who have a history of running away from home, or being "thrown away" (told to leave home by an adult caregiver or prevented from returning home without adequate alternative housing arrangement); a history of prior abuse, neglect, or other family dysfunction; or foster care placement.[6] Factors at the individual, family, community, and societal levels create vulnerability for CSEC (**Table 15-1**).

Table 15-1. Factors Creating Vulnerability to Sexual Exploitation[3,4,7-10]

Individual	Family	Community	Societal
— Runaway/throw-away status — History of maltreatment — Substance abuse — Mental health problems — Cognitive delay or other special needs — Gang involvement — Foster care placement	— Poverty — Caregiver substance abuse/mental health issues — Domestic violence — Child welfare involvement — Criminal activity/ adult prostitution in home — Members of socially marginalized group — Refugee status	— Poverty — Street prostitution by adults — Transient male populations — Community tolerance of adult-child sexual relationships and violence against children	— Gender bias — Glorification of "pimp culture" — Sexualization of girls — Political/social unrest, corruption, poverty — Social exclusion

Victims of commercial sexual exploitation may be recruited by strangers, acquaintances, family members or relatives, gang members, or peers.[4,11] Common sites of recruitment include shopping malls, bus stops or stations, schools, homeless shelters, and other areas where children may have limited supervision.[4] Deceit and manipulation are common methods of recruitment.[12] A child may be enticed by promises of romance or exciting opportunities (eg, modeling, acting), offered shelter and protection, or they may be promised employment with the opportunity to send money home to impoverished parents in their home country. Once involved with the exploitation, however, many experience extreme physical and sexual violence, emotional abuse, isolation, and deprivation.[12,13] Victims are at high risk of sexually transmitted infection, HIV/AIDS, physical injury, infertility from pelvic inflammatory disease or complications from abortion, drug addiction, posttraumatic stress disorder, major depression, chronic pain disorders, and suicide.[14-21]

The Protocol to Prevent, Suppress, and Punish Trafficking in Persons, Especially Women and Children, Supplementing the United Nations Convention Against Transnational Organized Crime (also called the Palermo Protocol)[22] was created to prevent and combat trafficking in persons, to protect and assist victims, and to promote cooperation among States Parties. With respect to prevention, the protocol calls upon countries to establish comprehensive policies, programs, and other measures to prevent trafficking. It directs countries to engage in research and disseminate information about human trafficking. It recommends developing social and economic initiatives to combat trafficking, and encourages collaboration between governmental and nongovernmental agencies and other stakeholders. The protocol calls for measures to alleviate conditions that contribute to trafficking and decrease the demand for sex trafficking. These recommendations may be generalized to child sexual exploitation, in general.

More recently, the United Nations General Assembly adopted a Global Plan of Action to Combat Trafficking in Persons.[23] This plan reiterates the international support for antitrafficking efforts. More importantly, it emphasizes the need to address all factors that create vulnerability to trafficking (from individual risk factors to regional socioeconomic and political problems, to cultural norms), and to do so using a human rights–based gender- and age-sensitive approach. As in the Palermo Protocol and other major documents,[24,25] the Global Plan stresses that transnational collaboration is essential to eradicating international human trafficking, as is coordination between government entities, private businesses, the media, and nongovernmental organizations (NGOs).

Central to the success of efforts to end child commercial sexual exploitation is the shift of focus from simply trying to prevent a negative event (child exploitation) to creating a positive social or economic change in communities, regions, or countries. These positive changes may include building a collective capacity to recognize and support high-risk children, reduce gender bias, provide opportunities for employment, or increase the knowledge of high-risk children and families regarding the dangers of CSEC.[26] (A multitude of prevention initiatives have been implemented by antitrafficking organizations and state or federal agencies. Some of these are described at the end of this chapter.) In addition, organizations whose mission does not specifically target human trafficking have created critical social and economic changes that ultimately serve to decrease the risk of trafficking. In its work to help victims of natural disaster, war, and other crises, the International Rescue Committee[27] has created programs that empower women and provide them with options that may obviate the need to migrate or engage in other activities that place them or their children at a high risk for sex trafficking. Vocational training, as well as increased access to credit and investment opportunities, has helped families recover from poverty and social strife; making their children less vulnerable to trafficking.

Challenges to Primary Prevention of CSEC

There are considerable challenges to successful CSEC prevention, not the least of which is the paucity of empirical research on the issues and difficulties in obtaining accurate statistics on incidence and prevalence.[5,24,28-30] In their review of English-language research-based literature on human trafficking, Gozdziak and Bump found that only 39 of 218 (18%) journal articles were based on empirical research, and of those 39, only 7 discussed children.[31] Of the 218 articles, only 1 specifically discussed boys. Much of the information regarding CSEC derives from studies of international human trafficking, small samples of survivors or exploiters, studies combining women and children subjects, and information obtained from professionals working with survivors.[14,21,31-33] There is a predominance of qualitative methodologies used in data collection, with relatively few studies and reports using quantitative methods.[31] Given the hidden and illegal nature of CSEC, it is likely that only a minority of victims are identified,[25,28] and these persons may differ in fundamental ways from the rest of the victim population, potentially limiting the generalizability of studies on survivor characteristics and experiences. However, an effective primary prevention program must be based on accurate data regarding the vulnerabilities of child victims, pathways of entry to CSEC, risk factors for youth and adults to become exploiters, behaviors and strategies used by exploiters, and the various factors related to buyer behavior, desires, and attitudes.

The dearth of research on commercial child sexual exploitation extends to a paucity of outcomes studies measuring the impact of the prevention programs now in existence.[30] Many programs have published no formal evaluation, and those that do cite data tend to focus on program output (eg, number of professionals educated, number of high-risk children participating in the program), with little or no attention paid to program outcomes and impact.[34] Such research is desperately needed in order to effectively reduce child sexual exploitation and to inform how limited public and private resources are used for prevention. While evaluation of CSEC prevention programs may be limited by any of the common problems associated with evaluation (eg, an unclear evaluation purpose or lack of time and funding for the evaluation) particular challenges related to CSEC projects may involve:

— Failure to recognize and address selection bias (eg, gathering and analyzing data only from known victims of human trafficking who are participating in case prosecution, but generalizing findings and conclusions to the whole population of CSEC youth)

— Poor operational definition of key concepts (ie, trafficking in persons, CSEC)

— Lack of clear and objective criteria to identify victims

— Confidentiality issues and protection of identity (programs may be reluctant to allow outside evaluators access to data on victims they serve)[34]

— Lack of accurate baseline prevalence statistics and difficulty determining program impact due to influence of other factors (ie, increased or decreased recognition and reporting of cases over time)

Other major challenges to primary prevention of commercial child sexual exploitation involve difficulties in establishing the necessary capacity to develop, implement, and monitor effective programs.[24] Such issues are present at the organizational, community, regional, national, and international levels. Funding is typically very limited, so prevention experts, victim service providers, and law enforcement may all be competing for the same dollars. In countries or regions with severe poverty, limited resources, or social unrest, there may be no solid infrastructure at the community or national level that would support a prevention program. In some areas, there may be few local or regional professionals with the expertise in CSEC to guide efforts. An important aspect of primary prevention involves education of key professionals on child sexual exploitation. To do this effectively, one needs stakeholders within those professions who are knowledgeable about CSEC and willing/able to commit time and resources to education.

When community financial resources are limited, there may be staff cutbacks and increased workloads, all of which can preclude those with expertise from being able to disseminate information to others in their field. There may be difficulties related to transnational cooperation between countries involved in a particular type of exploitation (eg, combating child trafficking in Greece involves working with the Albanian government, because many victims originate in that country). Efforts at transnational cooperation have been intensive in this case, and have included information sharing, multinational teams working in the field, and collaboration of efforts to return children across borders to the country of origin.[35] However, analogous efforts may be lacking in other areas of the world, especially if the countries involved have opposing political views or very different cultural beliefs. Comprehensive resources are available for designing effective programs,[26] for conducting program evaluations,[30] and for developing appropriate performance indicators.[36]

CSEC Prevention

To combat CSEC, the National Plan to Prevent the Sexual Abuse and Exploitation of Children[37] recommends focusing on 6 action areas:

1. Research into factors that motivate perpetration and perpetuation of exploitation and abuse, conditions placing children at risk, as well as testing prevention strategies for efficacy and impact.

2. Public awareness about the problem and extent of CSEC and abuse; as well as education of the public on social justice, healthy environments, relationship, and sexuality. The plan recommends use of a variety of communication strategies, including mass and social media, personal networks, and spheres of influence.
3. Efforts to end demand, including educating the general public and professionals about the need to perceive exploited children as "victims/survivors" rather than criminals and the need to hold those who exploit children accountable for their actions. The plan also promotes educating boys and men in prevention efforts and challenging the public to recognize and change the pervasive tendency to hypersexualize children.
4. Enhance evidence-based practices and policies targeting prevention of CSEC and other sexual harm toward children as well as treatment practices for individuals deemed at risk for becoming perpetrators of sexual abuse.
5. Encourage and support collaboration between agencies and organizations to maximize the use of resources and promote effective prevention strategies and policies. Collaboration should occur at the individual, organizational, community, and national levels and involve governmental agencies, nonprofit service providers, health care, industry, media and the arts, and faith-based organizations. Cross-collaboration with professionals and organizations in related areas (eg, intimate partner violence, children's rights) is encouraged.
6. Increase funding for prevention in the public and private sectors. Support measures that would include resources for CSEC prevention as part of larger policies or strategies that focus on sex crime punishment and prosecution.

Many nonprofit organizations seek to prevent CSEC by creating and implementing programs within a target community. In one study of community-based child protective programs around the world (targeting sex trafficking, and other forms of violence, exploitation, abuse, and neglect of children), results suggested that 7 factors may be important in successful community-based programs: (1) community ownership of the problem and the group efforts to address it, (2) recognizing and using pre-existing resources in the community, (3) support of formal and nonformal community leaders, (4) child participation in the project, (5) inclusion of diverse groups in the process and appropriate balance of power among participants, (6) adequate human and material resources, and (7) linkages with formal and nonformal systems in the community and district.[38] These factors may present considerable challenges, based in part on limited resources, reluctance to discuss and acknowledge a "taboo" practice in the community, reluctance to include marginalized populations in the project (typically women/children from minority groups who are being victimized), and lack of support from political leaders.

Prevention programs that seek to eliminate CSEC may use a variety of strategies.[26,37] Some may seek to reduce the supply side of the equation, working with all youth or those youth or families at high risk for child sexual exploitation. These programs may strive to educate youth about Internet safety, dangers of exploitation, and common recruiting practices.[39] They may teach or improve life skills for adolescents. They may work within impoverished communities to help families find alternative means of support so children do not need to be sent away to earn money and, thus, fall prey to traffickers.[35] Other programs focus on demand (ie, buyers of pornography, juvenile prostitution, sex tourism).[40] Some organizations may implement a zero-tolerance policy for sexual exploitation activities, even if they are legal in the country where the individual is employed. Some agencies may require government workers to undergo training to raise awareness of CSEC and the negative impact on children.[25] Programs may target young males to alter their perceptions of the sex industry, change their attitudes about sexualizing and objectifying girls, and educate them about commercial sexual exploitation.

Still other programs are directed toward third-party entities that may indirectly enable CSEC to occur, including members of the hospitality and tourist industries (eg, hotel staff, taxi drivers, airline companies).[41] Governmental policies and programs may seek broad social and economic changes to alleviate the conditions that drive CSEC (eg, poverty, social unrest, unemployment, marginalization of certain social groups). They may take measures to improve border control and reduce corruption of border guards and law enforcement. Even though an evidence base is lacking, the myriad programs being implemented across the globe show tremendous diversity. A few of these programs are described in the next section.

"My Life, My Choice"

The "My Life, My Choice" curriculum[39] was designed for any adolescent girl aged 12-18 years, for high-risk adolescent girls (ie, those with a history of maltreatment, exposure to family violence, substance abuse or those who live in areas disproportionately targeted by exploiters), and for victims/survivors of CSEC. Based on survivor knowledge and public health principles, the 10-session curriculum has been implemented in 21 states. Groups of participants are led by a pair of facilitators, including a trained CSEC survivor and a trained and licensed clinician or service provider. Through psycho-education, group interaction, and journaling, the sessions aim to change girls' attitudes about CSEC (ie, it's dangerous, not glamorous). They aim to increase their knowledge about victim vulnerability to CSEC, conditions in "the life" and common recruiting methods and teach them to recognize and avoid recruiting tactics. For those girls who are already victims of CSEC, the curriculum seeks to empower them to develop and use resources that will help them leave the exploitative environment. To date, over 1200 girls have completed the curriculum within a variety of settings (eg, Los Angeles County Probation Department, group homes for children in state custody, middle and high schools) (Lisa Goldblatt-Grace, oral communication). The majority of the participants have been youth deemed to be at high risk for commercial sexual exploitation (although some of these eventually disclose exploitation experiences in their pasts). Of the initial 40 girls involved in the curriculum, 38 had reported having been approached by a trafficker at some time, 3 had been commercially sexually exploited by a trafficker, and 6 had been exploited while living on the streets. Program evaluation includes pre- and postcurricula questionnaires, review of journal entries, and debriefing with program and school staff. There has been no formal empirically based research on outcomes to date (Lisa Goldblatt-Grace, oral communication); however, plans are in progress to launch a formal outcomes evaluation.

Informally, findings have been promising: 96% of participants reported being "very satisfied" with the curriculum. One of the most significant changes has been in participant understanding of common recruitment techniques. For example, the results of the program implemented at a group home indicated a substantial increase in the correct response (preprogram score 30% correct, postprogram score 90%) to the following prompt: "Name 3 signs that someone is trying to recruit you for prostitution." In 1 middle school, 30% of the girls were able to identify a "pimp" in a sample anecdote during the pretest, while 90% were able to do so after the training. Victims of CSEC have demonstrated an increased knowledge of available resources and a comfort level with the idea of reaching out to police or social workers.

End Child Prostitution, Child Pornography, and Trafficking of Children for Sexual Purposes

End Child Prostitution, Child Pornography, and Trafficking of Children for Sexual Purposes (ECPAT International) is a global network of organizations and individuals who are working toward elimination of child commercial sexual exploitation.[42] As of 2007, groups existed in over 70 countries. One of the many projects developed by ECPAT is the Code of Conduct for the Protection of Children from Sexual Exploitation in Travel and Tourism.[43] This project involves collaboration with stakeholders in the tourism industry in an effort to eradicate child sex tourism.

Participating entities agree to abide by the Code, which means they will[37]:

1. Establish a corporate ethical policy against CSEC.
2. Train personnel in the country of origin and travel destinations.
3. Introduce clauses in contracts with their suppliers, stating a common repudiation of CSEC.
4. Provide information about CSEC to travelers through catalogues, brochures, in-flight films, ticket-slips, Web sites, etc.
5. Provide CSEC information to local "key persons" at destinations.
6. Report annually on their activities.

The Code began as an ECPAT project in 1998 but currently is an independent organization funded by the Japan Committee for UNICEF and supported by the World Tourism Organization. As of March 2013, over 1100 signatories have joined the Code, from 45 countries across Europe, Asia, Africa, and the Americas.[41] The number of tourists affected by this program is estimated to be over 30 million annually.[44] Challenges faced by the Code include a lack of data on impact and success of the program, fear of company leaders that the campaign will "scare away" tourists or give the tourist destination a bad reputation, fear that the public would perceive the tourism industry as being somehow involved in the sex trade, difficulties convincing companies that adoption of the Code will benefit the company itself, and lack of commitment by large tourism companies (eg, airlines).[45] However, the program has been successful in raising awareness of CSEC at major child sex tourism locations and increasing reporting of suspected cases. An example of Code activity is the training of tuk-tuk (auto rickshaw) drivers in Cambodia and recruiting them to serve as watchdogs in the community. Elsewhere, the hotel staff of 1 company now asks for identification of all guests checking into the hotel, including the identification of children.[45]

Georgia's Not Buying It

The Georgia's Not Buying It campaign[40] provides an example of public-private collaboration to raise public awareness of child sex trafficking. The state Attorney General's office has partnered with law enforcement, the Governor's Office for Children and Families, and multiple nonprofit organizations to create a public service announcement featuring famous sports players in Atlanta. Their message extends beyond general information about trafficking to targeting potential buyers: "If you are buying, beware. Your secret is out. Georgia isn't buying the lie." The campaign is publicized through billboards and posters on public transportation vehicles. The Web site challenges reader to take the following pledge (**Box 15-1**):

Box 15-1. Georgia's Not Buying It Pledge

I pledge to:

—Walk in integrity by not purchasing sex.

—Exhibit courage by raising awareness, speaking out against CSEC, and reversing today's distorted perception of sex.

—Leave a legacy by mentoring the next generation to walk in integrity and exhibit the courage to eradicate CSEC from the face of the earth.

Within the first 4 months of the campaign, the Web site received nearly 450 pledges. The site also provides a tip line telephone number for those seeking to report information on suspected trafficking cases.

Not For Sale Red Card Campaign

In 2010, South Africa hosted the World Cup in soccer. Not For Sale,[46] a nonprofit anti-trafficking organization, recognized the opportunity to target potential buyers of sex who congregate at this major sporting event. They partnered with Martin/Williams Advertising to launch the "Red Card Campaign," which used the concept of the red card in soccer (a penalty given to players who commit major transgressions during the game). The campaign used the red card to call attention to human trafficking as a form of modern-day slavery and the greatest transgression of human rights. Volunteers dressed up as soccer players and referees handed out red cards educating the public about human trafficking. They distributed over 25 000 cards to fans in the stadiums and in the streets, customers at South Africa Pep stores, and to students and crowds at popular destinations.[47] They placed billboards and posters across the country. They conducted a radio interview, a public service announcement, and a YouTube video.[48]

Conclusion

The commercial sexual exploitation of children has gained international attention as a major human rights issue affecting one of society's most vulnerable populations. Efforts to prevent CSEC are being launched by individual advocates, faith-based groups, and community, national, and international NGOs and government agencies. Considerable challenges must be faced, including a lack of empirical research and accurate data on incidence and prevalence, lack of outcomes data on prevention strategies, and lack of resources. Nonetheless, there are growing numbers of innovative primary prevention programs targeting potential victims, buyers, and the general public. As knowledge of this type of child maltreatment gradually increases, sophisticated program evaluations will begin to identify successful programs and inform future work in prevention.

References

1. United Nations Children's Fund, United Nations Economic and Social Commission for Asia and the Pacific, End Child Prostitution in Asian Tourism. *Commercial Sexual Exploitation of Children and Child Sexual Abuse in the Pacific: A Regional Report.* Suva, Fiji: United Nations Children's Fund Pacific; 2006.

2. Greene JM, Ennett ST, Ringwalt CL. Prevalence and correlates of survival sex among runaway and homeless youth. *Am J Public Health.* 1999;89(9):1406-1409.

3. Williamson C, Prior M. Domestic minor sex trafficking: a network of underground players in the midwest. *J Child Adol Trauma*. 2009;2:1-16.
4. Estes RJ, Weiner NA. *The Commercial Sexual Exploitation of Children in the U.S., Canada and Mexico*. Philadelphia, PA: University of Pennsylvania, Center for the Study of Youth Policy; 2002.
5. Stansky M, Finkelhor D. *How Many Juveniles Are Involved in Prostitution in the U.S.?* Durham, NH: University of New Hampshire, Crimes Against Children Research Center; 2008.
6. Hammer H, Finkelhor D, Sedlak AJ. *Runaway/Thrownaway Children: National Estimates and Characteristics*. Washington, DC: US Department of Justice, Office of Justice Programs, Office of Juvenile Justice and Delinquency Prevention; 2002.
7. Clawson HJ, Dutch N, Solomon A, Grace LG. *Human Trafficking Into and Within the United States: A Review of the Literature*. Washington, DC: US Department of Health and Human Services; 2009.
8. Cusick L. Youth prostitution: a literature review. *Child Abus Rev*. 2002;11:230-251.
9. Gragg F, Petta I, Bernstein H, Eisen K, Quinn L. *New York Prevalence Study of Commercially Sexually Exploited Children: Final Report*. Rensselaer, NY: New York State Office of Children and Family Services; 2007.
10. Polaris Project. Overview of human trafficking. http://www.polarisproject.org/human-trafficking/overview. Accessed on January 24, 2013.
11. Curtis R, Terry K, Dank M, Dombrowski K, Khan B. *The Commercial Sexual Exploitation of Children in New York City, Volume 1: The CSEC Population in New York City: Size, Characteristics and Needs*. Washington, DC: US Department of Justice, National Institute of Justice; 2008.
12. Smith LA, Vardaman SH, Snow MA. *The National Report on Domestic Minor Sex Trafficking: America's Prostituted Children*. Vancouver, WA: Shared Hope International; 2009.
13. Zimmerman C, Yun K, Shvab I, et al. *The Health Risks and Consequences of Trafficking in Women and Adolescents: Findings From a European Study*. London, England: London School of Hygiene and Tropical Medicine; 2003.
14. Bortel A, Ellingen M, Ellison MC, Phillips R, Thomas C. *Sex Trafficking Needs Assessment for the State of Minnesota*. Minneapolis, MN: Advocates for Human Rights; 2008.
15. Burnette ML, Lucas E, Ilgen M, Frayne SM, Mayo J, Weitlauf JC. Prevalence and health correlates of prostitution among patients entering treatment for substance use disorders. *Arch Gen Psychiatry*. 2008;65(3):337-344.
16. Choi H, Klein C, Shin MS, Lee HJ. Posttraumatic stress disorder (PTSD) and disorders of extreme stress (DESNOS) symptoms following prostitution and child abuse. *Violence Against Women*. 2009;15(8):933-951.
17. Deb S, Mukhergee A, Mathews B. Aggression in sexually abused trafficked girls and efficacy of intervention. *J Interper Viol.* 2011;26(4):745-768.

18. Elam AL, Ray VG. Sexually related trauma: a review. *Ann Emerg Med.* 1986;15(5):576-584.

19. Silverman JG. Adolescent female sex workers: invisibility, violence and HIV. *Arch Dis Child.* 2011;96(5):478-481.

20. Yates GL, Mackenzie RG, Pennbridge J, Swofford A. A risk profile comparison of homeless youth involved in prostitution and homeless youth not involved. *J Adolesc Health.* 1991;12(7):545-548.

21. Zimmerman C. *Stolen Smiles: A Summary Report on the Physical and Psychological Consequences of Women and Adolescents Trafficked in Europe.* London, England: London School of Hygiene and Tropical Medicine; 2006.

22. United Nations. Protocol to Prevent, Suppress and Punish Trafficking in Persons, Especially Women and Children, Supplementing the United Nations Convention Against Transnational Organized Crime. New York, NY: United Nations; 2000. https://treaties.un.org/doc/publication/mtdsg/volume%20ii/chapter%20xviii/xviii-12-a.en.pdf. Accessed November 7, 2016.

23. United Nations. United Nations Global Plan of Action to Combat Trafficking in Persons. New York, NY: United Nations; 2010. https://www.unodc.org/documents/human-trafficking/United_Nations_Global_Plan_of_Action_to_Combat_Trafficking_in_Persons.pdf. Accessed November 7, 2016.

24. United Nations Office on Drugs and Crime. *Global Report on Trafficking in Persons 2012.* Vienna, Austria: United Nations Office on Drugs and Crime; 2012.

25. US Department of State. *Trafficking in Persons Report 2013.* Washington, DC: US Department of State; 2013.

26. Dottridge M. *A Handbook on Planning Projects to Prevent Child Trafficking.* Lausanne, Switzerland: Terre des Hommes; 2007.

27. International Rescue Committee. Where we focus: economic wellbeing. http://www.rescue.org/economic-recovery-development-technical-unit-erd. Accessed November 7, 2016.

28. Finklea KM, Fernandes-Alcantara AL, Siskin A. *Sex Trafficking of Children in the United States: Overview and Issues for Congress.* Washington, DC: Congressional Research Service; 2015.

29. Quayle E, Loo, L, Palmer T. Child pornography and sexual exploitation of children online: concept note. http://www.ecpat.net/worldcongressIII/PDF/Thematic/CHILD_ABUSE_IMAGES_concept_note.pdf. Accessed July 7, 2013.

30. Todres J. Moving upstream: the merits of a public health law approach to human trafficking. *North Carol Law Rev.* 2011;89(2):447-506.

31. Gozdziak EM, Bump MN. *Data and Research on Human Trafficking: Bibliography of Research-Based Literature.* Washington, DC: National Criminal Justice Reference Service; 2008.

32. Macy RJ, Graham LM. Identifying domestic and international sex-trafficking victims during human service provision. *Trauma Violence Abuse.* 2012;13(2):59-76.

33. Quayle E, Taylor M. Child pornography and the internet: perpetuating a cycle of abuse. *Deviant Behav.* 2002;23(4):331-361.

34. US Agency for International Development. *An Evaluation Framework for USAID-Funded TIP Prevention and Victim Protection Programs: Final Report.* Washington, DC: US Agency for International Development; 2009.

35. Shuteriqi M, Pippidou D, Stoecklin D. *Transnational protection of children: The case of Albania and Greece: 2000-2006.* Lausanne, Switzerland: Terre des Hommes; 2006.

36. International Organization for Migration. *Handbook on Performance Indicators for Counter-Trafficking Projects.* Washington, DC: International Organization for Migration; 2008.

37. National Coalition to Prevent Child Sexual Abuse and Exploitation. *National Plan to Prevent the Sexual Abuse and Exploitation of Children.* Washington, DC: National Coalition to Prevent Child Sexual Abuse and Exploitation; 2012.

38. Wessells M. *What Are We Learning About Protecting Children in the Community: An Inter-agency Review of Evidence on Community-based Child Protection Mechanisms in Humanitarian and Development Settings.* Fairfield, CT: Save the Children Fund; 2009.

39. Justice Resource Institute. Behavioral health clinics and truama services, community-based behavioral health services. http://jri.org/services/behavioral-health-and-trauma-services/community-based-behavioral-health-services/my-life-my-choice. Accessed November 7, 2016.

40. Georgia's Not Buying It. Home page. http://www.notbuyingit.org. Accessed November 7, 2016.

41. The Code. Home page. http://www.thecode.org. Accessed November 7, 2016.

42. End Child Prostitution Child Pornography and Trafficking of Children for Sexual Purposes. Vision. http://www.ecpat.net/ei/Ecpat_vision.asp. Accessed July 7, 2013.

43. End Child Prostitution Child Pornography and Trafficking of Children for Sexual Purposes. Code of conduct for the protection of children from sexual exploitation in travel and tourism: background and implementation examples. http://www.ecpat.net/ei/Publications/CST/Code_of_Conduct_ENG.pdf. Accessed June 6, 2013.

44. Hunter P. Human trafficking and business: good practices to prevent and combat human trafficking. http://www.ilo.org/sapfl/Informationresources/NonILOpublications/WCMS_142722/lang--en/index.htm. Accessed July 7, 2013.

45. Perrin B (moderator). Presentation on the code of conduct. http://www.ecpat.net/WorldCongressIII/PDF/Nov28/Code_of_Conduct.pdf. Accessed July 7, 2013.

46. Not For Sale Campaign. Stop them from scoring: NFS South Africa gives the red card. http://www.notforsalecampaign.org/news/2010/06/17/stop-them-from-scoring-nfs-south-africa-gives-the-red-card. Accessed July 7, 2013.

47. Martin Williams launches human trafficking awareness campaign at world cup. http://www.prnewswire.com/news-releases/martinwilliams-launches-human-trafficking-awareness-campaign-at-world-cup-96051199.html. Accessed July 5, 2013.

48. Manpower/not for sale: Red Card campaign against human trafficking. http://www.justmeans.com/blogs/Manpower-Not-For-Sale---Red-Card-Campaign-Against-Human-Trafficking/57.html. Accessed July 5, 2013.

Chapter 16

Community Violence Exposure Among Children and Youth: Considering Risk and Protective Factors and Prevention

Vanessa Vorhies Klodnick, LCSW, PhD
Neil Guterman, PhD

Introduction

Child and adolescent exposure to community violence has gained growing attention, particularly since the beginning of the 1990s when studies began documenting community violence exposure (CVE) as a problem of widespread proportions with major physical, psychological, psychosocial, and broader societal consequences. The notion of "community violence" remains a vague concept and is most appropriately conceived of as an omnibus term, encompassing a variety of types and manifestations of violence across a number of community settings. Much is known about the prevalence rates and subsequent outcomes of youth exposure to community violence, but less is known about effective methods to prevent it. Although recognized as a major public health concern,[1] CVE can be missed during assessments by health and social services professionals who, if screening for violence exposure, tend to focus on family violence and child maltreatment concerns. This chapter provides a comprehensive definition of CVE, explains why CVE must be addressed by health care and allied professionals, explores the prevalence and risk factors associated with CVE, describes select currently implemented prevention strategies, and proposes strategies to prevent youth CVE.

What Is Community Violence?

At its most basic, the term community violence denotes acts of interpersonal violence that occur in community settings, including neighborhoods, streets, schools, shops, playgrounds, or other community locales. These acts may include rape or sexual assault and random acts of violence between individuals who are unrelated and who may or may not know each other.[2] Macro-level violence (eg, social unrest or riots in community settings) as well as microlevel violence (eg, violence in the home) have also been included in some studies of community violence. Although the location and persons involved in the violence (ie, victims, perpetrators, and witnesses) often shape whether an act of violence is considered community violence, no clear consensus yet exists as to what boundaries demarcate community violence from other forms of violence. Different forms of violence may overlap with or even "spill over" into community violence and vice versa as community violence may be alternately labeled as domestic violence, crime, gang violence, or school violence depending on the victim, perpetrator, setting, and situation. Also, the victimization and perpetration of violence in the community are often intimately entwined and overlap with other types of violence in the home (eg, father to youth aggression).[3,4]

The lack of clear and precise demarcation of the term ***community violence*** makes it difficult to accurately track the magnitude of the problem, monitor changing trends over time, or identify risk and protective factors. Of further concern, the presently diffuse definition of the term also risks its politicization, or worse, lends itself to be used in a biased or pejorative way, such as to purvey racist, classist, or ageist stereotypes about "violent communities" or demographically defined groups. In reality, CVE is prevalent in urban, suburban, and rural areas across varying socioeconomic classes and cultures. There is much to be done to further our understanding of CVE. Although a concise definition of CVE does not currently exist, studies of prevalence can be explored that include varying levels and types of exposure, risk factors, and youth outcomes:

— ***Indirect exposure***: Possessing knowledge of others' victimization in the community

— ***Direct exposure***: Witnessing violence in the community

— ***Direct victimization***: Being directly victimized in the community

— ***Direct involvement in CVE***: Combined involvement as victim, perpetrator, and/or witness

— ***Frequent and/or continual exposure***: CVE through frequent exposure to the use of guns, knives, drugs, and random violence in the community

Why Prevention is Important: Outcomes of Community Violence Exposure for Children and Adolescents

Preventing youth CVE remains an urgent matter, given the broad array of detrimental effects CVE has on youth of all ages. The general understanding of CVE outcomes for children and adolescents is based predominantly on urban nonwhite samples who are at the greatest risk for experiencing violence across community, family, and intimate partner relations[5-7] as well as other challenging life experiences, such as poverty, discrimination, residential segregation, and lack of access to resources or quality schools.[8] Therefore, prevention methods aiming to decrease the rates of CVE and the numerous challenges facing urban minority youth may also serve to address many negative outcomes that are often associated with CVE.

Exposure to multiple and chronic stressors (eg, child maltreatment, poverty) as a child have been linked to changes in brain functioning, development of poor stress management systems, and an increased propensity for stress-related disorders and cognitive impairment.[9] Youth exposed to community violence exhibit increased states of physiological hypoarousal and hyperarousal, which can result in either desensitization to violence or increased levels of anxiety.[10,11] Violence exposure also interferes with many of the primary developmental tasks in childhood and adolescence, such as the acquisition of trust, the ability to differentiate between threat and safety, behavioral and emotional self-regulation, and the capacity to form and maintain social relationships.[12-14] This is extremely important as social support and a primary buffer for youth exposed to chronic life stress.[9]

Frequently documented are the significant mental health sequelae linked to CVE in youth. For youth of all ages, CVE is associated with internalizing symptoms, such as anxiety, depression, and somatic complaints (eg, sleep disturbances, stomachaches, increased asthma symptoms). The most notable symptom is posttraumatic stress disorder (PTSD), which is an anxiety disorder commonly manifested after exposure to a traumatic event.[15-20] CVE in children and adolescents is also associated with an array of externalizing behaviors, including increased aggressive behavior and violence perpetration,[18,21,22] greater HIV-related risk behaviors (eg, inconsistent condom use sex with multiple partners),[23,24] and increased use of alcohol and drugs.[25]

Evidence suggests that internalizing and externalizing symptoms and mental health conditions of youth exposed to community violence are associated with gender, age, type of CVE, location of CVE, frequency of CVE, relationship with victim, and length of time post CVE. Younger children are more likely to possess symptoms of internalizing symptoms compared to older children.[26]

Girls tend to exhibit more internalizing symptoms than boys, and girls also tend to exhibit aggression after community school violence exposure, but not after school violence exposure; boys are more likely to exhibit aggression after both school and community violence exposure.[27] The link between internalizing symptoms and CVE appears to be stronger for females than males, with no observed difference in the strength of the relationship between externalizing symptoms and CVE between males and females.[18]

Internalizing symptoms are more prevalent immediately following exposure to community violence, whereas externalizing behaviors are more prevalent as time passes and the child grows older.[28] A meta-analysis of 114 studies of CVE and mental health outcomes revealed that the link between PTSD and community violence is stronger for adolescents than it is for younger children.[18] Victimization through community violence had a significantly stronger impact on externalizing and internalizing problems when compared to only witnessing community violence.[18]

Witnessing multiple incidents of community violence and witnessing incidents where the victim was a known nonrelative was linked to PTSD in adolescents. Witnessing multiple incidents of community and in-home violence and fearing that they might be injured or killed was linked with meeting criteria for a major depressive episode.[25] Lambert, Boyd, Cammack and Ialongo also found that adolescents who witnessed community violence against a family member or a friend was linked with depression, violence against a stranger was linked to anxiety, and violence against familiar persons and strangers was linked to aggression.[29]

Future research is necessary to understand how timing, stage of development, and individual physiological responses mediate or moderate the relationship between violence exposure and subsequent symptomology for CVE prevention methods to be devised and implemented.

Prevalence of Community Violence Exposure

Youth are more likely to be exposed to violence than adults.[30] Federal data indicate that homicide is the fifth leading cause of death among children aged 5 to 14 years, after unintentional injuries, cancer, congenital disease (eg, birth defects), and suicide. For youth aged 15 to 19 years, homicide is the third leading cause of death, after unintentional injuries (eg, motor vehicle accidents) and suicide.[31] Homicide rates in US youth younger than 15 years were found to be 5 times as high as the total number of homicides in 25 countries that are comparable in terms of economic status (eg, gross national product) and size.[32] Rates of serious victimization, including sexual assault, rape, and aggravated assault, is higher for young people aged 12 to 24 than those 25 years and older.[33] Despite national homicide and CVE rates declining since 2002, the prevalence of community violence may be highly underestimated; reports suggest that approximately half of violence fails to be reported.[30,33]

Research utilizing self-report methodologies indicate a widespread problem. A large nationally representative survey of US high school students revealed that in 2011, 33% of students have been in a physical fight, 7% report having been threatened or injured with a weapon (eg, gun, knife, or club) 1 or more times on school property, and 4% were physically injured and needed medical treatment from at least 1 physical fight.[34] Among 12- to 17-year-olds in the 2005 National Survey of Adolescents-Replication study, witnessing community violence was reported by approximately 38% of youth.[25] Another large nationally representative sample of children aged 0 to 17 years (as reported by youth and their caregivers) revealed in 2008 that 61% have experienced at least 1 direct or witnessed victimization, 46% have experienced at least 1 physical assault, and 19% have witnessed an assault in the community.[35] Approximately 65% of these youth had 2 or more victimizations in the past year, while 12% had 5 or more exposures to violence in the past year.[35] Longitudinal studies suggest that violence exposure does not dissipate over time for children, but rather violence exposure tends to remain constant over time.[13,21,36]

Risk Factors for Community Violence Exposure

A number of factors increase the risk of youth CVE in the United States, including (but not limited to) possession of economic hardship, being male, affiliation with a gang, living in a high-crime neighborhood, prior history of violence exposure, and being Latino or African American.[6,37] Often, many of these risk factors are closely associated with one another, such as minority group status and impoverished living in an urban neighborhood. Given this, it is particularly challenging to determine which risk factors to identify in order to devise appropriate and effective prevention strategies. Risk factors that have been broadly identified as linked in some way to CVE include urbanicity and neighborhood characteristics, race/ethnicity, age, gender, and psychosocial and behavioral characteristics.

Urbanicity and Neighborhood Characteristics

CVE is associated with community settings characterized by high concentrations of poverty, as indicated by scarce resources, poor housing conditions, and high rates of residential instability.[38,39] Conditions in urban neighborhoods (eg, neighborhood stability, racial composition) are related to perceived social and environmental stress.[40] These stressors may be related to increased illicit activities, such as drug trafficking and gang involvement, from which violence may often originate.[41-43]

Rates of serious violent crime (eg, rape, sexual assault, aggravated assault) and simple assault decreased across urban, suburban, and rural youth from 1994 to 2010. However, urban youth in 2010 still report almost twice the rate of victimization through serious violence compared to suburban and rural youth.[44] In a large national study, urban youth were more likely to report at least 1 victimization in the past year (eg, threatened with weapon, hit by intimate partner) and having been in a fight in the past year as compared to suburban and rural youth.[45] Witnessing community violence in urban settings is also prevalent for urban youth, with rates of exposure estimated between 50% and 100%.[46,47]

Several studies indicate that youth living in middle-class suburban and rural settings also face significant risk for violence exposure outside the home.[48-50] In 2010, rates of simple assault were similar for urban and suburban youth, approximately 25 per 1000 and 22 per 1000 respectively.[44] Rates of death via firearms in youth aged 19 and younger does not differ between urban and rural youth from 1999 to 2006.[51] Yet, rural youth were slightly more likely to have carried a gun or carried any weapon to school in the last month,[45] and access to guns has been found to be related to increased likelihood of death by firearm.[52] Also, rates of witnessing are high in suburban adolescents. Among 184 suburban adolescents (94% Caucasian) in New York state, 86% had seen someone beaten up, 72% had seen someone being arrested, and 61% had seen drug deals.[53]

An important theory to explain the higher rates of CVE in urban communities is "collective efficacy." Collective efficacy of a neighborhood is characterized by the degree to which its residents perceive positive social cohesion among one another and the degree to which they exercise informal social control (eg, willingness to intervene in community) to maintain positive social norms.[54] Collective efficacy has been linked to variation in violence rates in the United States and other countries (eg, Australia and Sweden).[55,56]

Race and Ethnicity

A number of studies report that all ethnic groups experience CVE in the United States; yet, like the problem of poverty, the reported rates of CVE and victimization among ethnic minorities are disproportionately high.[57,58] Cross-sectional and longitudinal studies consistently find that African American youth are significantly more likely to be exposed to community violence compared to white and Latino youth.[59,60] In 2002 and 2010, compared to other racial and ethnic groups, African Americans experienced the highest levels of exposure to violent crimes in the United States.[33] From 1994 to 2010, the rates of violent victimization for African American youth (25.7 victimizations per 1000 youth) aged 12 to 17 years was more than twice the rates for white (11.7 per 1000) and Latino youth (11.3 per 1000).[44] From 2002, rates of serious violent crimes against white and Latino youth decreased (by 25% and 65% respectively)[44]; however, rates for African American youth remained the same. In 2009, homicide rates were highest among 15- to 19-year-old African American males (55.4 per 100 000), which was 5 times the rate of white males (13.2 per 100 000).[52] Less explored are rates of CVE among other ethnic groups in the United States (eg, Southeast Asian, American Indian). However, research suggests that CVE is prevalent among urban American Indian adolescents and Chinese American youth.[61,62]

Age

Most studies reveal an important relationship between age and rates of CVE, where personal victimization in the community is lower in younger children but higher in adolescents. Witnessing violence appears to be similar for both children and adolescents, especially in urban communities.[47] The most substantial difference between younger and older youth CVE is observed in homicide rates. Of homicides in 2009 across 16 states, 4.5% were comprised of children 5 years and younger, 1.8% were children aged 6 to 14, and 9.4% were adolescents aged 15 to 19.[63] There are disparities in CVE even among children who are close in age. For example, older youth in a sample of sixth to eighth grade middle school students reported significantly higher levels of CVE than younger youth.[20]

Of 12- to 17-year-olds in a national sample, 38% witnessed CVE (actually seeing someone else physically or sexually victimized).[25] One study found that 96% of urban youth (n=121) were exposed to community violence indirectly (eg, witnessing or hearing about less severe interpersonal violence), 81% had witnessed someone being beaten up, and 55% knew someone killed through community or school violence.[64] Nearly all mothers of preschool-aged children (n=471) living in an urban community reported co-witnessing gunshots on a weekly basis.[65] In a 1-year period, 42% of children witnessed at least 1 violent act and 21% had witnessed 3 or more violent acts.[66]

Gender

Mixed research exists regarding gender and CVE risk. Some research suggests that male children and adolescents are at an increased risk for experiencing and witnessing violent incidents in the community across socioeconomic gradients and ethnic groups as compared to females.[67,68] Other research suggests that there is not as wide of a gender gap in CVE, and other factors may interact with gender, such as age and type of exposure. Foster, Kuperminc, and Price[17] found no difference in witnessing or victimization through CVE in 11- to 16-year-old African American youth attending Boys and Girls Clubs in a metropolitan area in the Southeast United States. Shahinfar and colleagues found no gender differences in preschool children's CVE.[69] However, Attar and colleagues found that girls in elementary school reported higher rates of CVE than did boys of the same age, although those differences disappeared in a follow-up study conducted 2 years later.[41] Being female increases the risk for sexual assaults, while being male increases the risk of personally experiencing and witnessing physical violence.[17,70,71]

Psychosocial, Behavioral, and Developmental Factors

Understanding child behavior and characteristics in conjunction with peer and family characteristics are important for unpacking the CVE risk. Adolescents with aggressive behavior problems and deviant peer groups are at increased risk for CVE, particularly so for males with depressive symptoms.[36] Gang membership has also been found to be associated with higher rates of alcohol and drug use.[72] Exploring multiple factors related to CVE overtime, Lambert, Bradshaw, Cammack, and Ialongo found that aggression and behavior problems in children were associated with a lack of academic readiness, both of which contributed to subsequent peer rejection, conduct problems, and deviant peer association that ultimately resulted in an increased likelihood of CVE.[73]

Parental mental health and parental stress, as related to use of physical and abusive discipline, has been associated with adolescent CVE and negative youth outcomes to exposure.[64,74] Earlier research of developmental process models suggest CVE is associated with negative and harsh parenting that shapes the aggressive behavior of children and affects their socializing patterns to include delinquent peers.[75,76] However, more recent research suggests that the relationship between family processes is mediated by social network and child characteristics. For example, deviant friend groups and the child's behavior were found to mediate the relationship between parenting context, negative parenting, and both witnessing and being victimized through community violence.[6]

Protective Factors

Although few researchers have examined protective factors with direct relationships with CVE itself, many factors have been reported as serving a protective role in moderating the outcomes of youth exposed to community violence.

Neighborhood and School Context

Both the neighborhoods and schools in which youth reside and attend play an important role in the likelihood that they will encounter community violence. Among 12- and 15-year-olds participating in a longitudinal neighborhood study in Chicago, those who lived in neighborhoods that offered a greater variety of youth organizations were less likely to report exposure to community violence in the last year compared to neighborhoods with less variety in youth organizations.[77] Schools are also commonly thought to serve a protective function, but they are rarely studied as such with respect to CVE. For urban adolescents, it has been theorized that schools may function as a zone of relative safety for youth, but are also settings in which youth are victimized or engage in violence.[78]

In the United States and Europe, approximately 80% of youth report witnessing verbal aggression and 75% report witnessing physical aggression in schools.[79,80] Rates of being threatened or injured with a weapon on school property steadily decreased from 9.2% in 2003 to 7.4% in 2011 in a national sample of adolescents.[81] However, rates of being in a physical fight (12.8% to 12.0%) or carrying a gun (6.1% to 5.4%) on school property from 2003 to 2011 did not change significantly.[81] Of all homicides from 2009 to 2011 of 5- to 18-year-olds, less than 2% occurred on school property, suggesting that schools are protective from severe violence.[82] When measuring community violence, school violence is often included and not differentiated from community violence, which makes it challenging to determine differences in type or severity of violence exposure between school and community settings. However, there is evidence that schools are protective. Perceptions of safety associated with the school environment are associated with educational and psychological outcomes.[83] Higher levels of identification with one's school and higher levels of perceived teacher support were associated with increased hope independent of violence exposure in urban adolescents.[84] Teacher support has also been found to moderate the relationships between violence exposure and mental health in youth.[85] An understanding of the interactions between school, individual, family, and community level protective and risk factors is necessary to further determine if and how schools function as protection from community violence.

Family Context

Family cohesion and parental monitoring protect youth from CVE and moderate the effects of CVE on youth. Adolescents with low family cohesion who had witnessed CVE were nearly 2 times more likely to report behavior problems than those with high family cohesion who had not witnessed violence.[86] Also, the extent to which adolescents who had witnessed CVE but had high family cohesion showed no difference in reporting behavior problems than youth with high cohesion families who had not witnessed CVE.[86] Compared to those with less parental monitoring, Ceballo, Ramirez, Hearn, and Maltese found that increased parental monitoring was associated with less subsequent CVE and better psychological well-being (eg, less likely to have symptoms of depression) among fourth and fifth graders exposed to CVE.[87] Also, parental monitoring impacted the relationship between CVE and externalizing symptoms and depression in Italian adolescents and has been found to be protective of subsequent CVE in sixth to eighth grade males with aggression and anxiety, but not for males with aggression and depression.[36,88] This suggests that there is more research to be done to unpack the complex characteristics of family dynamics and their impact on youth with certain psychological responses to CVE.

Perceived parental support is also an important factor in mitigating the psychosocial impact of CVE on youth, depending on the extent of the exposure and mental health conditions. For instance, lower perceived maternal support was associated with increased depressive symptoms in youth as their overall exposure to violence increased.[85] Also, lower levels of guardian support was related to higher rates of anxiety and depression symptoms, but not related to higher rates of PTSD symptoms in adolescents exposed to community violence.[20] A significant relationship between CVE and committing violence was found in adolescent males with lower levels of perceived parental support, while no relationship was found between CVE and committing violent acts among adolescent males with high levels of perceived parental support.[89]

Youth characteristics, such as gender and mental health, appear to play an important role in relationship between CVE, parental support, and psychosocial outcomes. Bookmeyer and colleagues found that for females, the relationship between parental support and

CVE was nonsignificant whereas for males this relationship was significant.[89] Also, there was no relationship between CVE and committing acts of violence in females who possessed prosocial cognitions, while prosocial cognitions did not have the protective impact on male adolescents who were exposed to community violence.[89] Family dynamics, including the level of parental distress and the willingness of youth to tell family about their experience with community violence, impact the risk for CVE and subsequent outcomes. For instance, Margolin and colleagues found that a stronger relationship existed between CVE and parent-to-youth aggression for youth who had fathers with high rates of global distress compared to those who had fathers with low rates of global distress.[4] Youth with lower perceived constraints to discuss CVE are less likely to develop PTSD symptoms in the wake of CVE.[85]

CVE Pathways

It has been historically theorized that youth who are at highest risk for negative outcomes after CVE are those who already live in the context of accumulated risk, such as experience with domestic violence, poverty, or abuse.[90] Recent research has found evidence for this theory. The interrelationships among different kinds of CVE and trauma are often neglected, and once disentangled may also indicate risk pathways to exposure. For example, children abused by parents are more likely to be bullied at school.[91] Finkelhor and colleagues suggest that certain types of victimization may be "precursors" or "catalysts" for exposure to other types of violence.[92]

Polyvictimization is the term recently introduced by Finkelhor and colleagues to describe multiple traumas from varying arenas (eg, exposure to domestic violence, child maltreatment).[92] Polyvictimization increases the risk of persisting victimization.[93] For example, of youth who experienced at least 1 type of victimization in 1 year, 69% experienced another type of victimization in the same year.[93] When included in statistical models, polyvictimization eliminates the direct effects that individual types of victimization has on youth outcomes, meaning that exposure to multiple forms of victimization has a stronger association with youth outcomes than any individual type of victimization.[94]

Similarly, research suggests that the total amount of adverse circumstances, including CVE and other life experiences like poverty and parental divorce, has a stronger impact on youth psychosocial functioning than any individual adverse event.[95] Exposure to different types of violence is not static, rather exposure rates fluctuate.[4] For example, over 3 years 41% of adolescents reported mother-to-youth aggression and 10% reported CVE each year, while 82% reported mother-to-youth aggression and 50% reported CVE at least once in the 3 years.[4] Research that aims to untangle CVE from other types of violence increases the risk of misunderstanding the impact that violence and trauma have on youth functioning. It also limits any attempt at understanding how combinations of violence matter in relation to protective factors (eg, parental support) and specific mental health or behavioral outcomes (eg, PTSD, depression).[96]

Community Violence Exposure Prevention

Prevention of youth CVE is possible through a number of different routes: policy changes; community, school, and family violence prevention programs; and addressing youth perpetration of violence. However, little empirical evidence demonstrates the effectiveness of primary, secondary, or tertiary programs and strategies that target a reduction in youth CVE. At present, a number of scientific standards or "blueprints" of prevention strategies have been identified that are linked to significant reductions in the perpetration of violent behavior, crime, antisocial behavior, and substance use, which should directly predict the reduction of victimization by violent behavior.[97] Limbos and colleagues attribute the lack of knowledge about program effectiveness to reduce CVE to the complexity of the problem, the lack of adequate study designs, and inconsistent data collection between studies preventing model comparison.[98] Much more is known about the effectiveness of approaches that address youth violence perpetration, which can be indirectly beneficial in reducing CVE. However, a great deal of community youth victimization is not perpetrated by other youth. Roughly 55% of youth are victimized through adult perpetrators.[99] The following is a brief discussion of youth CVE and youth violence prevention strategies with evidence that either supports their efficacy or describes their promising trends.

Policy

The United States, along with other countries, has only very recently begun to consider utilizing proactive or preventative approaches instead of reactive approaches to addressing community violence.[100] Macro-level risk factors in the United States, such as cultural norms and laws implicitly or explicitly supporting violence and punishment, access to guns, and racial discrimination, increase the probability of youth violence.[101] For example, a review of research of state efforts to deter violence found that the practice of transferring juveniles convicted of person or property offences to adult courts is linked to increased arrest and jail recidivism when compared to those who stay in the juvenile court system.[102] Crime control policies are often set through political agendas, not scientific research.[103] Systematic reviews of violence prevention through community approaches reveal the glaring lack of evidence supporting the effectiveness of firearm policies directly or indirectly impacting violence.[104] The Centers for Disease Control and Prevention (CDC) approach to violence prevention includes focusing on preventing direct victimization; building the knowledge base of violence and associated factors through research and collaboration with a variety of disciplines, including health, criminal justice, social science, etcetera; and preventing violence across all populations in the United States. However, more research is necessary to explore the relationships between local, state, and federal policies and their effectiveness in decreasing youth CVE.

Community

Communities are important prevention targets with the capacity to develop, implement, and evaluate violence prevention efforts.[105] The collaboration between parents, schools, and communities is emphasized as crucial for preventing violence.[106] CVE rates are impacted by community efforts to foster and support social ties and increase community cohesion.[107] Coalition approaches to preventing violence, such as the PROSPER Project, require community organization of multiple parties (eg, school, families, human service agencies, university researchers) in applying evidence-based practices to foster youth development.[108] The PROSPER Project includes family psychoeducation, youth life skills training, and after school programs, all of which have been found to significantly improve family and individual level outcomes that are often linked to violence, substance use, aggression, and peer pressure.[109] Other promising community level interventions include Communities That Care (CTC) and CeaseFire.

CTC is a systems prevention approach aimed at decreasing youth violence and delinquency through engaging community stakeholders in forming a coalition to assess and address the community's unique needs. The coalition develops a plan tailored to their community to address the needs based on local data and evidence-based practices, implements the adopted intervention, and evaluates the intervention's impact using repeated measures of youth outcomes.[110] A randomized evaluation study found that youth risk factors (eg, substance use, delinquent behavior) were significantly lower in the communities where CTC was implemented (controlling for prior use and delinquent behavior) compared to communities where CTC was not implemented.[111] Community level prevention approaches like CTC do not produce results overnight, but rather result in changes on a community level and individual level overtime.[110]

CeaseFire is an evidence-based community violence prevention program that mobilizes communities through street level outreach, public education, and collaboration between spiritual leaders and law enforcement.[112] CeaseFire utilizes "violence interrupters" or individuals who typically have personal histories of gang involvement and criminal behavior to develop rapport and establish relationships with local gangs in order to stop the cycle of violence.[113] CeaseFire's Chicago implementation (now called Cure Violence) resulted in a 16% to 28% decrease in shootings, as well as forged meaningful relationships between at-risk youth and adults in their community.[113]

Cure Violence has been fully implemented in other communities and has demonstrated positive results, including substantial decreases in shootings and homicides.[114] However, findings are typically mixed, with some communities experiencing increases in homicides and nonfatal shootings after the intervention ceased.[115,116] Similarly, in Boston and Indianapolis where CeaseFire implementation was linked to substantial decreases in homicide rates (60% and 30% respectively). Over a decade later, homicide rates are on the rise.[114] Sustainability of community level programs must be addressed in order to maintain the desired lower levels of violence.

Papachristos cautions that although evaluations of these programs are ill conceived, findings are mixed, and negative results are often dismissed, high levels of funding and political agendas continue to endorse the programs.[115] Practitioners and program administrators need to carefully review study findings and be aware of the varying elements that are part of both CeaseFire and Cure Violence as they continue to be mixed and matched in various adaptation and evaluation efforts across the country.

School

A selection of school-based violence prevention programs document their success in decreasing youth violence rates. In a systematic review of 53 studies of school violence prevention programs across all grades (kindergarten through high school), on average youth violence decreased by 15% regardless of socioeconomic status or crime rate.[117] Additionally, not 1 specific prevention approach (eg, informational, cognitive/affective, and social skills building) was particularly more successful in decreasing violence, as all school approaches were all linked to decreases in youth violence.[118] Curriculum-based violence prevention programs are commonly implemented in schools. For example, Responding in Peaceful and Positive Ways (RiPP) includes 16 developmentally appropriate 50 minute lessons per year with sociocognitive-based activities aimed at increasing problem-solving skills and altering attitudes towards violence in middle schools.[119] Also, interventions aimed at altering school culture and attitudes about violence have been implemented in conjunction with curriculum-based programs. For example, the "Best Behavior Program" targets school policies and rules addressing violence in order to create a standardized and systematic approach to addressing and preventing violence.[120]

A meta-analysis of 26 randomized control trials of school-based violence prevention programs found the programs to be mildly successful (ie, overall small effective size) at decreasing aggressive and violent behavior in first through 12th grade students.[121] Also, the school-based programs aimed at younger children were more successful in decreasing aggressive and violence behaviors in youth, contrary to what the authors hypothesized and what previous research suggests, than programs aimed at adolescents.[121] Intervening even earlier for children is found to prevent violent behavior. Kellerman, Fuqua-Whitley, Rivara, and Mercy found interventions introduced in later childhood and adolescence intended to reduce violence are not as effective in preventing youth violence, as compared to those introduced between the prenatal period and 6 years of age.[122]

School-implemented programs have been developed that teach adolescents skills to address anger without violence (eg, Positive Adolescent Choices Training, PACT).[123] Also, peer mediation programs aim to build social, cognitive, or behavioral skills through classes, counseling, and group work.[124] Despite the type of treatment approach, aggressive behaviors commonly observed in schools, such as fighting, name-calling, intimidation, and other problematic interpersonal behaviors, generally decrease with adoption of peer mediation programs in school, especially for those students at increased risk for violence or exposure to violence.[124]

Family

Intervening with the family in order to prevent violence is often considered a key ingredient to multimodal community violence prevention approaches. However, research on family-focused interventions is mixed. Early childhood home visits are linked to decreases in child maltreatment, but there is insufficient evidence to conclude that home visitation prevents youth or domestic violence.[104] Studies were lacking in Bilukha and colleagues' 2005 review that specifically explored the link between home visits and subsequent CVE.[104] A review of person-to-person approaches, which involve direct contact between intervention staff and adolescent caregivers to mitigate adolescent risk behaviors through altering caregiver behavior, are found to be effective with 13- to 18-year-olds.[125] Of the 4 studies discussed that evaluated person-to-person approaches to addressing youth violence exposure, it was inconclusive as to the impact that the changes in parental behaviors (eg, increased parental monitoring) had on youth violence (eg, getting into a fight) pre or 1-year post intervention.[126]

Other family-centered models that aim to decrease violence in youth may indirectly decrease CVE, yet evaluation studies have not explored CVE as an outcome variable. For example, multiple family group (MFG) approaches aim to alter parental strategies and responses to youth behavior through providing psychoeducation, training, and opportunities to interact with other families in groups over a course of 8 to 12 weeks.[127] Programs like this increase family support and connections to the community, which may indirectly decrease youth violence exposure as social isolation is linked to community and family violence.[107] Two other evidence-based practices for addressing youth violence are multisystemic therapy (MST) and functional family therapy (FFT). MST engages both families and the community to address adolescent delinquency through therapy, education, and training to empower families, schools, and communities to alter practices that support negative youth outcomes.[128] FFT is a short-term family-based therapy approach that aims to build parenting skills and family communication while decreasing dysfunctional behavior patterns and adolescent delinquency.[129]

MST and FFT have been extensively studied across the world in child and adolescent populations with rigorous research designs. Compared to youth who received usual services across multiple sites and states, adolescents who received MST had lower rates of delinquency (eg, offense, arrests), were less likely to return to jail, and had fewer days of confinement.[128] These arrest, conviction, and incarceration rates were maintained at a 14- and 22-year follow-up, which suggests that MFT affects CVE rates if youth continue to not engage in violence as they enter adulthood.[130,131] FFT was found to be effective in reducing adolescent felony recidivism when implemented as intended (with program fidelity), but not when implemented with partial fidelity.[132] This suggests the importance of maintaining high fidelity for any impact to be had on violence-related crimes in youth. Huey and colleagues found that MST improved family relations, and family cohesiveness protects youth from CVE.[133] Family strength is supported by community factors, thus the importance of programs that target both families and communities are essential to prevent youth CVE.[106]

Youth

Before intervention, an emphasis must be placed on assessments that include multiple forms of CVE in addition to other forms of violence.[134] After exploring CVE and related youth struggles, determining a program or approach to treatment is necessary. Despite the numerous societal, contextual, and historical factors implicated in community violence, a variety of programs targeting youth who exhibit aggressive or violent tendencies are implemented and evaluated. These include early assessment and use of developmentally appropriate violence prevention methods, including individual and family counseling, mental health programs, and alternative education programs.[105] Programs targeting individual youth tend to focus on anger management, behavior modification, social perspectives, moral development, social skill building and problem-solving, and conflict resolution.[135] For example, Interpersonal Cognitive Problem Solving (ICPS) and Providing Alternative Thinking Strategies (PATHS) result in short-term changes in aggressive behavior and problem-solving skills.[136,137] Reduction in aggression and ADHD symptoms were maintained at a 2-year follow-up in Swiss children.[138]

Conclusion

Youth CVE is prevalent, is associated with many factors on numerous levels (eg, individual, family, and community), and can be prevented through community, school, and family collaboration. Current approaches to preventing CVE target known "violent" and "aggressive" children, which are secondary and tertiary approaches to violence prevention. These approaches are important to addressing violence and must be tailored to subpopulation characteristics (eg, age, race/ethnicity, rural or urban communities). Many Web sites provide information on community and youth violence prevention methods by specific population, situation, or location (**Table 16-1**). These approaches must emphasize community strengths and needs, as opposed to community "deficits," and move beyond a focus on individual outcomes to address societal trends, cultural norms, and biases in order to prevent violence.[106]

Table 16-1. Web sites for Addressing and Preventing CVE
Blueprints for Healthy Youth Development http://www.blueprintsprograms.com/ http://www.colorado.edu/cspv/blueprints/index.html
The Community Guide: Your Online Guide of What Works to Promote Health Communities http://www.thecommunityguide.org/violence/index.html
CDC Injury Prevention & Control: Division of Violence Prevention http://www.cdc.gov/ViolencePrevention/index.html
Institute for Community Peace: Integrating Research and Practice to Transform Community http://instituteforcommunitypeace.org/icp/
Communities That Care: http://communitiesthatcare.net/

Primary prevention of community violence is the key to preventing youth CVE. More work must be done to initiate and study primary prevention strategies that:

1. Increase awareness of factors that contribute to CVE

2. Foster accountability through the creation of organizations within communities that collaborate with schools, law enforcement, hospitals, and human service organizations

3. Create a shared set of principles that guide development, implementation, and evaluation of violence prevention efforts[106]

With technology and more complex longitudinal research designs, exploration of the interactions and bi-directional relationships of the multilevel factors associated with CVE is possible. Additionally, large-scale evaluation of prevention efforts that measure the effects of multilevel community intervention strategies will provide important insight into how to effectively address and ameliorate youth CVE.

References

1. Carmona RH. Family violence as a public health issue. http://www.surgeongeneral.gov/ news/speeches/violence08062003.htm. Published 2007. Accessed June 25, 2013.

2. Krug EG, Dahlberg LL, Mercy JA, Zwi AB, Lozano R, eds. *World Report on Violence and Health*. Geneva, Switzerland: World Health Organization; 2002.

3. Sheilds N, Nadasen K, Pierce L. A comparison of the effects of witnessing violence and direct victimization among children in Cape Town, South Africa. *J Interpers Violence*. 2008;24(7):1192-1208.

4. Margolin G, Vickerman KA, Ramos MC, et al. Youth exposed to violence: stability, co-occurrence, and context. *Clin Child Fam Psychol Rev*. 2009;12(1):39-54.

5. Buka SL, Stchick TL, Birdthistle I, Earles FJ. Youth exposure to violence: prevalence, risks, and consequences. *Am J Orthopsychiatry*. 2001;71(3):298-310.

6. Salzinger S, Ng-Mak DS, Feldman RS, Kam C, Rosario M. Exposure to community violence: Processes that increase risk for inner-city middle school children. *J Early Adolesc*. 2006;26:232-266.

7. Youngstrom E, Weist MD, Albus KE. Exploring violence exposure, stress, protective factors and behavioral problems among inner-city youth. *Am J Community Psychol*. 2003;32:115-129.

8. Johnson SD, Davis LE, Williams JH. Enhancing social work practice with ethnic minority youth. *Child and Adolescent Social Work Journal*. 2004;21:611-627.

9. Shonkoff JP, Garner AS; Committee on Psychological Aspects of Child and Family Health; Committee on Early Childhood, Adoption, and Dependent Care; Section on Developmental and Behavioral Pediatrics. The lifelong effects of early childhood adversity and toxic stress. *Pediatrics*. 2012;129(1):e232-e346.

10. Krenichyn K, Saegert S, Evans GW. Parents as moderators of psychological and physiological correlates of inner city children's exposure to violence. *J Appl Dev Psychol*. 2001;22:581-602.

11. Wilson D, Kliewer W, Teasley N, Plybon L, Sica D. Violence exposure, catecholamine excretion, and blood pressure non-dipping status in African-American male versus female adolescents. *Psychosom Med*. 2002;64:906-915.

12. Fox NA, Shonkoff JP. How persistent fear and anxiety can affect young children's learning, behaviour and health. *Early Childhood Matters*. 2011;116:8-14.

13. Margolin G, Gordis B. The effects of family and community violence on children. *Annu Rev Psychol.* 2000;51:445-479.

14. Sharkey P, Tirado-Strayer N, Papachristos AV, Raver CC. The effect of local violence on children's attention and impulse control. *Am J Public Health*. 2012;102(12):2287-2293.

15. Bailey BN, Delaney-Black V, Hannigan JH, Ager J, Sokol RJ, Covington CY. Somatic complaints in children and community violence exposure. *J Dev Behav Pediatr*. 2005;26(5):341-348.

16. Fitzpatrick KM, Piko BF, Wright DR, LaGory M. Depressive symptomatology, exposure to violence, and the role of social capital among African American adolescents. *Am J Orthopsychiatry*. 2005;75:262-274.

17. Foster JD, Kuperminc GP, Price AW. Gender differences in posttraumatic stress and related symptoms among inner-city minority youth exposed to community violence. *J Youth Adolesc*. 2004;33:59-69.

18. Fowler PJ, Tompsett CJ, Braciszewski JM, Jacques-Tiura AJ, Baltes BB. Community violence: a meta-analysis of the effect of exposure and mental health outcomes of children and adolescents. *Dev Psychopathol.* 2009;21:227-259.

19. Paxton KC, Robinson WL, Shah S, Schoeny ME. Psychological distress for African American adolescent males: Exposure to community violence and social support as factors. *Child Psychiatry Hum Dev*. 2004;34:281-295.

20. Rosario M, Salzinger S, Feldman RS, Ng-Mak DS. Intervening processes between youths' exposure to community violence and internalizing symptoms over time: The roles of social support and coping. *Am J Community Psychol.* 2008;41:43-62.

21. Gorman-Smith D, Henry DB, Tolan PH. Exposure to community violence and violence perpetration: the protective effects of family functioning. *J Clin Child Adolesc Psychol.* 2004;33(3):439-449.

22. Weaver CM, Borkowski JG, Whitman TL. Violence breeds violence: childhood exposure and adolescent conduct problems. *J Community Psychol.* 2008;36:96-112.

23. Voisin D. Victims of community violence and HIV sexual risk behaviors among African American males. *HIV/AIDS Education and Prevention for Adolescents and Children*. 2003;5(3):111-121.

24. Wilson HW, Woods BA, Emerson E, Donenberg GR. Patterns of violence exposure and sexual risk in low-income, urban African American girls. *Psychol Violence*. 2012;12(2):194-207.

25. Zinzow HM, Ruggiero KJ, Resnick H, et al. Prevalence and mental health correlates of witnessed parental and community violence in a national sample of adolescents. *J Child Psychol Psychiatry*. 2009;50(4):441-450.

26. Buckner JC, Beardslee WR, Bassuk EL. Exposure to violence and low-income children's mental health: direct, moderated, and mediated relations. *Am J Orthopsychiatry*. 2004;74:413-423.27.

27. O'Keefe M, Sela-Amit M. An examination of the effects of race/ethnicity and social class on adolescents' exposure to violence. *J Soc Serv Res*. 1997;22(3):53-71.

28. Schwab-Stone M, Chuansheng C, Ellen G, Silver D, Lichtman J, Voyce C. No safe haven II: the effects of violence exposure on urban youth. *J Am Acad Child Adolesc Psychiatry*. 1999;38(4):359-367.

29. Lambert S, Boyd R, Cammack N, Ialongo N. Relationship proximity to victims of witnessed community violence: Associations with adolescent internalizing and externalizing behaviors. *Am J Orthopsychiatry*. 2012;82(1):1-9.

30. Finkelhor D, Ormond R, Turner H, Hamby SL. The victimization of children and youth: A comprehensive, national survey. *Child Maltreatment*. 2005;10:5-25.

31. Hoyert DL, Xu J. Deaths: Preliminary data for 2011. *Natl Vital Stat Rep*. 2012;61(6):1-51.

32. Centers for Disease Control and Prevention. Rates of homicide, suicide, and firearm-related death among children – 26 industrialized countries. *MMWR*. 1997;46(05):101-105.

33. Truman JL, Planty M. *"Criminal Victimization, 2011." Bureau of Justice Statistics Bulletin*. Washington, DC: Bureau of Justice Statistics; 2012.

34. Centers for Disease Control and Prevention. Youth risk behavior surveillance study—United States, 2011. MMWR Surveill Summ. 2012;61(4):1-162.

35. Finkelhor D, Turner H, Ormond R, Hamby SL. Violence, abuse, and crime exposure in a national sample of children and youth. *Pediatrics*. 2009;124(5):1411-1423.

36. Lambert SF, Ialongo NS, Boyd RC, Cooley MR. Risk Factors for Community Violence Exposure in Adolescence. *Am J Community Psychol*. 2005;36:29-38.

37. Heron M. Deaths: leading causes for 2006. *Natl Vital Stat Rep*. 2010;58(14):1-100.

38. Berman S, Kurtines W, Silverman W, Serafini L. The impact of exposure to crime and violence on urban youth. *Am J Orthopsychiatry*. 1996;66:329-336.

39. Guerra NG, Williams KR. Ethnicity, youth violence, and the ecology of development. In: Guerra NG, Smith EP, eds. *Preventing Youth Violence in a Multicultural Society*. Washington, DC: American Psychological Association; 2006:17-45.

40. Schulz AJ, Zenk SN, Israel BA, Metnz G, Stokes C, Galea S. Do neighborhood economic characteristics, racial composition, and residential stability predict perceptions of stress associated with the physical and social environment? findings from a multilevel analysis in Detroit. *J Urban Health*. 2008;85(5):642-661.

41. Attar BK, Guerra NG, Tolan PH. Neighborhood disadvantage, stressful life events, and adjustment in urban elementary school children. *J Clin Child Psychol*. 1994;23:391-400.

42. Garbarino J, Dubrow N, Kostelny K, Pardo C. *Children in Danger: Coping With the Consequences of Community Violence*. San Francisco, CA: Jossey-Bass Social and Behavioral Science Series; 1992.

43. Neugebauer R, Wasserman GA, Fisher PW, Kline J, Geller PA, Miller LS. Darryl, a cartoon-based measure of cardinal post-traumatic stress symptoms in school-aged children. *Am J Public Health*. 1999;89:758-761.

44. White N, Lauritzen JL. *Violent Crime Against Youth*, 1994-2010. Washington, DC: US Department of Justice, Office of Justice Programs, Bureau of Justice Statistics; 2012.
45. Johnson AO, Mink MD, Harun N, Moore CG, Martin AB, Bennett KJ. Violence and drug use in rural teens: national prevalence estimates from the 2003 Youth Risk Behavior Survey. *J Sch Health.* 2008;70(10):554-561.
46. Barroso CS, Peters RJ, Kelder S, Conroy J, Murray N, Orpinas P. Youth exposure to community violence: association with aggression, victimization, and risk behaviors. *J Aggress Maltreat Trauma.* 2008;17(2):141-155.
47. Stein BD, Jaycox LH, Kataoka SH, et al. A mental health intervention for schoolchildren exposed to violence: a randomized controlled trial. *JAMA.* 2003;290:603-611.
48. Carlson KT. Poverty and youth violence exposure: experiences in rural communities. *Child Sch.* 2006;28(2):87-96.
49. Slovak K, Singer M. Gun violence exposure and trauma among rural youth. *Violence Vict.* 2001;16:389-400.
50. Sullivan TN, Kung EM, Farrell AD. Relation between witnessing violence and drug use initiation among rural adolescents: parental monitoring and family support as protectors. *J Clin Child Adoles Psychol.* 2004;33:488-498.
51. Nance ML, Carr BG, Kallan MJ, Branas CC, Wiebe DJ. Variation in pediatric and adolescent firearm mortality rates in rural and urban US counties. *J Pediatr.* 2010;130(5):e1416-e1423.
52. Dowd MD, Sledge RD. Firearm-related injuries affecting the pediatric population. *J Pediatr.* 2012;130(5):e1416-e1423.
53. Bradshaw CP, Rodgers CRR, Ghandour LA, Garbarino J. Social-cognitive mediators of the association between community violence exposure and aggressive behavior. *Sch Psychol Q.* 2009;24(3):199-210.
54. Sampson RJ, Morenoff JD, Gannon-Rowley T. Assessing "neighborhood effects": social processes and new directions in research. *Annu Rev Sociol.* 2002;28:443-478.
55. Browning C, Leventhal T, Brooks-Gunn J. Sexual initiation in early adolescence: the nexus of parental and community control. *Am Sociol Rev.* 2005;70:758-778.
56. Mazzerolle L, Wickes R, McBroom J. Community variations in violence: the role of social ties and collective efficacy in comparative context. *J Res Crime Delinq.* 2010;47(1):3-30.
57. Garbarino J, Hammond R, Mercy J, Yung BR. Community violence and children: preventing exposure and reducing harm. In: Maton KI, Schellenbach CJ, Leadbeater BJ, Solarz AL, eds. *Investing in Children, Youth, Families, and Communities.* Washington, DC: American Psychological Association; 2004:13-30.
58. Gibson C, Morris S, Beaver K. Secondary exposure to violence during childhood and adolescence: does neighborhood context matter? *Justice Q.* 2009;26(1):30-57.
59. Crouch JL, Hanson RF, Saunders BE, Kilpatrick DG, Resnick HS. Income, race/ethnicity, and exposure to violence in youth: results from the National Survey of Adolescents. *J Community Psychol.* 2000;28(6):625-641.

60. Milan S, Zona K, Acker J, Turcios-Cotto V. Prospective risk factors for adolescent PTSD: sources of differential exposure and differential vulnerability. *J Abnorm Child Psychol.* 2013;41:339-353.

61. West AE, Williams E, Suzukovich E, Strangeman K, Novins D. A mental health needs assessment for urban American Indian youth and families. *Am J Community Psychol.* 2012;49:441-453.

62. Chen W. Exposure to community violence and adolescents' internalizing behaviors among African American and Asian American adolescents. *J Youth Adolesc.* 2010;39:403-413.

63. Karch DL, Logan J, McDaniel D, Parks S, Patel N. Surveillance for violent deaths—national violent death reporting system, 16 States, 2009. *MMWR.* 2012;61(6):1-43.

64. Self-Brown SR, LeBlanc M, Kelly M, Hanson R, Laslie K, Wingate A. Effects of community violence exposure and parental mental health on the internalizing problems of urban adolescents. *Violence Vict.* 2006;21(2):183-198.

65. Farver JM, Xu Y, Eppe S, Fernandez A, Schwartz D. Community violence, family conflict, and preschoolers' socioemotional functioning. *Dev Psychol.* 2005;41(1):160-170.

66. Linares LO, Heeren T, Bronfman E, Zuckerman B, Augustyn M, Tronick E. A meditational model for the impact of exposure to community violence on early child behavior problems. *Child Dev.* 2001;72:639-652.

67. Kilpatrick DG, Saunders BE, Smith DW. Research in Brief: Youth Victimization: Prevalence and Implications. Washington, DC: US Department of Justice, National Institute of Justice; 2003.

68. Voison DR, Neilands TB. Community violence and health risk factors among adolescents on Chicago's southside: does gender matter? *J Adoles Health.* 2010;46(6):600-602.

69. Shahinfar A, Fox NA, Leavitt LA. Preschool children's exposure to violence: relation of behavior problems to parent and child reports. *Am J Orthopsychiatry.* 2000;70:115-125.

70. Hanson RF, Borntrager C, Self-Brown S, et al. Relations among gender, violence exposure, and mental health: The National Survey of Adolescents. *Am J Orthopsychiatry.* 2008;78:313-321.

71. Tolin DF, Foa EB. Sex differences in trauma and posttraumatic stress disorder: a quantitative review of 25 years of research. *Psychological Bulletin.* 2006;132(6):959-992.

72. Swahn MH, Bossarete RM, West B, Topalli V. Alcohol and drug use among gang members: experiences of adolescents who attend school. *J Sch Health.* 2010;80(7):353-360.

73. Lambert SF, Bradshaw CP, Cammack NL, Ialongo NS. Examining the developmental process of risk for exposure to community violence among urban youth. *J Prev Interv Community.* 2011;39(2):98-113.

74. Salzinger S, Feldman RS, Stockhammer T, Hood J. An ecological framework for understanding risk for exposure to community violence and the effects of exposure on children and adolescents. *Agress Violent Behav.* 2002;7:423-451.

75. Centers NL, Weist MD. Inner-city youth and drug dealing: a review of the problem. *J Youth Adolesc.* 1998;27:395-411.

76. Lauritsen JL, Laub JH, Sampson RJ. Convention and delinquent activities: implications for the prevention of violent victimization among adolescents. *Violence Vict.* 1992;7:91-108.

77. Gardner M, Brooks-Gunn J. Adolescents' exposure to community violence: are neighborhood youth organizations protective? *J Community Psychol.* 2009;37(4):505-525.

78. Kann L, Warren CW, Harris WA, et al. Youth risk behavior surveillance—United States, 1995. *J Sch Health.* 1996;66(10):365-377.

79. Flannery DJ, Wester KL, Singer MI. The impact of exposure to violence in school on child and adolescent mental health and behavior. *J Community Psychol.* 2004;32:559-573.

80. Geland B, Philipot P, Buidin G, et al. School violence in Belgium: differences between institutions and temporal evolution. *Rev Fr Pedagogie.* 2004;149:1-14.

81. Centers for Disease Control and Prevention. Trends in the prevalence of behaviors that contribute to violence on school property: national YRBS: 1991-2011. https://www.cdc.gov/healthyyouth/data/yrbs/pdf/trends/us_violenceschool_trend_yrbs.pdf. Published 2012. Accessed November 8, 2016.

82. Robers S, Kemp J, Truman J. *Indicators of School Crime and Safety: 2012.* Washington, DC: National Center for Education Statistics, US Department of Education, and Bureau of Justice Statistics, Office of Justice Programs, US Department of Justice; 2013.

83. Arum R. *Judging School Discipline: The Crisis of Moral Authority.* Cambridge, MA: Harvard University Press; 2003.

84. Ludwig KA, Warren JS. Community violence, school-related protective factors, and psychosocial outcomes in urban youth. *Psychology in the Schools.* 2009;46(10):1061-1073.

85. Ozer EJ, Weinstein RS. Urban adolescents' exposure to community violence: the role of support, school safety, and social constraints in a school-based sample of boys and girls. *J Clin Child Adolesc Psychol.* 2004;33(3):463-476.

86. Barr SC, Hanson R, Begle AM, et al. Examining the moderating role of family cohesion on the relationships between witnessed community violence and delinquency in a national sample of adolescents. *J Interpers Violence.* 2012;27(2):239-262.

87. Ceballo R, Ramirez C, Hearn KD, Maltese KL. Community violence and children's psychological well-being: does parental monitoring matter? *J Clin Child Adolesc Psychol.* 2003;32(4):586-592.

88. Bacchini D, Miranda MC, Affuso G. Effects of parental monitoring and exposure to community violence on antisocial behavior and anxiety/depression among adolescents. *J Interpers Violence.* 2010;26:269-292.

89. Brookmeyer KA, Henrich CC, Schwab-Stone M. Adolescents who witness community violence: can parent support and prosocial cognitions protect them from committing violence? *Child Dev.* 2005;76(4):917-929.

90. Garbarino J, Kostelny K. The effects of political violence on palestinian children's behavior problems: a risk accumulation model. *Child Dev.* 1996;67:33-45.

91. Perry DG, Hodges EVE, Egan SK. Determinants of chronic victimization by peers: a review and a new model of family influence. In: Juvonen J, Graham S, eds. *Peer Harassment in School: The Plight of the Vulnerable and Victimized.* New York, NY: Guilford Press; 2001:73-104.

92. Finkelhor D, Ormrod RK, Turner HA, Hamby SL. Measuring poly-victimization using the Juvenile Victimization Questionnaire. *Child Abuse Negl.* 2005;29:1297-1312.

93. Finkelhor D, Ormrod RK, Turner HA. Polyvictimization and trauma in a national longitudinal cohort. *Dev Psychopathol.* 2007;19:149-166.

94. Finkelhor D, Ormrod RK, Turner HA. Polyvictimization: a neglected component in child victimization. *Child Abuse Negl.* 2007;31:7-16.

95. Flaherty EG, Thompson R, Litrownik AJ, et al. Effect of early childhood adversity on child health. *Arch Pediatr Adolesc Med.* 2006;160(12):1232-1238.

96. Moore CF. An unhealthy start in life—what matters most? *Psychol Sci Public Interest.* 2005;6(3):i-ii.

97. Center for the Study and Prevention of Violence. *Blueprints for Violence Prevention: Overview and Model Programs, Boulder, CO.* www.colorado.edu/cspv/blueprinst/index.html. Published 2004. Accessed July 15, 2013.

98. Limbos AM, Chan LS, Warf C, et al. Effectiveness of interventions to prevent youth violence: a systematic review. *Am J Prev Med.* 2007;33(1):65-74.

99. Finkelhor D, Ormrod R. *Reporting Crimes Against Juveniles.* Washington, DC: US Department of Justice, Office of Justice Programs, Office of Juvenile Justice and Delinquency Prevention; 2000.

100. Junger M, Feder L, Clay J, et al. Preventing violence in seven countries: global convergence in policies. *Eur J Crim Policy Res.* 2007;13(3):327-356.

101. Hawkins JD, Herrenkohl TI, Farrington DP, et al. *Predictors of Youth Violence.* Washington, DC: US Department of Justice, Office of Justice Programs, Office of Juvenile Justice and Delinquency Prevention; 2000.

102. Redding RE. *Juvenile Justice Bulletin: Juvenile Transfer Laws: An Effective Deterrent to Delinquency?* Washington, DC: US Department of Justice, Office of Justice Programs, Office of Juvenile Justice and Delinquency Prevention; 2010.

103. Henggeler SW, Schoenwald SK. Evidence-Based interventions for juvenile offenders and juvenile justice: policies that support them. *Sharing Child and Youth Development Knowledge.* 2011;25(1):1-24.

104. Bilukha O, Hah RA, Crosby A, et al. The effectiveness of early childhood home visitation in preventing violence: a systematic review. *Am J Prev Med.* 2005;28(2S1):11-39.

105. Cunningham NJ, Sandhu DS. A comprehensive approach to school-community violence prevention. *Professional School Counseling.* 2000;4(2):126-133.

106. Family Strengthening Policy Center. Community violence prevention as a family strengthening strategy: a program of the National Human Services Assembly, Policy Brief No. 5. http://www.nassembly.org/fspc/practice/documents/vpdraft_2_.pdf. Published 2005. Accessed July 15, 2013.

107. Carter J. Domestic violence, child abuse, and youth violence: strategies for prevention and early intervention. http://www.mincava.umn.edu/link/documents/fvpf2/fvpf2.shtml. Published 2003. Accessed July 15, 2013.

108. Feinberg ME, Chilenski SM, Greenberg MT, Spoth RL, Redmond C. Community and team member factors that influence the operations phase of local prevention teams. *Prev Sci.* 2007;8(3):214-226.

109. Bird K. Message from the director. *Pennsylvania Statewide After School Development Network.* 2007;3:1-6, 110.

110. Hawkins JD, Brown EE, Oesterle S, Arthur MW, Abbott RD, Catalano RF. Early effects of Communities That Care on targeted risks and initiation of delinquent behavior and substance use. *J Adolesc Health.* 2008;43:15-22.

111. Hawkins JD, Oesterle S, Brown EC, Arthur MW, Abott RD, Catalano RF. Results of a type 2 translational research trial to prevent adolescent drug use and delinquency. a test of Communities That Care. *Arch Pediatr Adolesc Med.* 2009;163(9):789-798.

112. Skogan WG, Hartnett SM, Bump N, Dubois J. Evaluation of Ceasefire-Chicago. http://www.northwestern.edu/ipr/publications/ceasefire_papers/mainreport.pdf. Published 2008. Accessed July 15, 2013.

113. Ritter N. CeaseFire: a public health approach to reduce shootings and killings. http://www.ojp.usdoj.gov/nij/journals/264/ceasefire.htm. Published 2009. Accessed July 15, 2013.

114. McGarrell EF, Hipple NK, Bynum TS, et al. *Promising Strategies for Violence Reduction: Lessons From Two Decades of Innovation.* Washington, DC: Project Safe Neighborhoods; 2013.

115. Papachristos AV. Too big to fail: the science and politics of violence prevention. *Criminol Public Policy.* 2011;10:1053-1061.

116. Webster DW, Whitehill JM, Vernick JS, Parker EM. Evaluation of Baltimore's Safe Streets program: effects on attitudes, participants' experiences, and gun violence. Baltimore, MD: Johns Hopkins Center for Prevention of Youth Violence; 2012.

117. Hahn RH, Fuqua-Whitley D, Wethington H, et al. The effectiveness of universal school-based programs for the prevention of violent and aggressive behavior. a report on recommendations of the Task Force on Community Preventive Services. *MMWR Recomm Rep.* 2007;56:1-12.

118. School-based programs to reduce violence. www.thecommunityguide.org/violence/schoolbasedprograms.html. Published 2007. Accessed July 15, 2013.

119. Farrell AD, Meyer AL, Sullivan TN, Kung EM. Evaluation of the Responding in Peaceful and Positive Ways (RiPP) seventh grade violence prevention curriculum. *J Child Fam Stud.* 2003;12(1):101-120.

120. Silvia S, Blitstein J, Williams J, Ringwalt C, Dusenbury L, Hansen W. *Impacts of a Violence Prevention Program for Middle Schools: Findings From the First Year of Implementation.* Washington, DC: National Center for Education Evaluation and Regional Assistance, Institute of Education Sciences, US Department of Education; 2010.

121. Park-Higgerson HK, Perumean-Chaney SE, Bartolucci AA, Grimley DM, Singh KP. The evaluation of school-based violence prevention programs: a meta-analysis. *J Sch Health.* 2008;78(9):465-479.

122. Kellerman AL, Fuqua-Whitley DS, Rivara FP, Mercy J. Preventing youth violence: what works? *Annu Rev Public Health.* 1998;19:271-92.

123. Elias M. Sustainability of Social-Emotional Learning and related programs: lessons from a field study. *Int J Emot Educ.* 2010;2(10):17-33.

124. Wilson SJ, Lipsey MW. The Effectiveness of School-Based Violence Prevention Programs for Reducing Disruptive and Aggressive Behavior. http://www.ncjrs.gov/pdffiles1/nij/grants/211376.pdf. Published 2005. Accessed July 20, 2009.

125. Burrus B, Leeks KD, Sipe TA, et al. Person-to-person interventions targeted to parents and other caregivers to improve adolescent health. a community guide systematic review. *Am J Prev Med.* 2012;42(3):316-326.

126. Li X, Stanton B, Galbraith J, Burns J, Cottrell L, Pack R. Parental monitoring intervention: practice makes perfect. *Journal of the National Medical Association.* 2002;94(5):364-370.

127. DeVoe ER, Dean K, Traube D, McKay MM. The SURVIVE Community Project: a family-based intervention to reduce the impact of violence exposures in urban youth. *J Aggress Maltreat Trauma.* 2005;11(4):95-116.

128. Henggeler SW, Melton GB, Smith LA, Schoenwald SK, Hanley JH. Family preservation using multisystemic treatment: long-term follow-up to a clinical trial with serious juvenile offenders. *J Child Fam Stud.* 1993;2:283-293.

129. Sexton T, Turner CW. The effectiveness of functional family therapy for youth with behavioral problems in a community practice setting. *J Fam Psychol.* 2010;24(3):339-348.

130. Sawyer AM, Borduin CM. Effects of multisystemic therapy through midlife: a 21.9-year follow-up to a randomized clinical trial with serious and violent juvenile offenders. *J Consult Clin Psychol.* 2011;79(5):643-652.

131. Schaeffer CM, Borduin CM. Long-term follow-up to a randomized clinical trial of multisystemic therapy with serious and violent juvenile offenders. *J Consult Clin Psychol.* 2005;73(3):445-453.

132. Barnoski R. *Outcome Evaluation of Washington State's Research-Based Programs for Juvenile Offenders.* Olympia, WA: Washington State Institute for Public Policy; 2004.

133. Huey SJ, Henggeler SW, Brondino MJ, Pickrel SG. Mechanisms of change in multisystemic therapy: reducing delinquent behavior through therapis*t adherence and improved family and peer functioning.* J Consult Clin Psychol. 2000;68(3):451-467.

134. Lambert SF, Nylund-Gibson K, Copeland-Linder N, Ialongo NS. Patterns of community violence exposure during adolescence. *Am J Community Psychol.* 2010;46(3-4):289-302.

135. Guerra NG, Williams KR. *A Program Planning Guide for Youth Violence Prevention: A Risk-Focused Approach*. Boulder, CO: University of Colorado, Center for the Study and Prevention of Violence; 1996.

136. Curtis C, Norgate R. An evaluation of the Promoting Alternative Thinking Strategies curriculum at key stage 1. *Educ Psychol Pract*. 2007;23:33-44.

137. Domitrovich CE, Cortes RC, Greenberg MT. Improving young children's social and emotional competence: a randomized trial of the preschools "PATHS" curriculum. *J Prim Prev*. 2007;28:67-91.

138. Malti T, Ribeaud D, Eisner MP. The effectiveness of two universal preventive interventions in reducing children's externalizing behavior: a cluster randomized controlled trial. *J Clin Child Adolesc Psychol*. 2011;40(5):677-692.

Chapter 17

Children Exposed to Domestic Violence: Prevention Approaches With Mothers and Fathers

Tova B. Walsh, PhD
Jeffrey L. Edleson, PhD
Richard M. Tolman, LMSW, PhD

Introduction

Over the last 2 decades researchers, policymakers, and practitioners have increasingly recognized that exposure to domestic violence may disrupt children's experiences of consistent safety and care, and this disruption can lead to serious developmental difficulties, including emotional and behavioral problems and academic difficulties.[1-7] Consequently, social interventions to help alleviate the traumatic effects of exposure to domestic violence on children are expanding.[8-10] In this chapter the protective and risk factors that affect how children respond to adult domestic violence exposure are first examined. The focus is then on ***universal***, ***selective***, and ***indicated*** prevention strategies aimed at minimizing risk factors and maximizing protective factors for children, with a specific focus on the role of parents.

Understanding Child Exposure to Domestic Violence

Defining Domestic Violence

The American Psychological Association's (APA) Task Force on Male Violence Against Women defined interpersonal violence as[11]:

> Physical, visual, verbal, or sexual acts that are experienced by a woman or a girl as threat, invasion, or assault and have the effect of hurting her or degrading her and/or taking away her ability to control contact (intimate or otherwise) with another individual.

One subcategory of interpersonal violence is relationship or domestic violence defined as "committed by one partner against the other in a relationship."[12] Note that intimate partner violence (IPV) is the preferred, more precise terminology of the Centers for Disease Control and Prevention, recognizing that within the domestic setting there can also be child abuse, elder abuse, and animal abuse as forms of violence. For purposes of this chapter, the terms DV (ie, domestic violence) and IPV can be considered synonymous.

In recent years, there has been great debate about the relevance of gender to conceptualization of domestic violence, with some concluding that there exists "gender symmetry" in the experience of domestic violence in intimate relationships (ie, that men's experiences of violence in the domestic setting are the same as women's).[13] However, as

Hamby has pointed out, men commit over 90% of sexual violence, create higher levels of fear in their partners, and injure and murder their partners at much higher rates than do women.[14] This is not to say that women do not commit violent acts against their partners; however, it is at a much lower rate than men and appears to be less severe.[14] Stanko identifies gender as vitally relevant to how domestic violence is conceptualized, spoken of, and challenged.[15] They note that, "to lose sight and insight by ignoring how gender matters impoverishes any analyses of violence."[15]

Thus, in this chapter the focus is on the impact of domestic violence used by men against women, but recognizing that a child's exposure to any violence may have detrimental effects on his or her current physical and mental health as well as the child's long-term development.

Defining Exposure

Several different terms have been used to define children's exposure to adult domestic violence. The terms ***witnesses*** or ***observers*** of violence have frequently been used, but these terms are being replaced with an expanded terminology referring to child exposure to domestic violence.[16,17] Exposure usually refers to a wide variety of experiences of children in homes where 1 adult is using violent actions to control another adult.[8,16] For example, Kitzmann et al expanded the definition of witnessing violence to include hearing the violence and observing the aftermath of abuse[17]; for example, bruises on their mother's body or moving to a shelter. In some instances of exposure, children may respond by becoming involved in the violent incident. Child involvement may vary from becoming actively involved in the conflict to distracting him or herself and the parents.[18,19] For example, children in homes in which violence was occurring were 9 times more likely to verbally or physically intervene in parental conflicts than comparison children from homes in which no violence occurred.[20] Similarly, based on the reports of 111 battered mothers, Edleson et al found that 36% of the children frequently or very frequently yelled to stop violent conflicts, 11.7% frequently or very frequently called someone for help during a violent event, and 10.8% frequently or very frequently physically intervened to stop the violence.[21]

In this chapter, child exposure will refer to this expanded range of child experiences. Exposure will be considered seeing, hearing, and becoming involved in the violent incidents, as well as experiencing the multiple events that both lead up to and follow violence in homes.

Incidence of Exposure

A 2008 national survey of 4549 children aged 0 to 17 found that 6.2% of US children were exposed to DV in the past year. The same survey found 16.3% of children of all ages were exposed to DV since birth, but when asking older children with more life experience (ie, those 14 to 17 years of age) over a third (34.6%) reported they were exposed to DV in their lifetime.[22]

A study of police responses to DV in 5 US cities found that younger children are more likely to be present than older children when police arrive at homes where DV has occurred.[7] Children of all ages are often exposed to extreme violence. For example, a study of intimate partner homicides and attempted homicides involving 237 children in 10 US cities found that children were frequently present during these extremely violent events. Of 146 children whose mothers were murdered, 35% witnessed their mother's death and 37% found their murdered mothers. Of 91 children in families with an attempted homicide, 62% witnessed the violent event and 28% found their mothers afterwards.[23]

Children exposed to domestic violence may also be direct victims of physical and sexual maltreatment. Reviews examining the co-occurrence of documented child maltreatment and adult domestic violence revealed a 41% median co-occurrence of child maltreatment and adult domestic violence, with the majority of studies finding a 30% to 60% overlap.[24-28]

It appears that large numbers of children are exposed to domestic violence each year and over their lifetimes, which raises a question about the impact of this exposure on their child and adult development.

Impact of Child Exposure

Children can be harmed by exposure to violence even when they are not themselves direct targets of physical or sexual violence.[5,29] The co-occurrence of child exposure to domestic violence and other detrimental experiences (eg, direct child maltreatment) gives rise to a methodological challenge of separating out the impact of domestic violence exposure; many noted associations are thus correlational and not established as direct effects of domestic violence exposure. Studies of children who are both victims of violence and exposed to parental violence show that each experience uniquely and independently contributes to behavior problems.[30] Children's experiences and expectation of consistent safety and care may be disrupted and replaced by an environment characterized by instability and vulnerability.[1] This disruption can lead to serious developmental difficulties, including emotional and behavioral problems and academic difficulties.[2-7]

The impact of exposure to adult domestic violence has been well documented.[8,16,17,31-33] The frequency of adult domestic violence in a home is highly associated with children's behavioral problems, including externalizing behavior such as aggression and disobedience and internalizing behavior such as depression, sadness, and lack of self-confidence.[32] In general, children exposed to domestic violence demonstrate lower cognitive functioning and reduced skills for resilience, including lower capacity in the areas of social competence, problem-solving, autonomy, and self-efficacy.[24,34,35] In a review by Margolin and Gordis, the consequences of being exposed to violence in a child's home included both short- and long-term impacts on the child.[33] Short-term impacts included aggression and delinquency; emotional and mood disorders; posttraumatic stress symptoms such as exaggerated startle, nightmares, and flashbacks; health-related problems and somatic symptoms such as sleep disturbances; and academic and cognitive problems. Long-term impacts included an increased likelihood that a child will become either a victim or perpetrator of aggression later in life.

Overall, meta-analyses by Kitzmann, Gaylord, Holt, and Kenny; Wolfe, Crooks, Lee, McIntyre-Smith, and Jaffe; and Evans, Davies, and DiLillo drawing from 2 decades of studies have shown children exposed to domestic violence exhibit significantly worse social and behavioral problems than children not so exposed, but the size of this effect is relatively small (Zr=.28 in Wolfe et al).[17,36,37] Exposed children were not, however, significantly different than children who were physically abused or who were both physically abused and exposed to violence.[17]

The harm of exposure to domestic violence begins even prior to birth. Estimates of the prevalence of violence against pregnant women vary widely. In an early review, Gazmararian et al synthesized findings across studies from 1963 to 1995 and found prevalence rates ranging from 0.9% to 20.1%.[38] Campbell cited previous year prevalence estimates of 2.5% of pregnant women in the UK, 6% in Canada, 7% in South Africa, and 11% in Sweden.[39] Violence that occurs during pregnancy can be seen as a form of exposure for the developing fetus, as domestic violence during pregnancy causes harm not only to the woman being abused but also to her baby. Among the potential consequences of violence during pregnancy are low birth weight, premature labor, miscarriage, fetal trauma, and fetal death.[40-56] Additional studies confirm a positive association between domestic violence during pregnancy and delayed prenatal care and substance abuse, which may increase risk for negative pregnancy outcomes.[57-59] Physical and psychological abuse during pregnancy is also associated with increased risk of postpartum depression, decreased breastfeeding, and increased substance abuse, all of which also confer subsequent risk for children.[60-64]

Recent research on child exposure to trauma indicates that exposure to violence in childhood alters brain development and, particularly, that the abnormalities are more prominent if the traumatic exposure is early in life, severe, and chronic.[65] Young children's exposure to domestic violence is therefore particularly concerning because of the neurobiological changes that may occur and shape lifelong development and capacities. Specifically, traumatizing experiences may overstimulate the neural pathways that control the fear response, leaving children in an ongoing heightened state of fear or anticipation, even in the absence of traumatizing stimuli. Importantly, child physiology can rebound to relatively normal levels with restorative experiences. For example, reestablishing regular routines helps children to feel safe and promotes recovery.[66-70]

Approximately half of children exposed to domestic violence are in the clinical range of internalizing behavioral problems (eg, depression, anxiety, withdrawal) and externalizing behavioral problems (eg, aggressive or delinquent behavior, impulsivity, hyperactivity), many with overlapping diagnoses.[71,72] However, Graham-Bermann points out that many exposed children show no greater problems than children not so exposed.[73] Several studies found that approximately half of the exposed children studied appeared similar to nonexposed children on a variety of measures.[71,74,75] Given these varying impacts, a logical question is how does the differential presence of both protective and risk factors in children's lives moderate the impact of violence exposure on a child's development?

Patterns of Risk and Protection for Battered Mothers and Their Children

In examining how mothers may provide protection from or contribute to the risk their children experience from exposure to domestic violence, a number of factors may be considered. Maternal depression, parenting stress, and aggressive parenting have been shown to elevate children's risks for developing internalizing and externalizing symptoms.

Depression is a characteristic response of children to disruptions in their social environment, but the greatest risk factor predicting depression and internalizing symptoms in children exposed to domestic violence is maternal depression.[76,77] The majority of women who experience domestic violence have diagnosable levels of depression, and studies have found an intergenerational connection of parent and child depression.[39,78,79] Jarvis and Novaco found an association between maternal depression and internalizing symptoms in children following their stay in a domestic violence shelter.[80] Morrel et al studied a population of primarily African American children aged 4 to 6 and their mothers and found that the mother's own depression mediated the relationship between maternal victimization and maternal reports of children's internalizing symptoms.[81] Similarly, Levendosky and Graham-Bermann found that maternal mental health predicted the adjustment of violence-exposed children.[82] Jones, Forehand, and Neary studied a diverse sample of children over the course of a 2-year period.[83] They also found that maternal levels of depression prospectively predicted children's development of depressive symptoms, regardless of the quality of the parenting relationship.

Parenting effectiveness, particularly including the ability to parent well through stressful family circumstances, is a protective factor for children exposed to domestic violence. Mothers who reported lower levels of parenting stress and higher levels of mastery reported that their children had significantly lower levels of externalizing behavior problems.[84] Similarly, Boney-McCoy and Finkelhor found that strong parent-child relationships mitigated the effects of exposure to violence on children, though effects were not eliminated.[85] Levendosky and Graham-Bermann reported that greater parenting effectiveness reduced the negative effects of violence on children's internalizing and externalizing behavior problems.[82] A series of other studies also found a connection between family conflict and child problems.[81,86,87]

Patterns of Risk and Protection for Abusive Fathers and Their Children

More data are available on battered mothers and their caregiving than on perpetrators and their caregiving. Unfortunately, at times the overreliance on data collected from and about battered mothers may lead to partial or inaccurate conclusions. For example, it may be that the perpetrator's behavior is the key to predicting the emotional health of a child. By not collecting data about the perpetrators, we may incorrectly conclude that it is the mothers' problems and not the perpetrators' violent behavior that is creating negative outcomes for the children.

Several studies show that violent men directly impact the parenting of mothers. For example, Holden et al found that battered mothers, when compared to other mothers, more often altered their parenting practices in the presence of the abusive male.[88] Mothers reported that this change in parenting was made to minimize the men's irritability. A survey of 95 battered mothers living in the community also indicated that their abusive partners undermined the mothers' authority with their children, making effective parenting more difficult.[89] In an earlier qualitative study of 1 child support and education group program, Peled and Edleson found that fathers often pressured their children not to attend counseling when mothers were seeking help for their children.[90]

The relationship between the child and the adult perpetrator also appears to influence how the child is affected by exposure. A study of 80 mothers residing in shelters and 80 of their children revealed that an abusive male's relationship to a child directly affects the child's well-being, without being mediated by the mother's level of mental health.[75] Violence perpetrated by a biological father or stepfather was found to have a greater impact on a child than the violence of nonfather figures (ie, partners or ex-partners of the mother who played a minimal role in the child's life).

Some research suggests that men who batter may be more likely to use negative childrearing practices and less likely to use positive parenting.[91,92] There is mixed evidence about whether they spend less time with their children. Holden and Ritchie and Sternberg, Lamb, Greenbaum, Dawud, Cortes, and Lorey found abusive men were less involved with their children, but Fox and Benson found they did not differ from other fathers in time spent with their children.[91-93] Abusive men may display more negative affect and anger towards their children.[88,94] For example, in an observational study, Margolin and John found that men who were abusive towards their partners were less supportive, warm, and nurturing and used more power assertion towards their children.[95]

It cannot be assumed that separation from an abusive father will end violence against the mother or mitigate the negative effects of children's exposure to that violence. Domestic violence frequently continues after separation.[96-99] Continuing threats and violence towards mothers can be a factor in child visitation.[100,101] For example, Saunders, Sullivan, Tolman, and Grabarek found that 43% of mothers involved in supervised visitation reported continued direct contact with their ex-partners, even though such contact was prohibited.[102] Over a one-month period, of those who did not want this direct contact, 33% reported their ex-partners threatened them with violence or abuse, 61% reported threats involving their children, and 59% were stalked.[102] Similarly, in an early Canadian study, one quarter of women reported threats by a perpetrator during child visitations.[101]

As Perel and Peled point out, the literature has generally focused solely on the negative aspects of the batterers' parenting.[103] This tendency may obscure the potential for positive change that can prevent children's subsequent exposure to violence and increase the probability of fathers' positive influence upon their children's well-being. Qualitative studies have begun to explore domestic violence perpetrators as fathers in richer detail. Interviews conducted by Fox, Sayers, and Bruce revealed that recognizing the impact of their violence upon their children may motivate abusers to change.[104] Perel and Peled's interviews with 14 men who were abusive toward their partners showed their attitudes toward parenting were basically positive and that they worked toward being (and considered themselves) good fathers.[103] However, they also identified constraints to their parenting, eg, they believed their own experiences with their fathers did not properly prepare them for fatherhood.

This more complex picture of domestic violence perpetrators has also been supported by some quantitative research. Fox and Benson, using US national survey data, found domestic violence perpetrators spent as much time with their children and applied similar monitoring standards and actions as nonviolent men.[92] However, as cited previously, they also found that violent men were more likely to be punitive and less likely to use positive parenting behaviors when compared to nonabusive men. The promise of prevention strategies focused on violent fathers is explored later in this chapter.

Other Protective and Risk Factors

Additional protective and risk factors may impact the degree to which a child is affected by exposure. One likely factor that leads to differences in children's experiences is the great variation in ***severity***, ***frequency***, and ***chronicity*** of violence. Other factors also play a role in children's exposure and interact with each other creating unique outcomes for different children. For example, many children exposed to domestic violence are also exposed to other adverse experiences. In a study of 17 421 patients within a large health maintenance organization, Dube, Anda, and colleagues found that increased exposure to adult domestic violence in a child's life was positively associated with increasing "adverse childhood experiences" (eg, exposure to substance abuse, mental illness, incarcerated family members and other forms of abuse or neglect).[105] Problems associated with exposure vary based on gender and age of a child, but not race or ethnicity.[105-110] For example, younger children appear to be present more often during domestic violence. Fantuzzo and colleagues examined data on police and victim reports of domestic assault incidents in 5 cities and found children ages 0 to 5 years were significantly more likely to be present during single and recurring domestic violence incidents.[7] Interesting, the longer it has been since exposure to a violent event also appears to be associated with lessening problems.[111]

Summary

The definitions of child exposure to domestic violence have expanded to include not just seeing but also hearing violence, becoming involved in violent events, and experiencing additional events leading up to and following the outbreak of violence. Best estimates find millions of American children exposed to adult domestic violence in these varied ways every year. Research results suggest that such exposure may lead to negative behavioral, social, and physiological developmental changes in a child's life; but the effect of exposure is both moderated and mediated by a variety of risk and protective factors.

Prevention Approaches With Mothers and Fathers

In this section, ways in which practitioners have addressed the needs of children exposed to adult domestic violence are reviewed, and how such exposure may be prevented in the first place is explored. There are many approaches to the prevention of domestic violence, prevention of children's exposure to domestic violence, and intervention with exposed children; but the central focus here is on efforts that engage mothers or fathers and their children.

Prevention Continuum

A commonly accepted continuum of prevention includes ***universal***, ***selective***, and ***indicated*** prevention efforts.[112] Prevention efforts with parents may be universal (ie, aimed at improving parenting in the entire population and thus preventing domestic violence and exposure to it among other ills). Programs may alternatively be selective or targeted to parents at key transition points (ie, right before or after the birth of a child). Finally, programs may be indicated (ie, directed to parents currently experiencing stressors such as domestic violence).

Little data exists on the effectiveness of programs at any of these prevention levels to reduce the exposure of children to domestic violence. Promising practices and what evidence does exist to support their adoption will be highlighted, and other possible preventive efforts will be considered where major gaps in existing services are identified (**Table 17-1**).

Table 17-1. Prevention Continuum

	Universal	Selective	Indicated
Birth to 5 Years Old	Programs with expectant and new parents to promote positive parenting, including home visiting and center-based programs	Home visiting and community-based programs with families identified as high risk	Home visiting and community-based programs with victims of domestic violence and their children, providing specialized services
School-age Children	School-based programs addressing violence awareness and prevention, mediation, and conflict resolution skills	School- or community-based intervention with children following signs of possible exposure; may include education or therapy	Individual or group treatment, including crisis support, education and therapy. Appropriate treatment for indicated emotional or behavioral problems
Adolescents	School-based program targeting violence prevention and conflict resolution skills AND programs with specific focus on prevention of dating violence	School- or community-based intervention following signs of possible exposure; reinforce education about respectful adolescent dating relationships	Individual or group treatment, including crisis support, education, and therapy; appropriate treatment for indicated emotional or behavioral problems
Adults	Public education and media campaigns challenging gender stereotypes and social norms that support domestic violence; attributing universal responsibility for reducing violence	Community-based intervention upon indication of possible exposure	Multidisciplinary services to assist victims of chronic violence, inclusive of social support, medical treatment, police intervention legal advocacy, counseling

Universal Prevention Efforts

A key advantage of universal approaches to prevention is the large number of individuals who can be reached. Applied across a population, even an intervention that generates modest effects can have a widespread impact. Universal prevention programs involve changing social norms, behaviors, and policies that directly and indirectly contribute to domestic violence; and as such, universal prevention is intrinsically part of a broad-based, long-term agenda. As the responsibility for violence prevention lies with the perpetrator, and mothers are more frequently the victims of domestic violence, the larger part of this discussion of universal prevention is dedicated to efforts focused on fathers.

Universal Prevention Programs

Universal prevention programs include both education and media programs. Education programs that can be considered primary prevention in the area of child exposure to domestic violence include both programs to promote positive parenting and programs to build relational skills, such as effective communication and conflict management. Research demonstrates that parenting has a powerful effect on children's well-being, that parenting can be improved through intervention programs, and that improving parenting contributes to enhanced outcomes for children.[113-127] Universal parenting programs, by improving parenting practices and parental understanding of children's developmental needs, can be seen as a mechanism for preventing child exposure to domestic violence. Brooks-Gunn and Markman note that parenting programs in the United States are typically targeted to poor families, and thus serve disproportionate numbers of minority families, whereas in several countries all new mothers receive a series of home visits after the birth of a child.[128,129] Preventive effects of parenting programs are, on the whole, not distributed evenly across the population in the United States.

Universal programs aimed at shifting beliefs and attitudes about violence and building communication and conflict resolution skills are another approach to preventing the onset of domestic violence, thus preventing child exposure. Several studies demonstrate the efficacy of school-based programs to prevent dating violence.[36,130,131] Several longitudinal studies find that early conduct disorder/generalized violence predicts dating violence perpetration, which suggests that prevention and intervention in the area of conduct problems can also be seen as preventive of dating violence.[31,132-135]

There is little research on programs to prevent partner violence outside of school settings. One study of a community-based communication and conflict management skills program offered to couples planning to marry found that up to 4 years after program completion, participants reported better communication and less physical violence in their relationships compared to a control group; but by the 5-year follow-up, the only lasting effect was in the area of men's use of communication skills.[136]

A number of promising community-based efforts in the United States to prevent domestic violence altogether have been discussed in the literature.[137-139] In Australia, the state government of Victoria supports a statewide media awards program aimed at influencing community attitudes toward violence against women by encouraging journalistic quality in the reporting and characterization of family violence.[140]

Universal Prevention With Mothers

Victims of domestic violence do not bear responsibility for preventing the violence to which they are victim. Therefore, universal prevention with mothers builds awareness of personal rights within the context of a partner relationship, ability to recognize domestic violence, and knowledge of community resources. An example of such an effort was a collaboration with children's museums across the United States. The Ameriquest

Mortgage Company and the Family Violence Prevention Fund offered a program to[141]:

> ...coach mothers in sound investments, encourage them to build and manage assets, and invest in their financial future...[The aim of the program is to reach out to mothers] in non-threatening settings and encourage their financial independence... [so that they] will have the tools they need to protect themselves and their children if family violence occurs.

There has not yet been evidence to demonstrate benefits of this approach. Programs of prenatal and infancy home visitation increasingly consider domestic violence prevention in comprehensive service provision, and these are discussed elsewhere in this book.[142]

Universal Prevention With Fathers

At the most universal level, numerous authors have noted that the conceptualization of fatherhood is changing.[143,144] Expectations for fathers' roles seem to have shifted from ones emphasizing material support to more engaged roles. Fathers have probably benefited from this increased permission to develop close, emotionally satisfying relationships with their children, but a large gap remains between cultural support and clarity for fathers' positive involvement with their children. Interventions that promote the positive involvement of fathers with their children may help to prevent both abuse of women and exposure of children to domestic violence. This is an emergent area of research and to date there exists limited evidence to support universal strategies targeting fathers. The authors are part of a team of researchers who are working to develop and test a series of interventions aimed at engaging expectant and new fathers in violence prevention. The project, titled the Global Research Program on Mobilizing Men for Violence Prevention, is a joint project of the Universities of Michigan, Minnesota, and Washington.

Many efforts have emerged recently for engaging fathers in prevention of violence. Broadly construed, 1 approach has been to engage nonviolent men as allies to end domestic violence. These efforts can presumably help to reduce the risk of abuse by men who participate, but also change the culture that might support other men's behavior. A number of authors have argued that male involvement in campaigns to end violence against women can undermine beliefs, attitudes, and power relationships that support violence and transform the culture to support constructions of masculinity that lead to respectful and nonviolent relationships with women.[145,146]

Crooks et al have identified elements of universal prevention campaigns that are specifically directed towards fathers that can promote their effectiveness.[147] First, programs should provide information to fathers that can help to improve their involvement and positive parenting participation. Second, campaigns should create motivation through group membership. Third, campaigns should include specific skills that will help fathers take action.

The Family Violence Prevention Fund (FVPF) has sponsored 2 widely disseminated campaigns that contain these elements. Family Violence Prevention Fund (FVPF) has is aimed at recruiting men who explicitly denounce violence against women and children and promote a culture of respect by men towards women. One activity includes publishing an annual ad on Father's Day in *The New York Times* demonstrating men's concern about the issue of partner violence and soliciting additional participation by other men. An international registry of men who have supported the campaign is maintained. Participants are encouraged to take the campaign into their workplaces with brochures, cards, and other materials that can be distributed to raise awareness and engage others into joining the campaign.

Another prevention program developed by the FVPF is Coaching Boys into Men. It is a media campaign that uses public service announcements and other ads that promote the idea that men should deliver messages to boys that violence against women is unacceptable. A related program is the Coaching Boys Into Men Leadership Program for sports coaches that attempts to engage athletic coaches (many of whom are fathers themselves) into having conversations with their team members to promote respect for women and girls and erode support for violence as a defining characteristic of masculinity. The program distributes a "playbook" that provides a curriculum for presenting this information and finding teachable moments to promote these ideas. There is also a more structured weekly curriculum available and a newly developed Coaches' Training Kit. Coaches are encouraged to be involved in community outreach and other change efforts as well. Via a Web site, coaches have access to program materials and tips from fellow coaches on how to implement the program.

While formal evaluation of these programs has not been undertaken, the FVPF cites some support for the potential of such programs to influence public opinion and attitudes. A national telephone survey of 1020 men commissioned by the FVPF demonstrated that a majority of men surveyed were aware of domestic violence as a problem (67% thought domestic violence was at least fairly common).[148] Fifty-six percent believed they know someone who was involved in a domestic violence or sexual assault situation and 57% believed that they could make at least some difference in preventing domestic violence and sexual assault. Of fathers with children under 18, 64% said they could make at least some difference in prevention and 83% believed they could promote healthy, respectful, nonviolent relationships among young people. These survey findings point to the promise of primary prevention efforts to build upon men's current beliefs and expand the number of men who believe that violence is a problem and that they can do something about it.

Selective Prevention Efforts

Selective prevention efforts target groups identified as being at elevated risk for becoming a victim or perpetrator of domestic violence. First, selective prevention efforts with mothers will be discussed followed by selective prevention efforts with fathers. Bridging the discussion of selective prevention with mothers and fathers, the period of pregnancy and new parenthood is identified as a critical time for targeted prevention with all parents.

Selective Prevention by Screening Mothers in Health Care Settings

Although many victims of domestic violence do not seek treatment for acute injuries, many enter the health care system presenting with gynecological symptoms, gastrointestinal symptoms, or stress-related disorders.[40] These presenting problems are among a number of consistent, health-related risk markers exhibited by victims of domestic violence.[149,150] The consistency of these risk markers suggests an opportunity for medical professionals to selectively screen for domestic violence. Asking questions about violence can help to identify new victims, assess the current level of safety of previously identified victims, and increase awareness of the problem of domestic violence among all patients.

Screening allows medical professionals to provide support and referrals to patients who reveal domestic violence, decreasing the likelihood of exposure of children to violence and reducing long-term health effects.[151] Two studies have demonstrated that screening for domestic violence and providing a wallet-sized referral card to patients who report violence is associated with reduced physical violence over time, compared to the level of violence reported at the time of the initial screening.[152,153] Research indicates that introducing protocols and screening tools, as many health care institutions have now done, increases identification and documentation rates of domestic violence in medical settings.[154-157]

Selective Prevention With Expectant and New Mothers

When medical and other service providers meet with pregnant women, there is an opportunity to screen for domestic violence and to intervene if necessary to prevent the violence from occurring or progressing and to prevent subsequent child exposure to violence.

Macy et al tracked physical, psychological, and sexual abuse across the perinatal period.[158] For women who had been physically abused prior to pregnancy, the first 6 months of pregnancy saw a sharp increase in risk for physical abuse. Important for prevention efforts, their results showed an increased risk of sexual and psychological abuse in the first month after birth for women whose partners had not previously abused them either during pregnancy or before. Adolescent mothers are consistently at heightened risk for domestic violence and at especially high risk for experiencing domestic violence during the postpartum period.[159] Prevalence of violence was highest at 3 months' postpartum (21%) and lowest at 24 months (13%). Seventy-five percent of mothers who reported violence during pregnancy also reported violence in the postpartum period, 78% of mothers who experienced violence during the first 3 postpartum months had not reported violence before delivery. These data point to the need for screening at multiple points, since efforts aimed only at those known to be abusive prior to pregnancy would not be effective in preventing abuse that emerges postnatally.

Promising screening and violence prevention approaches integrated into existing services, such as home visiting programs and family planning programs, for women of childbearing age were recently identified in 2008.[160] Importantly, these programs screen for violence at least once during pregnancy and at least once during the postpartum period, as well as screening at times when a significant life change occurs (eg, a death, job change, relationship change, or move). Screening rates have increased among those who receive home visiting services due to adoption of a shorter and more frequent screening protocol, and attention to sources of additional stress for families.[160] Another notable example is the Nurse-Family Partnership home visitation program. The program offers an array of services, and screening for domestic violence is embedded in an early, comprehensive risk assessment. Mothers-to-be who report domestic violence are provided with support and referrals, and Olds et al determined that 2 years after home visitation services had ended, nurse-visited women in Denver reported less domestic violence in comparison with women who did not receive home visitation.[161] However, a corresponding effect on domestic violence was not found in a study of women in Memphis, 4 years after cessation of home visiting services.

Prevention With Expectant Fathers

As discussed previously, preventing domestic violence during pregnancy is necessary for eliminating potentially harmful effects of exposure to the developing fetus during pregnancy, and may also make subsequent violence exposure to infants and older children less likely as well. Men may have increased motivation for positive change during pregnancy and this may make efforts to prevent or stop domestic violence more effective. Additionally, this may be a key time to address issues such as positive partnering and parenting.

Despite these potentially beneficial outcomes, there do not appear to be any violence prevention programs specifically focused on expectant fathers that have established their efficacy through rigorous evaluations. However, other prevention efforts that have been used to promote positive transitions in this stage might be useful for reducing domestic violence as well. For example, parenting preparation might reduce stress, which could increase the probability of subsequent partner or child abuse.

However, a number of efforts have been developed to engage fathers who are at risk in various ways (eg, adolescent fathers, unemployed, and those with a criminal history) and some of these include expectant and new fathers among their targeted groups. One of the best-known programs for fathers experiencing stressors is the Baltimore Responsible Fatherhood Project (BRFP).[162] Participants in this program are primarily non-custodial fathers. Most are unemployed, have not graduated high school, and may have been involved in the criminal justice system and/or used illegal drugs. The program assists these low-income fathers with seeking employment, providing child support, taking steps to reduce recidivism, learning skills for effective parenting, and maintaining healthy relationships. While these fathers clearly are experiencing multiple stressors and have a number of risk factors, they do not participate in the program due to domestic violence or child abuse. However, BRFP actively works to identify domestic violence if it has occurred and motivates men to seek help for their abusive behavior if identified. They have established a cooperative relationship with a batterer intervention program at House of Ruth to provide cross-training and service referrals.

Another program that targets fathers at risk is the Con Los Padres program affiliated with the National Latino Fatherhood and Family Institute (NLFFI) of Bienvenidos Family Services.[163,164] The program helps young and expectant fathers aged 16 to 25 to develop positive relationships with their children through 20 weekly classes. Case management services are available for young fathers who need additional support to develop appropriate interaction with their children. The program screens for domestic violence and other forms of family and community violence and can refer men to a more structured program that attempts to address aggression. This aggression program is based on the principles of "Un Hombre Noble" (a noble man). Un hombre noble is a man of "palabra," a man who keeps his word as the foundation of respectful relationship with his children and others in his life. As the NLFFI curriculum describes[164]:

> Through the process of sitting in a circle with other men who collectively reflect the reality of their gifts and their baggage, men can begin to acknowledge and accept that aggression and violence is not acceptable and realize it causes irreparable damage to themselves and others.

These programs in Maryland and California highlight the need for prevention efforts to be culturally specific. This specificity may increase the probability of successful engagement of fathers into the programs. Cultural specificity may also increase the effectiveness of intervention by delivering messages that are more readily received by participants, but comparative studies are needed to confirm if these hypotheses are correct.

Specific components aimed at mothers and fathers who are identified through screening, are already known to be aggressive towards family members, or are the targets of such aggression leads to the final category of prevention: indicated efforts to aid mothers, fathers, and their children where domestic violence is known to have occurred.

Indicated Prevention Efforts

Chalk and King state that[165]:

> In all areas of family violence, after-the-fact services predominate over preventive interventions...For domestic violence, interventions designed to treat victims and offenders and defer future incidents of violence are more common [than services aimed at prevention].

In terms of intervening with children after intimate partner violence has already occurred, this indicated prevention may also be considered selective prevention as it can reduce the possibility that those children will grow up to be perpetrators themselves. People exposed as children are more likely to perpetrate intimate partner violence themselves as adults.[166,167] For example, Whitfield et al found that among 8629 HMO patients studied, men exposed to physical abuse, sexual abuse, and adult domestic violence as a child were 3.8 times more likely than other men to perpetrate domestic violence as adults.[168]

Working With Battered Women and Their Children

As mentioned previously, time away from violence was found to lessen the impacts of exposure,[111] thus providing a child and his or her primary caregiver with safe shelter and longer-term supports may end or limit future exposure and its negative impacts. Interventions for children exposed to domestic violence have been offered in shelters for over 30 years.[169,170] Child-oriented programs recently have become more widespread in their availability in nonshelter, community settings, most often in the form of individual treatment for trauma, individual intervention with parent-child dyads, and separate group support and education programs for children and for their mothers.[73,171-175]

This section of the chapter will review evidence-based practices that have been found to improve outcomes for children exposed to domestic violence. Four specific intervention programs are reviewed, about which much has been written. These intervention programs are seen as forms of indicated prevention in that they respond to exposed children, but may also be viewed as primary prevention in that they may prevent exposure in the next generation of children.

Child-Parent Psychotherapy

Child-Parent Psychotherapy for Family Violence (CPP-FV) focuses on strengthening the parent-child relationship and repairing the damage done to the child's developmental trajectory.[10] CPP-FV is intended for early intervention, that is with children 5 years old and younger in situations where baseline physical safety has been established and domestic violence is not ongoing.[10] Child-parent attunement is the bedrock of the treatment, as CPP-FV views attachment as critical to both general healthy development and recovery from the trauma of exposure to domestic violence.[10] The CPP-FV model integrates psychodynamic, attachment, trauma, cognitive-behavioral, and social-learning theories into a dyadic treatment approach aimed at rebuilding the relationship between child and parent, as well as to restoring damage to the child's developmental and mental health progression incurred by the exposure to domestic violence. Treatment centers on 3 therapeutic goals: to improve the child-parent relationship, to help parent and child to more effectively modulate their feelings, and to help the parent better understand the child's experience so that the parent can become more effectively protective.[10] The CPP-FV model involves 12 months of weekly, hour-long, joint child-parent psychotherapy sessions. Typically sessions take place in an office playroom (in a clinical setting); but where it is safe, sessions may be held in the home. Two studies have demonstrated the effectiveness of CPP-FV. Results of a study of 75 mother-child dyads, comparing the efficacy of CPP-FV with case management plus treatment as usual in the community, demonstrated significantly improved outcomes in the areas of children's total behavior problems, traumatic stress symptoms, and diagnostic status, as well as mothers' avoidance symptoms, PTSD symptoms, and general distress.[176] An investigation of the durability of improvement in maternal and child symptoms 6 months after termination of CPP-FV demonstrated the durability of effects on the mothers' general distress and the children's total behavior problems.[177]

Kids Club and Moms Parenting Empowerment Program

The Kids Club and Moms Parenting Empowerment Program is an intervention that includes both mothers who have experienced domestic violence and their children who are in treatment.[178,179] The 10-session, manualized Kids Club intervention is described by Graham-Bermann as targeting children's emotional adjustment by addressing attitudes and beliefs about families and violence, helping children to identify and process feelings associated with their experiences of violence, and enhancing children's coping behaviors.[178,179] Groups are age-graded and include boys and girls together. The program provides an environment for children to discover that they are not alone in their exposure to violence, to share their experiences, and to discuss the responsibility for and learn new strategies for coping with violence exposure. Activities designed to identify family strengths are incorporated, and only after relationships among group participants and leaders are well established do children's group leaders allow for discussion of the specifics of violence in the family.

Concurrent with each children's group, mothers meet in a separate group to share their experiences, concerns, and support related to parenting. Graham-Bermann[178,179] describes the Moms Parenting Empowerment Program as a 10-session intervention based on goals of enhancing mothers' social and emotional adjustment and improving mothers' repertoire of parenting and disciplinary skills, and thereby reducing the behavioral and adjustment difficulties of their children.

An efficacy trial compared child-only intervention, child-plus-mother intervention, and a wait list, treatment as usual comparison group.[179] Participants consisted of 181 children aged 6 to 12 and their mothers exposed to domestic violence during the preceding year. Children showed the greatest improvement over time when the child and mother both participated in the intervention. Improvements were demonstrated for all 3 measured outcomes: internalizing behavior problems, externalizing behavior problems, and change in attitude and beliefs.

Child Witness to Violence Project

The Child Witness to Violence Project (CWVP) at Boston Medical Center provides trauma-focused clinical intervention to children 8 years old and younger who have been exposed to violence in their family or community. CWVP addresses disrupted attachment between parent and child, conflict between parent and child, parental lack of understanding of the impact of trauma on children, trauma associated with being a victim of domestic violence, and particularly maladaptive symptoms in the child (eg, aggression, sleep disturbances, learning difficulties, and difficult peer relationships).[180] Groves and Zuckerman identify 3 focal points in the work of CWVP: reestablishing a sense of order and routine in the home, explaining violent events to children, and responding to children's fears and worries in an honest and reassuring manner.[181] Principles of trauma-focused cognitive behavioral therapy and child-parent psychotherapy are integrated in the intervention model.[176,177,182] CWVP recommends weekly sessions of 1 to 1.5 hours for at least 5 months.[9] Services are typically offered in an outpatient clinic but are in some cases home-based, and services are offered in English or Spanish.

Along with individual child psychotherapy and dyadic therapy, the intervention provides parent guidance, case management, and advocacy. CWVP works in collaboration with domestic violence, law enforcement, child protection, and other community agencies to help families secure safety and receives referrals from throughout the community. The CWVP offers a promising approach to intervention with trauma-exposed children as evidenced by clinical experience, but there are currently no published, peer-reviewed research studies for the model.

Supportive Advocacy With Mothers and Children

Some community-based support programs for battered women and their children also include an advocacy component. Sullivan, Bybee, and Allen and McDonald, Jouriles, and Skopp have evaluated strengths-based support and advocacy interventions and determined that these programs effectively reduce the harmful effects of children's exposure to domestic violence.[183,184] Sullivan, Bybee, and Allen utilized a longitudinal, experimental design, and over the course of 8 months assessed children's exposure to abuse and their self-competence, maternal experience of abuse, and maternal well-being.[183] The experimental intervention involved advocacy for mothers and their children, as well as a 10-week support and education group for the children. Study participants included 80 mothers and their children. Findings indicated that children in the experimental condition endorsed significantly higher self-competence in several domains as compared to children in the control group, and mothers in the experimental condition demonstrated improvement in depression and self-esteem over time as compared to mothers in the control group. McDonald, Jouriles, and Skopp evaluated a project to provide services to women and children upon their departure from a domestic violence shelter.[184] Participating families had at least 1 child aged 4 to 9 exhibiting clinical levels of conduct problems. At 2 years post treatment, 15% of children in families who had received support and advocacy services exhibited clinical levels of conduct problems, as compared to 53% in the comparison condition. Mothers of children who had received the additional support also reported their children to be happier, to have better social relationships, and to have lower levels of internalizing problems versus the comparison condition.

Summary

The programs reviewed here show promise for intervening to prevent future domestic violence by working with battered mothers and their children who are already exposed to domestic violence.

Working With Men Who Batter and Their Children

Applying these findings to prevention, domestic violence perpetrators would benefit from efforts to improve their parenting, especially in terms of decreasing punitive behavior and expression of negative affect. On the other hand, the evidence of these men's involvement with and positive motivation for fathering supports the possibility that investment in fathering may be a positive motivation for cessation of domestic violence. Perel and Peled note that models of intervention with men who batter as fathers can be distinguished by the extent to which they see the issue of fathering as an end in itself or as an entry point into the men's inner world and into other potential areas of change, such as the violent behavior.[103] However, these need not be mutually exclusive.

There are several examples of emerging programs specifically designed for training perpetrators to parent without violence, yet most of these have been established only the in last decade or so. These programs can be classified into 2 types: parenting programs are supplementary sessions within existing batterer intervention programs or separate curricula that are offered to men once they have completed a traditional batterer intervention group curriculum.

One of the best documented programs is the Caring Dads program.[185] Caring Dads uses a range of approaches including motivational interviewing, psychoeducation, cognitive-behavioral techniques, confrontation, and shame work. The program seeks to address 4 goals: engaging men to examine their fathering by developing trust and motivation; increasing awareness and application of child-centered fathering; increasing awareness of, and responsibility for, abusive and neglectful fathering and domestic violence; and rebuilding children's trust in the men's fathering and planning for the future.

A preliminary evaluation of the Caring Dads program compared pre-to post-intervention measures for 23 participants.[186] Using self-reports on the Parenting Stress Index, fathers' hostility, denigration, and rejection of child all decreased significantly, as did angry arousal to child and family situations.[187] Self-reported partner abuse decreased, but not significantly. They also attained a low attrition rate for participants (34 of 42 completed).

Another well-described and widely disseminated program is the Fathering After Violence program, developed by the FVPF.[188] The curriculum is aimed for incorporation into existing batterer intervention programs and is based on exercises that create empathy for children's experience of domestic violence, identify behaviors that constitute positive modeling by fathers for their children and support the mother's parenting, and increase understanding of father's roles in the process of repairing a damaged relationship with their children.

Fleck-Henderson conducted an initial evaluation of the Fathering After Violence program.[189] Data was gathered on about 60 participants in 3 programs in the Boston area. Staff and participants' self-reports provided some support that the curriculum was engaging and readily integrated into the batterer intervention program. The exercises appeared to result in improvements in the 3 goal areas noted previously. Although attempts to contact partners were not very successful, the majority of those reached (about half) did report positively on the participants' behavior towards their children and were positive about the program.

One prevention strategy for reducing children's exposure to domestic violence may be limiting visitation rights of abusers. Screening might focus on high conflict divorces.[190] Targeting men who are already abusive may be viewed as a prevention strategy even if separation ends the exposure of violence for their existing children. It is likely these men will have children from other partners in their past or future relationships and may continue to have contact with his children despite court orders to the contrary.[191]

The last decade has brought a growing recognition of the potential of interventions that directly focus on the prevention harm to children by promoting positive involvement of fathers in their children's lives. However, this work has primarily been done in the context of programs that actively seek to end partner abuse, and this remains a core condition for the reduction of the harm of exposure.

Conclusion

The findings reviewed in this chapter come from the growing but still small number of studies on children's exposure to intimate partner violence and the approaches that seek to prevent exposure and its subsequent harm. These findings provide a foundation for understanding the effects of exposure to domestic violence on children; the risk and protective factors that help to explain the extent to which exposed children experience negative developmental outcomes; and the important elements of appropriate, effective interventions to support children's recovery. The research work that has been done to date points to important directions for future research. Given that the early years of life are a period of rapid change in degree of cognitive, emotional, and behavioral maturation, further study is indicated to evaluate if and how to effectively intervene with children at various ages and how to modify manualized approaches (ie approaches to intervention that offer a prescriptive approach based on manuals and specialized training) to meet individual developmental needs. It is known that some trauma symptoms may only emerge long after the precipitating trauma; longitudinal studies are necessary both to evaluate long-term durability of treatment outcomes and to assess potential association between treatment and lifespan trauma symptoms.

Similarly, if the outcomes of universal prevention efforts are to come to fruition, both long-term investment in such approaches, as well as longitudinal research, will be necessary. Enormous progress has been made in the past 30 years in identifying and addressing intimate partner violence as a social concern and threat to public health and safety. Future work that reduces the harm to adult survivors and their children and promotes healthy and positive relationships between adult partners and between parents and their children will be welcome.

References

1. Gewirtz A, Edleson J. Young children's exposure to adult domestic violence: Towards a developmental risk and resilience framework for research and intervention. *J Fam Violence.* 2007;22(3):151-163.

2. Skopp NA, McDonald R, Jouriles EN, Rosenfield D. Partner aggression and children's externalizing problems: Maternal and partner warmth as protective factors. *J Fam Psychol.* 2007;21(3):459-467.

3. Turner HA, Finkelhor D, Ormrod R. The effect of lifetime victimization on the mental health of children and adolescents. *Soc Sci Med.* 2006;62(1):13-27.

4. Bogat GA, DeJonghe E, Levendosky AA, Davidson WS, von Eye A. Trauma symptoms among infants exposed to intimate partner violence. *Child Abuse Negl.* 2006;30:109-125.

5. Carlson BE. Children exposed to intimate partner violence: research findings and implications for intervention. *Trauma Violence Abuse.* 2000;1(4):321-340.

6. Scheeringha MS, Gaensbauer TJ. Posttraumatic stress disorder. In: Zeanah CH, Jr, ed. *Handbook of Infant Mental Health.* 2nd ed. New York, NY: Guilford Press; 2000:369-381.

7. Fantuzzo JW, Brouch R, Beriama A, Atkins M. Domestic violence and children: prevalence and risk in five major U.S. cities. *J Am Acad Child Adolesc Psychiatry.* 1997;36:116-122.

8. Edleson JL. A response system for children exposed to domestic violence: public policy in support of best practices. In: Feerick M, Silverman GB, eds. *Children Exposed to Violence.* Baltimore, MD: Brookes; 2006:191-211.

9. Groves BM. *Children Who See too Much: Lessons From the Child Witness to Violence Project.* Boston, MA: Beacon Press; 2002.

10. Lieberman AF, Van Horn P. *Don't Hit My Mommy!: A Manual for Child-Parent Psychotherapy With Young Witnesses of Family Violence.* Washington, DC: Zero to Three Press; 2005.

11. Koss M, Goodman L, Browne A, Fitzgerald L, Keita GP, Russo NF. *No Safe Haven: Male Violence Against Women at Home, at Work, and in the Community.* Washington, DC: American Psychological Association; 1994.

12. APA Intimate Partner Abuse and Relationship Violence Working Group. Intimate partner abuse and relationship violence. http://www.apa.org/about/division/activities/partner-abuse.pdf. Published 2002. Accessed November 10, 2016.

13. Dutton DG, Nicholls TL. The gender paradigm in domestic violence research and theory: part 1 - the conflict of theory and data. *Aggress Violent Behav.* 2005;10(6):680-714.

14. Hamby SL. The gender debate on intimate partner violence: solutions and dead ends. *Psychol Trauma.* 2009;1(1):24-34.

15. Stanko EA. Theorizing about violence: observations from the economic and social research council's violence research program. *Violence Against Women.* 2006;12(6):543-555.

16. Fantuzzo JW, Mohr WK. Prevalence and effects of child exposure to domestic violence. *Future Child.* 1999;9:21-32.

17. Kitzmann KM, Gaylord N, Holt A, Kenny E. Child witnesses to domestic violence: a meta-analytic review. *J Consult Clin Psychol.* 2003;271:339-352.

18. Garcia O'Hearn H, Margolin G, John RS. Mothers' and fathers' reports of children's reactions to naturalistic marital conflict. *J Am Acad Child Adolesc Psychiatry.* 1997;36:1366-1373.

19. Peled E. The experience of living with violence for preadolescent witnesses of woman abuse. *Youth Soc.* 1998;29:395-430.

20. Adamson JL, Thompson RA. Coping with interparental verbal conflict by children exposed to spouse abuse and children from nonviolent homes. *J Fam Violence.* 1998;13:213-232.

21. Edleson JL, Mbilinyi LF, Shetty S. *Parenting in the Context of Domestic Violence.* San Francisco, CA: Judicial Council of California; 2003.

22. Finkelhor D, Turner HA, Ormrod RK, Hamby SL. Violence, crime, and exposure in a national sample of children and youth. *Pediatrics.* 2009;124(5):1411-1423.

23. Lewandowski LA, McFarlane J, Campbell JC, Gary F, Barenski C. "He killed my mommy!" murder or attempted murder of a child's mother. *J Fam Violence.* 2004;19:211-220.

24. Appel AE, Holden GW. The co-occurrence of spouse and child abuse: a review and appraisal. *J Fam Psychol.* 1998;12:578-599.

25. Edleson JL. Children's witnessing of adult domestic violence. *J Interpers Violence.* 1999;14(8):839-870.

26. Holden GW. Children exposed to domestic violence and child abuse: terminology and taxonomy. *Clin Child Fam Psychology Rev.* 2003;6(3):151-160.

27. Lee LC, Kotch JB, Cox CE. Child maltreatment in families experiencing domestic violence. *Violence Vict.* 2004;19(5):573-591.

28. McGuigan WM, Pratt CC. The predictive impact of domestic violence on three types of child maltreatment. *Child Abuse Negl.* 2001;25(7):869-883.

29. Rossman BBR, Hughes HM, Rosenberg MS. *Children and Inter-Parental Violence: The Impact of Exposure.* Philadelphia, PA: Brunner/Mazel; 2000.

30. Litrownik AJ, Newton R, Hunter WM, English D, Everson MD. Exposure to family violence in young at-risk children: a longitudinal look at the effects of victimization and witnessed physical and psychological aggression. *J Fam Violence.* 2003;18:59-73.

31. Ehrensaft MK, Cohen P, Brown J, Smailes E, Chen H, Johnson JG. Intergenerational transmission of partner violence: a 20-year prospective study. *J Consult Clin Psychol.* 2003;71:741-753.

32. Jouriles EN, Norwood WD, McDonald R, Vincent JP, Mahoney A. Physical violence and other forms of marital aggression: links with children's behavior problems. *J Fam Psychol.* 1996;10:223-234.

33. Margolin G, Gordis EB. Children's violence exposure in the family and community. *Curr Dir Psychol Sci.* 2004;13:152-155.

34. Rossman BBR. Descartes's error and posttraumatic stress disorder: gognition and emotion in children who are exposed to parental violence. In: Holden GW, Geffer R, Jouriles EN, eds. *Children Exposed to Marital Violence: Theory, Research, and Applied Issues*. Washington, DC: American Psychological Association; 1988:223-256.

35. Graham-Bermann SA, Edelson JL. *Domestic Violence in the Lives of Children: The Future of Research, Intervention, and Social Policy*. Washington, DC: APA; 2001.

36. Wolfe DA, Crooks CV, Lee V, McIntyre-Smith A, Jaffe PG. A meta-analysis of the effects of children's exposure to domestic violence: the need for a developmental framework. *Clin Child Fam Psychol Rev*. 2003;(6):171-187.

37. Evans SE, Davies C, DiLillo D. Exposure to domestic violence: a meta-analysis of child and adolescent outcomes. *Aggress Violent Behav*. 2008;13:131-140.

38. Gazmararian JA, Lazorick S, Spitz AM, Ballard TJ, Saltzman LE, Marks JS. Prevalence of violence against pregnant women. *JAMA*. 1996;275(24):1915-20.

39. Campbell J. Health consequences of interpersonal violence. *J Lancet*. 2002;359(9314):1331-1336.

40. Campbell J, Torres S, Ryan J, et al. Physical and nonphysical partner abuse and other risk factors for low birth weight among full term and preterm babies. *Am J Epidemiol*. 1999;150(7):714-726.

41. Curry MA, Harvey SM, eds. *Stress Related to Domestic Violence During Pregnancy and Infant Birth Weight (Vol. 9)*. Thousand Oaks, CA: Sage; 1998.

42. Fernandez FM, Krueger PM. Domestic violence: effect on pregnancy outcome. *J Am Osteopath Assoc*. 1999;99(5):254-256.

43. Bullock L, McFarlane J. The birth-weight/battering connection. *Am J Nurs*. 1989;89(9):1153-1155.

44. Parker B, McFarlane J, Soeken K. Abuse during pregnancy: effects on maternal complications and birth weight in adult and teenage women. *Obstet Gynecol*. 1994;84(3):323-328.

45. Rosen D, Seng JS, Tolman RM, Mallinger G. Intimate partner violence, depression, and posttraumatic stress disorder as additional predictors of low birth weight infants among low-income mothers. *J Interpers Violence*. 2007;22(10):1305-1314.

46. Sharps PW. Intimate partner violence and the childbearing year: maternal and infant health consequences. *Trauma Violence Abuse*. 2007;8(2):105.

47. Renker PR. Physical abuse, social support, self-care, and pregnancy outcomes of older adolescents. *J Obstet Gynecol Neonatal Nurs*. 1999;28:377-388.

48. El Kady D, Gilbert WM, Xing G, Smith LH. Maternal and neonatal outcomes of assaults during pregnancy. *Obstet Gynecol*. 2002;105:357-363.

49. Cokkinides VE, Coker AL, Sanderson M, Addy C, Bethea L. Physical violence during pregnancy: maternal complications and birth outcomes. *Obstet Gynecol*. 1999;93(5):661-666.

50. Shumway J, O'Campo P, Gielen A, Witter FR, Khouzami AN, Blakemore KJ. Preterm labor, placental abruption, and premature rupture of membranes in relation to maternal violence or verbal abuse. *J Materna Fetal Med*. 1999;8(3):76-80.

51. Morland LA, Leskin GA, Block CR, Campbell JC, Friedman MJ. Intimate partner violence and miscarriage: examination of the role of physical and psychological abuse and posttraumatic stress disorder. *J Interpers Violence*. 2008;23:652-669.

52. Rachana C, Suraiya K, Hisham A, Abdulaziz A, Hai A. Prevalence and complications of physical violence during pregnancy. *Eur J Obstet Gynecol Reprod Biol.* 2002;103:26-29.

53. Jacoby M, Gorenflo D, Black E, Wunderlich C, Eyler AE. Rapid repeat pregnancy and experiences of interpersonal violence among low-income adolescents. *Am J Prev Med.* 1999;16(4):318-321.

54. Connolly A, Katz VL, Bash KL, McMachon MJ, Hansen WF. Trauma and pregnancy. *Am J Perinatol.* 1997;14(6):331-336.

55. Berrios DC, Grady D. Domestic violence: risk factors and outcomes. *West J Med.* 1991;155:133-135.

56. Webster J, Chandler J, Battistutta D. Pregnancy outcomes and health care use: effects of abuse. *Am J Obstet Gynecol.* 1996;174(2):760-767.

57. Dietz PM, Gazmararian JA, Goodwin M, Bruce FC, Johnson CH, Rochat R. Delayed entry into prenatal care: effect of physical violence. *Obstet Gynecol.* 1997;90(2):221-224.

58. Goodwin M, Gazmarian J, Johnson C, Gilbert B, Saltzman L. Pregnancy intendedness and physical abuse around time of pregnancy: findings from the Pregnancy Risk Assessment Monitoring System, 1996-1997. *Matern Child Health J.* 2000;4:85-92.

59. Bailey BA, Daugherty RA. Intimate partner violence during pregnancy: incidence and associated health behaviors in a rural population. *Matern Child Health J.* 2007;11(5):495-503.

60. Tiwari A. The impact of psychological abuse by an intimate partner on the mental health of pregnant women. *BJOG.* 2008;115(3):377.

61. Espinosa L, Osborne K. Domestic violence during pregnancy: implications for practice. *J Midwifery Womens Health.* 2002;47(5):305-317.

62. Lau Y, Chan KS. Influence of intimate partner violence during pregnancy and early postpartum depressive symptoms on breastfeeding among Chinese women in Hong Kong. *J Midwifery Womens Health.* 2007;52(2):e15-e20.

63. Silverman JG, Decker MR, Reed E, Raj A. Intimate partner violence around the time of pregnancy: association with breastfeeding behavior. *J Womens Health (Larchmt).* 2006;15(8):934-940.

64. Kendall-Tackett KA. A new paradigm for postpartum depression: the role of inflammation, stress, fatigue, pain and trauma. *Int Breastfeed J.* 2007;(2)6. doi: 10.1186/1746-4358-2-6.

65. Perry BD. The neurodevelopmental impact of violence in childhood. In: Schetky D, Benedek E, eds. *Textbook of Child and Adolescent Forensic Psychiatry*. Washington, DC: American Psychiatric Press, Inc; 2001:221-238.

66. Blaufarb H, Levine J. Crisis intervention in earthquake. *Soc Work.* 1972;17:16.

67. Gordon R, Wraith R. Responses of children and adolescents to disaster. In: JP Wilson, B Raphael, eds. *International Handbook of Traumatic Stress Syndromes*. New York, NY: Plenum; 1993:561-575.

68. Prinstein MJ, La Greca AM, Vernberg EM, Silverman WK. Children's coping assistance: how parents, teachers, and friends help children cope after a natural disaster. *J Clin Child Psychol.* 1996;25:463-464.

69. Terr L. *Unchained Memories: True Stories of Traumatic Memories, Lost and Found.* New York, NY: Basic Books; 1994.

70. Vogel J, Vernberg EM. Children's psychological response to disaster. *J Clin Child Psychol.* 1993;22:470-484.

71. Grych JH, Jouriles EN, Swank PR. Patterns of adjustment among children of battered women. *J Consult Clin Psychol.* 2000;68(1):84-94.

72. McFarlane JM, Gross JY, O'Brien JA, Watson K. Behaviors of children who are exposed and not exposed to intimate partner violence: an analysis of 330 black, white and Hispanic children. *Pediatrics.* 2003;112(3):202-207.

73. Graham-Bermann SA. Evaluating interventions for children exposed to family violence. *J Aggress Maltreat Trauma.* 2000;4(1):191-216.

74. Hughes HM, Luke DA. Heterogeneity in adjustment among children of battered women. In: Holden GW, Geffner R, Jouriles EN, eds. *Children Exposed to Marital Violence.* Washington, DC: American Psychological Association; 1998:185-221.

75. Sullivan CM, Juras J, Bybee D, Nguyen H, Allen N. How children's adjustment is affected by their relationships to their mothers' abusers. *J Interpers Violence.* 2000;15(6):587-602.

76. Farruggia SP, Greenberger E, Chen C, Heckhausen J. Perceived social environment and adolescents' well-being and adjustment: comparing a foster care sample with a matched sample. *J Youth Adolesc.* 2006;35(3):349-358.

77. Dawson G, Hessl D, Frey K. Social influences on early developing biological and behavioral systems related to risk for affective disorder. *Dev Psychopathol.* 1994;6:759-779.

78. Todd RD, Botteron KN. Is attention deficit hyperactivity disorder an energy deficiency syndrome? *Biol Psychiatry.* 2001;50(3):151-158.

79. Goodman SH, Gotlib IH. Risk for psychopathology in the children of depressed mothers: a developmental model for understanding mechanisms of transmission. *Psychol Rev.* 1999;106(3):458-490.

80. Jarvis KL, Novaco RW. Postshelter adjustment of children from violent families. *J Interpers Violence.* 2006;21(8):1046-1062.

81. Morrel TM, Dubowitz H, Kerr MA, Black MM. The effect of maternal victimization on children: a cross-informant study. *J Fam Violence.* 2003;18(1):29-41.

82. Levendosky AA, Graham-Bermann SA. Parenting in battered women: a trauma theory approach. *J Aggress Maltreat Trauma.* 2001;3(1):25-36.

83. Jones DJ, Forehand R, Neary EM. Family transmission of depressive symptoms: replication across Caucasian and African American mother-child dyads. *Behav Ther.* 2001;32(1):123-138.

84. Kalil A, Tolman RM, Rosen D, Gruber G. Domestic violence and children's behavior in low-income families. *Journal of Emotional Abuse*. 2003;3:75-102.

85. Boney-McCoy S, Finkelhor D. Is youth victimization related to trauma symptoms and depression after controlling for prior symptoms and family relationships? a longitudinal, prospective study. *J Consult Clin Psychol.* 1996;64(6):1406-1416.

86. Rice F, Harold GT, Shelton KH, Thapar A. Family conflict interacts with genetic liability in predicting childhood and adolescent depression. *J Am Acad Child Adolesc Psychiatry*. 2006;45(7):841-848.

87. Katz LF, Low SM. Marital violence, co-parenting, and family-level processes in relation to children's adjustment. *J Fam Psychol.* 2004;18(2):372-382.

88. Holden GW, Stein JD, Ritchie KL, Harris SD, Jouriles EN. Parenting behaviors and beliefs of battered women. In: Holden GW, Geffner R, Jouriles EN, eds. *Children Exposed to Marital Violence: Theory, Research, and Practice.* Washington, DC: American Psychological Association; 1998:289-336.

89. Levendosky AA, Lynch S, Graham-Bermann SA. Maternal perceptions of the impact of violence on their parenting strategies. *Violence Against Women*. 2000;6:247-271.

90. Peled E, Edleson JL. Process and outcome in small groups for children of battered women. In: Peled E, Jaffe PG, Edleson JL, eds. *Ending the Cycle of Violence: Community Responses to Children of Battered Women.* Newbury Park, CA: Sage; 1995.

91. Holden G, Ritchie K. Linking extreme marital discord, child rearing and child behaviour problems: evidence from battered women. *Child Dev.* 1991;62(2):311-327.

92. Fox GL, Benson ML. Violent men, bad dads? fathering profiles of men involved in intimate partner violence. In: Lamb ME, Day RD, eds. *Conceptualizing and Measuring Father Involvement.* Mahwah, NJ: Lawrence Erlbaum Associates; 2004:359-384.

93. Sternberg KJ, Lamb ME, Greenbaum C, Dawud S, Cortes RM, Lorey F. The effects of domestic violence on children's perceptions of their perpetrating and nonperpetrating parents. *Int J Behav Dev.* 1994;17:779-795.

94. Margolin G, John RS, Ghosh CM, Gordis EB. Family interaction process: an essential tool for exploring abusive relations. In: Cahn DD, Lloyd SA, eds. *Family Abuse: A Communication Perspective.* Newbury Park, CA: Sage; 1996:37-58.

95. Margolin G, John RS. Children's exposure to marital aggression: direct and mediated effects. In: Kaufman Kantor G, Jasinski J, eds. *Out of the Darkness: Contemporary Research Perspectives on Family Violence.* Thousand Oaks, CA: Sage; 1997:90-104.

96. Hardesty JL. Separation assault in the context of postdivorce parenting: an integrative review of the literature. *Violence Against Women.* 2002;8(5):593-621.

97. Jaffe P, Lemon N, Poisson S. *Child Custody and Domestic Violence: A Call for Safety and Accountability.* London, England: Sage Publications; 2002.

98. Fleury RE, Sullivan CM, Bybee DI. When ending the relationship doesn't end the violence: women's experiences of violence by former partners. *Violence Against Women.* 2000;6(12):1363-1383.

99. Liss MB, Stahly GB. Domestic violence and child custody. In: Hansen M, Harway M, eds. *Battering and Family Therapy: A Feminist Perspective.* Thousand Oaks, CA: Sage; 1993.
100. Sheeran M, Hampton S. Supervised visitation in cases of domestic violence. *Juvenile and Family Court Journal.* 1999;50(2):13-26.
101. Leighton B. *Spousal Abuse in Metropolitan Toronto: Research Report on the Response of the Criminal Justice System.* Ottawa, Ontario: Solicitor General of Canada; 1989.
102. Saunders D, Sullivan C, Tolman RM, Grabarek M. Domestic abuse survivors perceptions of safety and reports of abuse in the context of supervised visits and exchanges. Paper presented at: Society for Social Work Research; January 11-14, 2007; San Francisco, CA.
103. Perel G, Peled E. The fathering of violent men: constriction and yearning. *Violence Against Women.* 2008;14(4):457-482.
104. Fox GL, Sayers J, Bruce C. Beyond bravado: redemption and rehabilitation in the fathering accounts of men who batter. *Marriage Fam Rev.* 2001;32(3/4):137-163.
105. Dube SR, Anda RF, Felitti VJ, Edwards VJ, Williamson DF. Exposure to abuse, neglect, and household dysfunction among adults who witnessed intimate partner violence as children. *Violence Vict.* 2002;17(1):3-17.
106. Carlson BE. Outcomes of physical abuse and observation of marital violence among adolescents in placement. *J Interpers Violence.* 1991;6:526-534.
107. Hughes HM. Psychological and behavioral correlates of family violence in child witness and victims. *Am J Orthopsychiatry.* 1988;58:77-90.
108. O'Keefe M. Linking marital violence, mother-child/father-child aggression, and child behavior problems. *J Fam Violence.* 1994;9:63-78.
109. Spaccarelli S, Sandler IN, Roosa M. History of spouse violence against mother: correlated risks and unique effects in child mental health. *J Fam Violence.* 1994;9:79-98.
110. Stagg V, Wills GD, Howell M. Psychopathology in early childhood witnesses of family violence. *Topics Early Child Spec Educ.* 1989;9:73-87.
111. Wolfe DA, Zak L, Wilson S, Jaffe P. Child witnesses to violence between parents: critical issues in behavioral and social adjustment. *J Abnorm Child Psychol.* 1986;14:95-104.
112. Chamberlain L. *A Prevention Primer for Domestic Violence: Terminology, Tools, and the Public Health Approach.* Harrisburg, PA: VAWnet; 2008.
113. Bornstein MH, ed. *Children and Parenting.* 2nd ed. Mahwah, NJ: Lawrence Erlbaum Associates; 2002.
114. Bornstein MH, ed. *Biology and Ecology of Parenting.* 2nd ed. Mahwah, NJ: Lawrence Erlbaum Associates; 2002. *Handbook of Parenting*; vol 2.
115. Bornstein MH, ed. *Status and Social Conditions of Parenting.* 2nd ed. Mahwah, NJ: Lawrence Erlbaum Associates; 2002. *Handbook of Parenting*; vol 3.

116. Bornstein MH, ed. *Applied Parenting*. 2nd ed. Mahwah, NJ: Lawrence Erlbaum Associates; 2002. *Handbook of Parenting*; vol 4.

117. Bornstein MH, ed. *Practical Parenting*. 2nd ed. Mahwah, NJ: Lawrence Erlbaum Associates; 2002. *Handbook of Parenting*; vol 5.

118. Maccoby EE, Martin JA. Socialization in the context of the family: parent-child interaction. In: Mussen PH, Hetherington EM, eds. *Socialization, Personality, and Social Development*. 4th ed. New York, NY: Wiley; 1983:1-101. *Handbook of Child Psychology*; vol 4.

119. Brooks-Gunn J, Berlin L, Fuligni AS. Early childhood intervention programs: what about the family? In: Shonkoff JP, Meisel SJ, eds. *Handbook of Early Childhood Intervention*. 2nd ed. New York, NY: Cambridge University Press; 2000.

120. Brooks-Gunn J, Fuligni AS, Berlin LJ, eds. *Early Child Development in the 21st Century: Profiles of Current Research Initiatives*. New York, NY: Teachers College Press; 2003.

121. Brooks-Gunn J. Intervention and policy as change agents for young children. In: Chase-Lansdale PL, Kiernan K, Friedman RJ, eds. *Human Development Across Lives and Generations: The Potential for Change*. New York, NY: Cambridge University; 2004:293-340.

122. Bakermans-Kranenburg MJ, van IJzendoorn MH, Juffer F. Less is more: meta-analyses of sensitivity and attachment interventions in early childhood. *Psychol Bull.* 2003;129(2):195-215.

123. Barnett WS. Long-term effects of early childhood programs on cognitive and school outcomes. *The Future of Children*. 1995;5(3):25-50.

124. Currie J. Early Childhood education programs. *J Econ Perspec.* 2001;15(2):213.

125. Cunningham CE, Bremner R, Boyle M. Large group community-based parenting programs for families of preschoolers at risk for disruptive behaviour disorders: utilization, cost effectiveness, and outcome. *J Child Psychol Psychiatry.* 1995;36(7):1141-1159.

126. Magnuson K, Waldfogel J. Pre-school enrollment and parents' use of physical discipline. *Infant Child Dev.* 2005;14(2):177-198.

127. Tucker S, Gross D, Fogg L, Delaney K, Lapporte R. The long-term efficacy of a behavioral parent training intervention for families with 2-year-olds. *Res Nurs Health.* 1998;21(3):199-210.

128. Brooks-Gunn J, Markman L. The contribution of parenting to ethnic and racial gaps in school readiness. *Future Child.* 2005;15(1):139-168.

129. Kamerman SB. Early childhood education and care (ECEC): an overview of developments in OECD countries. *Int J Educ.* 2000;33:7-29.

130. Jaffe P, Sudermann M, Reitzel D, Killip SM. An evaluation of a secondary school primary prevention program on violence in relationships. *Violence Vict.* 1992;7:129-146.

131. Weisz A, Black B. Sexual assault and dating violence prevention with urban youth: assessing effectiveness. *Soc Work Res.* 2001;25(2):89-102.

132. Lavoie F, Hebert M, Tremblay R, Vitaro F, Vezina L, McDuff P. History of family dysfunction ad perpetration of dating violence by adolescent boys: a longitudinal study. *J Adolesc Health.* 2002;30(5):365-383.

133. Capaldi DM, Owen LD. Physical aggression in a community sample of at-risk young couples: gender comparisons for high frequency, injury, and fear. *J Fam Psychol.* 2001;15(3):425-440.

134. Magdol L, Moffitt TE, Caspi A, Silva PA. Developmental antecedents of partner abuse: a prospective-longitudinal study. *J Abnorm Psychol.* 1998;107:375-389.

135. Brendgen M, Vitaro R, Tremblay RE, Lavoie F. Reactive and proactive aggression: predictions to physical violence in different contexts and moderating effects of parental monitoring and caregiving behavior. *J Abnorm Child Psychol.* 2001;29(4):293-304.

136. Markman HJ, Renick MJ, Floyd FJ, Stanley SM, Clements M. Preventing marital distress through communication and conflict management training: a four and five year follow-up. *J Consult Clin Psychol.* 1993;62(1):70-77.

137. Bowen LK, Gwiasda V, Brown M. Engaging community residents to prevent violence. *J Interpers Violence.* 2004;19(3):356-367.

138. Graffunder CM, Noonan RK, Cox P, Wheaton J. Through a public health lens. preventing violence against women: an update from the US Centers for Disease Control and Prevention. J Womens Health. 2004;13(1):5-14.

139. Mitchell-Clark K, Autry A. *Preventing Family Violence: Lessons from the Community Engagement Initiative.* San Francisco, CA: Family Violence Prevention Fund; 2004.

140. Victorian Health Foundation. Violence against women: funded projects. http://www.vichealth.vic.gov.au/~/media/ProgramsandProjects/MentalHealthandWellBeing/DiscriminationandViolence/Attachments/VAW_FundedProjectsevidence_3.ashx. Accessed December 9, 2009.

141. Family Violence Prevention Fund. Ameriquest and leading violence prevention group to encourage economic independence for young mothers. http://endabuse.org/content/press_room/detail/504/. Accessed December 9, 2009.

142. Olds D, Hill P, Mihalic S, O'Brien R. *Blueprints for Violence Prevention, Book Seven: Prenatal and Infancy Home Visitation by Nurses.* Boulder, CO: Center for the Study and Prevention of Violence; 1998.

143. Marsiglio W, Amato P, Day RD, Lamb ME. Scholarship on fatherhood in the 1990s and beyond. *J Marriage Fam.* 2000;62:1173-1191.

144. Pleck EH, Pleck JH. Fatherhood ideals in the United States: historical dimensions. In: Lamb ME, ed. *The Role of the Father in Child Development.* 3rd ed. New York, NY: Wiley; 1997:33-48.

145. Crooks CV, Goodall GR, Baker LB, Hughes R. Preventing violence against women: engaging the fathers of today and tomorrow. *Cog Behav Pract.* 2006;13:82-93.

146. Flood M. Men's collective struggles for gender justice: the case of anti-violence activism. In: Kimmel M, Hearn J, Connell RW, eds. *The Handbook of Studies on Men and Masculinities.* Thousand Oaks, CA: Sage; 2005:458-465.

147. Crooks CV, Goodall GR, Hughes R, Jaffe PG, Baker LL. Engaging men and boys in preventing violence against women: applying a cognitive-behavioral model. *Violence Against Women*. 2007;13(3):217-239.

148. Peter Hart Research Associates Poll. Founding Fathers poll, April 23-May 3, 2007. http://www.endabuse.org/content/news/detail/945. Accessed December 9, 2009

149. Crowell NA, Burgess AW. *Understanding Violence Against Women*. Washington, DC: National Academy Press; 1996.

150. Saunders DG, Hamberger LK, Hovey M. Indicators of woman abuse based on a chart review at a family practice center. *Arch Fam Med.* 1993;2(5):537-43.

151. Chrisler JC, Ferguson S. Violence against women as a public health issue. *Ann N Y Acad Sci*. 2006;1087:235-249.

152. McFarlane J, Soeken K, Wiist W. An evaluation of interventions to decrease intimate partner violence to pregnant women. *Public Health Nurs*. 2000;17(6):443-451.

153. McFarlane J, Groff JY, O'Brien JA, Watson K. Secondary prevention of intimate partner violence: a randomized controlled trial. *Nurs Res*. 2006;55:52-61.

154. Covington DL, Dalton VK, Diehl SJ, Brent DW, Piner HM. Improving detection of violence among pregnant adolescents. *J Adolescent Health*. 1997;21:18-24.

155. McLeer S, Anwar R. Identification of abuse in emergency departments. *Am J Public Health*. 1989;79:65-66.

156. McFarlane J, Parker B, Soeken K, Bullock L. Assessing for abuse during pregnancy. *JAMA*. 1992;267:3176-78.

157. McFarlane J, Parker B. Preventing abuse during pregnancy: an assessment and intervention protocol. *Am J Matern Child Nursing*. 1994;19:321-322.

158. Macy RJ, Martin SL, Kupper LL, Casanueva C, Guo S. Partner violence among women before, during, and after pregnancy: multiple opportunities for intervention. *Womens Health Issues*. 2007;17(5):290.

159. Harrykissoon SD, Rickert VI, Wiemann CM. Prevalence and patterns of intimate partner violence among adolescent mothers during the postpartum period. *Arch Pediatr Adolesc Med*. 2002;156(4):325-330.

160. National Association of County & City Health Officials (NACCHO). Issue brief: intimate partner violence among pregnant and parenting women. local health department strategies for assessment, intervention, and prevention. http://www.naccho.org/topics/HPDP/mch/upload/IPV-Issue-Brief-6-11-08.pdf. Accessed December 9, 2009

161. Olds D, Kitzman H, Cole R, et al. Effects of nurse home visiting on maternal life course and child development: age 6 follow-up results of a randomized trial. *Pediatrics*. 2004;114(6):1550-1559.

162. Center for Urban Families. Baltimore Responsible Father Project. http://www.cfuf.org/BRFP. Published 2009. Accessed December 9, 2009.

163. Carillo R, Tello J. Fathers in recovery. In: Edleson JL, Williams OJ, eds. *Parenting by Men Who Batter: New Directions for Assessment and Intervention*. New York, NY: Oxford University Press; 2007:131-136.

164. National Latino Fatherhood and Family Institute. Fatherhood lessons. http://www.nlffi.org. Published 2003. Accessed December 9, 2009.

165. Chalk R, King PA, eds. *Violence in Families: Assessing Prevention and Treatment Programs*. Washington DC: National Academy Press; 1998.

166. Delsol C, Margolin G. The role of family-of-origin violence in men's marital violence perpetration. *Clin Psychol Rev*. 2004;24:99-122.

167. Holtzworth-Munroe A, Bates L, Smutzler N, Sandin E. A brief review of the research on husband violence. part I: Maritally violent versus nonviolent men. *Aggress Violent Behav*. 1997;2:65-99.

168. Whitfield CL, Anda RF, Dube SR, Felitti VJ. Violent childhood experiences and the risk of intimate partner violence in adults: assessment in a large health maintenance organization. *J Interpers Violence*. 2003;18:166-185.

169. Illinois Coalition Against Domestic Violence. *Annual Report—FY 1995*. Springfield, IL: Illinois Coalition Against Domestic Violence; 1996.

170. New Jersey Coalition for Battered Women. *Annual Report—1991*. Trenton, NJ: New Jersey Coalition for Battered Women; 1992.

171. Groves BM. Mental health services for children who witness domestic violence. *Future Child*. 1999;9:122-132.

172. Silvern L, Karyl J, Landis TY. Individual psychotherapy for the traumatized children of abused women. In: Peled E, Jaffe PG, Edleson JL, eds. *Ending the Cycle of Violence: Community Responses to Children of Battered Women*. Thousand Oaks, CA: Sage; 1995:43-76.

173. Van Horn P, Best S, Lieberman AF. Breaking the chain: preventing the transmission of trauma in children of battered women through parent child psychotherapy. Paper presented at: 14th Annual Meeting of the International Society for Traumatic Stress Studies; November 21, 1998; Washington, DC.

174. Sudermann M, Marshall L, Loosely S. Evaluation of the London (Ontario) community group treatment programme for children who have witnessed woman abuse. In: Geffner RA, Jaffe PG, Sudermann M, eds. *Children Exposed to Domestic Violence*. New York, NY: Haworth; 2000:127-160.

175. Peled E, Davis D. *Groupwork With Children of Battered Women*. Thousand Oaks, CA: Sage; 1995.

176. Lieberman AF, Van Horn P, Ghosh Ippen C. Toward evidence-based treatment: child-parent psychotherapy with preschoolers exposed to marital violence. *J Am Acad Child Adolesc Psychiatry*. 2005;44(12):1241-1248.

177. Lieberman AF, Van Horn P, Ghosh Ippen C. Child-parent psychotherapy: six-month follow-up of a randomized control trial. *J Am Acad Child Adolesc Psychiatry*. 2006;45(8):913-918.

178. Graham-Bermann SA. *The Kids' Club: A Preventive Intervention Program for Children of Battered Women*. Ann Arbor, MI: University of Michigan; 1992.

179. Graham-Bermann SA, Lynch S, Banyard V, Devoe E, Halabu H. Community-based intervention for children exposed to intimate partner violence: an efficacy trial. *J Consult Clin Psychol*. 2007;72(2):199-209.

180. Groves B, Gewirtz A. Interventions and promising approaches for children exposed to domestic violence. In: Feerick M, Silverman G, eds. *Children Exposed to Domestic Violence*. Baltimore, MD: Brookes Publishing; 2006.

181. Groves BM, Zuckerman B. Interventions with parents and caregivers of children who are exposed to violence. In: Osofsky JD, ed. *Children in A Violent Society*. New York, NY: Guilford; 1997:183-201.

182. Cohen JA, Mannarino AP, Staron VR. A pilot study of modified cognitive-behavioral therapy for childhood traumatic grief (CBT-CTG). *J Am Acad Child Adolesc Psychiatry*. 2006;45(12):1465-1473.

183. Sullivan CM, Bybee DI, Allen NE. Findings from a community-based program for battered women and their children. *J Interpers Violence*. 2002;17(9):915-936

184. McDonald R, Jouriles EN, Skopp NA. Reducing conduct problems among children brought to women's shelters: intervention effects 24 months following termination of services. *J Fam Psychol*. 2006;20(1):127-136.

185. Scott K, Francis K, Crooks C, Kelly T. Caring Dads: *Helping Fathers Value Their Children*. Victoria, British Columbia: Trafford Victoria; 2006.

186. Scott KL, Crooks CV. Preliminary evaluation of an intervention program for maltreating fathers. *Brief Treatment and Crisis Intervention*. 2007;7:224-238.

187. Abidin RR. *Parenting Stress Index*. 3rd ed. Odessa, FL: Psychological Assessment Resources, Inc; 1995.

188. Arean JD, Davis L. Working with fathers in batterer intervention programs: lessons from the Fathering After Violence project. In: Edleson JL, Williams OJ, eds. *Parenting by Men Who Batter: New Directions for Assessment and Intervention*. New York, NY: Oxford University Press; 2007:118-130.

189. Fleck-Henderson A. Application of theoretical frameworks for domestic violence. In: Danis F, Lockhart L, eds. *Breaking the Silence in Social Work Education: Domestic Violence Modules for Foundation Courses*. Washington, DC: Council on Social work Education; 2004.

190. Jaffe PG, Crooks CV. Visitation and child custody issues in the case of domestic violence. In: Williams O, Edleson J, eds. *Parenting by Men Who Batter*. London, England: Oxford University Press; 2006:45-64.

191. Edleson JL, Williams OJ. *Introduction: Involving Men Who Batter in Their Children's Lives*. New York, NY: Oxford University Press; 2007.

Chapter 18

Prevention of Psychological Maltreatment

Marla R. Brassard, PhD
Lisa R. Melmed, PhD

Introduction

In a seminal article written in 2004, Guterman[1] articulated emerging strategies and issues in advancing prevention research on child abuse, youth violence, and domestic violence. Defining prevention as "the averting of violent events before they occur," he identified 3 particularly important domains that pose critical challenges for researchers if they are to gather valid, rigorous, and useful information to move prevention knowledge forward. These challenges include:

1. Addressing measurement and conceptual issues in defining violence so that there is a way to assess the effectiveness of prevention efforts
2. Designing research studies that advance the capacity to assess risk of violence and to predict future violence
3. Applying research so that it drives the development of intervention practices to prevent violence

These challenges, or goals, are consistent with a public health model and are similar to the objectives of the National Center for Injury Prevention and Control (NCIPC) at the Center for Disease Control and Prevention (CDC).[2]

This chapter will use the Guterman framework to address these challenges in the area of psychological maltreatment (PM), also known as emotional abuse and neglect. The status of definitions/conceptual frameworks and surveillance tools will be reviewed in regard to efficiency in identifying PM in the general population as well as high-risk groups so that researchers can:

— Evaluate the effectiveness of prevention efforts

— Review select prevention programs that have shown to be effective in enhancing interpersonal relationships and reducing violence to assess how well they target PM or could be modified to do so

— Recommend next steps to move prevention research forward in the area of PM

While the primary focus of the chapter is on PM by parents and other caregivers in the home, psychological abuse by peers in the form of bullying and dating violence, and by other adults such as teachers, is also addressed in the review of surveillance tools and prevention programs.

Defining Psychological Maltreatment

Guterman[1] argues that definitional issues have been a struggle regarding practices, policy, and research aimed at preventing child abuse, youth violence, and domestic violence because attention is focused most often on "the most egregious forms of interpersonal violence," contributing to a common misperception that violence is a "you-know-it-when-you-see-it" phenomena.[1] However, from a prevention standpoint, more inclusive definitions of violence are useful for establishing and predicting levels of risk and directing prevention efforts. He also notes that while there is a great deal of consensus around what is an extremely violent act, there is less consensus around "less extreme and more commonly occurring behaviors, particularly given differing definitions and meaning of 'violence' among individuals involved, across cultures, historical epochs, and service systems."[1] Guterman argues that advancing violence prevention practices and policies makes the development of consensus around scientifically valid and practically useful definitions particularly consequential. Consensus involves a negotiated settlement between science and professional expertise on the one hand, and community values and culture on the other hand. Considerable progress in this regard has been made in the last 30 years for all forms of maltreatment, including PM.[3-6]

In the 1980s, lack of definitions was the major impediment to progress in understanding psychological maltreatment. The 1983 International Conference on Psychological Abuse, held to integrate and facilitate research in this area, led to considerable work on refining and elaborating the subtypes of PM.[7-11] Operational definitions of PM were also developed by Baily and Baily, McGee and Wolfe, Glaser, and Barnett et al in their Maltreatment Classification System for coding child protective service records.[12-15] This research culminated in the 1995 Guidelines for Psychosocial Evaluation of Suspected Psychological Maltreatment of Children and Adolescents,[16] published by the American Professional Society on Abuse of Children, which were based on the Hart and Brassard definition of PM with input from most PM researchers.[17] The guidelines begin with a broad definition: "'Psychological maltreatment' means a repeated pattern of caregiver behavior or extreme incident(s) that convey to children that they are worthless, flawed, unloved, unwanted, endangered, or only of value in meeting another's needs."[16] The Guidelines then define 6 subtypes of PM:

1. Spurning
2. Terrorizing
3. Isolating
4. Exploiting/corrupting
5. Denying emotional responsiveness
6. Mental health, medical, and educational neglect

(**Table 18-1** contains the detailed definitions of the 6 subtypes of PM.)

Table 18-1. Psychological Maltreatment Forms
A repeated pattern or extreme incident(s) of the conditions described in this list constitute PM. Such conditions convey the message that the child is worthless, flawed, unloved, endangered, or only valuable in meeting someone else's needs. ***Spurning (hostile rejecting/degrading)*** includes verbal and nonverbal caregiver acts that reject and degrade a child. Spurning includes: — Belittling, degrading, and other nonphysical forms of overtly hostile or rejecting treatment — Shaming and/or ridiculing the child for showing normal emotions such as affection, grief, or sorrow — Consistently singling out 1 child to criticize and punish, to perform most of the household chores, or to receive fewer rewards — Public humiliation *(continued)*

Table 18-1. Psychological Maltreatment Forms *(continued)*

Exploiting/corrupting includes caregiver acts that encourage the child to develop inappropriate behaviors (eg, self-destructive, antisocial, criminal, deviant, or other maladaptive behaviors). Exploiting/corrupting includes:

— Modeling, permitting, or encouraging antisocial behavior (eg, prostitution, performance in pornographic media, initiation of criminal activities, substance abuse, violence to or corruption of others)

— Modeling, permitting, or encouraging developmentally inappropriate behavior (eg, parentification, infantilization, living the parent's unfulfilled dreams)

— Encouraging or coercing abandonment of developmentally appropriate autonomy through extreme overinvolvement, intrusiveness, and/or dominance (eg, allowing little or no opportunity or support for child's views, feelings, and wishes; micromanaging child's life)

— Restricting or interfering with cognitive development

Terrorizing includes caregiver behavior that threatens or is likely to physically hurt, kill, abandon, or place the child or child's loved ones/objects in recognizably dangerous situations. Terrorizing includes:

— Placing a child in unpredictable or chaotic circumstances

— Placing a child in recognizably dangerous situations

— Setting rigid or unrealistic expectations with threat of loss, harm, or danger if they are not met

— Threatening or perpetrating violence against the child

— Threatening or perpetrating violence against a child's loved ones or objects

Denying emotional responsiveness (ie, ignoring) includes caregiver acts that ignore the child's attempts and needs to interact (eg, failing to express affection, caring, and love for the child) and showing no emotion in interactions with the child. Denying emotional responsiveness includes:

— Being detached and uninvolved through either incapacity or lack of motivation

— Interacting only when absolutely necessary

— Failing to express affection, caring, and love for the child

Isolating includes caregiver acts that consistently deny the child opportunities to meet needs for interacting/communicating with peers or adults inside or outside the home. Isolating includes:

— Confining the child or placing unreasonable limitations on the child's freedom of movement within his or her environment

— Placing unreasonable limitations or restrictions on social interactions with peers or adults in the community

Mental health, medical, and educational neglect includes unwarranted caregiver acts that ignore, refuse to allow, or fail to provide the necessary treatment for the mental health, medical, and educational problems or needs for the child. Mental health, medical, and educational neglect includes:

— Ignoring the need for, failing, or refusing to allow or provide treatment for serious emotional/behavioral problems or needs of the child

— Ignoring the need for, failing, or refusing to allow or provide treatment for serious physical health problems or needs of the child

— Ignoring the need for, failing, or refusing or allow or provide treatment for services for serious educational problems or needs of the child

Adapted from Hart SN, Brassard MR.[17]

Readers might wonder why this specific list. Why is rejection not listed as a category, especially given the large research literature that uses this term?[18] Why are exploiting and corrupting merged into 1 category? In the mid-1980s, Hart and Brassard engaged in a series of multidimensional scaling studies using social workers, school psychology graduate students, teachers, and psychologists.[19] These individuals were asked to sequentially sort descriptions of constructive parenting and 6 subtypes of PM (rejection, exploiting, corrupting, isolating, terrorizing, denying emotional responsiveness) into (a) categories they generated, (b) the 6 Hart and Brassard categories and constructive parenting, and (c) the 16 categories of PM developed by Baily and Baily.[12,17] They found that rejecting descriptions were reliably separated by sorters into either a hostile rejecting of the child category or the emotionally unavailable category. This separation surprised them, but was consistent with the cross-cultural findings of Rohner and Rohner.[18] As a result, the category of rejecting was dropped and spurning was selected from a thesaurus as the best descriptor of the behaviors included in the hostile rejection category. The rejecting items that were not actively hostile sorted into the denying emotional responsiveness category. They also found that descriptions of exploiting and corrupting parental behavior could not be discriminated by sorters, no matter how the items were modified. They concluded that it was impossible to exploit without corrupting or corrupt without exploiting, and so they settled on a merged category for the 2 concepts. With the refinement of categories into the first 5 listed in **Table 18-1** (the 6th category was added later), sorters had no difficulty reliably classifying items. (See Brassard and Donovan for a comprehensive review of major definitional systems of PM, their congruence and discrepancies, and the empirical support for each category at each developmental period.)[20]

The APSAC definitions of PM are consistent with other definitional systems (eg, National Incidence Study,[4,21] Brassard and Donovan[20]) can be used to reliably code child protection records, are based on research that documents the damage caused by this form of maltreatment, are cross-culturally valid, and are consistent with definitions used by governments and other professional organizations (eg, Singapore, American Academy of Pediatrics, American Humane Association).[18,20-29]

Research on PM has utilized a combination of clinical, community, and community/clinical samples. The majority of the studies have used correlational designs but there is a sizable subgroup of longitudinal studies. Causal inferences are therefore based on replication of findings across studies and over time, the ruling out of competing hypotheses, and, increasingly, experimental studies with animals.

PM victimization has been empirically tied to 5 general problem categories.[23,25] These include:

1. Problems of intrapersonal thoughts, feelings, and behaviors, such as low self-esteem, anxiety, depression, and negative cognitive styles that increase vulnerability to depression and suicidal thoughts and behaviors (eg, negative life views, self-criticism, immature defenses)[18,30-53]

2. Emotional symptoms, such as substance abuse and eating disorders, emotional and borderline instability, impulse control problems, unresponsiveness, and more impaired functioning among individuals diagnosed with bipolar disorder[18,29,35,54-64]

3. Social competency problems and antisocial functioning, such as impaired social competency, social phobia, low empathy, attachment insecurity/disorganization, self-isolating behavior, non-compliance, dependency, sexual maladjustment, aggression and violent behavior, and delinquency or criminality[18,28,30,33,35-37,41-43,48,58,60,63,65-80]

4. Learning problems, such as impaired learning, academic problems and lower achievement test results, decline in IQ over time, lower measured intelligence, noncompliance and lack of impulse control at school, and impaired development of moral reasoning[18,20,33,35,37,48,68,75,76,81-88]

5. Physical health problems, such as high infant mortality rates, delays in almost all areas of physical and behavioral development; allergies, asthma, and other respiratory ailments; deviant adrenocortical responding and amygdala reactivity; white matter tract abnormalities, hypertension, and somatic complaints[58,89-104]

These outcomes are found across community and clinical samples around the world, suggesting that the harmful correlates or effects of PM are widespread among those who experience it and not limited to certain subgroups.

There is a high degree of agreement among researchers, government agencies, and the public about what PM is and the strong evidence that it is harmful for children, which makes PM an ideal target for prevention efforts. PM is a very common parenting practice; however, there is not a clear consensus on the degree of severity or how many instances of psychologically aggressive or neglectful behaviors are required to constitute PM and be counted in governmental surveillance efforts. For example, a telephone survey conducted by Straus and Field revealed that 90% of American parents reported using more than 1 form of psychological aggression by the time the child was 2 years of age, and by age 5, 98% reported using more than 1 form of verbal aggression.[105] The *National Incidence Study of Child Abuse and Neglect (NIS-4)*—a survey of 10 791 professionals from 1094 agencies (eg, schools, hospitals, shelters, police) and 126 Child Protective Services (CPS) agencies in 2005 and 2006—collected data on children that these professionals encountered who had either experienced maltreatment that has caused harm (The Harm Standard) or maltreatment that had not yet caused harm (The Endangerment Standard).[21] Emotional abuse was found to occur in 337 500 children (0.5% of the US child population) according to the Harm Standard, and 1 044 000 children (1.4% of the US child population) according to the Endangerment Standard. Emotional neglect was found to occur in 312 500 children (0.4% of the US child population) according to the Harm Standard, and 1 508 000 children (2% of the US child population) according to the Endangerment Standard.

Measuring the percent of CPS reports from 49 states that were screened-in for investigation that included PM, the *Child Maltreatment Annual Report by the National Child Abuse and Neglect Data System (NCANDS)*[106] identified 52 532 incidents of PM per year, which is 7.6% of the total number of abused or neglected children investigated by CPS. However, PM is likely to be considerably underrepresented in CPS calls due to lack of physical evidence, difficulty for untrained observers to distinguish between PM and poor parenting, and great variability in state laws. Additionally, a number of studies have collected data regarding the prevalence of childhood histories of 1 or more dimensions of PM by retrospectively surveying adults about their childhood experiences.[40,107-109] Binggeli, Hart, and Brassard reviewed this literature and estimated that PM may have been a significant presence in the childhood histories of over one-third of the general adult population of the United States.[23] Internationally, psychologically aggressive/abusive parenting practices are extremely common, as well.[29,110] Zolotor et al, utilizing a surveillance survey for children ages 11 to 19 that live with their parents, found that psychological abuse (parental and older sibling) was reported by 64% of children surveyed in Colombia, 72% in India, 81% in Russia, and 48% in Iceland.[111] Clearly, psychological maltreatment is widespread.

The APSAC definition includes 6 overarching forms of psychological maltreatment, each with 3 or more subtypes and 21 subtypes in total (see **Table 18-1**). Even the best parent exhibits some of these behaviors on occasion. What constitutes maltreatment is the pervasiveness of these forms of parenting, not their presence/absence on a single occasion, unless the behavior is extreme. Psychological maltreatment is recognizable when observed, harmful even at low levels when experienced over time, and a precursor to physical violence, making it an ideal target for prevention.[112,113]

Surveillance of Psychological Maltreatment

Guterman[1] notes that the mounting of large-scale surveillance systems to aid in determining the degree to which prevention strategies are helpful and to monitor trends in violent behavior over time requires not only uniform operational definitions, but there also needs to be practical tools that can be widely and easily applied. While the issue of definition has been largely resolved, practical tools for assessing most forms of PM are available but have not been widely deployed. At this point in time there is no surveillance system in place that frequently and accurately assesses PM.

Brassard and Donovan[20] reviewed existing measures of parental PM of children and adolescents broken down by format (eg, observational, questionnaire) and source (eg, collateral report, youth self-report) on the following characteristics: comprehensiveness in covering all subtypes of PM, ages covered, and psychometric properties of the measure. In line with other researchers, they concluded that multisource information was best. Other than record reviews, which have well-known limitations as a source of information, all other formats needed further development because of problems with comprehensiveness of content covered (questionnaires), appropriateness of items for all ages (questionnaires), and ease of use (observational forms). Other problematic measurement issues identified by Guterman[1] for all forms of violence include the tendency of victims to underreport their experiences. This may stem from cognitive minimization strategies or deliberate strategies to keep violent events secret in order to protect themselves, perceptive biases that are linked to memory recall and reporting of violent events, and the ability of perpetrators to distort the perception of victims so that they do not self define violent events as violent.

Cases Known to Mandated Reporters

The national incidence studies conducted by the United States (eg, the National Incidence Studies in 1980, 1988, 1996, 2010, Sedlak et al[21]) and other developed countries are expensive, technically sophisticated studies with nationally representative samples (in some countries) that include all cases known to mandated reporters.[114] They do not identify cases not known to professionals, such as those known or unrecognized within a family. They can provide periodic, accurate portraits of a nation regarding the incidences of child maltreatment, its perpetrators, its victims, and their context, but do not provide the timely information that policymakers, researchers, and interventionists need to assess the effectiveness of policies and targeted prevention and intervention efforts in reducing abuse and neglect.

Annual data collection systems based on reports to child protective services, like the US National Child Abuse and Neglect Data System (NCANDS), are of limited use for prevention unless standard reporting criteria are used.[115] The NCANDS is an aggregation of cases that have been officially reported within all 50 states. Since states define maltreatment in different ways (especially PM) and have different criteria for screening in and substantiating cases, results are not comparable from state to state.

Parent Reports

The model for obtaining parents' reports of psychologically aggressive/abusive behavior by parents toward children comes from the landmark studies in the United States by Straus and his colleagues using the Psychological Aggression Subscale from the Parent-Child Conflict Tactics Scale (CTSPC).[116] The CTSPC is the only nationally normed measure of psychological and physical aggression for spousal and parent to child conflict and has been used in over 300 empirical studies. The 5-item psychological aggression scale on the CTSPC asks the child how often each conflict resolution tactic (eg, "called me dumb or lazy or some other name like that") is used by each of his or her parents, and is then measured on a 7-point scale that assesses frequency of occurrence over an immediately previous time segment (eg, "in the past year"). The strengths of the CTSPC are that the instructions normalize parent-child conflict and the items are behavioral descriptions of parental behavior. Its weakness is its lack of comprehensiveness of PM subtypes, only covering spurning ("shouted, yelled, or screamed at him or her," "swore or cursed at him/her," "called him or her dumb or lazy or some other name like that") and terrorizing ("threatened to spank or hit him/her but did not actually do it," "said you would send him/her away or kick him/her out of the house"). Nonetheless, it has reasonable reliability and validity for a screening measure and thus has been widely used. It provided the model for a series of tools developed for international use that are described in the following section.

The Multiple Indicator Cluster Survey (MICS) is an internationally comparable household survey for countries to evaluate country level progress of children and women in low and middle income countries in different regions of the world,[117,118] contains 2 items of psychological aggression in its section on childrearing discipline and violence ("shouted, yelled at, or screamed at the child" and "called the child dumb, lazy, or another name like that"), as well as items on physical abuse (items are very similar to those on the Parent-Child Conflict Tactics Scale). In nationally representative surveys of 24 developing countries, name calling was 1 of only 2 out of 11 items (the other was hit with an object) that were correlated negatively with all 3 measures of a country's Human Development Index: life expectancy, economic well-being, and educational attainment.[119] The use of an internationally comparable survey that includes items of PM creates the possibility of regular (albeit narrow) surveillance on an international level.

Parent, Child, and Young Adult Reports

Recently, the International Society for the Prevention of Child Abuse and Neglect (ISPCAN) developed a set of 3 screening instruments to assess lifetime victimization as part of a United Nations effort to study violence against children worldwide. They are:

1. The 15-item ISPCAN Child Abuse Screening Tool Retrospective Version for young adults ages 18-26 (ICAST-R)[27]
2. The 40-item ICAST-P for parents with children in the home[29]
3. The 38-item (home) and 44-item (institution) ICAST-C for children ages 12-17 to assess all forms of victimization[111]

The measures were developed through focus group discussions with international experts, and then a Delphi study in 2 waves to determine the perceived importance and ease with which items can be translated into multiple languages. This was followed by field testing in 7 countries for the young adult version (Russia, Egypt, Columbia, India, Lebanon, Malaysia, and Kyrgyzstan) with convenience samples of 842 young adults, 4 countries for the adolescent version (Russia, Columbia, India, and Iceland) with convenience samples of 571 teens ages 12 to 17, and 7 countries for the parent version (Congo, Russia, Egypt, Columbia, India, Lebanon, Malaysia) with convenience samples of 697. The PM items chosen for each of the scales are similar to those on the CTS-PC in that they primarily assess spurning and terrorizing (eg, told [they] wish you were never born or were dead, threatened to be hurt or killed) although the parent version includes a isolating and a denying emotional responsiveness item (eg, locked in dark room, refused to speak). They have a reasonable degree of internal consistency for scales with 5 to 11 items: alphas of .63, .77, and .78, respectively. Respondents on the retrospective and child versions were allowed to choose a range of perpetrators (eg, mother, father, older sister, boy at school) for each item. Teachers were reported almost as often as parents for PM and peers were also mentioned frequently, including fellow students, boys in the neighborhood, and siblings, reinforcing the importance of targeting all forms of PM in prevention efforts. The brevity, ease of comprehension, lack of SES and cultural bias, universality of the behaviors listed, lack of missing data, and acceptability of the psychometric characteristics make these measures promising for gathering surveillance data in North America and internationally, especially if items representing all forms of PM were added to the tools.

Youth Report

While the ICAST-C would be the best existing surveillance tool to administer to youth internationally, doing so annually or biannually to a nationally representative sample would require an enormous, expensive, and long-term effort. A more promising approach might be adding items on PM to existing surveillance systems, such as the biannual Youth Risk Behavior Surveillance Survey (YRBSS) conducted by the US Center for Disease Control and Prevention (CDC) since 1991. Administered in schools to a nationally representative sample of public school students in grades 9 through 12, items cover risk behaviors that contribute to unintentional injury and violence in the form of dating violence that is sexual or physical, bullying on school property or electronically and includes psychological aggression, and being forced to have intercourse or being injured in a physical fight. However, the YRBSS is produced under great constraint in terms of the number and types of items that can be included, given the 45-minute single class period in which it is administered and the number of federal and state agencies involved in reviewing and selecting items. These constraints may be the reason that items on psychological violence by dating partners were omitted form the survey and why the CDC chose to focus on health risk behaviors rather than what they consider the determinants of those behaviors (eg, knowledge, attitudes, beliefs, and skills), which would be powerfully shaped by the family environment and the presence or absence of child maltreatment. Even if only 6 items representing the 6 subtypes of PM were to be included it would allow for biannual youth reports of their experiences of PM in parent-child and peer relationships and provide real-time information that can be more closely tied to specific prevention efforts nationally and in individual states.

Another youth report tool that shows promise in surveillance of PM is the Global Student Health Survey (GSHS) developed by the World Health Organization (WHO) and the CDC for ages 11 to 16 and older, but is primarily used with 13- to 15-year-olds. This school-based tool has been in use since 2003. It has a core and expanded questionnaire for protective factors; the expanded questionnaire covers many of the forms of PM. These including bullying by other students (eg, "how many days in the last month were you made fun of because of your race, religion, or color?") and parental disrespect of individuality and worth (eg, items covering spurning such as "ridicule or put you down"; denying emotional responsiveness, such as "ignore you, walk away from you, or not pay attention"; exploiting and corrupting such as "try to make you feel guilty"; "expect too much of you"). It also includes items on protective factors which are positive parental behaviors, the absence of which may constitute emotional neglect (eg, support and encourage you, show you affection, etc), and physical neglect (eg, provide for necessities). Adding just a few items on isolating, terrorizing, and mental health/ medical/educational neglect would make this measure a comprehensive screen for PM.

A reasonable approach to surveillance of PM in North America would come from (a) the NIS and CIS programs (Canada has the Canadian Incidence Study on Reported Child Abuse and Neglect), which are sophisticated and representative of the US population but infrequent, combined with (b) strategies to obtain parent reports (using the CTS-PC or the ICAST-P) and youth reports (the 2 versions of the ICAST, modifications of the YRBSS, or the GSHS) administered to nationally representative samples in the schools and communities biannually. Researchers could then focus their efforts on tracking the relationship of PM to local and/or state/province-wide prevention efforts that target its reduction, as well as to validation studies to assess the accuracy of the surveillance systems by calibrating them with more sensitive measures of self-report. For example, Guterman[1] recommended the use of computer-assisted self-interviewing to maximize a sense of privacy in the administration of questionnaires and the use of prospective logs of violence experience kept by study respondents over specified periods of time, because they appear to substantially reduce memory decay. Improving surveillance systems of PM will require use of brief comprehensive measures that capture all forms of PM, the use of multiple informants/sources, and the use of methodologies that increase the validity of the data obtained.

Strategies for Prevention of PM

The field of child protection is in the midst of a major paradigm shift, from one of protecting children from immediate harm (typically after the fact) with narrowly focused interventions that are often limited to only some aspects of child needs and have the potential to do more harm than good,[120,121] to one of promoting children's short- and long-term holistic well-being. Much of the impetus for this change has come from international children's rights organizations and the worldwide adoption (except for the United States) of the legally binding human rights treaty in 1989, the Convention on the Rights of the Child.[122] The Convention asserts children's rights to survival, dignity, well-being, health, and development. Article 19 of the Convention is the right of the child to protection from all forms of violence and maltreatment. Researchers around the world are using the Convention to frame their research on the relationship of country level indicators with children's well-being and freedom from violence (eg, Britto, Ulkuer[123]; Hendricks, Lansford, Deater-Deckard, Bornstein[124]; Svevo-Cianci, Hart, Rubinson[125]).

International Prevention Strategies

The report to the UN General Assembly of the UN Secretary General's Study on Violence Against Children[122] is the most significant international child protection event of recent history. It provides a global picture of violence against children and makes recommendations to address the issue. At the March 2008 meeting of the International Child Protection and Rights Consortium, the primary goal of all child protection efforts was declared as "the well-being, development and health of the child."[126] The ISPCAN Global Summit on Protecting Children from Violence, Abuse, and Neglect (held April 2008 in Chicago) reached a similar conclusion and recognized that the promotion of well-being, development, and health deserved to be given high priority in all child protection work. ISPCAN and IICRD joined forces to develop a position paper on *A Child Rights Approach to Child Protection* with the intent of guiding professional preparation, policy, and services for child protection. These 2 organizations drafted General Comment 13 for

Article 19 of the UN Convention on the Rights of the Child,[127] which was adopted by the General Assembly in 2011. These efforts demonstrate the international concern for preventing all forms of violence against children, including PM (labeled mental violence in the UN Convention), and encouraging positive child development in the context of familial and community relationships. Professional groups, like school psychology, have been using the UN Convention and Article 19 to reconceptualize their training and practice models from a child rights perspective, including what child protection means in schools.[128] PM is likely to get significantly more attention from this orientation.

National Prevention Strategies

Sweden serves as a model for the prevention of mental and physical punishment of children with the passage of the Parents Code prohibiting all forms of corporal punishment of children in 1979 and granting children the right to quality of care and personal dignity.[129] Building on a series of prior legislative efforts since the 1920s to restrict corporal punishment of children, the Parents' Code stated that "Children are entitled to care, security and a good upbringing. Children are to be treated with respect for their person and individuality and may not be subjected to physical punishment or other injurious or humiliating treatment."

Not only did Sweden prohibit these behaviors, but they also took active steps to make children's environments safe from violence and danger in a variety of ways. For example, they prohibited the sale of violent toys to children, restricted violence in media watched by children, made new housing projects traffic-free so that parents would not be tempted to spank children for running out into traffic, and required a barrier in the front of stoves so children could not reach up and pull hot food down.[130] Their efforts were successful: they altered public attitudes toward the use of physical and mental punishment, reduced the use of mental and physical violence by parents, decreased child fatalities, increased early identification of children at risk for abuse, and promoted earlier and more supportive intervention to families without an increase in prosecution rates of parents. In addition, these changes were followed by significantly reduced youth violence, delinquency, and substance abuse.[129,131] Sweden's social policy exemplifies the paradigmatic shift to a children's rights approach from a child protection approach, and the research of Durrant and others provides a model for evaluating the effects of a shift in national social policy if other countries were to move in this direction. Many countries have since passed similar legislation, including Germany, Finland, Denmark, Latvia, Austria, Israel, and Croatia.[132]

Prevention Programs in the United States

While a national social policy designed to prevent PM and other forms of maltreatment is ideal, federal law in the United States is limited to psychological maltreatment in the form of discrimination by race, gender, or disability. However, 49 of 50 states have enacted anti-bullying laws and 14 states include specific cyberbullying laws, indicating a willingness at the state level to prohibit psychological victimization in a variety of settings. Surveillance systems are needed to assess the impact of these laws and policies and to identify the characteristics of perpetrators, victims, and the contexts in which victimization is most likely, so that prevention efforts can be effectively employed and evaluated.

Additionally, a positive trend is that researchers and governments are increasing pressure on educators and clinicians to only implement rigorously evaluated interventions,[133,134] and those with implementation frameworks that maximize the possibility that an intervention will be implemented with integrity are especially valuable.[135] Most empirically supported programs use a social-ecological framework based on the assumption that a child is affected by multiple factors in the environment, including his or her family, peer group, school, community, and culture.[136] Implementing change in multiple components of the system is typically more effective than an individual approach.[137] For example, Swearer and Espelage[136] promote systematic change to address bullying in schools because individual students' behavior is greatly impacted by the school culture and community norms. Instituting a schoolwide policy that punishes aggressive behavior and rewards positive behaviors creates social-ecological change.[138] Often abusive parents rely on schools and the community to compensate for their shortcomings.[139] Programs that involve a child's entire ecosystem (ie, home, school, community) and focus on increasing social competence and decreasing parental abuse, teacher abuse, and peer victimization are the most promising for preventing PM. Examples of programs that target multiple systems are The Incredible Years program,[140] which has a universal parent prevention program, a classroom social skills intervention targeted at children, and a classroom intervention targeted at teachers, and the Olweus Bullying Prevention Program[141] that targets students, teachers, and parents.

Universal Parenting Programs

Parenting programs for community families may be an avenue for preventing PM in the general population if they improve parent-child relationships and educate parents about PM, the different forms it can take, the damage it can cause, and where the line is between acceptable parenting and PM. What is not known is whether universal parenting programs are already addressing the core concepts related to PM, or whether a new program would need to be created to meet that need. To date, programs focused on specifically preventing parental PM have not been established. Baker et al[142] reviewed 10 widely used, empirically supported and manualized, universal group-based parenting programs (eg, Incredible Years,[140] Strengthening Families[143]) to assess the degree to which they covered each of the APSAC subtypes of PM, both in terms of what not to do (PM) and what to do (positive parenting). They found that only spurning in the form of belittling was covered well by each of the programs, both for what to do and what not to do. Each of the 10 programs also included what to do in terms of promoting cognitive development, a subcategory of exploiting/corrupting, and all 3 subcategories of denying emotional responsiveness: being emotionally involved, interacting frequently, and expressing affection. At least 7 of the 10 programs adequately addressed the what to do behaviors of promoting emotions (subcategory: spurning), using positive discipline (subcategory: terrorizing), and encouraging prosocial behavior (subcategory: exploiting/corrupting). The remaining subcategories included in the APSAC definition of PM were only rarely dealt with adequately from either perspective. Out of the 18 PM subcategories reviewed, the number of concepts covered by these programs ranged from a low of 1 to a high of 7 covered adequately for what not to do and from 7 to 15 for what to do, with medians of 2.5 and 9.5 respectively. Overall, the programs reviewed provided more content on what to do than on what not to do. Altogether, Incredible Years[140] covered the most PM content for both what to do and what not to do (15 and 7 respectively) while Triple P,[144] the program for which there is the most evidence of efficacy in reducing child maltreatment,[145] covered the least with 7 subcategories covered for what to do and one for what not to do.

These evidenced-based programs are well established and considered effective. That limited content on PM that was found was not a criticism of their curricula according to Baker et al,[142] as the programs were not developed for the purpose of reducing PM. The authors acknowledged that before calling for the development of PM specific education, research is needed to determine the prevalence of PM behavior in community parents and whether new programs with specific PM content are even necessary. It is possible that participation in 1 of the reviewed programs may reduce PM behaviors without direct instruction. However, given the high rates of PM as a parental control strategy, a universal prevention program for parents may well need specific curriculum on PM in addition to typical modules in these empirically supported programs on building a positive relationship, giving clear commands, rewarding positive behavior, and constructive discipline.

School-Based Programs

Effective prevention of PM must address it in all of a child's relationships. How well do school-based violence prevention programs cover PM categories for what not to do (PM) and what to do instead (promote positive relationships, social competence)? In general, these programs have peer interpersonal violence as their primary target, but they also address the roles of adults working with youth in school settings in regard to their responsibility to protect children from interpersonal violence and to not use PM towards children themselves. They cover positive ways to deal with interpersonal conflict and promote positive social interaction as will be seen in our review of 2 of the evidence-based programs following.

To evaluate the degree to which each program adequately covers PM a similar methodology to Baker et al[142] was used. First, the 18 subtypes were reviewed to see if they were relevant when evaluating curricula targeting peer bullying and dating violence as well as adult responsibilities in regard to protecting children and not engaging in PM. The exploiting/corrupting subtype, restricting or interfering with cognitive development, was not coded because it is not a responsibility of peers or dating partners. While it is a responsibility of teachers in their teaching role per se, it is not part of the role of school personnel in protecting children from peer or adult violence at school or in the community. Second, empirically supported, widely used, manualized programs were identified in each of 2 categories: (1) school-based bullying prevention programs and (2) school-based dating violence prevention programs. One exemplar program from each category was chosen to evaluate. Third, independent ratings were made of the degree to which each of the 17 concepts was covered both in terms of what not to do (PM) and what to do (positive treatment). Overall, all of the PM subcategories were addressed, at least in part, by each of the Olweus and Safe Dates programs, except for the interaction subcategory of denying emotional responsiveness. (See **Table 18-2** and **Table 18-3** for more detail on the degree to which the selected programs currently cover each of the APSAC categories.) In this section, 2 selected prevention programs are reviewed that (a) are universally applicable to a major component of a child's ecosystem, (b) focus on both what not to do (PM) in relationships as well as what to do to promote closer relationships or foster competence, (c) are evidence-based, and (d) have the potential to be extended or enhanced to explicitly include PM.

Olweus Bullying Prevention Program

Peer victimization and bullying are forms of PM experienced by children. Verbal taunting, name-calling, and emotional abuse are common in schools.[138] In the National Crime Victimization Study conducted during the 2006-2007 school year, 31.7% of students ages 12 to 18 reported being bullied and 3.7% reported being cyberbullied.[146]

The Olweus Bullying Prevention Program was designed using the socioecological approach to prevent aggressive behavior and protect students from being victimized. Developed in Norway, the Olweus Bullying Prevention program is the best-researched and most widely used intervention for bullying.[147] Its goals are to reduce existing bullying behavior, prevent the development of bullying, and improve peer relations. Olweus utilizes a school-wide approach involving students, parents, teachers, and school staff. The school environment is considered an essential aspect of the program because its

Table 18-2. Olweus and Safe Dates Approaches to APSAC Categories of Psychological Maltreatment

APSAC categories of psychological maltreatment	Subcategories of parental/caregiver behavior toward child—What not to do (-)	Subcategories of parental/caregiver behavior toward child—What to do (+)	Olweus (bullying prevention)		Safe Dates (dating violence prevention)	
			-	+	-	+
Spurning	Belittling, denigrating, or other rejecting	Nonphysical forms of accepting, praising, appreciating, admiring, or commending	X	X	X	X
	Ridiculing for showing normal emotions	Accepting, promoting, coaching child's expression of normal emotions		X		X
	Singling out	Treating fairly in relation to siblings	X	X		
	Humiliating in public	Encouraging rather than discouraging when struggles in public	X		X	
Terrorizing	Placing child in unpredictable/chaotic circumstances	Placing child in safe and predictable psychological environment		X	X	
	Placing child in recognizably dangerous situations	Placing child in safe and predictable environment, protecting child from danger	X	X		X
	Having rigid/unrealistic expectations accompanied by threats if not met	Help teach and allow child to struggle to achieve them			X	
	Threatening/perpetuating violence against child	Not threatening or perpetrating violence against child, using positive discipline	X	X	X	
	Threatening/perpetuating violence against child's loved ones/objects (includes exposure to domestic violence)	Respecting child's feelings for other people and valued objects	X		X	

(continued)

Table 18-2. Olweus and Safe Dates Approaches to APSAC Categories of Psychological Maltreatment *(continued)*

APSAC categories of psychological maltreatment	Subcategories of parental/caregiver behavior toward child—What not to do (-)	Subcategories of parental/caregiver behavior toward child—What to do (+)	Olweus (bullying prevention)		Safe Dates (dating violence prevention)	
			-	+	-	+
Isolating	Confining within environment	Allowing child freedom of movement within controlled environment			X	
	Restricting social interactions in community	Encouraging age-appropriate social interactions and prosocial behavior	X	X	X	
Exploiting/ corrupting	Modeling, permitting, or encouraging antisocial behavior	Modeling, permitting, or encouraging prosocial behavior	X	X	X	X
	Modeling, permitting, or encouraging developmentally inappropriate behavior	Modeling, permitting, or encouraging developmentally appropriate behavior			X	X
	Restricting/ undermining psychological autonomy	Allowing and encouraging child to strive for developmentally appropriate autonomy			X	X
	Restricting/ interfering with cognitive development	Promoting and encouraging cognitive development				
Denying emotional responsive-ness	Having/exhibiting incapacity or lack of motivation	Being emotionally involved and interested	X			
	Interacting only when necessary	Interacting frequently and spontaneously				
	Failing to show affection/ caring/love	Expressing affection, care, and love with words, touch, and behavior		X		

Table 18-3. How Many of the Two Programs Were Coded as "Yes" on "What Not to Do" and "What to Do" for Each of the 17 Psychological Maltreatment Variables

Variable	What Not To Do	What To Do
Spurning: belittling	2	2
Spurning: shaming for emotions	0	2
Spurning: singling out	1	1
Spurning: public humiliation	2	0
Terrorizing: chaotic	1	1
Terrorizing: dangerous	1	2
Terrorizing: threats re expectations	1	0
Terrorizing: threaten violence	2	1
Terrorizing: harm loved one	2	0
Isolating: limit movement	1	0
Isolating: limit socialization	2	1
Exploiting: antisocial	2	2
Exploiting: developmentally inappropriate	1	1
Exploiting: abandon autonomy	1	1
Exploiting: cognitive development	omitted	omitted
DER: lack of attention	1	0
DER: infrequent attention	0	0
DER: lack of warmth and affection	0	0

positive structure can counteract the lack of supervision, inconsistent rules, and harsh punishments at home, which are known risk factors for bullying.[147] Studies by Olweus and replications in the United States have found the program to be effective in reducing bullying and antisocial behavior and in improving the school climate.[147] Bauer et al[148] conducted a study of the Olweus program across 10 middle schools in Washington State measuring changes in psychological as well as physical aggression. While the results were not significant for other races, white students exhibited a 28% decrease in relational aggression in addition to a 37% decrease in physical aggression.[148]

Safe Dates: An Adolescent Dating Abuse Prevention Curriculum

Physical and sexual abuse, especially in romantic relationships, is often accompanied by psychological abuse. Programs created to prevent dating violence include protecting individuals from verbal and emotional abuse. Safe Dates[149] is an effective approach to reducing partner aggression and empowering victims by encouraging help-seeking behavior. It is a primary and secondary prevention program that involves schools, communities, and families to protect adolescents from dating violence.

A classroom curriculum and school activities (eg, a poster contest) help to change views about acceptable dating behavior, teach conflict management skills, and inform students of support services. In the community, support groups and a crisis line encourage students to seek assistance. The program author implemented Safe Dates for eighth and ninth graders for 5 months and found a 25% decrease in psychological abuse, a 60% decrease in sexual violence, and a 60% decrease in dating violence.[150] Safe Dates was then evaluated using a randomized trial with 5 waves of data collection to examine the effects of the program over time. Adolescents exposed to the program in the eighth or ninth grade, as compared with controls, reported less moderate physical dating violence victimization and less psychological, moderate physical, and sexual dating violence perpetration at all 4 follow-up periods. The evaluation also compared adolescents who had not been involved in dating violence with those who are already showing signs of those problems.[151] It seemed most effective with adolescents who are already involved in dating violence and appeared to be equally effective for males and females and for whites and nonwhites.

Families for Safe Dates, a randomized, self-administered program mailed to the home with follow-up health educator telephone contact, was effective in reducing barriers to parent involvement in dating violence prevention based on pre and post testing of the caregivers and physical dating violence victimization based on youth report.[152]

Evaluation of Programs for Psychological Maltreatment Content

Olweus and Safe Dates were evaluated for PM content, both the negative components what not to do and the opposite what to do. The extent to which these programs covered the 17 subcategories of PM can be found in **Table 18-2** and **Table 18-3**. Similar to the findings of Baker et al,[142] belittling/accepting (subcategory: spurning) was present in both programs. In addition, Olweus and Safe Dates both include the positive and negative forms of encouraging antisocial/prosocial behavior (subcategory: exploiting/corrupting). The programs differed in several ways as well. Safe Dates did not address any of the denying emotional responsiveness subcategories for adults involved with teens in the program, while Olweus presented some material on emotional involvement and affection on the part of teachers. Olweus covered singling out (subcategory: spurning) in both the positive and negative forms, but did not include content on encouraging developmentally inappropriate behaviors (subcategory: exploiting/corrupting) or psychological autonomy (subcategory: exploiting/corrupting), which were found in the Safe Dates program. Also, Safe Dates, but not Olweus, touched on what not to do in terms of unrealistic expectations (subcategory: terrorizing) and confining (subcategory: isolating). Olweus and Safe Dates were found to adequately include negative and positive aspects of PM content (Olweus: 9 of 17 what not to do, 9 of 17 what to do; Safe Dates: 11 of 17 what not to do, 6 of 17 what to do).

Neither of these peer-focused programs, like the surveillance tools reviewed previously, adequately addresses psychological neglect (denying emotional responsiveness). The 1 exception is that some material in the Olweus program encourages teachers to interact in a friendly way with students. While being ignored by peers, a boss, a teacher, or a dating partner can be intensely painful, it is hard to require that others pay attention and demonstrate caring and warmth outside of family relationships. Given the high rates of teacher PM in some schools in North America[153,154] and in the ICAST studies cited previously, it would be worthwhile to develop a prevention program on PM for school personnel. While a fair amount is known on teacher and student characteristics that are related to closer and more conflictual teacher-student relationships,[155] it would be beneficial to conduct research to determine if teachers would benefit from interactive exercises tying concepts into one's personal experiences similar to those available for students in the Safe Dates and Olweus programs.

Conclusions and Summary

PM is an ideal target for prevention efforts because it is very common; because there is a high degree of agreement among researchers, public, and government agencies and the general public about what PM is; because there is conclusive evidence that it is harmful for children even at low levels; and because it is a precursor of physical abuse. Preventing PM and encouraging its opposite, positive interpersonal relationships, can prevent considerable misery and further the goal of positive child well-being.

Recommendations that will improve prevention research on PM in the future include:

1. In regard to creating surveillance systems to assess the effectiveness of PM policies and prevention programs, brief, regular surveillance of parent and youth reported PM, coupled with the infrequent but sophisticated and in-depth NIS and CIS systems using mandated reporters, allows for both frequent anonymous community screening of all PM experiences as well as periodic in-depth assessment of severe known cases of parental PM. In our opinion, the ICAST model of surveying parents, young adults, and children living at home and in institutions is sound, especially as the child/youth versions assesses PM from all sources.[27,29,111] The surveys conducted by the Family Violence Laboratory at the University of New Hampshire provide a model of how to survey parents. The CDC Youth Risk Behavior Surveillance Systems Violence Survey provides a model for surveying children in schools.
2. Researchers should assess the validity of parent and youth report information on PM obtained as suggested by Guterman[1] and described previously.
3. As international and national institutions move from a stance of protecting children from violence toward adopting a child rights orientation toward child protection that includes promoting child well-being, researchers play a key role in ensuring that surveillance instruments cover both psychologically abusive behavior towards children and youth on the part of parents, teachers, other family members and peers. The presence of enhancing activities on the part of caregiving adults that research has shown to be critical to the development of emotional and social competence. The opposite of which, if extreme, is psychological neglect (eg, showing a child affection, protecting a child from harm from others). The GSHS looks promising in regard to assessing enhancing activities. This type of surveillance data can inform the development and implementation of prevention programs and policies and can be used to monitor effects on public beliefs and PM behaviors over time.
4. Programs that involve a child's entire ecosystem (ie, home, school, community) and focus on increasing social competence and decreasing parental abuse, teacher abuse, and peer victimization are the most promising for preventing PM. There is a need for an evidenced-based PM prevention program for typical and high-risk parents; one that augments already established programs might produce the best results. A parent program that could be integrated with peer-focused PM prevention programs like the Olweus Peer Bullying Prevention Program and Safe Dates would be ideal. There is a similar need for a PM prevention program for teachers and other school personnel.

References

1. Guterman N. Advancing prevention research on child abuse, youth violence, and domestic violence: emerging strategies and issues. *J Interpers Violence.* 2004;19(3):299-321.
2. Tharp AT, Simon TR, Saul J. Preventing violence against children and youth. *J Safety Res.* 2012;43(4):291-298.

3. National Research Council. *Understanding Child Abuse and Neglect.* Washington, DC: National Academies Press; 1993.

4. Feerick MM, Knutson JF, Trickett PK, Flanzer SM, eds. *Child Abuse and Neglect: Definitions, Classifications, and a Framework for Research.* Baltimore, MD: Paul Brookes; 2006.

5. Heyman RE, Slep AMS. Creating and field testing diagnostic criteria for partner and child maltreatment. *J Fam Psychol.* 2006;20(3):397-408.

6. Heyman RE, Slep AMS. Reliability of family maltreatment diagnostic criteria: 41 site dissemination field trial. *J Fam Psychol.* 2009;23(6):905-910.

7. Brassard MR, Hart SN, Hardy DB. The psychological maltreatment rating scales. *Child Abuse Negl.* 1993;17:715-729.

8. Garbarino J, Guttman E, Seeley J. *The Psychologically Battered Child: Strategies for Identification, Assessment and Intervention.* San Francisco, CA: Jossey-Bass; 1986.

9. Hart SN, Brassard MR. *Developing and Validating Operationally Defined Measures of Emotional Maltreatment: A Multimodal Study of the Relationship Between Caretaker Behaviors and Children Characteristics Across Three Developmental Levels.* Washington, DC: Department of Health and Human Services, National Conference on Child Abuse and Neglect; 1986.

10. Hart SN, Brassard MR. *Developing and Validating Operationally Defined Measures of Emotional Maltreatment: A Multimodal Study of the Relationship Between Caretaker Behaviors and Children Characteristics Across Three Developmental Levels.* Washington, DC: Department of Health and Human Services, National Conference on Child Abuse and Neglect; 1989-1991.

11. Hart SN, Germain RB, Brassard M. The challenge: to better understand and combat psychological maltreatment of children and youth. In: Brassard MR,Germain R, Hart SN, eds. *Psychological Maltreatment of Children and Youth.* New York, NY: Pergamon; 1987:3-24.

12. Baily TF, Baily WH. *Operational Definitions of Child Emotional Maltreatment: Final Report.* Washington, DC: US Government Printing Office; 1986.

13. McGee RA, Wolfe DA. Psychological maltreatment: towards an operational definition. *Dev Psychopathol.* 1991;3:3-18.

14. Glaser D. Emotional abuse and neglect (psychological maltreatment): a conceptual framework. *Child Abuse Negl.* 2000;26:697-714.

15. Barnett D, Manly JT, Cicchetti D. Continuing toward an operational definition of psychological maltreatment. *Dev Psychopathol.* 1991;3:19-29.

16. American Professional Society on the Abuse of Children (APSAC). *Guidelines for Psychosocial Evaluation of Suspected Psychological Maltreatment of Children and Adolescents.* Chicago, IL: American Professional Society on the Abuse of Children; 1995.

17. Hart SN, Brassard MR. Definition of psychological maltreatment. Indianapolis, IN: Office for the Study of the Psychological Rights of the Child; Indiana University School of Education; 1991-2001.

18. Rohner RP, Rohner EC. Antecedents and consequences of parental rejection: a theory of emotional abuse. *Child Abuse Negl.* 1980;4:189-198.

19. Hart SN, Brassard MR. Psychological maltreatment: progress achieved. *Dev Psychopathol.* 1991;3:61-70.

20. Brassard MR, Donovan KL. Defining psychological maltreatment. In: Feerick MM, Knutsoon JF, Trickett PK, Flanzer SM, eds. *Child Abuse and Neglect: Definitions, Classifications, and a Framework for Research.* Baltimore, MD: Paul H. Brookes; 2006:151-197.

21. Sedlak AJ, Mettenburg J, Basena M, et al. *Fourth National Incidence Study of Child Abuse and Neglect (NIS-4): Report to Congress.* Washington, DC: US Department of Health and Human Services, Administration for Children and Families; 2010.

22. Trickett PK, Mennen FE, Kim K, Sang J. Emotional abuse in a sample of multiply maltreated, urban young adolescents: issue of definition and identification. *Child Abuse Negl.* 2009;33:27-35.

23. Binggeli NJ, Hart SN, Brassard MR. *Psychological Maltreatment: A Study Guide.* Thousand Oaks, CA: Sage, 2001.

24. Hart SN, Binggeli NJ, Brassard MR. Evidence of the effects of psychological maltreatment. *J Emot Abuse.* 1998;1(1):27-58.

25. Hart SN, Brassard MR, Davidson HA, Rivelis E, Diaz-Thompson V, Binggelli N. Psychological maltreatment. In: Myers JEB, American Professional Society on the Abuse of Children, eds. *The APSAC Handbook on Child Maltreatment.* 3rd ed. Newbury Park, CA: Sage; 2011:125-144.

26. Wright MO, ed. Childhood *Emotional Abuse: Mediating and Moderating Processes Affecting Long-Term Impact.* Binghamton, NY: Haworth; 2008.

27. Dunne MP, Zolotor AJ, Runyan DK, et al. ISPCAN child abuse screening tools retrospective version (ICAST-R): Delphi study and field-testing in seven countries. *Child Abuse Negl.* 2009;33:815-825.

28. Rohner RP. *They Love Me, They Love Me Not: A Worldwide Study of the Effects of Parental Acceptance and Rejection.* New Haven, CT: Human Relations Area Files Press; 1975.

29. Runyan DK, Dunne MP, Zolotor AJ, et al. The development and piloting of the ISPCAN child abuse screening tool-parent version (ICAST-P). *Child Abuse Negl.* 2009;33:826-832.

30. Briere J, Runtz M. Multivariate correlates of childhood psychological and physical maltreatment among university women. *Child Abuse Negl.* 1988;12:331-341.

31. Briere J, Runtz M. Differential adult symptomatology associated with three types of child abuse histories. *Child Abuse Negl.* 1990;14:357-364.

32. Caples HS, Barrera M. Conflict, support and coping as mediators of the relation between degrading parenting and adolescent adjustment. *J Youth Adolesc.* 2006;35(4):603-615.

33. Claussen AH, Crittenden PM. Physical and psychological maltreatment: relations among types of maltreatment. *Child Abuse Negl.* 1991;15:5-18.

34. Courtney EA, Kushwaha M, Johnson JG. Childhood emotional abuse and risk for hopelessness and depressive symptoms during adolescence. *J Emot Abuse.* 2008;8(3):281-298.

35. Crittenden PM, Claussen AH, Sugarman DB. Physical and psychological maltreatment in middle childhood and adolescence. *Dev Psychopathol.* 1994;6:145-164.

36. Donovan KL, Brassard MR. Trajectories of maternal verbal aggression across the middle school years: associations with negative view of self and social problems. *Child Abuse Negl.* 2011;35(10):814-830.

37. Egeland B, Erickson M. Psychologically unavailable caregiving. In: Brassard MR, Germain R, Hart SN, eds. *Psychological Maltreatment of Children and Youth*. New York, NY: Pergamon; 1987:110-120.

38. Finzi-Dottan R, Karu T. From emotional abuse in childhood to psychopathology in adulthood: a path mediated by immature defense mechanisms and self-esteem. *J Nerv Ment Dis*. 2006;194(8):616-621.

39. Gibb BE, Chelminski I, Zimmerman M. Childhood emotional, physical, and sexual abuse, and diagnoses of depressive and anxiety disorders in adult psychiatric patients. *Depress Anxiety*. 2007;24:256-263.

40. Gross AB, Keller HR. Long-term consequences of childhood physical and psychological maltreatment. *Aggress Behav*. 1992;18:171-185.

41. Herrenkohl RC, Herrenkohl EC, Egolf BP. Circumstances surrounding the occurrence of child maltreatment. *J Cons Clin Psychol*. 1983;51:424-431.

42. Herrenkohl EC, Herrenkohl RC, Toedter L, Yanushefski AM. Parent-child interactions in abusive and nonabusive families. *J Am Acad Child Psychiatry*. 1984;23(6):641-648.

43. Herrenkohl RC, Herrenkohl EC, Egolf BP, Wu P. The developmental consequences of child abuse: the Lehigh longitudinal study. In: Starr RH, Wolfe DA, eds. *The Effects of Child Abuse and Neglect: Issues and Research*. New York, NY: Guilford Press; 1991:57-80.

44. Herrenkohl RC, Egolf BP, Herrenkohl EC. Preschool age antecedents of adolescents' assaultive behavior: results from a longitudinal study. *Am J Orthopsychiatry*. 1997;67(3):422-432.

45. Kashani JH, Burbach DJ, Rosenberg TK. Perception of family conflict resolution and depressive symptomatology in adolescents. *J Am Acad Child Adolesc Psychiatry*. 1988;27(1):42-48.

46. Kim IJ, Ge X, Brody GH, Conger RD, Gibbons FX. Parenting behaviors and the occurrence and co-occurrence of depressive symptoms and conduct problems among African-American children. *J Fam Psychol*. 2003;17(4):571-583.

47. Lipschitz D, Winegar RP, Nicolaou AL, Hartnick E, Wolfson M, Southwick SM. Perceived abuse and neglect as risk factors for suicidal behavior in adolescent inpatients. *J Nerv Ment Dis*. 1999;187(1):32-39.

48. Naughton AM, Maguire SA, Mann MK, et al. Emotional, behavioral, and developmental features indicative of neglect or emotional abuse in preschool children: a systematic review. *JAMA Pediatrics*. 2013;167(8):769.

49. Ney PG, Fung T, Wickett AR. The worst combinations of child abuse and neglect. *Child Abuse Negl*. 1994;18(9):705-714.

50. Ney PG, Moore C, McPhee J, Trought P. Child abuse: a study of the child's perspective. *Child Abuse Negl*. 1986;10:511-518.

51. Padilla Paredes P, Calvete E. Cognitive vulnerabilities as mediators between emotional abuse and depressive symptoms. *J Abnorm Child Psychol*. 2014;42(5):743-753.

52. Sachs-Ericsson N, Verona E, Joiner T, Preacher KJ. Parental verbal abuse and the mediating role of self-criticism in adult internalizing disorders. *J Affect Disord*. 2006;93(1-3):71-78.

53. Steinberg JA, Gibb BE, Alloy LB, Abramson LY. Childhood emotional maltreatment, cognitive vulnerability to depression, and self-referent information processing in adulthood: reciprocal relations. *J Cogn Psychother.* 2003;17(4):347-358.

54. Braver M, Bumberry J, Green K, Rawson R. Childhood abuse and current psychological functioning in a university counseling center population. *J Couns Psychol.* 1992;39(2):252-257.

55. Engels ML, Moisan D. The psychological maltreatment inventory: Development of a measure of psychological maltreatment in childhood for use in adult clinical settings. *Psychol Rep.* 1994;74:595-604.

56. Garno JL, Goldberg JF, Ramirez PM, Ritzler BA. Impact of childhood abuse on the clinical course of bipolar disorder. *Brit J Psychiatry.* 2005;186(2):121-125.

57. Johnson JG, Cohen P, Smailes EM, Skodol AE, Brown J, Oldham JM. Childhood verbal abuse and risk for personality disorders during adolescence and early adulthood. *Compr Psychiatry.* 2001;42(1):16-23.

58. McCord J. A forty-year perspective on effects of child abuse and neglect. *Child Abuse Negl.* 1983;7:265-270.

59. Kong S, Bernstein K. Childhood trauma as a predictor of eating psychopathology and its mediating variables in patients with eating disorders. *J Clin Nurs.* 2009;18(13):1897-1907.

60. Mullen PE, Martin JL, Anderson JC, Romans SE, Herbison GP. The long-term impact of the physical, emotional, and sexual abuse of children: a community study. *Child Abuse Negl.* 1996;20(1):7-21.

61. McLewin LA, Muller RT. Attachment and social support in the prediction of psychopathology among young adults with and without a history of physical maltreatment. *Child Abuse Negl.* 2006;30(2):171-191.

62. Moran PB, Vuchinich S, Hall NK. Associations between types of maltreatment and substance use during adolescence. *Child Abuse Negl.* 2004;28:565-574.

63. Rorty M, Yager J, Rossotto E. Childhood sexual, physical, and psychological abuse in bulimia nervosa. *Am J Psychiatry.* 1994;151(8):1122-1126.

64. Rosenkranz SE, Muller RT, Henderson JL. Psychological maltreatment in relation to substance use problem severity among youth. *Child Abuse Negl.* 2012;36(5):438.

65. Brown SE. Social class, child maltreatment, and delinquent behavior. *Criminology.* 1984;22:259-278.

66. George C, Main M. Social interactions of young abused children: approach, avoidance, and aggression. *Child Dev.* 1979;50:306-318.

67. Glueck S, Glueck E. *Unraveling Juvenile Delinquency.* New York, NY: Harper & Row; 1950.

68. Hughes HM, Graham-Bermann SA. Children of battered women: impact of emotional abuse on adjustment and development. *J Emot Abuse.* 1998;1(2):23-50.

69. Kim MJ, Tajima EA, Herrenkobl TI, Huang B. Early child maltreatment, runaway youths, and risk of delinquency and victimization in adolescence: a mediational model. *Soc Work Res.* 2009;33(1):19-28.

70. Kuo JR, Goldin PR, Werner K, Heimberg RG, Gross JJ. Childhood trauma and current psychological functioning in adults with social anxiety disorder. *J Anxiety Disord.* 2011;25(4):467-473.

71. Lavoie F, Hebert M, Tremblay R, Vitaro F, Vezina L, McDuff P. History of family dysfunction and perpetration of dating violence by adolescent boys: a longitudinal study. *J Adolesc Health.* 2002;30(5):375-383.

72. Lefkowitz M, Eron L, Walder L, Huesman L. *Growing Up to Be Violent: A Longitudinal Study of the Development of Aggression.* New York, NY: Pergamon; 1977.

73. Loeber R, Strouthamer-Loeber M. Family factors as correlates and predictors of juvenile conduct problems and delinquency. In: Tonry M, Morris N, eds. *Crime and Justice: An Annual Review of the Research.* Chicago, IL: University of Chicago Press; 1986;7:29-149.

74. Loos ME, Alexander PC. Differential effects associated with self-reported histories of abuse and neglect in a college sample. *J Interpers Violence.* 1997;12(3):340-360.

75. Main M, George C. Responses of abused and disadvantaged toddlers to distress in agemates: a study in the day care setting. *Dev Psychol.* 1985;21(3):407-412.

76. Main M, Goldwyn R. Predicting rejection of her infant from mother's representation of her own experience: implications for the abuse-abusing intergenerational cycle. *Child Abuse Negl.* 1984;8:203-217.

77. Martin MJ, Schumm WR, Bugaighis MA, Jurich AP, Bollman SR. Family violence and adolescents' perceptions of outcomes of family conflict. *J Marriage Fam.* 1987;49:165-171.

78. Shaffer A, Yates TM, Egeland BR. The relation of emotional maltreatment to early adolescent competence: developmental processes in a prospective study. *Child Abuse Negl.* 2009;33(1):36-44.

79. Taussig HN, Culhane SE. Emotional maltreatment and psychosocial functioning in preadolescent youth placed in out-of-home care. *J Aggress Maltreat Trauma.* 2010;19(1):52-74.

80. Vissing YM, Straus MA, Gelles RJ, Harrop JW. Verbal aggression by parents and psychosocial problems of children. *Child Abuse Negl.* 1991;15:223-238.

81. Bilbro T, Boni M, Johnson B, Roe S. *The Relationship of Parental Acceptance Rejection to the Development of Moral Reasoning.* Mansfield, CT: University of Connecticut, Center for the Study of Parental Acceptance-Rejection; 1979.

82. Chan J. Correlates of parent-child interaction and certain psychological variables among adolescents in Hong Kong. In: Dawson JLM, et al, eds. *Perspectives in Asian Psychology.* Lisse: Swets & Zeitlinger; 1981.

83. Erickson MF, Egeland B, Pianta R. The effects of maltreatment on the development of young children. In: Cicchetti D, Carlson V, eds. *Child Maltreatment: Theory and Research on the Causes and Consequences of Child abuse and Neglect.* New York, NY: Cambridge University Press; 1989:647-684.

84. Hoffman ML. Moral development. In: Mussen PH, ed. *Carmichael's Manual of Child Psychology.* Vol 2. New York, NY: John Wiley; 1970.

85. Manley R. Parental warmth and hostility as related to sex differences in children's achievement orientation. *Psychol Women Quart.* 1977;1:229-246.

86. Sheintuch G, Lewin G. Parents' attitudes and children's deprivation: child rearing attitudes of parents as a key to the advantaged-disadvantaged distinction in preschool children. *Int J Behav Dev.* 1981;4(125):142.

87. Solomon C, Serres F. Effects of parental verbal aggression on children's self-esteem and school marks. *Child Abuse Negl.* 1999;23(4):339-351.

88. Starkey SL. The relationship between parental acceptance-rejection and the academic performance of fourth and fifth graders. *Behav Sci Res.* 1980;15:67-80.

89. Bos PA, Montoya ER, Terburg D, van Honk J. Cortisol administration increases hippocampal activation to infant crying in males depending on childhood neglect. *Hum Brain Map.* 2014;35(10):5116-5126.

90. Bowlby J. Maternal care and mental health. *Bull World Health Organ.* 1951;31:355-533.

91. Bugental DB, Martorell GA, Barraza V. The hormonal costs of subtle forms of infant maltreatment. *Horm Behav.* 2003;43:237-244.

92. Burlingham D, Freud A. *Infants Without Families.* London, England: Allen & Unwin; 1944.

93. Carpenter LL, Tyrka AR, Ross NS, Khoury L, Anderson GM, Price LH. Effects of childhood emotional abuse and age on cortisol responsivity in adulthood. *Bio Psychiatry.* 2009;66:69-75.

94. Choi J, Jeong B, Rohan ML, Polcari AM, Teicher MH. Preliminary evidence for white matter abnormalities in young adults exposed to parental verbal abuse. *Bio Psychiatry.* 2009;65:227-234.

95. Coleman R, Provence SA. Developmental retardation (hospitalism) in infants living in families. *Pediatrics.* 1957;19:285-293.

96. Goldfarb W. Psychological privation in infancy and subsequent adjustment. *American J Orthopsychiatry.* 1945;102:247-255.

97. Jacobs M, Spilken A, Noeman M. Perception of faulty parent-child relationships and illness behavior. *J Consult Clin Psychol.* 1972;39:49-55.

98. Krugman RD, Krugman MK. Emotional abuse in the classroom. *Am J Dis Child.* 1984;138:284-286.

99. McGinn NF. Perceptions of parents and blood pressure. *Diss Abstr.* 1963;24:872.

100. Miller H, Baruch DW. Psychosomatic studies of children with allergic manifestations: I, maternal rejection: a study of 63 cases. *Psychosom Med.* 1948;10:275-278.

101. Prugh DG, Harlow RG. Masked deprivation in infants and young children. In: Bowlby J, ed. *Deprivation of Maternal Care: A Reassessment of Its Effects.* Geneva: World Health Organization; 1962:201-221.

102. Puckering C, Pickles A, Skuse D, Heptinstall E, Dowdney L, Zur-Szpiro S. Mother-child interaction in the cognitive and behavioral development of 4 year old children with poor growth. *J Child Psychol Psychiatry.* 1995;36(4):573-595.

103. Spitz RA. Hospitalism; an inquiry into the genesis of psychiatric conditions in early childhood. *Psychoanal Study Child.* 1945;1:53-74.

104. White MG, Bogdan R, Fisher PM, Muñoz KE, Williamson DE, Hariri AR. FKBP5 and emotional neglect interact to predict individual differences in amygdala reactivity. *Genes Brain Behav.* 2012;11(7):869-878.

105. Straus MA, Field CJ. Psychological aggression by American parents: national data on prevalence, chroncity, and severity. *J Marriage Fam.* 2003;65:795-808.

106. US Department of Health and Human Services. *Child Maltreatment 2006.* Washington, DC: US Government Printing Office; 2008.

107. Buntain-Ricklefs JJ, Kemper KJ, Bell M, Babonis T. Punishments: what predicts adult approval? *Child Abuse Negl.* 1994;18(11):945-955.

108. Hemenway D, Solnick S, Carter J. Child-rearing violence. *Child Abuse Negl.* 1994;18(12):1011-1020.

109. Moeller TP, Bachman GA, Moeller JR. The combined effects of physical, sexual, and emotional abuse during childhood: long-term health consequences for women. *Child Abuse Negl.* 1993;17:623-640.

110. Krug EG, Dahlberg LL, Mercy JA, Zwi AB, Lozano R, eds. *World Report on Violence and Health.* Geneva, Switzerland: World Health Organization; 2002.

111. Zolotor AJ, Runyan DK, Dunne MP, et al. ISPCAN child abuse screening tool children's version (ICAST-C). *Child Abuse Negl.* 2009;33:833-841.

112. Murphy CM, O'Leary KD. Psychological aggression predicts physical aggression in early marriage. *J Consult Clin Psychol.* 1986;57:579-582.

113. O'Leary KD, Malone J, Tyree A. Physical aggression in early marriage: pre-relationship and relationship effects. *J Consult Clin Psychol.* 1994;62:594-602.

114. AlEissa MA, Fluke JD, Gerbaka B, et al. A commentary on child maltreatment surveillance systems: examples of progress. *Child Abuse Negl.* 2009;33:809-814.

115. US Department of Health and Human Services; Admistration for Children and Families; Administration on Children, Youth and Families; Children's Bureau. *Child Maltreatment 2007.* Washington, DC: US Government Printing Office; 2009.

116. Straus MA, Hamby SL, Boney-McCoy S, Sugarman DB. The revised conflict tactics scales: development and preliminary psychometric data. *J Fam Issues.* 1996;17(3):283-316.

117. Bornstein MH, Britto PR, Nonoyama-Tarumi Y, Ota Y, Petrovic O, Putnik DL. Child development in developing countries: introduction and methods. *Child Dev.* 2012;83(1):16-31.

118. United Nations Children's Fund. *Multiple Indicator Cluster Survey Manual 2005: Monitoring the Situation of Children and Women.* New York, NY: United Nations Children's Fund; 2006.

119. Lansford JE, Deater-Deckard K. Childrearing discipline and violence in developing countries. *Child Dev.* 2012;83(1):62-75.

120. Lawrence CR, Carlson EA, Egeland B. The impact of foster care on development. *Dev Psychopathol.* 2006;18(1):57-76.

121. Melton GB. Mandated reporting: a policy without reason. *Child Abuse Negl.* 2005;29(1):9-18.

122. United Nations General Assembly. *Adoption of a Convention on the Rights of the Child.* New York, NY: United Nations General Assembly; 1989.

123. Britto PR, Ulkuer N. Child development in developing countries: child rights and policy implications. *Child Dev.* 2012;83(1):92-103.

124. Hendricks C, Lansford JE, Deater-Deckard K, Bornstein MH. Associations between child disabilities and caregiver discipline and violence in low- and middle-income countries. *Child Dev.* 2014;85(2):513-531.

125. Svevo-Cianci KA, Hart SN, Rubinson C. Protecting children from violence and maltreatment: a qualitative comparative analysis assessing the implementation of U.N. *Child Abuse Negl.* 2010;34(1):45-56.

126. International Institute for Child Rights and Development. *Annual Report 2008-2009.* Victoria, Canada: International Institute for Child Rights and Development; 2009.

127. Bennett S, Hart SN, Svevo-Cianci KA. The need for a General Comment for Article 19 of the UN Convention on the rights of the Child: toward enlightenment and progress for child protection. *Child Abuse Negl.* 2009;33(1):783-790.

128. Fiorvanti CM, Brassard MR. Advancing child protection through respecting children's rights: A shifting emphasis for school psychology. *School Psychol Rev.* 2014;43(4):349-366.

129. Durrant JE. Evaluating the success of Sweden's corporal punishment ban. *Child Abuse Negl.* 1999;23:435-448.

130. Durrant J.E, Olson GM. Parenting and public policy: contextualizing the Swedish corporal punishment ban. *J Soc Welf Fam Law.* 1997;19(4):443-461.

131. Durrant JE, Janson S. Legal reform, corporal punishment and child abuse: the case of Sweden. *Int Rev Vict.* 2005;12:139-158.

132. Durrant JE. Legal reform and attitudes toward physical punishment in Sweden. *Int J Child Rights.* 2003;11:147-174.

133. Chaffin M, Friedrich B. Evidence-based treatment of child abuse and neglect. *Child Youth Serv Rev.* 2004;26:1097-1113.

134. No Child Left Behind Act of 2001, Pub L No. 107-110, 115 Stat 1425 (2002).

135. Sanders MR, Kirby JN, Tellegen CL, Day JJ. The Triple P-Positive Parenting Program: a systematic review and meta-analysis of a multi-level system of parenting support. *Clin Psychol Rev.* 2014;34(4):337-357.

136. Swearer SM, Espelage DL. Introduction: a social-ecological framework of bullying among youth. In: Espelage DL, Swearer SM, eds. *Bullying in American Schools: A Social-Ecological Perspective on Prevention and Intervention.* Mahwah, NJ: Lawrence Erlbaum Associates; 2004:1-12.

137. Horne AM, Orpinas P, Newman-Carlson D, Bartolomucci CL. Elementary school bully busters program: understanding why children bully and what to do about it. In: Espelage DL, Swearer SM, eds. *Bullying in American Schools: A Social-Ecological Perspective on Prevention and Intervention.* Mahwah, NJ: Lawrence Erlbaum Associates; 2004:297-326.

138. Orpinas P, Horne AM, Staniszewski D. School bullying: changing the problem by changing the school. *Sch Psychol Rev.* 2003;32(3):431-444.

139. Daro D, Donnelly AC. Prevention of child abuse. In: Myers JEB, Berliner L, Briere J, Hendrix CT, Jenny C, Reid TA, eds. *The APSAC Handbook on Child Maltreatment.* 2nd ed. Thousand Oaks, CA: Sage; 2002:79-103.

140. Webster-Stratton C. *The Incredible Years: A Troubleshooting Guide for Parents of Children Aged 3 to 8.* Seattle, WA: The Incredible Years; 1992.

141. Olweus D. *Bullying at School: What We Know and What We Can Do.* Cambridge, UK: Blackwell; 1993.

142. Baker A, Brassard MR, Schneiderman M, Donnelly LJ. How well do evidence-based group parenting programs teach high-risk or maltreating parents about psychological maltreatment? a program review. *Child Abuse Negl.* 2011;35(10):855-865.

143. Kupfer K. *The Strengthening Families Program 6 - 11 Parents' Skills Training. Group Leader's Manual.* Salt Lake City, UT: Lutra Group SP; 2006.

144. Markie-Dadds C, Turner MT, Sanders M. *Every Parent's Group Workbook.* Queensland, Australia: Triple P International Pty, Ltd; 2003.

145. Prinz RJ, Sanders MR, Shapiro CJ, Whitiker DJ, Lutzker JR. Population-based prevention of child maltreatment: the U.S. Triple P system population trial. *Prev Sci.* 2009;10:1-2.

146. US Department of Justice. *School Crime Supplement (SCS) to the National Crime Victimization Survey (NCVS), Bureau of Justice Statistics.* Washington, DC: US Department of Justice; 2007.

147. Limber SP. Implementation of the Olweus Bullying Prevention Program in American schools: lessons learned from the field. In: Espelage DL, Swearer SM, eds. *Bullying in American Schools: A Social-Ecological Perspective on Prevention and Intervention.* Mahwah, NJ: Lawrence Erlbaum Associates; 2004:351-363.

148. Bauer N, Lozano P, Rivara FP. The effectiveness of the Olweus Bullying Prevention Program in public middle schools: a controlled trial. *J Adolesc Health.* 2007;40(3):266-274.

149. Foshee V, Langwick S. *Safe Dates: An Adolescent Dating Abuse Prevention Curriculum.* Center City, MN: Hazelden Foundation; 2004.

150. Foshee VA, Bauman KE, Arriaga XB, Koch GG, Linder GF. An evaluation of Safe Dates, an adolescent dating violence prevention program. *Am J Pub Health.* 1998;88(1):45-50.

151. Foshee VA, Bauman KE, Ennett ST, Linder GF, Benefield T, Suchindran C. Assessing the long term effects of the Safe Dates Program and a booster in preventing and reducing adolescent dating violence victimization and perpetration. *Am J Pub Health.* 2004;94:619-624.

152. Foshee VA, Reyes HLM, Ennett ST, Cance JD, Bauman KE, Bowling JM. Assessing the effects of Families for Safe Dates, a family-based teen dating abuse prevention program. *J Adolesc Health.* 2012;51:349-356.

153. Brendgen M, Wanner B, Vitaro F. Verbal abuse by the teacher and child adjustment from kindergarten through grade 6. *Pediatrics.* 2006;117(5):1585-1598.

154. Twemlow SW, Fonagy P, Sacco FC, Brethour JR. Teachers who bully students: a hidden trauma. *Int J Soc Psychiatry.* 2006;52(3):87-198.

155. Murray C, Murray KM. Child level correlates of teacher-student relationships: an examination of demographic characteristics, academic orientations, and behavioral orientations. *Psychol Sch.* 2004;41:751-762.

Chapter 19

Preventing Cyber Sexual Solicitation of Adolescents

Sandy K. Wurtele, PhD

Introduction

Information and communication technologies (ICTs), particularly the Internet and Internet-enabled devices, have rapidly become an integral part of adolescent life. Today's youth, a cohort dubbed digital natives,[1,2] use the Internet to conduct school research and do homework, access worldwide media, play interactive games, watch videos, download music, get health and medical information, shop, and communicate with friends and family. Digital media and online technologies have the potential for enormous benefits, and may promote cognitive skills including creativity, improve visual-spatial skills and vocabulary, reduce social isolation, promote identity development, and help to empower youth (particularly disadvantaged and marginalized adolescents).[3,4] Internet-enabled handheld devices (eg, smartphones) promote social connection and support and allow access to the Web. Together, these ICTs provide adolescents new tools with which to master normal developmental tasks, make social connections, exercise independence and autonomy, and explore identity issues (including their sexual identity).

Along with benefits, there are also hazards associated with ICTs. Potential risks of the Internet include threats to privacy and security of personal information, risks of commercial exploitation, risks of being subjected (or subjecting others) to cyber-bullying or online harassment, excessive time spent online especially while gambling and gaming, hypertexting, exposure to sexually explicit material or violent content, and the focus of this chapter—the potential for online sexual solicitation by adults. Online sexual solicitation includes requests by adults to a child or adolescent to engage in sexual talk or activities either online, offline, or both.[5] Similarly, using a mobile phone is important for maintaining friendships and intimate relationships, but cell phone usage also comes with risks, especially for young people. Some teens use their smartphones to send sexually explicit images to each other (ie, "sexting"). Like the Internet, smartphones provide adults who have sexual interests in children and youth with opportunities for sexual solicitation. As will be seen in the examples provided in this chapter, some of these offenders are adults in positions of authority in youth-serving organizations, like schools and sports groups, where they use digital communication to solicit sex with minors in their care.

Along with these sexual risks, the new media technologies are also exacerbating the tensions between societal obligations to protect minors without infringing on their rights to information, privacy, and freedom of expression. The United Nations Convention on the Rights of the Child is the most widely ratified international human rights treaty, establishing the civil, political, economic, educational, and cultural rights of children. The CRC addresses the child's well-being in 40 articles and establishes certain rights and protections. It protects children under age 18 from all forms of violence, exploitation, abuse, and discrimination. Article 34 was written to protect children from sexual exploitation and abuse. The Convention also established that all children have rights to obtain appropriate information, to freedom of thought and expression, and to privacy. Specifically, Article 13 protects children's right to seek out information and ideas of all kinds, as provided in writing, print, art, or any other media.[6]

In the United States the balance seems to have tilted to protecting minors against the supposed harms of the Internet. Protection from online sexual exploitation has come in the form of federal regulations designed to safeguard minors from exposure to indecent material and from online predators (eg, Child Online Protection Act of 1998, Children's Internet Protection Act of 2000, Deleting Online Predators Act [DOPA] of 2006).[7] These federal and state regulatory initiatives have been criticized for the overly broad restrictions they place on students' access to social networking Web sites and chat rooms in public schools and libraries. For example, the American Library Association opposed DOPA, as it would inadvertently limit library computer users' access to beneficial sites. In addition, a variety of software programs have been developed purportedly to allow parents to limit or restrict where their children go online. The challenge is to protect online users from infrequent harms for the few without limiting access for the majority. Instead of restricting children's rights to access digital information or regulating their freedom to explore sexual identity and interest, protection from technology-initiated sexual exploitation must come in the form of safety education and awareness campaigns for teenagers and their parents, along with development and implementation of risk-management strategies in youth-serving organizations.

The aim of this chapter is to describe the risks and benefits associated with today's online ICTs, with a specific focus on the risks associated with sexual victimization of adolescents by adults. First, youth Internet and mobile phone activity will be described, and risky online sexual behaviors will be examined through the lens of adolescent development. A review of the characteristics of victims and adult offenders of online sexual solicitations will follow. The use of mobile phones and the Internet as electronic tools to sexually groom youth will be described. Finally, the chapter concludes with recommendations for educators, parents, and youth-serving organizations to prevent technology-initiated sexual victimization of youth.

Extent of Internet and Smartphone Usage Among Youth

Surveys indicate that a majority of youth use the Internet on a regular basis, starting at a young age. According to Gutnick and colleagues,[8] 80% of children under age 5 are on the Internet at least once weekly, and by the age of 8 more than two-thirds of children are on the Internet daily. They access the Internet through computers, mobile devices, and gaming consoles. Teenagers and "tweens" ages 11 to 14 are particularly likely to use the Internet. In the United States, 95% percent of teenagers aged 12 to 17 report using the Internet, and they use it often—two-thirds of teenagers go online daily.[9] In another study, 95% of tweens accessed the Internet using a mobile device and 80% accessed the Internet using their gaming consoles while playing at home.[10] Computers and Internet access are available in nearly all public schools and libraries and in a significant percentage of households with children.

In the United States, the majority (78%) of adolescents ages 12 to 17 have a cell phone, and almost half (47%) own smartphones.[9,11] Ownership increases with age, as 58% of 12-year-olds, 73% of 13-year-olds, 76% of 14-year-olds, and 87% of teens ages 14 to 17 have mobile devices.[11] Mobile phones let youth be in "constant contact"[12] with their peers, allow parents to give their children more freedom, and facilitate adolescents' emancipation from their parents.[13,14] This Net generation also use smartphones and other Internet-enabled handheld devices (eg, gaming consoles, tablets) to go online. Adolescent smartphone owners in the lowest household income category are most likely to access the Internet via mobile devices, possibly because they do not have computers in their homes.[15] These devices provide valuable opportunities for youth to communicate with others using different tools such as chats, social networking sites, online interactive game sites, e-mail, text message, and instant messenger (IM) services.

Understanding Adolescent Internet Activity From a Developmental Framework

A key developmental task for adolescents is identity formation.[16] Identity formation involves a search for and commitment to various goals and values in several areas including religious, political, vocational, and sexual identity. Social networking sites (SNSs), such as MySpace and Facebook, may function as an important medium for self-discovery and identity development. SNSs serve as a means of self-expression, where teenagers can express their thoughts, interests, and opinions; and thus provide opportunities to construct a digital identity, or even multiple identities.[17,18] SNSs are extremely popular with teenagers, especially adolescent girls.[19] A 2014 survey of 7500 US teens conducted by Jaffray found that 95% were using social networks.[20] Today's teenagers use a wide variety of social media networks, including Instagram, Twitter, Snapchat, YouTube, Flickr, Bebo, Google+, Tumblr, Pinterest, and Vine.[20,21] Profiles on SNSs can include pictures and a personal description including age and birth date, interests, hobbies, and other personal information (including addresses of school, and home and phone numbers). Many youth, especially boys, reveal personal and contact information (including email address, mobile phone number, sexual orientation) in their public profiles.[22-24] From 2006 to 2013, the number of teenagers who reported posting pictures of themselves jumped from 79% to 91%, posting hometown jumped from 61% to 71%, and posting cell phone numbers rose from 2% to 20%.[23] This same survey found that 40% do not keep their SNS profiles private.

Separation and autonomy are important developmental tasks of the adolescent years, as teenagers shift their emotional valence from family to peer group.[25,26] Mobile phones and SNSs provide valuable opportunities for youth to expand their social networks. Posting, friending, texting, and IMing provide ways of staying constantly connected with others.[27] Some youth make connections in online interactive game sites. Others participate in blogs or discussion groups held in chat rooms, which are "virtual places to facilitate discussion of a specific subject or to bring together people with similar interests."[28] Some chat rooms have monitors to ensure that the forum is not being misused, but other chat rooms are not moderated. The anonymous nature of chat rooms allows adolescent users to create their own cyber identities and to have frank discussions about sensitive and embarrassing topics, including sexuality. In chat rooms, teenagers can explore their emerging sexuality in positive ways, especially when they communicate in monitored chat rooms.[29]

Facilitating Sexual Self-exploration

When 84% of US schools offer abstinence-based sexual education curricula,[30] youth must look elsewhere for information about sexuality. Adolescents look to parents, peers, and the media as alternative sources of information.[31] It is no surprise they are turning to the Internet to find health information, including information about sexual development and sexual activities. According to a Kaiser Family Foundation Survey,[32]

75% of online youth used the Internet to find health information, and 44% looked up sexual health information (eg, pregnancy, birth control, and HIV/AIDS or other STIs). Given that the Internet offers privacy and access to unlimited information, it is emerging as a prime resource for youth on issues of sexuality.[26,33-37] The Internet is being increasingly used by adolescents to facilitate their sexual self-exploration. Sexual identity is a critical part of a young person's self-definition, and individuals in their early and middle adolescence are in a period of establishing such identities.[38] The biological and physical changes during pubescence also lead to a flood of emotions, with sexual interest, energy, and drives typically peaking during adolescence.[39,40] From a developmental perspective, adolescents are at an age where they are starting to explore their sexuality offline, so it is natural for digital natives to do so online as well.

The Internet is particularly important to sexual-minority youth, as it can provide an important venue for sexual self-exploration in a relatively safe testing ground. Adolescents, especially same-sex attracted young people, prefer exploring sensitive sexual issues on the Internet, given the easy accessibility and anonymity.[37,41,42] Anonymous online forums provide sexual-minority adolescents with a safe haven for sexual exploration without the harassment and discrimination that gay, lesbian, and bisexual adolescents often face from peers and adults.[16] Sexual-minority youth in Craig and McInroy[43] described how new media enabled them to access resources, explore multiple identities, learn from the journeys of other LGBTQ youth online, and come out digitally prior to coming out offline.

Teenagers commonly report engaging in online sexual and romantic activities such as flirting, looking for a boyfriend/girlfriend, or visiting chat rooms involving discussions about sex.[44] In one study, half of the teenagers surveyed said they used SNSs to make new friends and about 1 in 5 stated they used them to "flirt."[45] Boys seem particularly fond of using digital communications to flirt. As one boy shared, "it's easier to message them than talk to them in the real world...because in the real world they're always with their friends or always in a group."[36] To make romantic connections, some adolescents use dating Web sites (eg, MyLOL.net).[46] Other teenagers "flirt" by sending each other sexually explicit messages and/or images, known as "sexting." Adolescents struggling to make sense of their nascent sexuality have always used media and peers as primary information resources, and this is a potential explanation for why some adolescents sext.[31]

Sexting

Sending sexually explicit messages, pictures, or videos via a mobile device (eg, cellular phones, tablets, computers, Web cams) is referred to as sexting—a combination of the words "sex" and "texting." Teen-to-teen sexting is a way for teenagers to explore their sexuality, and is often used as a form of sexual expression between adolescents who are already sexually active with one another or in lieu of sexual activity. In these cases of teen-to-teen sexting, the sexual photos are shared consensually and intended to be viewed only by the boyfriend or girlfriend.[47] Youth-produced sexual images have been positively viewed as "teen sexual speech"[48] and "visual love notes,"[49] or more negatively by some prosecutors as "youth-produced child pornography."[50]

Why do teenagers sext? Both males and females say the main reason they sext is to be "fun or flirtatious."[51] Sending nude or seminude photographs/videos or sexually suggestive text messages is increasingly used as a high-tech way of flirting—a courtship ritual to express or confirm romantic interest in another person.[31,52,53] As one participant in Lippman and Campbell's focus group explained, "if a girl and a guy want to have sex this is a somewhat normal thing to do."[31] Sexting is also driven by the desire to gain attention, status, and popularity with peers. Among a large study of Flemish teenagers, Vanden Abeele et al[54] found that teenagers with a greater need for popularity were more likely to send a sext. Motivations also vary by gender, with girls reporting feeling more pressure to be "sexy" and to send or post sexual images, whereas boys gain peer acceptance and popularity by having a collection of sexual images.[54] A sexual double standard exists regarding sexting. Girls are often criticized for their sexting practices (regardless of whether or not they sext), whereas boys appear immune from such criticism.[31]

How often do teenagers sext? Determining the exact prevalence of sexting is difficult, with prevalence estimates varying by sample, methodology, and definitions of sexting. Researchers have defined sexting in different ways; some definitions include sexually explicit text messages, others combine sending and receiving sexts, and some ask about sending "sexually suggestive" or "nearly-nude images," which could include a picture taken in a bathing suit. Given the many ways that sexting is defined and measured, it is not surprising that prevalence rates of youth sexting vary widely. In 2008, The National Campaign to Prevent Teen and Unplanned Pregnancy and CosmoGirl.com conducted an online survey of 653 minors and young adults (ages 13 to 19), and found that 39% of teenagers had sent or posted sexually suggestive messages (including text and images). This finding, along with scores of major newspapers and television news reports, led parents, school officials, and prosecutors to believe that sexting had reached "epidemic" proportions.[55] Other surveys have found lower rates. In a 2009 study conducted by the Pew Research Center, 4% of cell phone-owning youth (ages 12 to 17) reported they had sent a sexually suggestive nude or nearly-nude photo or video of themselves to someone else.[56] A 2010 survey of 4400 students found that 8% had sent naked or seminude images of themselves to others.[57]

Other studies find higher rates of sexting. Among a sample of young adolescents interviewed at home over landlines, 15% of youth (ages 15 to 17) reported sending images of themselves using the Internet.[58] Peskin et al[59] assessed over 1000 ethnic minority youth (15- and 16-year-old tenth grade students) and found that 21% reported sending a nude or seminude picture or video or sexually explicit text message (via email or cell phone). Another study of 606 high school students found that nearly 20% of participants (18% of males and 17% of females) had sent a sexually explicit cell phone picture.[60] Finally, a recent review of sexting studies found a mean prevalence of 12% of adolescents sending photos.[61]

In summary, between 10% to 20% of adolescents report sending or posting sexually explicit images. With increasing age and sexual experience, young people's involvement in sexting steadily increases with sexting being much more common among young adults than among minors. Interestingly, sexting among adults is viewed as a healthy form of intimate communication in romantic and sexual relationships; whereas in most of the mainstream media coverage, adolescent sexting has been framed as a type of deviant sexualized behavior, associated with many risks and significant long-term consequences.[62] The negative perspective on teen-to-teen sexting has many features of a "media panic," where discussion of a new media technology is framed by social anxieties (related to adolescent sexuality) rather than reason.[63]

Having private sexts become public has been linked to such emotional outcomes as embarrassment, humiliation, depression, and (in extreme cases) even suicides (eg, the tragic cases of Jessica Logan, Amanda Todd, and Hope Witsell). In schools, consequences for sexting have taken the form of expulsion or suspension, restitution to the victim, and mandatory education.[64] There are potentially serious legal consequences associated with sending and/or receiving sexts. Prosecutors in many states view "youth-produced sexual images" as child pornography under state statutes and have charged teenagers who have sent, received, forwarded, or saved such images with penalties ranging from fines, community service, misdemeanors, to felonies.[53,65,66] In some cases, teenage sexters (like Phillip Alpert of Florida)[67] have been subjected to registration requirements under the Sex Offender Registration and Notification Act (SORNA) within the Adam Walsh Child Protection and Safety Act of 2006.[68] Legal scholars have argued that the consequences of sex offender registration are so severe that they make this punishment for sexting teenagers unfit for the crime and caution against assigning severe penalties in teen-to-teen sexting cases.[69-72] According to Eraker, "the mainstream criminal justice system, and penalties created for serious sex offenses, is far too blunt an instrument to resolve a problem that reflects modern teenage life more than a cyber-crime epidemic."[69] In response, several states have introduced legislation to address sexting among minors.[73]

A similar criticism can be made about sexting warnings given to parents and their teenagers. Some prosecutors and media commentators have warned minors who sext that child pornographers "will hunt them down."[62] A digital safety Web site for parents claims that "tens of thousands of explicit self-portraits taken by teenagers are ending up on Web sites viewed by pedophiles."[74] With sexting portrayed as resulting in such devastating consequences as suicide and criminal convictions, some characterize these fear-based messages as a type of moral panic and warn that these sensationalistic messages can backfire.[55,75,76] In reality, these extreme consequences (eg, suicide, felony convictions, sex offender registration) are very uncommon. One study of over 3000 sexting cases handled by US law enforcement agencies found that most youth who produce or transmit images are not being treated as offenders or child pornographers.[77] Tension arises between legislative authority to regulate a minor's First Amendment right to engage in sexual speech and attempts to criminalize teen-to-teen sexting.[46] Although the debate continues whether teen-to-teen transmission of sexually explicit images constitutes criminal behavior, adult-to-teen sexting is indisputably illegal and the next section describes how adult-minor sexting is often found in cases of cyber sexual victimization.

Sexual Risks Associated With Digital Technology

Despite the positive value and many benefits, there are growing concerns about mobile and online risks, especially risks of online sexual solicitations and abductions of youth. One of parents' greatest fears concerning online safety is the potential risk their children will encounter online "cyber predators," a fear possibly fueled by the popular TV show *To Catch a Predator*.[78] News accounts and even alerts from the Federal Bureau of Investigation (FBI) warn parents about cyber predators who troll through online profiles and SNSs looking for young victims. Claims are also made about the magnitude of the problem. "It is believed that more than half a million pedophiles are online every day," according to an FBI report.[79] Predators are often portrayed as strangers contacting naïve young children, using deception to cover up their ages and sexual intentions, and then luring unsuspecting victims into meetings or stalking and abducting them.[80,81] News accounts of highly traumatized victims alarm the public, and policymakers have reacted by instituting draconian solutions typical of a moral crusade.[76] Parents have taken these grave "stranger danger" warnings seriously. Parents report high levels of concern that their children would interact or meet with online strangers.[82-84] The following section addresses the accuracy of these claims by examining the evidence regarding online solicitation of minors.

Online Sexual Solicitations

Online sexual solicitation includes requests to talk about sex; being asked for personal information, like what their bodies look like or what they do sexually; or requests to do something sexual online (eg, strip or masturbate using a Web cam, send or receive nude pictures). As part of the sexual solicitation, there can be requests to meet in person, but some adults limit their sexual exploitation to the online environment and do not cross-over to the offline environment. Studies of the frequency of online sexual solicitation vary by settings, sample sizes, survey methodology (eg, youth self-report, law enforcement data, newspaper reports of Internet-initiated sexual assault), survey questions, and identification of offenders (youth vs. adult).

Three US surveys have determined the extent to which youth receive online sexual solicitations from strangers. The First Youth Internet Safety Survey (YISS-1) was conducted in 2000 with 1501 youth Internet users and found that 19% of surveyed youth had received an online request to engage in sexual activities or sexual talk or to give personal sexual information to an adult.[85] Five years later, YISS-2 was conducted with 1500 youth Internet users, and found that online sexual solicitations had decreased to about 1 in 7 youth (13%),[86] with only 5% talking to the unknown individual about sex and 4% receiving requests to meet offline.[87] YISS-3 showed that Internet-based sexual solicitations had declined to 9% in 2010.[88] Thus, unwanted sexual solicitations declined over the 3 time points, from 19% to 13% to 9%. Of the 3001 participants in YISS-1 and YISS-2, 2 reported being sexually assaulted through Internet solicitation. Wolak and colleagues[89] estimated there were 52 sexual assaults per 100 000 adolescents aged 12 to 17 years from 2000 to 2001.

A study in upstate New York found that 11% of seventh to ninth grade students reported that they had been asked (mostly by other adolescents) to talk about sexual things online; 12% of offenders identified themselves as being an adult.[90] Prevalence rates of unwanted online sexual solicitation of 5.6% for male adolescents and 19.1% for female adolescents were found among Dutch adolescents.[91] One study in the United Kingdom, based on records of law enforcement agencies, found that 2% of all cases of child sexual abuse reported to police services were cases of online-initiated sexual solicitation.[92] There were 812 US adolescent sexual assault victims identified in newspaper reports across 12 years from 1996 to 2007, with 50 assaults per 100 000 adolescents for years 2004 to 2006.[93] Taken together, these findings suggest that, fortunately, only a minority of adolescent Internet users report being sexually solicited by adults.

Similarly, few teenagers go online to meet strangers for dating, romance, or sexual liaisons, and even fewer have face-to-face meetings with unknown online "friends."[36] According to a survey of young adolescents, only 4% reported ever considering meeting someone in person whom they had only talked to online,[10] whereas 8% of middle-school students said they had met face-to-face with an online stranger.[94] The EU Kids Online survey found that 9% of European 9- to 16-year-olds had gone to a meeting face-to-face with someone they first met online.[95]

One of parents' greatest fears concerning online safety is the risk their children will be abducted by online "predators."[78] Rather than being abducted, many teenagers who meet their online adult "friends" go willingly, a common characteristic of what retired FBI Special Agent Kenneth Lanning[96] refers to as "compliant victims." This term is used to describe teenagers who cooperate and/or participate in their own victimization, often because they have developed intense and passionate feelings for the offender. When these teenagers arrange to meet adults, they plan on having sex with someone they "know" and who "cares" about them. Hinduja and Patchin[97] describe several cases of young adolescent girls (aged 14 to 16) who had face-to-face contacts with men they had met on social networking sites. In all cases, the girls voluntarily went to meet them, fully aware of the fact that they were adult men, and in all cases the girls were sexually victimized. Studies from the United States on offline sex crimes committed against youth subsequent to an initial online contact show the same pattern.[87,89] In a study from the United Kingdom, all of the girls who had experienced online grooming to the point of offline sexual abuse considered their abusers to be a "boyfriend" at some point during the contact.[98] In a recent US case, a Colorado man initially met his victim (a 14-year-old girl from Connecticut) on a Disney-run Web site, and after a 2-year online "dating relationship" he met and sexually assaulted the girl.[99]

In summary, although there is considerable heterogeneity in the frequency estimates of online sexual solicitation by adults, extant research suggests that only a minority of youth receive requests from adults to engage in sexual activities or sexual talk. Fortunately, most youth never receive such requests and the number of those who are solicited who then agree to meet offline is likely to be relatively small.[100] The next section addresses characteristics of those youth who appear most vulnerable to technology-related sexual solicitation.

Characteristics of Youth at Risk for Technology-Initiated Sexual Victimization

What kinds of youths are at risk for technology-initiated solicitation and victimization? Although ethnicity does not appear to be a significant factor in these crimes,[101] youth victims have varied in terms of age, gender, on- and off-line behaviors, and emotional problems.

Age

Contrary to media portrayals of naïve and innocent young children being at risk, the reality is that risk for online victimization increases with age, with older youth being much more likely to become targets of Internet-related sexual victimization. The vast majority of cases of online grooming and sexual solicitation involve young adolescents (primarily between ages 12 to 17), as opposed to prepubescent children.[91,100,102,103] Risk appears to peak in early to mid-adolescence. Almost all (99%) of the victims in the National Juvenile Online Victimization (N-JOV) study were between 13- and 17- years-old, none was younger than 12, and most were aged between 13 and 15.[89] Of 378 victims of online sexual grooming reported to police in Sweden, the largest age group was ages 13 to 14 (39% of all cases; the mean age of all victims was 13.3 years), with only 8% of victims being under 11.[100] The median age of the 812 US adolescent sexual assault victims identified in newspaper reports was 14 years, with incidence of assaults greatest among adolescents aged 13 to 15 years old for both females and males.[93] Similarly, the 3 middle school students who reported offline sexual assaults by online strangers were either 13 or 14 years old in Dowdell,[94] and the onset of online grooming for 8 young victims happened when they were between 12 and 14 years in Whittle et al.[98]

Developmentally, young adolescents are at higher risk than children for technology-related sexual victimization. Young children do not possess as many digital media skills as older youth and do not engage in as much complex and interactive Internet use.[104] Younger children use the Internet in less interactive ways, preferring instead to visit Web sites or look up information. Additionally, younger children tend not to take as many risks with revealing their personal identities (school name, photos or videos, email address, cell phone number), nor are they as likely to engage in sexually risky behaviors online or to communicate with unknown people. In contrast, adolescents spend more time on the Internet and, given their sexual curiosity, they are much more likely to engage in risky sexual behaviors while online.[23,105] One large-scale survey of Dutch adolescents found that online risky sexual behaviors began increasing during early adolescence (ages 12 to 14) and peaked during middle adolescence (ages 15 to 16).[106] Gaining sexual compliance is also easier with young adolescents, given their natural curiosity about sex, struggles about sexual identity, insecurity about attractiveness to others (and vulnerability to flattery about their "specialness"), quest for independence, propensity toward sensation-seeking and impulsivity, and desire for romantic connections.[107] Other characteristics that make teenagers more vulnerable to sexual exploitation include that they are generally curious, adventuresome, trusting, and eager for attention and affection.[87,108]

Gender

Regarding gender, girls are more at risk than boys for online solicitation and victimization. The sex ratio seems to be 2 to 4 girls for every boy, which is similar to the gender ratio reported for offline sexual abuse.[109] Girls who reach puberty earlier than their peers and become sexually active during early adolescence are at higher risk.[110] Although girls are at higher risk than boys for Internet-initiated sex crimes, boys constituted 15% to 25% of self-reported victims in the N-JOV studies.[89,111] Of the 812 US adolescent sexual assault victims identified in newspaper reports, 21% were male.[93] Boys are also more likely than girls to engage in online risky sexual behaviors, including seeking out pornography.[106,112] Among a large sample of Swedish youth, boys were more likely than girls to report posting pictures or films of themselves when partially undressed, along with masturbating and having sex with someone and showing it via Web cam or a mobile phone.[113]

Sexual-minority adolescents (LGBTQ youth) are more at risk for online sexual victimization. LGBTQ youth may be at higher risk to receive unwanted sexual contact online as they are often marginalized, harassed, isolated, and might not have family support like nonsexual minority youth do.[36] For these marginalized young people, the Internet allows them to meet and connect with other people like themselves who might not be available in their offline environments. Boys who identify themselves as gay or those who are unsure about their sexual orientation appear to be especially susceptible to online victimization.[87,114] Wolak et al[89] found that sexual minority teenagers were more vulnerable to Internet-initiated sex crimes because of the frequency with which they searched sex-related sites. Using the Internet to find answers to their questions about sexuality or to meet romantic partners increases their risk for being exploited by adults who appear to offer help and support.

Troubled Youth

It seems that teenagers who are "at risk" offline are also at higher risk online. The link between offline and online victimization is well supported. For example, 96% of respondents who reported online victimization also reported offline victimization.[115] High-risk youth—those who reported experiencing sexual abuse, physical abuse, or high parental conflict in the past year—were 8.6 times more likely to report receiving an aggressive sexual solicitation than those who were not considered high risk.[116] Wolak, Finkelhor, Mitchell, and Ybarra[87] conclude that youth who are vulnerable to online grooming tend to be high-risk youth with a history of prior sexual abuse. Similarly, Noll and colleagues found that adolescent girls who had been sexually abused were more likely to receive online sexual solicitations and to have met someone offline.[117,118] Much like offline abuse, adolescents who live with single parents or in reconstituted families are at greater risk.[15,92] These findings suggest that youth who have problems at home are particularly vulnerable to an online groomer's flattery, attention, and emotional manipulation, including false promises of "love."

Similar findings were obtained by Wolak et al.[119] These researchers examined youth Internet users who formed close relationships with people they met on the Internet. For both girls and boys, being highly troubled (a composite variable of high levels of depression and peer victimization) and being alienated from parents (defined as high levels of conflict with parents for girls and low levels of communication with parents for boys) predicted close online relationships. Youth with these problems showed a trend toward more online relationships and face-to-face meetings. In addition, youth who do not get along well with their parents spend more time with media, including online media.[19] Lack of close parent-child relationships may increase their loneliness and need for contact, resulting in more time spent online, which in turn appears to increase vulnerability to forming online relationships.

Other psychosocial factors have been highlighted as increasing vulnerability to sexual solicitation, although it remains unclear from correlational studies whether these were pre-existing problems or resulted from their online victimization. Some researchers have suggested that young people who suffer from sadness, loneliness, or depression; who are shy or struggle with face-to-face social interactions; and who have low self-esteem are more vulnerable to online sexual solicitations.[120,121] These lonely, shy, and socially-anxious youth may use online chat rooms to establish emotional connections with others, which in turn puts them at risk of becoming victims of online sexual abuse. In a qualitative study of young people who had been sexually groomed online, Quayle, Jonsson, and Loof[122] quote 1 victim as saying, "I was feeling good about what was happening between him and me, because it was fun and I kind of got the attention I felt that I had been missing."[122] As will be explained following, use of chat rooms puts young people at risk of sexual approaches.[87] In 1 study, youth who revealed in chat rooms that they had emotional difficulties were at risk for being targeted.[123] In another study, Dutch adolescents with low self-esteem were more likely to meet with online contacts.[124] Livingstone and Helsper[125] found that youth with lower life satisfaction ratings were more likely to engage in risky communication online.

Several studies find youth who engage in high-risk interactive behavior have high rates of a variety of offline problems, including sensation seeking, conduct problems, or rule-breaking behaviors. For example, among a sample of middle-school students, Dowdell[95] found that all 3 students who reported offline sexual assault by an online stranger also reported that they had stolen something within the past 6 months. Girls who were high or average substance users (tobacco, alcohol, or drugs) were more likely to receive unwanted online sexual solicitation than girls who were low or nonusers.[126] In their review of online risks, Livingstone and Smith[96] note that sensation seekers and youth who experience psychological problems take more risks offline and online and are more likely to receive online sexual messages.

Risky Online Sexual Behaviors

Certain online behaviors increase the likelihood of serious online sexual solicitation. Risky online behaviors include interacting online with unknown people, having unknown people on a buddy list, accessing adult pornographic Web sites, using profanity, being rude or nasty online, entering adult chat rooms, searching for someone online to talk about sex, sending a sexually explicit photo or video to someone they know only online, and (especially) discussing sex online with strangers.[87,91,103,127,128] Teenagers who are interested in and curious about sexual issues find it easy to flirt or have sexual conversations in chat rooms and during IM sessions. But these types of risky online sexual behaviors increase the risk of online sexual solicitation[86,129] Chat rooms and IMs take place instantly and in real time and may encourage more impulsive and risk-taking behavior.[130] The likelihood of communicating with strangers online also appears to depend on both the frequency and intensity of using the Internet—the more youth using the Internet, the more online opportunities they take up, and thus the more online risks they encounter.[132] High Internet consumers are at greater risk for sexual solicitation online.[87,91,109,113] Sexting nude photos or videos to people known only online, although rare (eg, 2% of youth in Baumgartner et al[89] reported sexting to unknown people), is commonly found among victims of online sexual solicitation.[98,99,132]

Whether in chat rooms or SNSs, having "provocative" personal profiles that are set for public (vs. private) viewing also increase risk. Online sexual perpetrators report looking for minors posting provocative profiles.[133] Provocative or risky personal profiles include having a sexually suggestive screen name (eg, Hottie4U, lil_kitty14) or self-descriptor such as "Will go all the way"; posting pictures that are sexually suggestive (eg, posing in swimsuits or underwear); and including references to smoking, substance use, violence, or sexual activities or interests.[97,123,134] Alarmingly, 1 analysis of MySpace profiles found that 54% of youth included risky content.[135] One quarter (24%) of the profiles referenced sexual behaviors, 41% referenced substance use, and 14% referenced violence. Profiles including risky and sexual content were more likely to be from girls and from those reporting their sexual orientation as other than straight. In contrast, sexual references were mostly posted by Dutch boys in a sample of Facebook profiles analyzed by Doornwaard et al.[136] In their analysis of 752 public profiles on the teen dating site MyLOL.net, Pujazon-Zazik et al[46] found that 28% of profiles indicated involvement in risky behavior, with the most prevalent being sex related (16%). Referencing sexual or risky behaviors put youth at increased risk for online sexual solicitations. According to Malesky, "The most common characteristic of potential online victims was their willingness to make sexual comments or discuss sexually related issues or topics."[133] In addition, perpetrators report looking for youth who mention sex, in any fashion, in their online interactions. Likewise, Wolak et al[87] conclude that adolescents were more likely to experience sexually explicit interactions if they had sent personal information and talked about sex with online "friends." Among their sample of online perpetrators, Malesky[133] found that almost all (97%) reported engaging in sexually explicit conversations with their victims.

Although parents are often told to warn their children about posting personal information on SNSs,[137] research shows that posting personal information per se is not associated with online sexual solicitation.[138] Indeed, Wolak et al[87] reported that they knew of no case of a sex offender stalking and abducting a minor on the basis of information posted on SNSs. Instead, online offenders "seek youths who are susceptible to seduction."[87] These authors conclude that "vulnerability appears to be distinguished more by interactive behavior than by online location or the posting of personal information."[87]

Another risky online behavior is seeking out sexually explicit online material (SEOM). SEOM is quickly becoming an important agent of sexual socialization for youth. In their survey of US adolescents between 10 and 17 years of age, Ybarra and Mitchell[139] found that 8% of youth reported intentionally searching online for pornographic material. In a survey of Swiss adolescents, 10.5% of males and less than 1% of females were frequent (daily) users of online pornography.[140] Similar findings were obtained in a survey of Dutch adolescents by Peter and Valkenburg,[141] who found that 10% of males and 2% of females were frequent users of SEOM. In a large survey of Swedish adolescents, Jonsson et al[113] found that boys and girls who were high consumers of online pornography were also more likely to produce and distribute sexually explicit photos and videos of themselves using Web cams or mobile phones, putting them at risk for cyber sexual victimization.

Intentional SEOM-seekers have been noted to have other characteristics that might indirectly heighten their risk for cyber victimization. They report poorer relationships with their caregivers, to be living with only one parent, to hold fewer pro-social attitudes, to have less attachment to school, and to have low levels of parental control and regulation.[109,139,142,143]

As mentioned previously, sexual-minority youth or youth questioning their sexual orientation are at increased vulnerability for sexual solicitation, and they are also more likely to seek out SEOM. Two studies found that adolescents who were not exclusively heterosexual used SEOM more often than exclusively heterosexual adolescents.[141,144]

Risky Offline Sexual Behaviors

Teenagers who engage in these types of online risky sexual behaviors are also at higher risk of engaging in offline risky sexual behaviors. In their longitudinal study of 1762 Dutch adolescents, Baumgartner et al[106] measured online sexual risk behavior with 4 questions. Participants were asked whether they had:

1. Searched for someone on the Internet to talk about sex
2. Searched for someone on the Internet to have sex
3. Sent a photo or video in which they were partly naked to someone they knew only online
4. Sent an address or telephone number to someone they knew only online

They also assessed self-reported prevalence of offline sexual risk behaviors based on participants' responses to 2 questions asking whether in the past 6 months they had sexual intercourse with someone they had just met and unprotected sexual intercourse with someone they had just met. A small group of adolescents (6%) reported high levels of online risky sexual behaviors, and these were also the adolescents who engaged in offline sexually risky behaviors. These findings suggest that some adolescents use the Internet and their smartphones to experiment with their sexuality online, which in turn leads to engagement in offline sexual activities; future research is needed to disentangle the causal relationship between online and offline sexual risk behavior.

Three recent studies have also found strong associations between sexting and offline sexual risk-taking behaviors among US adolescents.[114,145,146] Houck et al[145] reported that teenagers who sexted were between 4 and 7 times more likely to have engaged in a variety of sexual behaviors, including oral and vaginal sex. Sexting photos was associated with greater likelihood of early sexual activity. In Rice et al,[146] sexting youth were over 7 times more likely to have ever engaged in sexual intercourse and nearly twice as likely to engage in unprotected sex compared to nonsexters. Likewise, Temple et al[114] found that among girls, the prevalence of having started dating, having had sexual intercourse, having multiple sex partners, and using alcohol or drugs before sex were all higher among those who sexted. In addition, boys who sent a sext and asked for a sext were more likely to report a history of sexual intercourse. These researchers suggest that for both boys and girls, sexting serves as an invitation to engage in sexual activities (ie, high-tech flirting). Taken together, these results suggest that sexting may serve as a fairly reliable indicator of offline unsafe sexual behaviors, but whether sexters are at heightened risk of online sexual victimization has yet to be adequately determined. Peskin et al[59] found that sexters were much more likely to send sexually explicit photos or messages via email or cell phones than to post them online. This suggests the need to measure the relationships between different sexting behaviors (eg, messages, photos, videos) transmitted via different technologies (eg, cell phones, SNSs, blogs) and experiences of online sexual solicitations.

Based on limited research, youth who are most at risk of online sexual solicitation appear to be young adolescents who engage in a variety of sexual and other high-risk behaviors, both online and offline. In addition, youth with psychological problems are more vulnerable, as are females, sexual minority youth, and female victims of childhood sexual abuse. Potential victims seem to need attention and affection; appear distressed, depressed, submissive, or lonely; and are alienated from friends and family. These youth may turn to the Internet for connections and support they are not able to obtain in the offline world.

Characteristics of Adult Online Offenders

Offline and online child sexual offenders share many similarities. Like in-person sexual abuse, most perpetrators of Internet-initiated sex crimes are adult men.[87,100,102] However, as will be described in the cases occurring in youth-servicing organizations, both men and women use communication technologies (eg, computers, cell phones, SNSs) to sexually groom and exploit youth in their care.[147] Male victims of Internet-initiated sexual assault were more likely to have female offenders in Canders et al.[93] Also similar to offline child sexual offenders, most are young adults, often in their 20s and 30s. In 2 studies of incarcerated male online solicitation offenders, the average age was 35.[133,148] In Canada, an analysis of incidents of child luring on the Internet showed that the accused were most often males between the ages of 18 to 34.[149] According to Lanning,[150] situational computer offenders are often curious and impulsive young men in their late teens or early 20s looking to connect with younger girls. For example, in a United States study of arrests for Internet-facilitated sex crimes against minors, about half were aged 25 years or younger.[111] Based on their analysis of newspaper reports of Internet-initiated sexual assault of adolescents, Canders et al[94] reported a median age of 30 years for male offenders (n = 736) and 27 years for the female offenders (n = 10). In a study of cases reported to Swedish police, 59% involved men between the ages of 18 and 34.[100] In other studies, online offenders were more likely to be single and not living with partners, and few had prior arrests for sexual offenses.[111,151,152]

In contrast to the image of predators masquerading as teenagers, most research suggests that few offenders lie about their age or gender. Wolak et al[89] reported that only 5% of offenders presented themselves as teenagers; in a later study, 15% of online offenders deceived their victims by claiming to be younger than 18.[111] One case of a man pretending to be a teen was Chad Geyen, who allegedly lured 6 boys aged 13 years or younger through a phony Facebook persona—that of Maddi Ray, a 13-year-old girl.[153] Although they usually present themselves as adults, offenders sometimes misrepresent their age, by describing themselves as "a few years younger." For example, Katie was 13 when she met 23-year-old Mark in a chat room for teenagers. He gained her trust, professed love, and convinced her to meet him while she was at an out-of-state swim meet. Mark turned out to be 41-year-old Francis Kufrovich, an investment funds company president.[154] Likewise, 1 victim in Briggs et al[152] felt betrayed because her offender had claimed to be 25 years old when in fact he was 35 years old.

Similar to offline offenders, few online offenders are strangers. The vast majority of adult sexual solicitors are persons who know their victims from offline contexts, and are most likely to be friends of the family, acquaintances (including authority figures), family members, or neighbors.[111] Most of these known offenders use the Internet to communicate privately with the youth. Although MySpace and Facebook users are told to set their profile to "private," which allows only friends on their list to access it, this safety tip may be creating a false sense of security.[97] A potential perpetrator could be among that "buddy list" as the majority of victimizations against youths are committed by friends and acquaintances, not strangers. Additionally, about one-third of youths surveyed included someone in their "buddy list" who they had only met online, not in person.[128] Middle-school students in Dowdell[94] also reported that they "friended" people who were introduced to them by a friend who had shared the student's contact information. Thus, they did not believe they were communicating with strangers, "but with friends of friends."[94]

E-Grooming

There is limited research exploring how adults use ICTs to identify, contact, and sexually groom their minor victims. Sexual grooming refers to the dynamic process of manipulation where an offender prepares the youth for sexual abuse or sets up opportunities to abuse the child.[155,156] Sexual grooming of youth can occur both offline and online. Electronic grooming (ie, E-grooming)[157] occurs when an offender uses ICTs (ie, Internet and mobile phones) to contact a youth and prepare the child for sexual contact.

E-grooming of adolescents typically begins with establishing a friendship and/or relationship by expressing enjoyment of similar interests and activities, making the teenager feel "special" through compliments and flattery, promising love or romance, or by offering a sympathetic "ear" to the adolescent's concerns (eg, sexual orientation) or frustrations (eg, school problems, parent conflict). In an analysis of investigative interviews with victims of Internet-related child sexual abuse, Katz[158] describes how the rapport building creates close emotional bonds. "He is very caring, asking me about my day at school and I told him everything, he really understood me with my teacher and everything," noted 1 child.[158] The liberal use of flattery and compliments make the child feel special and appreciated [eg, "U r sweet and u r a beautiful girl. Lots of guys must like u at your school" (from transcript in Williams, Elliott, and Beech)].[159] Using a range of manipulation styles, the offender can use technology in multiple ways (eg, email, text message, IM, cell phone) resulting in the young person becoming highly accessible around the clock.[160]

The grooming process may continue for days or weeks before the online offender begins to introduce sexual content into the conversation,[79] although the duration of grooming varies according to the offender's motivations.[152,160-162] Online interactions lasted a month or more among two-thirds of offenders in Wolak and Finkelhor.[111] Once sexual content has been introduced, then the offender escalates sexually related conversation. Online sexualization may take many forms. Sexual solicitation can involve sexual talk, requests for personal information, offers to educate victims about sex or provide sexual "advice," or invitations to engage in sexual activity.[159,163] Online offenders might present or exchange pornographic material for the purpose of desensitizing the teen to sexual material.[123] For example, half (52%) of the online offenders in Malesky[134] used child pornography to groom and seduce potential victims. Many sent nude photos of themselves to victims and/or project themselves in sex acts via Web cams. Most the offenders convicted of Internet-initiated offenses in Briggs et al[152] sent their victims nude photos of themselves along with images of themselves engaging in a sex act (eg, masturbation). "At the beginning, he asked me about my body and breasts, then he asked me if I had ever seen a penis...then he showed me his penis on the web camera" reported 1 youth in Katz.[158] Some request photos or videos of victims, even offering to pay for these images. Many of the men arrested for Internet-related crimes in Wolak and Finkelhor[111] solicited victims to create and send sexual images of themselves (ie, youth-produced sexual images). All but 1 victim in Whittle et al[99] created sexual photos and/or videos for their abusers, and all said "these received positive responses, which made them feel good."[98]

For those online solicitors who arrange face-to-face meetings, their goal is to have sex with the minor. Briggs et al[152] refer to these as contact-driven offenders (compared to fantasy-driven offenders who engage adolescents in online cybersex without intent to meet offline). One case in the author's hometown involved an offender sending text messages to solicit sex with a female high-school student. The 27-year-old offender made arrangements to meet the girl at a nearby convenience store.[164] The student reported it to school staff who informed law enforcement, and an officer posing as the student agreed to meet him at the store. The "student" was a detective on a sting operation as part of an Internet Crimes Against Children (ICAC) Task Force and the man was apprehended. As of 2007, each state now has an ICAC Task Force to investigate and coordinate cases involving computer-facilitated sex crimes against minors.[28]

Another category of offenders includes men and women, often serving in positions of trust, who use electronic communications as a way of facilitating sexual contacts with youth. Although no study has documented the extent to which offenders are using ICTs to solicit and groom youth, media reports and headlines around the country suggest E-grooming is alarmingly common.[165] Many of these cybersex cases occur between youth and adult authority figures working in youth-serving organizations, including schools. "Cells, Texting Give Predators Secret Path to Kids" by CNN writer Oglesby[166] and "Sex Abuse in Schools: Prosecutors Say Manipulation Often Begins With a Text or Email" by staff writers Layton and Diskin[167] are just 2 of the many headlines describing this alarming trend. Digital communications provide access to and privacy with youth around the clock. Offenders groom youth through social networking sites, call or text adolescents via cell phones, and email sexually explicit photos or videos. One such example is when an assistant principal of a Florida high school sent a topless photo of herself to a 14-year-old boy.[168]

These media cases describe how adults use mobile devices to entice and groom youth. Law enforcement use evidence from cell phones to build a case against an alleged offender.[169] For example, during 1 investigation of a high school teacher in Pennsylvania, troopers say they recovered "thousands of text messages and dozens of pictures" exchanged between a teacher and a male student.[170] In another case, a 30-year-old male coach and teacher in San Francisco was arrested on sexual assault charges based on sexual text messages found on the 14-year-old girl's cell phone.[171] Likewise, parents can use cell phone texting history to inform authorities, like when one boy's mother found hundreds of calls and texts from a 27-year-old female teacher on her son's cell phone. The last text read, "erase your phone."[172]

In conclusion, the media portrayal of the Internet as the new "pedophile's playground" is largely inaccurate.[173] Instead of pedophiles (ie, individuals with sexual interests in children) preying on young children, most Internet-initiated sex crimes involve young adults (mostly men) who target and seduce teenagers into sexual encounters. Although the exact number of youth victimized online has not been determined and is likely to be small, from known cases it appears that certain adolescents are more vulnerable than others. At-risk teenagers include youth with histories of sexual or physical abuse, those who experience conflict with and/or alienation from their parents and/or guardians, boys who are gay or questioning their sexual orientation, and those who talk online about sex with unknown people or engage in patterns of offline risk-taking.

Policy and Prevention Recommendations

In response to the risks of technology-related solicitation and victimization of teenagers, several prevention efforts have emerged to address perceived online dangers. Responses have included teen-focused safety education programs, educational efforts to support parents and caregivers, and guidelines for youth-serving organizations. Because of a lack of high quality research, many of these Internet safety efforts have been based on "panic-driven recommendations" or built on untested assumptions about online risks.[174]

Adolescent-Focused Education

Internet safety Web sites targeted at teenagers contain fairly consistent messages about how to prevent online sexual victimization. One theme cautions teenagers about risky sites and modes of communication. For example, www.GetNetWise.org tells users to "avoid chat rooms or discussion areas that look sketchy or provocative." A second theme is about keeping their identities private: "Never share full name, mailing address, telephone number, or name of school." Taking this recommendation for complete anonymity even further, an online safety campaign produced by the National Center for Missing and Exploited Children recommends using a nickname that does not identify one's gender or age. Third, most recommend that teenagers never get together with virtual friends unless they meet in a public place and bring along a friend or an adult, even a parent. MTV's online safety campaign also suggests that users get proof of identity through video chatting and asking for some form of identification before meeting an online friend in person. Very few address adolescents' risky online behaviors that are shown to be related to cyber sexual solicitation. Although Connectsafely.org tells teenagers not to "talk about sex with strangers. Don't lead them on—you don't want to be the target of a predator's grooming," this message may not be effective with youth having online "relationships" with adults who would not be perceived as either a stranger or a predator.

A number of official sexting education campaigns have also appeared on the Internet. As reviewed by Doring,[175] such campaigns typically address several different types of sexting risks including legal repercussions of sexting, risks associated with bullying by peers, exclusion from educational and career opportunities should the sext be widely distributed, the risk of sexual solicitation and victimization, and the potential negative emotional consequences of sexting. Although the presence of such Internet safety sites is potentially a good idea, the extent to which teenagers are accessing them is unknown, and few have been evaluated.[123,175] In addition, some sexting campaigns have been criticized for relying on scare tactics, overemphasizing the risk of bullying and criminal prosecution, perpetuating female victim blaming, and recommending complete abstinence from sexting.[175] Furthermore, most of the advice provided in these Web sites (eg, not to post personal information) or their suggested restrictions (eg, avoid chat rooms or blogging; sexting abstinence) are contrary to the motivations of adolescents (ie, to aid in identity formation and sexual development) and inconsistent with the research. Abstinence messages, for example, may be in direct opposition to adolescent developmental needs and circumstances including responsible romantic or sexual technology-related behavior.[175,176] Warnings to avoid posting on SNSs is also inconsistent with respect to online sexual victimization. Lenhart[45] found that teenagers who have a SNS profile or post pictures of themselves online are no more likely than other youth to be contacted by online strangers. Likewise, Ybarra and Mitchell[140] found that only 4% of youth reported an incident on a SNS. As noted previously, solicitations are more commonly reported via IM and in chat rooms. Others have cautioned that restricting teenagers' access to SNS might hamper other educational and psychosocial benefits: more support from friends, more honest communication, and less shyness both online and offline.[84,177] These types of recommendations appear to stem more from public fears, perhaps driven by sensationalistic media accounts of a few rare but egregious crimes.[178]

Youth-focused Internet safety messages must place more emphasis on their online risky behaviors, especially interacting with adults first met online and communicating via text and images about risky topics (ie, sexuality, substance use, violence, etc). In addition, youth-focused prevention efforts should move from abstinence strategies (ie, "just say no to sexting") to greater emphasis on safer strategies.[175,179] Sexting abstinence messages are likely to be as ineffective as abstinence-only education.[62,180] Few teenagers need education on the risks of sexting, given that most youth know that there can be serious legal consequences and that they especially fear reputational damage.[31,181] Instead, teenagers need practical strategies for deciding what to send (eg, "When it comes to sending or posting photos or videos online, here's a good rule of thumb. Never send or post a pic that you wouldn't want your mom or dad to see. Because once a photo goes public, it floats around the Internet forever"), resisting pressure to sext (eg, "When you pressure me for nude pics, I throw up in my mouth a little"), reducing unauthorized distribution of their sexual selfies (eg, "don't send, share in person, on your device only"), and what to do if they receive sexts (delete if from a teen; report if from an adult). Prevention efforts should recognize that some technology-related sexual behaviors may be beneficial, and therefore, a risk-assessment approach may be helpful in empowering youth to make informed decisions about their risk and appropriate responses.[179] In addition, sexting safety campaigns need to incorporate normative education messages emphasizing that only a minority of their peers actually engage in risky sexual online behaviors.[91]

Educational efforts would also benefit from including the voices of youth about technology-related risks and responses. Although the value of involving youth in the development and delivery of online safety approaches is not developed well, their perspective could be valuable.[175,179] Given that adolescents typically view sexting within the context of their romantic relationships as an expression of trust and intimacy, peer educators could facilitate discussions about important issues associated with sexting such as the rules, 'netiquette,' safety, and ethics of sexting.[75,175,179] This approach would treat breaches of consent, rather than sexual expression itself, as the actual problem.[31]

Awareness-building strategies could help youth recognize that there are emotionally manipulative adults, whether online or in person, who will exploit their sexual curiosity and take advantage of their normal needs for affection, intimacy, and companionship. It would also be useful for youth to hear from victims of online abusers about how easy it was to become enmeshed in the relationship and the variety of manipulation techniques used throughout the grooming process. Shannon[100] describes how victims were seduced by offers of payment for sexual services or the promises of modeling work. It is also important to counter the belief that only girls are targeted and victimized online.[182] Young people also need to recognize that adult-teen sexual relationships (ie, statutory rape) are punishable crimes, regardless of whether the teen is "in love" with the offender and "consents" to the sexual relationship.[183] The warning signs of E-grooming need to be described, covering such inappropriate sexual advances as being asked personal questions, talking about sex, being asked to send or receive sexually explicit images, or being told to keep the relationship a secret.[107] In addition to knowing how to recognize inappropriate sexual advances, young people need instruction on how to respond to these solicitations, and especially to report such incidents.[111] Alarmingly, teenagers rarely inform their parents when they receive sexual solicitations online.[85,184] Teenagers are often afraid that their computers or mobile devices will be taken away from them if they disclose receiving inappropriate messages to their parents. However, youth often tell their friends about these secret online relationships.[98,158] If informed on how to respond to disclosures of online relationships, these friends could intervene and advise against offline meetings. Chat room users could also be recruited to become "cyber-bystanders,"[185] and encouraged to warn the adolescent, the chat room monitor, Internet Service Provider (ISP), or even law enforcement about the possibility of E-grooming.

Educators can assist students in preventing online victimization by integrating sexting prevention into lessons about cyberbullying, health, and sex education, with specific strategies for students who may be at higher risk for online victimization.[53,186] For educators, DVDs are available, showing the dangers of cyberbullying and sexting and can be used to stimulate in-class discussions about digital privacy, consent, respect, and the ethics of unauthorized image sharing. (See Bilmes[187] for a review of DVDs.)

There are also Internet Safety Education (ISE) curricula including I-SAFE, IKeepSafe, Netsmartz, and Web Wise Kids; although a review of these programs suggests that few incorporate research-based messages, skill-based learning objectives, or opportunities for youth to practice new skills.[188] Many of these ISE programs convey messages with questionable protective logic (eg, that sending sexts is due to impulsivity, leading to the message "Think before you click"). Instead of offering stand-alone Internet safety programs, some experts recommend infusing technology safety instruction into other evidence-based prevention programs (eg, targeting broader social and safety problems including sexual abuse, dating violence, bullying, drug abuse, and sexual risk taking).[189-191] In addition, given that online risky behaviors peak in mid-adolescence, it would be important to implement prevention efforts in early adolescence, since middle school students are beginning risky behaviors on the Internet.[94]

How might this information be conveyed to today's tech-savvy adolescents? Studies show that the Internet is being used as a source of information about sexuality for both adults and adolescents.[33-37,192,193] Since we know youth are seeking information about sex and sexuality online, sites that cover such topics could include educational information about safe Internet use and the potential of being solicited online. This would allow youth who do not want to seek this sexuality information from parents or professionals to be exposed to safety information while remaining anonymous. Similarly, Twitter and YouTube are also used as health information sources,[194] and could be used to disseminate sexuality information and educational messages designed to safeguard youth online.

Parenting in a Digital World: Keeping Tech-Savvy Kids Safe

Media reports and parent-focused educational materials often exaggerate the risks associated with the Internet, especially about Internet predator abductions and the extent of and dangers associated with sexting. For example, Angelides[55] describes an information campaign in Australia that stresses to parents the catastrophic and damaging consequences that can result from sexting, including "criminal prosecution, sexual assault, humiliation, psychic trauma, cyberbullying, along with serious damage to university and job prospects."[55] Similarly, the US Web site www.Netsmartz.org advises parents to "talk to your child about the possible social, academic, and legal consequences of sexting. They could face humiliation, lose educational opportunities, and get in trouble with the law." Parents are also advised to scrutinize their children's Internet usage. Suggestions often include monitoring their children's Internet use by sharing this time with them, being in the same room as the child when the computer is in use, and placing the home computer or laptop in a public part of the house where they can monitor use at all times. Although these recommendations may be appropriate for young children, they are less useful for adolescents who access the Internet away from home and from their mobile devices.

Another frequently recommended safety strategy is to install software filters. Between half and two-thirds of surveyed parents say they have installed software or use other means of blocking, filtering, or monitoring their children's online activities.[83,195] These cyber security measures can create a false sense of security that their children are safe from online predators.[196] Likewise, this recommendation is limited to home computers, and perhaps younger, less tech-savvy children; but is not as useful with adolescents who might disable or circumvent monitoring software on the home computer or who access the Internet outside the home or via handheld devices. Nor do software filters for home computers block IM activity, which is a common way adult offenders communicate with teenagers.[94]

Along with being informed about the limitations of relying exclusively on blocking or monitoring software, parents and/or guardians need advice and guidance for talking to their children about how to be safe, responsible, and respectful digital citizens. When trying to protect their adolescents from online sexual solicitations, parents struggle finding a balance between using overly restrictive strategies and also respecting their privacy and needs for independence and autonomy. Helpful guidelines for discussing responsible use of the Internet and mobile devices are available on Web sites (eg, ConnectSafely.org, CovenantEyes.com, bewebaware.ca), books,[14,107,197,198] and in journal articles.[134,186,196] According to findings of the EU Kids Online survey, parents prefer to receive information about Internet safety from their child's school, leading to the suggestion to strengthen such home-school initiatives as training programs, workshops, and information dissemination.[199] Parents are advised to consider whether their children should have cell phones, tablets, or laptops that have texting and photographic capability. Having these digital devices is a privilege, and with this privilege comes responsibilities. Before these devices are purchased, parents may want to develop responsible-use-of-technology contracts, specifying acceptable and unacceptable uses of the device. Also, it is important that parents discuss the dangers of meeting a new Internet friend offline, how to handle receiving sexually explicit images, messages, or emails especially when sent to them by adults, and how to recognize and respond to E-grooming tactics, including "exit strategies"[177] to adopt if they are being sexually solicited online by an adult. Parents are also encouraged to talk about online risky behaviors (eg, flirting and having sexual conversations with strangers, posting provocative pictures, sexting, visiting pornography sites, etc).

The potential of enhancing parent-adolescent communication about technology-initiated sexual exploitation remains a promising but underutilized and under-researched area. Parents are viewed as the primary teachers of Internet safety by several groups, including teachers, pediatricians, adolescents, and parents themselves,[200] and studies are appearing showing that parental guidance does matter. For example, children who live in homes that limit media opportunities spend less time with media, including computers.[19] Adolescents surveyed by Liau, Khoo, and Ang[201] were less likely to have face-to-face meetings with strangers when parents set a rule never to meet with someone who is first met online. In their review of young people's vulnerabilities to online grooming, Whittle and colleagues[121] concluded that young people whose parents oversee their Internet use experience fewer negative online events, suggesting that a parent's involvement and monitoring of their children's Internet use appears to be a protective factor. Similarly, adolescents surveyed in Australia reported being more safety conscious when their parents had discussed Internet safety with them.[202] Adolescents who report positive relationships with their parents, including closeness, open communication, and parental monitoring, engage in fewer risky sexual behaviors, both online and offline.[203] Parenting style is also associated with teen online behavior. Rosen et al[84] found that teenagers with indulgent parents (parents who are warm but low in control) were more likely to meet someone offline whom they had met online, whereas adolescents with authoritative parents (parents who are warm, consistently apply standards, and are willing to reason with their children) exhibited the fewest risky or negative MySpace behaviors. As with any of the other risks teenagers face today (eg, drinking, drugs, sex) the best protection comes when parents give love but set limits, monitor their activities, and have open and honest dialogue, so their children have the right set of values to take along with them as they travel through cyberspace.

Guidance for Youth-Serving Organizations

The sexual exploitation of minors occurring in youth-serving organizations (YSOs), including schools, sporting groups, and faith-based institutions, is a serious and pervasive problem. YSOs can reduce the risk of staff sexual misconduct by strengthening appropriate formal structures (eg, risk-management policies and procedures) and informal structures, particularly providing clear codes of conduct and training on avoiding sexual boundary transgressions. Staff sexual boundary violations occur in many ways and across different types of boundaries. Communication boundaries can be crossed when a staff member has sexually-oriented conversations with a youth or sends sexual messages or images to a minor.[157] Professional boundaries need to be maintained in all forms of communication, including electronic communication (eg, text messaging, cell phone usage) and online social media.

Recognizing that youth are vulnerable to E-grooming, YSOs must develop and implement responsible use of technology policies, outlining the acceptable and unacceptable uses of digital devices and electronic communications, including guidelines for communication between staff and youth on SNSs and via cell phones. For example, the New York City Department of Education (DOE) publishes their Social Media Guidelines for both employees and students. The Spring 2013 guidelines recommended that DOE employees maintain separate professional and personal SNSs and email accounts and that they only communicate with students through school-based professional social media sites and professional email accounts. However, the guidelines do not address one-to-one communication via cell phones and text messaging between teachers and students, which have been more widespread and problematic.[204] In contrast, the Board of Education in Paramus, NJ set stricter restrictions on employees using SNSs and cell phones, including a prohibition against teachers giving out cell phone numbers to students or calling students under the age of 18 on their cell phones without the authorization of a parent. Some have noted that stricter E-communication guidelines are meeting resistance from some teachers because of the increasing importance of technology as a teaching tool and of the benefits of social media for engaging with students.[165] Schools have also addressed sexting by banning the behavior in their Student Code of Conduct. For example, the Houston Independent School District implemented a ban on using a cell phone or other personal communication device to send or possess text or email messages containing sexually explicit images while at school or at a school-related function.[205] Other schools and school districts have implemented additional restrictions by banning the use of cell phones all together. Partial or complete cell phone bans have been put in place in high schools in Los Angeles, Detroit, New York City, Milwaukee, and Toronto, Canada.[18,206]

In addition to schools, other youth-serving organizations are developing and implementing policies to limit digital contact between staff and youth in their care. For example, the Boy Scouts of America publish their social media guidelines, which emphasize that all communication between adult leaders and Scouts should be via public, not private, social media channels. The document specifies that "there should be no private messages and no one-on-one direct contact through email, Facebook messages, Twitter direct messaging, chats, Instant Messaging, or other similar messaging features." Similarly, in its Safe Sport Handbook, USA Swimming provides a model policy for electronic communication.[207] That policy states that electronic communication with swimmers should be "transparent, accessible, and professional," and not contain references to drugs or alcohol use, sexual language or activity, personal or relationship problems, or include inappropriate or sexually explicit pictures. Like the Boy Scouts of America, USA Swimming prohibits using any device capable of recording or transmitting visual images in showers, restrooms, or other areas where privacy is expected by participants, and also prohibits the taking or sending of sexually explicit photos or videos by cell phone or Web cams.

Conclusion

Sexuality is a major developmental issue for adolescents, and smartphones and the Internet are allowing them to express and explore this sensitive issue without the embarrassment of face-to-face contact. These technologies are being viewed as integral to youth sexual identities, relationships, agency, and entertainment, and as possibly providing much-needed information to youth about their bodies and their sexual health.[36,62] Unfortunately, it is this very natural developmental need of adolescents to explore their emerging sexual feelings and curiosity and develop their sexual identities that may put some youth at risk for online sexual victimization. Rather than restricting access through regulation, findings support the need for education of youth (and their parents) about the risks, but also the benefits, of the new technologies. Furthermore, to satisfy their normal curiosity about sexuality, more attention should be paid to the development of Web-based healthy sexuality education programs for adolescents tailored to the specific needs of unique groups (eg, sexual-minority youth; youth with developmental disabilities). Recognizing that youth are vulnerable to E-grooming, especially by adults in authority positions in youth-serving organizations, YSOs must develop and implement responsible-use-of-technology policies, outlining the acceptable and unacceptable uses of digital devices and electronic communications between authority figures and youth.[157]

Technology is tightly woven into the fabric of 21st century society. Since Internet and mobile media use is growing exponentially, particularly among youth, professionals need to develop ways to educate them about safe uses of these digital technologies, while being respectful of their rights to freedom of expression and access to information of all kinds, including sexuality information. It is imperative that developmentally appropriate online safety interventions be created and evaluated to prepare youth to navigate the ever-changing landscape of cyberspace. Youth should be involved in the development of these safety efforts, and all online safety education must be based on high-quality research, not speculation or rare high-profile cases. Although ideally parents are the best educators for their children on such topics, this approach may not always be feasible, particularly when parents and their children have difficulty communicating about sexual topics or when other victimization issues are present in a family. Encouragingly, there is evidence that having online safety discussions with other adults (ie, teachers) is also associated with less risky online behaviors, including fewer offline meetings.[208] Thus, the joint efforts of parents, educators, health care professionals, law enforcement, researchers, policymakers, private sector entities (eg, ISPs, developers), and digital natives themselves are needed to help keep young people safe in cyberspace. A multi-stakeholder approach is essential to uphold children's rights to access information but also their fundamental rights to live free of violence, including in the virtual world.

References

1. Palfrey J, Gasser U. *Born Digital: Understanding the First Generation of Digital Natives*. New York, NY: Basic Books; 2008.
2. Prensky M. Digital natives, digital immigrants. *On the Horizon*. 2001;9(5):1-6.
3. Greenfield PM. Technology and informal education: what is taught, what is learned. *Science*. 2009;323:69-71.
4. Guan SA, Subrahmanyam K. Youth Internet use: risks and opportunities. *Curr Opin Psychiatry*. 2009;22:351-356.

5. Marcum CD. Interpreting the intentions of internet predators: an examination of online predatory behavior. *J Child Sex Abuse*. 2007;16(4):99-114.

6. Wold T. Protection and access: to regulate young people's internet use. *International Journal of Media and Cultural Politics*. 2010;6(1):63-80.

7. Yan Z. Differences in high school and college students' basic knowledge and perceived education of Internet safety: Do high school students really benefit from the Children's Internet Protection Act? *J Appl Dev Psychol*. 2009;30:209-217.

8. Gutnick AL, Robb M, Takeuchi L, Kotler J. *Always Connected: The New Digital Media Habits of Young Children*. New York, NY: Joan Ganz Cooney Center at Sesame Workshop; 2011.

9. Madden M, Lenhart A, Duggan M, Cortesi S, Gasser U. Teens and Technology 2013. http://www.pewinternet.org/Reports/2013/Teens-and-Tech.aspx. Accessed December 30, 2014.

10. Cox Communications. Tween Internet survey. http://ww2.cox.com/wcm/en/aboutus/datasheet/takecharge/tween-internet-safety-survey.pdf. Published June, 2012. Accessed December 30, 2014.

11. Lenhart A. Teens, smartphones and texting. http://pewinternet.org/Reports/2012/Teens-and-smartphones.aspx. Published 2012. Accessed December 30, 2014.

12. Clark LS. The constant contact generation: exploring teen friendship networks online. In: Mazzarella S, ed. *Girl Wide Web*. New York, NY: Peter Lang; 2005:203-222.

13. Bond E. The mobile phone = bike shed? children, sex and mobile phones. *New Media and Society*. 2010;13(4):587-604.

14. Gold J. Screen-smart parenting. New York, NY: Guilford Press; 2015.

15. Mitchell KJ, Finkelhor D, Wolak J. Use of social networking sites in online sex crimes against minors: an examination of national incidence and means of utilization. *J Adolesc Health*. 2010;47:183-190.

16. Erikson EH. *Identity: Youth and Crisis*. New York, NY: Norton; 1968.

17. Jewkes Y. Much ado about nothing? representations and realities of online soliciting of children. *J Sex Aggress*. 2010;16(1):5-18.

18. Subrahmanyam K, Greenfield P. Online communication and adolescent relationships. *Fut Child*. 2008;18(1):119-146.

19. Rideout VJ, Foehr UG, Roberts DF. Generation M2: media in the lives of 8- to 18-year-olds. http://www.kff.org/other/report/generation-m2-in-the-lives-of-8-to-18-year-olds/. Published 2010. Accessed December 30, 2014.

20. Bosker B. Teens are leaving Facebook for Facebook. http://www.huffingtonpost.com/2014/04/11/teens-facebook_n_5127455.html#es_share_ended. Published April 11, 2014. Accessed December 30, 2014.

21. Guarini D. New study shows teens are sooo over Facebook. http://www.huffingtonpost.com/2014/01/16/facebook-teenager_n_4610870.html. Accessed December 30, 2016.

22. Livingstone S. Taking risky opportunities in youthful content creation: teenagers' use of social networking sites for intimacy, privacy and self-expression. *New Media and Society*. 2008;10:459-477.

23. Madden M, Lenhart A, Cortesi S, et al. Teens, social media, and privacy. http://pewinternet.org/Reports/2013/Teens-Social-Media-And-Privacy.aspx. Published 2013. Accessed December 30, 2014.

24. Taraszow T, Aristodemou E, Shitta G, Laouris Y, Arsoy A. Disclosure of personal and contact information by young people in social networking sites: an analysis using Facebook profiles as an example. *International Journal of Media and Cultural Politics.* 2010;6(1):81-102.

25. Rafla M, Carson NJ, DeJong SM. Adolescents and the Internet: what mental health clinicians need to know. *Curr Psychiatry Rep.* 2014;16(472):1-10.

26. Valkenburg PM, Peter J. Online communication among adolescents: an integrated model of its attraction, opportunities, and risks. *J Adolesc Health.* 2011;48:121-127.

27. Reich SM, Subrahmanyam K, Espinoza G. Friending, IMing, and hanging out face-to-face: overlap in adolescents' online and offline social networks. *Dev Psychol.* 2012;48(2):356-368.

28. Broughton DD. Internet child sexual exploitation. In: Jenny C, ed. *Child Abuse and Neglect: Diagnosis, Treatment, and Evidence.* Saint Louis, MO: Elsevier; 2011:142-146.

29. Subrahmanyam K, Smahel D, Greenfield P. Connecting developmental constructions to the Internet: identity presentation and sexual exploration in online teen chat rooms. *Dev Psychol.* 2006;42(3):395-406.

30. Guttmacher Institute. Facts on American teens' sources of information about sex. http://www.guttmacher.org/pubs/FB-Teen-Sex-Ed.html. Published 2012. Accessed December 30, 2014.

31. Lippman JR, Campbell SW. Damned if you do, damned if you don't...if you're a girl: relational and normative contexts of adolescent sexting in the United States. *J Child Media.* 2014;8(4):1-16.

32. Rideout VJ. Generation RX.com: how young people use the Internet for health information. http://kaiserfamilyfoundation.files.wordpress.com/2001/11/3202-genrx-report.pdf. Published 2001. Accessed December 30, 2014.

33. Daneback K, Mansson S, Ross MW, Markham CM. The Internet as a source of information about sexuality. *Sex Educ.* 2012;12(5):583-598.

34. Doring NM. The Internet's impact on sexuality: a critical review of 15 years of research. Comput Human Behav. 2009;25:1089-1101.

35. Levine D, McCright J, Dobkin L, Woodruff AJ, Klausner JD. SEXINFO: a sexual health text messaging service for San Francisco youth. *Am J Pub Health.* 2008;98(3):393-395.

36. Pascoe CJ. Resource and risk: youth sexuality and new media use. *Sex Res Soc Pol.* 2011;8:5-17.

37. Selkie EM, Benson M, Moreno M. Adolescents' views regarding uses of social networking websites and text messaging for adolescent sexual health education. *Am J Health Educ.* 2011;42(4):205-212.

38. DeLamater J, Friedrich WN. Human sexual development. *J Sex Res.* 2002;39(1):10-14.

39. Shulman S, Davila J, Shachar-Shapira L. Assessing romantic competence among older adolescents. *J Adolesc.* 2011;34:397-406.

40. Wurtele SK, Kenny MC. Normative sexuality development in childhood: implications for developmental guidance and prevention of childhood sexual abuse. *Counsel Hum Dev.* 2011;43(9):1-24.

41. Priebe G, Svedin CG. Online or off-line victimisation and psychological well-being: a comparison of sexual-minority and heterosexual youth. *Eur Child Adolesc Psychiatry.* 2012;21(10):569-582.

42. Hillier L, Harrison L. Building realities less limited than their own: young people practising same-sex attraction on the Internet. *Sexualities.* 2007;10(1):82-100.

43. Craig SL, McInroy L. You can form a part of yourself online: the influence of new media on identity development and coming out for LGBTQ youth. *J Gay Lesbian Ment Health.* 2014;18:95-109.

44. Sorbring E, Skoog T, Bohlin M. Adolescent girls' and boys' well-being in relation to online and offline sexual and romantic activity. *Cyberpsychology: Journal of Psychosocial Research on Cyberspace.* 2014;8(1):Article 7. doi:10.5817/CP2014-1-7.

45. Lenhart A, Madden M, MacGill A, Smith A. Teens and social media. http://www.pewinternet.org/PPF/r/230/report_display.asp. Published December 19, 2007. Accessed December 30, 2014.

46. Pujazon-Zazik MA, Manasse SM, Orrell-Valente JK. Adolescents' self-presentation on a teen dating Web site: a risk-content analysis. *J Adolesc Health.* 2012;50:517-520.

47. Dowdell EB, Burgess AW, Flores JR. Online social networking patterns among adolescents, young adults, and sexual offenders. *Am J Nurs.* 2011;111(7):28-36.

48. McLaughlin JH. Exploring the first amendment rights of teens in relationship to sexting and censorship. *Univ Mich J Law Reform.* 2012;45(2):315-350.

49. Wood RH. The first amendment implications of sexting at public schools: a quandary for administrators who intercept visual love notes. *J Law Pol.* 2010;18:1-34.

50. Richards RD, Calvert C. When sex and cell phones collide: inside the prosecution of a teen sexting case. *Hastings Communications and Entertainment Law Journal.* 2009;32:1-39.

51. National Campaign to Prevent Teen and Unplanned Pregnancy. Sex and tech: Results from a survey of teens and young adults. http://www.thenationalcampaign.org/sextech/PDF/SexTech_Summary.pdf. Accessed December 30, 2016.

52. O'Sullivan LF, Ronis ST. Virtual cheating hearts: extradyadic and poaching interactions among adolescents with links to online sexual activities. *Can J Behav Sci.* 2013;45(3):175-184.

53. Van Ouytsel J, Walrave M, Van Gool E. Sexting: between thrill and fear--how schools can respond. *Clearing House.* 2014;87:204-212.

54. Vanden Abeele M, Campbell SW, Eggermont S, Roe K. Sexting, mobile porn use, and peer group dynamics: boys' and girls' self-perceived popularity, need for popularity, and perceived peer pressure. *Media Psychol.* 2014;17:6-33.

55. Angelides S. 'Technology, hormones, and stupidity': the affective politics of teenage sexting. *Sexualities.* 2013;16(5/6):665-689.

56. Lenhart A. Teens and sexting. http://www.pewinternet.org/~/media//Files/Reports/2009/PIP_Teens_and_Sexting.pdf. Published 2009. Accessed December 30, 2014.

57. Patchin JW, Schafer JA, Hinduja S. Cyberbullying and sexting. http://www.fbi.gov/stats-services/publications/law-enforcement-bulletin/2013/june/cyberbullying-and-sexting. Published June 2013. Accessed December 30, 2014.

58. Mitchell KJ, Finkelhor D, Jones LM, Wolak J. Prevalence and characteristics of youth sexting: a national study. *Pediatrics*. 2012;129(1):13-20.

59. Peskin M, Markhan C, Addy R, Shegog R, Thiel M, Tortolero S. Prevalence and patterns of sexting among ethnic minority urban high school students. *Cyberpsychology, Behavior, and Social Networking*. 2013;16:454-459.

60. Strassberg DS, McKinnon RK, Sustaita MA, Rullo J. Sexting by high school students: an exploratory and descriptive study. *Arch Sex Behav*. 2013;42:15-21.

61. Klettke B, Hallford DJ, Mellor DJ. Sexting prevalence and correlates: a systematic literature review. *Clin Psychol Rev*. 2014;34:44-53.

62. Hasinoff AA. Sexting as media production: rethinking social media and sexuality. *New Media and Society*. 2012;15(4):449-465.

63. Draper NRA. Is your teen at risk? discourses of adolescent sexting in United States television news. *J Child Media*. 2012;6:221-236.

64. McEachern AG, McEachern-Ciattoni RT, Martin F. Sexting: new challenges for schools and professional school counselors. *J Sch Counsel*. 2012;10(20):1-26.

65. Klein R. Bloomberg's school cell phone ban will most likely be reversed when he leaves office. http://www.huffingtonpost.com/2013/04/29/bloomberg-cell-phone-ban-new-york-schools_n_3179336.html. Published April 29, 2013. Accessed December 30, 2014.

66. Mattey B, Diliberto GM. Sexting—it's in the dictionary. *NASN Sch Nurse*. 2013;28(2):94-98.

67. Mabrey V, Perozzi D. 'Sexting': should child pornography laws apply. http://abcnews.go.com/Nightline/phillip-alpert-sexting-teen-child-porn/story?id=10252790. Published April 1, 2010. Accessed December 30, 2014.

68. Forbes SG. Sex, cells, and SORNA: applying sex offender registration laws to sexting cases. *William Mary Law Rev*. 2011;52(5):1717-1746.

69. Eraker EC. Stemming sexting: sensible legal approaches to teenagers' exchange of self-produced pornography. *Berkeley Technol Law J*. 2010;25:555-596.

70. Shah K. Sexting: risky or [f]risky? an examination of the current and future legal treatment of sexting in the United States. *Faulkner Law Review*. 2010;2:193-216.

71. Szymialis JJ. Sexting: a response to prosecuting those growing up with a growing trend. *Indiana Law Rev*. 2010;44(1):301-339.

72. Zhang X. Charging children with child pornography--using the legal system to handle the problem of "sexting." *Computer Law and Security Review*. 2010;26:251-259.

73. National Conference of State Legislatures. Sexting legislation in 2013. http://www.ncsl.org/research/telecommunications-and-information-technology/2013-sexting-legislation.aspx. Published 2013. Accessed December 30, 2014.

74. Woda S. How teens' 'sexting' photos end up on pedophile websites. http://resources.uknowkids.com/blog/bid/320731/How-teens-sexting-photos-end-up-on-pedophile-websites. Published October 17, 2013. Accessed December 30, 2014.

75. Oravec JA. The ethics of sexting: issues involving consent and the production of intimate content. In: Heider D, Massanari AL, eds. *Digital Ethics: Research and Practice*. New York, NY: Peter Lang Publishing, Inc; 2012.

76. Weitzer R. The social construction of sex trafficking: ideology and institutionalization of a moral crusade. *Polit Soc*. 2007;35(3):447-475.

77. Wolak J, Finkelhor D, Mitchell KJ. How often are teens arrested for sexting? data from a national sample of police cases. *Pediatrics*. 2012;129(1):4-12.

78. Marwick AE. To catch a predator? the MySpace moral panic. *First Monday*. 2008;13(6). http://www.firstmonday.dk/ojs/index.php/fm/article/view/2152/1966. Accessed November 17, 2016.

79. Federal Bureau of Investigation. Child predators. the online threat continues to grow. http://www.fbi.gov/news/stories/2011/may/predators_051711. Published May, 2011. Accessed December 30, 2014.

80. Minaya Z. Pedophiles trolling in MySpace raise alarm. http://www.chron.com/business/technology/article/Pedophiles-trolling-in-MySpace-raise-alarm-1476607.php. Published March 3, 2006. Accessed December 30, 2014.

81. Rawe J. How safe is MySpace? http://www.time.com/time/magazine/article/0,9171,1207808,00.html. Published July 3, 2006. Accessed December 30, 2014.

82. Boyd D, Hargittai E, Schultz J, Palfrey J. Why parents help their children lie to Facebook about their age: unintended consequences of the 'Children's Online Privacy Protection Act.' *First Monday*. 2011;26(11). http://firstmonday.org/ojs/index.php/fm/article/view/3850/3075. Accessed December 30, 2014.

83. Madden M, Cortesi S, Gasser U, Lenhart A, Duggan M. Parents, teens, and online privacy. http://pewinternet.org/Reports/2012/Teens-and-Privacy.aspx. Published 2012. Accessed December 30, 2014.

84. Rosen LD, Cheever NA, Carrier LM. The association of parenting style and child age with parental limit setting and adolescent MySpace behavior. *J Appl Dev Psychol*. 2008;29:459-471.

85. Finkelhor D, Mitchell KJ, Wolak J. *Online victimization: A report on the nation's youth*. Alexandria, VA: National Center for Missing and Exploited Children; 2000.

86. Wolak J, Mitchell KJ, Finkelhor D. *Online Victimization: 5 Years Later*. Alexandra, VA: National Center for Missing and Exploited Children; 2006.

87. Wolak J, Finkelhor D, Mitchell KJ, Ybarra ML. Online "predators" and their victims: myths, realities, and implications for prevention and treatment. *Am Psychol*. 2008;63(2):111-128.

88. Priebe G, Mitchell KJ, Finkelhor D. To tell or not to tell? youth's responses to unwanted Internet experiences. *Cyberpsychology: Journal of Psychosocial Research on Cyberspace*. 2013;7(1):Article 6. doi: 10.5817/CP2013-1-6.

89. Wolak J, Finkelhor D, Mitchell K. Internet-initiated sex crimes against minors: implications for prevention based on findings from a national study. *J Adolesc Health*. 2004;35(5):424.e11-424e20.

90. McQuade SC, Sampt N. Survey of Internet and at-risk behaviors. http://scholarworks.rit.edu/article/1424. Published 2008. Accessed December 30, 2014.

91. Baumgartner SE, Valkenburg PM, Peter J. Unwanted online solicitation and risky sexual online behavior across the lifespan. *J Appl Dev Psychol.* 2010;31:439-447.

92. Gallagher B, Fraser C, Christmann K, Hodgson B. *International and Internet Child Sexual Abuse and Exploitation.* Huddersfield, UK: Centre for Applied Childhood Studies; 2006.

93. Canders CP, Merchant RC, Pleet K, Fuerch JH. Internet-initiated sexual assault among U.S. adolescents reported in newspapers, 1996-2007. *J Child Sex Abuse.* 2013;22:987-999.

94. Dowdell EB. Risky Internet behaviors of middle-school students. *CIN: Computers, Informatics, Nursing.* 2011;29(6):362-359.

95. Livingstone S, Smith PK. Annual research review: harms experienced by child users of online and mobile technologies: the nature, prevalence and management of sexual and aggressive risks in the digital age. *Annual Research Review.* 2014;55(6):635-654.

96. Lanning KV. Compliant child victims: confronting an uncomfortable reality. http://www.abusewatch.net/Compliant%20Child%20Victims.pdf. Published 2005. Accessed December 30, 2014.

97. Hinduja S, Patchin JW. Personal information of adolescents on the Internet: a quantitative content analysis of MySpace. *J Adolesc.* 2008;31:125-146.

98. Whittle HC, Hamilton-Giachritisis CE, Beech AR. "Under his spell": victims' perspectives of being groomed online. *Soc Sci.* 2014;3:404-426.

99. Mason A. Kidnapper met Hartford teen on Disney-run site. http://www.nbcconnecticut.com/news/local/Missing-Hartford-Teen-Found-Safe-274676481.html. Published September 12, 2014. Accessed December 30, 2014.

100. Shannon D. Online sexual grooming in Sweden: online and offline sex offences against children as described in Swedish police data. *J Scand Stud Criminol Crime Prev.* 2008;9:160-180.

101. Schrock A, Boyd D. Online threats to youth: solicitation, harassment, and problematic content. http://cyber.law.harvard.edu/sites/cyber.law.harvard.edu/files/RAB_Lit_Review_121808_0.pdf. Published 2008. Accessed December 30, 2014.

102. Biegler S, Boyd D. Risky behaviors and online safety: a 2010 literature review. http://cyber.aw.harvard.edu/node/6228. Published 2010. Accessed December 30, 2014.

103. Soo K, Bodanovskaya Z. Risk factors of becoming a victim of Internet related sexual abuse. In: Ainsaar M, Loof L, eds. *Online Behaviour Related to Child Sexual Abuse: Literature Report.* Stockholm, Sweden: Council of the Baltic States; 2011.

104. Livingstone S. Drawing conclusions from new media research: reflections and puzzles regarding children's experience of the Internet. *The Information Society.* 2006;22:219-230.

105. Livingstone S, Bober M, Helsper E. Active participation or just more information? young people's take-up of opportunities to act and interact on the Internet. *Inf Commun Soc.* 2005;8(3):287-314.

106. Baumgartner SE, Sumter SR, Peter J, Valkenburg PM. Identifying teens at risk: developmental pathways of online and offline sexual risk behavior. *Pediatrics.* 2012;130(6):1489-1496.

107. Wurtele SK. *Safe Connections: A Parent's Guide to Protecting Young Teens from Sexual Exploitation.* Seattle, WA: Parenting Press; 2012.

108. Kierkegaard S. Cybering, online grooming and ageplay. *Computer Law and Security Report.* 2007;24:41-55.

109. Svedin CG. Research evidence in to behavioural patterns which lead to becoming a victim of sexual abuse. In: Ainsaar M, Loof L, eds. *Online Behaviour Related to Child Sexual Abuse: Literature Report.* Stockholm, Sweden: Council of the Baltic States; 2011.

110. Bobkowski PS, Brown JD, Neffa DR. Hit me up and we can get down. *J Child Media.* 2012;6:119-134.

111. Wolak J, Finkelhor D. Are crimes by online predators different from crimes by sex offenders who know youth in-person? *J Adolesc Health.* 2013;53:736-741.

112. Peter J, Valkenburg PM. Adolescents' exposure to sexually explicit material on the Internet. *Commun Res.* 2006;33(2):178-204.

113. Jonsson LS, Priebe G, Bladh M, Svedin CG. Voluntary sexual exposure online among Swedish youth—social background, Internet behavior and psychosocial health. *Comput Hum Behav.* 2014;30:181-190.

114. Temple JR, Paul JA, van den Berg P, Le VD, McElhany A, Temple BW. Teen sexting and its association with sexual behaviors. *Arch Pediatr Adolesc Med.* 2012;166(9):828-833.

115. Mitchell KJ, Finkelhor D, Wolak J, Ybarra ML, Turner H. Youth internet victimization in a broader victimization context. *J Adolesc Health.* 2011;48:128-134.

116. Mitchell KJ, Finkelhor D, Wolak J. Youth Internet users at risk for the most serious online sexual solicitations. *Am J Prev Med.* 2007;32(6):532-537.

117. Noll JG, Shenk CE, Barnes JE, Haralson KJ. Association of maltreatment with high-risk Internet behaviors and offline encounters. *Pediatrics.* 2013;131(2):e510-e517.

118. Noll JG, Shenk CE, Barnes JE, Putnam FW. Childhood abuse, avatar choices, and other risk factors associated with Internet-initiated victimization of adolescent girls. *Pediatrics.* 2009;123(6):e1078-e1083.

119. Wolak J, Mitchell KJ, Finkelhor D. Escaping or connecting? characteristics of youth who form close online relationships. *J Adolesc.* 2003;26:105-119.

120. Bonetti L, Campbell MA, Gilmore L. The relationship of loneliness and social anxiety with children's and adolescents' online communication. *Cyberpsychol Behav Soc Netw.* 2010;13(3):279-285.

121. Whittle H, Hamilton-Giachritsis C, Beech A, Collings G. A review of young people's vulnerabilities to online grooming. *Aggression and Violent Behav.* 2013;18:135-146.

122. Quayle E, Jonsson L, Loof L. *Online Behaviour Related to Sexual Abuse: Interviews with Affected Young People.* Stockholm, Sweden: Council of the Baltic Sea States; 2012.

123. Dombrowski SC, LeMasney JW, Ahia CE, Dickson SA. Protecting children from online sexual predators: technological, psychoeducational, and legal considerations. *Prof Psychol Res Prac.* 2004;35(1):65-73.

124. Van den Heuvel A, Van den Eijnden RJJM, Van Rooij AJ, Van de Mheen D. Meeting online contacts in real life among adolescents: the predictive role of psychosocial wellbeing and internet-specific parenting. *Comput Hum Behav.* 2012;28:465-472.

125. Livingstone S, Helsper EJ. Taking risks when communicating on the Internet: the role of offline social-psychological factors in young people's vulnerability to online risks. *Inf Commun Soc.* 2007;10:619-644.

126. Ybarra ML, Leaf PJ, Diener-West M. Sex differences in youth-reported depressive symptomatology and unwanted internet sexual solicitation. *J Med Internet Res.* 2004;6(1):e5.

127. Steeves V, Webster C. Closing the barn door: The effect of parental supervision on Canadian children's online privacy. *Bull Sci Tech Soc.* 2007;28(4):4-19.

128. Ybarra ML, Mitchell KJ, Finkelhor D, Wolak J. Internet prevention messages: targeting the right online behaviors. *Arch Pediatric Adolesc Med.* 2007;161:138-145.

129. Sengupta A, Chaudhuri A. Are social networking sites a source of online harassment for teens? evidence from survey data. *Child Youth Serv Rev.* 2011;33(2):284-290.

130. Harvard Mental Health Letter. *Protecting children and teens from cyber-harm.* www.health.harvard.edu. Published July 2008. Accessed December 30, 2014.

131. Livingstone S, Helsper E. Balancing opportunities and risks in teenagers' use of the Internet: the role of online skills and Internet self-efficacy. *New Media and Society.* 2010;12(2):309-329.

132. Leander L, Christianson SA, Granhag PA. Internet-initiated sexual abuse: adolescent victims' reports about on- and off-line sexual activities. *Appl Cog Psychol.* 2008;22:1260-1274.

133. Malesky LA, Jr. Predatory online behavior: modus operandi of convicted sex offenders in identifying potential victims and contacting minors over the Internet. J Child Sex Abuse. 2007;16:23-32.

134. Wurtele SK, Kenny MC. Preventing online sexual victimization of youth. *The Journal of Behavior Analysis of Offender and Victim Treatment and Prevention.* 2010;2(1):63-73.

135. Moreno MA, Parks MR, Zimmerman FJ, Brito TE, Christakis DA. Display of health risk behaviors on MySpace by adolescents. *Arch Pediatr Adolesc Med.* 2009;163(1):27-34.

136. Doornwaard SM, Moreno MA, van den Eijnden RJJM, Vanwesenbeeck I, ter Bogt TFM. Young adolescents' sexual and romantic reference displays on Facebook. *J Adolesc Health.* 2014;55:535-541.

137. Wishart J. Internet safety in emerging educational contexts. *Comput Educ.* 2004;43:193-204.

138. Mitchell KJ, Wolak J, Finkelhor D. Are blogs putting youth at risk for online sexual solicitation or harassment? *Child Abuse Negl.* 2008;32:277-294.

139. Ybarra ML, Mitchell KJ. Exposure to Internet pornography among children and adolescents: a national survey. *Cyberpsychology and Behavior.* 2005;8(5):473-486.

140. Svedin CG, Akerman I, Priebe G. Frequent users of pornography. a population based epidemiological study of Swedish male adolescents. *J Adolesc.* 2011;34:779-788.

141. Peter J, Valkenburg PM. The use of sexually explicit Internet material and its antecedents: a longitudinal comparison of adolescents and adults. *Archives Sex Behav.* 2011;40:1015-1025.

142. Mesch GS. Social bonds and Internet pornographic exposure among adolescents. *J Adolesc.* 2009;32:601-618.

143. Sinkovic M, Stulhofer A, Bozic J. Revisiting the association between pornography use and risky sexual behaviors: the role of early exposure to pornography and sexual sensation seeking. *J Sex Res.* 2013;50(7):633-641.

144. Luder MT, Pittet I, Berchtold A, Akre C, Michaud PA, Suris JC. Associations between online pornography and sexual behavior among adolescents: myth or reality? *Arch Sex Behav.* 2011;40:1027-1035.

145. Houck CD, Barker D, Rizzo C, Hancock E, Norton A, Brown LK. Sexting and sexual behavior in at-risk adolescents. *Pediatrics.* 2014;133(2):e276-e282.

146. Rice E, Rhoades H, Winetrobe H, et al. Sexually explicit cell phone messaging associated with sexual risk among adolescents. *Pediatrics.* 2012;130(4):667-673.

147. Elliott IA, Ashfield S. The use of online technology in the modus operandi of female sex offenders. *J Sex Aggress.* 2011;17(1):92-104.

148. Seto MC, Wood JM, Babchishin KM, Flynn S. Online solicitation offenders are different from child pornography offenders and lower risk contact sexual offenders. *Law Hum Behav.* 2012;36(4):320-330.

149. Loughlin J, Taylor-Butts A. Child luring through the Internet. http://www.statcan.gc.ca/pub/85-002-x/2009001/article/10783-eng.pdf/ Published March 2009. Accessed December 30, 2014.

150. Lanning KV. Cyber "pedophiles:" a behavioral perspective. In: Borgeson K, Kuehnle K, eds. *Serial Offenders: Theory and Practice.* Sudbury, MA: Jones and Bartlett Learning, LLC; 2012:71-78.

151. Babchishin KM, Hanson R, Hermann CA. The characteristics of online sex offenders: a meta-analysis. *Sex Abuse.* 2011;23(1):92-123.

152. Briggs P, Simon WT, Simonsen S. An exploratory study of Internet-initiated sexual offenses and the chat room sex offender: has the Internet enabled a new typology of sex offender? *Sex Abuse.* 2011;23(1):72-91.

153. Levy P. Charges: man may have used Facebook to lure young sex-assault victims. http://www.startribune.com/local/north/239633961.html. Published January 10, 2014. Accessed December 30, 2014.

154. Burke L. Memoirs of a pedophile's victim. http://www.wired.com/culture/lifestyle/news/2000/04/35843. Published April 4, 2000. Accessed December 30, 2014.

155. Craven S, Brown S, Gilchrist E. Sexual grooming of children: review of literature and theoretical considerations. *J Sex Aggress.* 2006;12:287-299.

156. McAlinden AM. "Setting 'em up": personal, familial and institutional grooming in the sexual abuse of children. *Soc Leg Studies.* 2006;15(3):339-362.

157. Wurtele SK. Prevention the sexual exploitation of minors in youth-servicing organizations. *Child Youth Serv Rev.* 2012;34:2442-2453.

158. Katz C. Internet-related child sexual abuse: what children tell us in their testimonies. *Child Youth Serv Rev.* 2013;35:1536-1542.

159. Williams R, Elliott IA, Beech AR. Identifying sexual grooming themes used by Internet sex offenders. *Dev Behav.* 2013;34:135-152.

160. Whittle H, Hamilton-Giachritsis C, Beech A, Collings G. A review of online grooming: characteristics and concerns. *Aggression and Violent Behavior.* 2013;18:62-70.

161. Kloess JA, Beech AR, Hrakins L. Online child sexual exploitation: prevalence, process, and offender characteristics. *Trauma Violence Abuse.* 2014;15(2):126-139.

162. O'Connell R. *A Typology of Child Cybersexploitation and Online Grooming Practices.* Lancashire, UK: Cyberspace Research Unit, University of Central Lancashire; 2003.

163. Seto M. *Pedophilia and Sexual Offending Against Children: Theory, assessment, and Intervention.* Washington, DC: American Psychological Association; 2008.

164. Ruiz T. Colorado Springs police pose as student to catch accused child predator. http://www.fox21news.com/news/story.aspx?id=997557#. Published January 22, 2014. Accessed December 30, 2014.

165. Preston J. Rules to stop pupil and teacher from getting too social online. *New York Times.* December 17, 2011. http://www.nytimes.com/2011/12/18/business/media/rules-to-limit-how-teachers-and-students-interact-online.html. Accessed December 30, 2014.

166. Oglesby C. Cells, texting give predators secret path to kids. http://www.cnn.com/2008/CRIME/01/11/teachers.charged/index.html. Published January 11, 2008.

167. Layton MJ, Diskin C. Sex abuse in schools: prosecutors say manipulation often begins with a text or email. http://www.northjersey.com/news/138307709_Sex_abuse_in_school__Rise_in_arrests_is_a_troubling_trend.html. Published January 30, 2012. Accessed December 30, 2014.

168. Michael M. Police say assistant principal sent nude pics to teen. http://www.wtsp.com/news/local/story.aspx:storyid=132470#. Published 2010. Accessed December 30, 2014.

169. McCartan KF, McAlister R. Mobile phone technology and sexual abuse. *Inf Commun Tech Law.* 2012;21(3):257-268.

170. Joas J. Nicole Kurowski, Tulpehocken teacher, had sexual relationship with school senior, police say. WFMZ-TV 69 News Web site. http://www.wfmz.com/news/news-regional-berks/nicole-kurowski-tulpehocken-teacher-had-sexual-relationship-with-school-senior-police-say/-/121418/22835418/-/l51ct7z/-/index.html. Published November 6, 2013. Accessed December 30, 2014.

171. Ramirez D, Jr. Frisco coach faces sexual assault charge. http://www.star-telegram.com/2014/01/23/5509032/frisco-coach-faces-sexual-assault.html. Published January 23, 2014. Accessed December 30, 2014.

172. Buettner R. Queens teacher accused of sex with boy, 14. *New York Times.* May 29, 2009. http://www.nytimes.com/2009/05/29/nyregion/29statutory.html?_r=0. Accessed December 30, 2014.

173. Wurtele SK, Miller-Perrin C. Preventing technology-initiated sexual victimization of youth: a developmental perspective. In: Kenny MC, ed. *Sex Education: Attitude of Adolescents, Cultural Differences and Schools' Challenges.* New York, NY: Nova Publishers; 2014.

174. Finkelhor D, Wolak J, Mitchell KJ. Online safety: why research is important. http://publius.cc. Published June 11, 2010. Accessed December 30, 2014.

175. Doring N. Consensual sexting among adolescents: risk prevention through abstinence education or safer sexting? *Cyberpsychology: Journal of Psychosocial Research on Cyberspace.* 2014;8(1):Article 9. doi:10.5817/CP2014-1-9.

176. Albury K, Crawford K. Sexting, consent and young people's ethics: beyond Megan's story. *Continuum.* 2012;26:463-473.

177. Tynes BM. Internet safety gone wild? sacrificing the educational and psychosocial benefits of online social environments. *J Adolesc Res.* 2007;22:575-584.

178. Associated Press. Lincoln man, 20, charged with child sex assault. http://www.1011now.com/home/headlines/Lincoln-man-charged-with-child-sex-assault-234920831.html. Published December 8, 2013. Accessed December 30, 2014.

179. Atkinson C, Newton D. Online behaviors of adolescents: victims, perpetrators and Web 2.0. *J Sex Aggress.* 2010;16(1):107-120.

180. Alford S. Abstinence-only-until-marriage programs: ineffective, unethical, and poor public health. www.advocatesforyouth/PUBLICATIONS/policybrief/pbabonly.pdf. Published 2012. Accessed December 30, 2014.

181. Jolicoeur M, Zedlewski E. *Much Ado About Sexting.* Washington, DC: National Criminal Justice Reference Service; 2010.

182. Davidson JC, Martellozzo E. Protecting vulnerable young people in cyberspace from sexual abuse: raising awareness and responding globally. *Police Pract Res.* 2008;9(4):277-289.

183. Oudekerk BA, Farr RH, Reppucci ND. Is it love or sexual abuse? young adults' perceptions of statutory rape. *J Child Sex Abuse.* 2013;22(7):858-877.

184. Livingstone S, Bober M. U.K. children go on line: final report of key project findings (Economic and Social Research Council). http://www.lse.ac.uk/collections/children-go-online/UKCGOfinalReport.pdf. Published 2005. Accessed December 14, 2016.

185. Palasinski M. The roles of monitoring and cyberbystanders in reducing sexual abuse. *Comput Hum Behav.* 2012;28:2014-2022.

186. Burrow-Sanchez JJ, Call ME, Zheng R, Drew CJ. How school counselors can help prevent online victimization. *J Counsel Dev.* 2011;89:3-10.

187. Bilmes D. The realities of sexting (you can't unsend!). *School Library Journal.* 2011;57(2):54-55.

188. Jones LM, Mitchell KJ, Walsh WA. *Evaluation of Internet Child Safety Materials Used by ICAC Task Forces in School and Community Settings, Executive Summary.* Washington, DC: National Criminal Justice Reference Service; 2012.

189. Finkelhor D. Commentary: cause for alarm? youth and internet risk research: a commentary on Livingstone and Smith (2014). *J Child Psychol Psychiatry.* 2014;55(6):655-658.

190. Jones LM. The future of Internet safety education: critical lessons from four decades of youth drug abuse prevention. http://publius.cc/printpdf/future_internet_safety_education_critical_lessons_four_decades_youth_drug_abuse_prevention. Published 2010. Accessed December 30, 2014.

191. Wurtele SK. Preventing sexual abuse of children in the 21st century: Preparing for challenges and opportunities. *J Child Sex Abuse.* 2009;18:1-18.

192. Boies SC, Knudson G, Young J. The Internet, sex, and youths: implications for sexual development. *Sex Addict Compulsivity.* 2004;11:343-363.

193. Borzekowski DLG. Adolescents' use of the Internet: a controversial, coming-of-age resource. *Adolescence Medical Clinic.* 2006;17(1):205-216.

194. Gill HK, Gill N, Young SD. Online technologies for health information and education: a literature review. *J Consum Health Internet.* 2013;17(2):139-150.

195. Dowdell EB. Use of the Internet by parents of middle school students: Internet rules, risky behaviours and online concerns. *J Psychiatr Ment Health Nurs.* 2013;20:9-16.

196. Dombrowski SC, Gischlar KL, Durst T. Safeguarding young people from cyber pornography and cyber sexual predation: a major dilemma of the Internet. *Child Abuse Rev.* 2007;16(3):153-170.

197. Wurtele SK, Berkower F. *Off Limits: A Parent's Guide to Keeping Kids Safe from Sexual Abuse.* Brandon, VT: Safer Society Press; 2010.

198. Yan Z. Useful resources, important messages: The explosion of parenting books on adolescents and social networking sites. *J Appl Dev Psychol.* 2008;29:472-474.

199. O'Neill B, McLaughlin S. *Recommendations on Safety Initiatives.* London, UK: EU Kids Online; 2010.

200. Moreno MA, Egan KG, Bare K, Young HN, Cox ED. Internet safety education for youth: stakeholder perspectives. *BMC Publ Health.* 2013;13(543):1-6.

201. Liau AK, Khoo A, Ang PH. Factors influencing adolescents engagement in risky Internet behavior. *Cyberpsychology and Behavior.* 2005;8(6):513-520.

202. Fleming MJ, Greentree S, Cocotti-Muller D, Elias KA, Morrison S. Safety in cyberspace: adolescents' safety and exposure online. *Youth Soc.* 2006;38(2):135-154.

203. Wildsmith E, Barry M, Manlove J, Vaughn B. Dating and sexual relationships. http://www.childtrends.org/wp-content/uploads/2013/10/2013-04DatingSexual Relationships.pdf. Published October 2013. Accessed December 30, 2014.

204. Chen DW, McGeehan P. Social media rules limit New York student-teacher contact. *New York Times.* May 1, 2012. http://www.nytimes.com/2012/05/01/nyregion/social-media-rules-for-nyc-school-staff-limits-contact-with-students.html. Accessed December 30, 2014.

205. Billups A. School districts paint dark picture of 'sexting' danger. *Washington Times.* July 23, 2009. http://www.washingtontimes.com/news/2009/jul/23/school-districts-hope-students-get-the-picture-abo/. Accessed December 30, 2014.

206. Klein R. West Virginia bans sexting between juveniles while creating educational diversion program. http://www.huffingtonpost.com/2013/05/13/west-virgina-sexting-law-educational-diversion-program_n_3266643.html. Published May 13, 2013. Accessed December 30, 2014.

207. USA Swimming. *Safe Sport Handbook.* Colorado Springs, CO: USA Swimming; 2013.

208. Berson IR, Berson MJ, Ferron JM. Emerging risks of violence in the digital age: lessons for educators from an online study of adolescent girls in the United States. *J Sch Violence.* 2002;1:51-72.

Section IV

Conclusion

Chapter 20

Future of Child Abuse Prevention

Randell Alexander, MD, PhD

Introduction

What exactly is child abuse prevention? Can child abuse even be eliminated, significantly reduced, or marginally impacted? Considering the multiple approaches to child abuse prevention that already exist, what are the best approaches at this time? What is the balance between approaches that emphasize short-term successes and long-term impact? Significantly, what are the factors that help to shape the answers to these questions? Building on the understanding of child abuse prevention to date, this chapter proposes key issues that should form the basis for a more coherent approach to preventing the problem, and research that would help advance the field.

Negative Perception of Child Abuse

That child abuse is undesirable does not seem to be seriously in question. Even by 1999, Prevent Child Abuse America in its annual survey was able to show that:

1. Physical punishment and repeated yelling and swearing were viewed as detrimental by most respondents.
2. Parents reported using less physical punishment than 11 years earlier.
3. Decreases in physical punishment cut across all demographic groups.
4. Almost two-thirds of parents said they would take action if they observed an act of abuse or neglect.
5. Actual and potential recipients of home visitation services endorsed the approach and "overwhelmingly support government investment in strategies to support newborns and their parents."[1]

Even if physical punishment actually remained the same and the parents were more embarrassed to admit to it, this represents a significant attitudinal shift. While there may be differences of opinion over specific practices between different segments of society over issues such as corporal punishment in schools and homes, sexual boundaries, whether certain practices constitute neglect (eg, pool drownings with toddlers), and what verbal practices are emotionally damaging; there seem to be no significant arguments about more extreme forms of abuse (eg, severe beatings, sex with young children, more torturous confinement or chronic verbal assaults). Thus, the concept of child abuse now enjoys more universal condemnation (eg, the UN Declaration on the Rights of the Child) than in centuries past.

The perception that child abuse is bad is an important precursor to prevention. It is difficult to effect change if most parents fail to recognize the problem even exists.

Difficult as it sometimes may be to generate excitement and change with current child abuse prevention approaches, hundreds of years ago such thoughts would not have been seriously entertained. Hundreds of years ago there were no programs to prevent child abuse. For much of human history, children have been treated as property, and one can do no wrong to property.

However, for the last several centuries there have been positive changes in the perception of children. One advance has been the increase in children living to adulthood, in part through improvements in sanitation. This may enable greater attachment by parents to children. Children are more likely to have legal protections such as mandatory schooling and being kept outside of the workplace in many countries. Another change is the perception of abuse itself. In the 1860s, Ambroise Tardeau was the head of pathology in Paris, France.[2] While he described many of the findings recognized today as physical abuse and correctly said that parents abused children, he was about 100 years early for public acceptance. Thus, his efforts did not result in significant practice changes. Likewise, until there is some agreement that child abuse is a problem and is preventable, there is unlikely to be any emphasis to prevent it. Fortunately the tide of history has altered public perceptions about child abuse, aided by specific efforts by many groups, such as Prevent Child Abuse America, the American Academy of Pediatrics, the media, and others. Even with awareness and agreement about child abuse being wrong, the public and decisions-makers may not believe it is preventable, that it is just "bad parents" who need to be fixed, and that it does not affect them personally.

Rationale for Child Abuse Prevention

Nearly 100 years after Tardieu,[2] child abuse recognition was catapulted to national attention in the United States by Dr. Henry Kempe (pediatrician) and his 4 colleagues (3 specialized in radiology, psychiatry, and obstetrics) in the 1962 publication "The Battered Child Syndrome" in the *Journal of the American Medical Association*.[3] The timing in human history (at least for the United States) was ripe. As a result of this publication, all 50 states adopted child abuse reporting laws in 5 years. A host of other changes in the United States also occurred. In 1974, the Child Abuse Prevention and Treatment Act (CAPTA) was passed by Congress and it enabled billions of dollars to be spent on child abuse services, but did not fund robust primary prevention efforts, including funding for evaluation. Despite the multidisciplinary health approach represented by the authors of "The Battered Child Syndrome," until recently child abuse practice and research has been better funded in social and justice arenas than health. In the last decade, the Centers for Disease Control and Prevention (CDC) has taken a lead by funding several research projects on child abuse prevention (eg, shaken baby prevention research, primary sexual abuse prevention). But most child abuse prevention occurs at the state level through children's trust/prevention funds or their equivalent.

Social services interventions have been the bulwark of child protection for the last half century. Only a small fraction of cases seen by child protective services actually end up in court, usually juvenile court or its equivalent. Even though only a small fraction of cases are seen by child protective services (CPS) and even less end up in court, child abuse recognition and intervention has been primarily seen as and approached as a social service and justice problem to solve. However, many more children are abused who never come to the attention of authorities, perhaps 3 to 4 times as many. Each of these children also represents a health concern.

When proposing a social, justice, or health intervention, it is best to identify as precisely as possible what the actual harm exists that is being addressed. This is a product of both individual harm and collective cost to society. Saying that child abuse is bad or illegal begs the question, why are there laws about sexual abuse, and what is the reasoning behind them? Once the harms are better understood, then perhaps the prevention can be better focused prevention.

For example, sexual abuse of young children is illegal and widely perceived as immoral. But what are the harms beyond its illegality? Sometimes it is perceived that a young child suffers a physical injury and suffers as a consequence. Yet only about 5% of prepubescent girls (and even fewer boys) have an injury on medical examination by trained personnel.[4] Not only are the vast majority of instances of sexual abuse without physical injury, but sometimes magnification with special cameras is needed to see what are very small injuries. Such injuries usually need to be seen quickly or they will heal before the examiner can document them. If physical genital injury is the criterion, it is not a compelling rationale for stringent laws about sexual abuse. Ownership could be another rationale for such laws. If a child is perceived in a society as belonging to a parent, sexual abuse represents a concomitant assault against the parent. In a society that puts a high value on virginity, violation of a girl especially may represent an economic loss, consign the girl to an inferior societal status, and be seen as a matter of honor. These represent social and emotional harms. And in a society that is child focused, such laws might represent the observation that children are harmed by sexual abuse—emotionally in the short term, behaviorally and with changes in life trajectory in the long term.

There is now a considerable amount of research on the health harms of adverse childhood experiences (ACEs), much of which is child abuse.[5,6] This dovetails with other studies and clinical experience that indicates that child abuse often has a lasting impact. Problems such as substance abuse and alcoholism appear to represent self-treatment of childhood traumas, whereas some use legal and illegal prescriptions to achieve the same results. The health harms into adulthood of child abuse are intense and extensive.

Child abuse prevention has multiple justifications. If child abuse were to be prevented, there are at least 5 main consequences:

1. Reduction of child abuse would reduce violent crime.[7] It is conservatively estimated that child abuse results in an additional 35 000 violent criminals and more than 250 murderers in the United States each year. Considering that much crime is drug related and that many victims of child abuse "treat" themselves with legal and legal substances, the number of criminals and costs are undoubtedly much higher.
2. It would save money, at least $124 billion in the United States each year.[8] Over 69% of this savings would be for lost productivity. Health care costs more directly associated with child abuse are approximately 20% of this total, with special education, criminal justice, and child welfare costs estimated as being between 3% to 4% each. In comparison, the costs of the combined Afghanistan and Iraq wars were estimated by the Congressional Research Service to be about $131.7 billion in fiscal year 2012.[9]
3. Child abuse prevention would reduce health care costs throughout the lifespan.[5] Child abuse is the major predictor of substance abuse and mental health in adulthood, as victims of abuse suffer from their past and try to treat it. The burden of years lost, medications, and lost quality of life have yet to be fully calculated.
4. Child abuse prevention would reduce changes in the brain for many victims. A child who grows up with some form of child abuse lives in a different perceptual

world than one who has a safe, stable, stimulating, and nurturing environment. Neurochemical pathways develop in response to the world the child actually experiences, and brain architecture develops or fails to develop accordingly.[10] These alterations in brains and functions sometimes manifest with health, crime, and behavioral consequences.

5. Prevention would reduce the humanitarian burden of pain, suffering, and death. Most parents probably regard newborns as full of promise and anticipate years of amiable companionship. Few probably have babies with the intent to sexually abuse them, beat them, or to neglect them.

The goal of child abuse prevention is not only to reduce the harms perpetrated on children, but to encourage the positive development of creating better brains and healthier bodies. While social and justice concerns are ongoing problems, the health consequences are becoming increasingly evident. Media attention for cases of abuse is high compared to 50 years ago. Regardless of what might motivate a single individual, the awareness of child abuse and the rationale for its prevention seems to have gained societal traction.

Methods to Prevent Child Abuse Must Be Made at Multiple Levels

If a single intervention radically reduced child abuse, it could be argued that after 50 years of child abuse prevention efforts, such an intervention would be known and widely disseminated. While this is in part an *a posteriori* argument, the reality is that even if there is a decrease in child abuse, it does not seem to be the result of any known program. This does not, however, negate the possibility of a local effect.

Child abuse prevention inherently means that adult behaviors must change or that acceptable behaviors be taught where little currently exists.

1. There appears to be no strong argument that characteristics of a child are so compelling to elicit abuse.

2. Almost always, adults do not have a knowledge deficit but a motivational deficit. While some pregnancies might not be planned, it is unlikely that adults have children with the intent of having someone to hit, sexually abuse, or to neglect.

3. Many adults are reluctant to change. Interventions require personal effort for caregivers who may have many other demands or difficulties in their lives. Child abuse prevention can also seem discordant with adults' personal beliefs.

4. Often there is no long-standing community expectation for an intervention and the effort may feel unnatural to the intended recipient. Home visitation could seem this way in some countries, whereas in England, even royalty has home visitors.

While adult change might be accomplished in a one-to-one manner, there is too much abuse and too few resources to imagine this will make substantial change. Rather, efforts directed at key levels that build upon each other might have the potential of changing a segment of society. If a shift in community thinking and behaviors begins to occur, the hope is that this will snowball into a more widespread effect. This is not unreasonable. The Back to Sleep campaign by the American Academy of Pediatrics benefits beyond the one-to-one encounters of the pediatrician and parent. This has been adopted by many in the community and the message transcends the pediatric contribution to the effort. If sufficient numbers of people conform to the expected behaviors, this might achieve a self-perpetuating process of attitudinal and behavioral change. The hope is that like "herd immunity," only some subset of people need to be changed to propagate the desired population result. This means not only altering individual parents but altering the social and economic conditions that make some children and families more at risk of abuse/abusing.

Prevention can occur at different levels:

1. Primary prevention targets a large nonselected population before abuse occurs. Safety messages about unsafe sleep are universal.
2. Secondary prevention targets at-risk populations before abuse occurs. Some home visitation works with families who have been screened as being at a higher risk.
3. Tertiary prevention aims at reabuse, in which the target audience has already abused and the effort is to stop it from occurring again. An example might be parenting classes for those who have hurt a child.

An alternative formulation is:

1. ***Universal***: Everyone regardless of risk
2. ***Targeted***: Those most at risk
3. ***Indicated***: Those who have already committed abuse

Child abuse professionals also consider the social ecology level of the strategy: individual, community, or societal. None of these levels are exclusive of the other, and it is likely best that all be considered.

Figure 20-1 depicts a variety of levels and potential interventions. Efforts at the top require the most individual effort and affect the least number of people. In general, and if possible, the widest impact would be to change societal norms, rather than try to solve the problem by individual interventions. Interventions earlier in life (eg, prenatal, in infancy) make more of a long-term impact than those later in life. However, this does not mean that intimate partner violence or elder abuse are not important or deserving; rather, the pyramid suggests a more optimal balance to prevention based on likely impact.

Figure 20-1. *Health impact of different levels of intervention. Adapted from Frieden T.*[11]

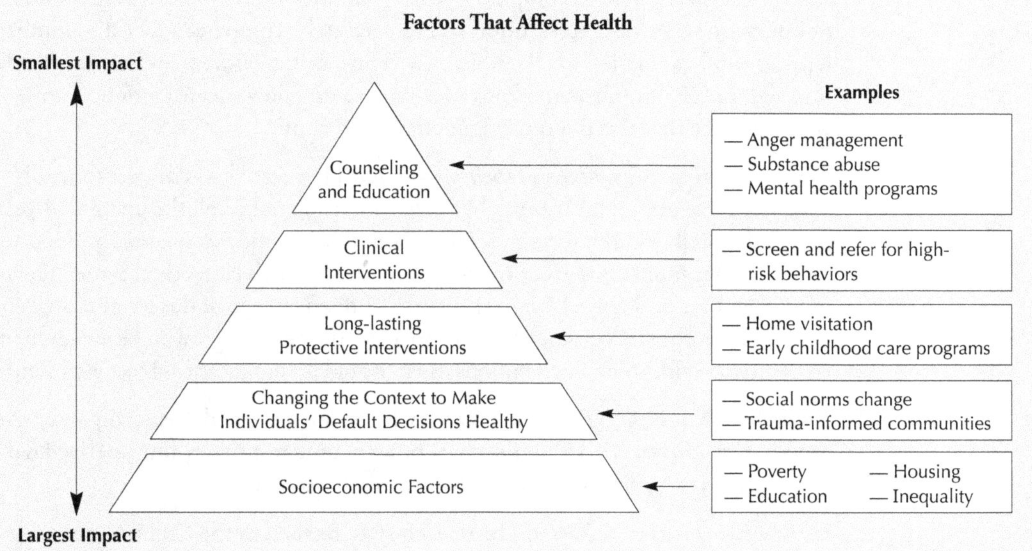

Figure 20-1

Assessment of Prevention

Currently there is significant disagreement about whether child abuse is decreasing or remaining the same. National Child Abuse and Neglect Data System (NCANDS) data, which relies on reports by individual states, has shown a decrease in sexual abuse and an apparent decrease in physical abuse.[12] These findings have been criticized as overly reliant on child protective services reports which are dependent on state definitions which can change to make it seem like there is less child abuse. However, neglect is more likely than sexual abuse to be susceptible to such interpretations and neglect rates have remained about the same. The *Fourth National Incidence Study of Child Abuse and Neglect (NIS-4)* has shown similar results.[13] Others have shown that serious physical abuse has increased.[14] It has been pointed out that Internet child pornography did not exist prior to 1995, and that this should be factored in when discussing any reported decrease in sexual abuse (S. Cooper, personal communication). While there may not be agreement about the course of child abuse statistics, and while it may take surveys of adults conducted years from now looking backwards to give the most complete picture, such numbers, with their limitations, may serve as useful benchmarks to see if child abuse prevention is making an impact.

A truism in many professions is that if it is not documented it did not occur. Likewise, if prevention is not tested, it cannot be safely said that it actually prevented anything. For funders and policy makers there may be a bottom line of proof that will eventually be required. There is also an ethical obligation to volunteers and those working in the field at low salaries because they believe in the work. For them, it is important that the mission is helping children and not wasting their time. Thus, assessment is not a process added onto a program but a vital, integral part of the entire process. This means that planning the assessment should occur simultaneously with the development of the proposal itself. For community efforts this may require collaboration with universities or other organizations with statistical skills. This may be facilitated by a statewide organization or through a collaborative of like-minded groups.

To assess prevention success requires careful development of exactly what is being measured. Is the outcome less child abuse? This might be measured in distinctly different ways:

1. ***Decrease in CPS numbers***: But the intervention would need to be taken to scale if state numbers are used to compare 1 year vs. another, or certain catchment areas of intervention vs. nonintervention would need to be compared. Yet CPS numbers represent only a fraction of all child abuse. Thus, this measurement more correctly is to reduce CPS numbers (perhaps over-representing low socioeconomic status) with the hope that this is a proxy for actual child abuse.

2. ***Decrease in reports by adults of their own abuse***: However, this is subject to recall bias. The most important bias might be that adults do not recall the first 3 or 4 years of their life well, and numbers they report would be an underestimation of the true incidence. Yet numbers derived by this approach are much larger than those known to CPS and are probably closer to the truth.[5] A disadvantage of this longitudinal approach is that it takes considerable time to allow the child to grow to be an adult and report back. With some interventions, there would be significant subject attrition.

3. ***An approach akin to NIS-4***: This is a very labor-intensive and financially intensive process that improves on CPS numbers but still underestimates adult-derived data. It is probably beyond the possibilities of most assessments.

4. ***Child abuse proxies***: This could be scoring systems such as the Child Abuse Potential Inventory or similar measures. The difficulty is that such measures do not actually measure abuse or all types of abuse.

Alternative measures could be to look at well-being, improved behaviors, and health behaviors; reduced negative parenting (by report or observation), such as less hitting; and better measures of the child. Reduction of hospital admissions for selected forms of child abuse is probably resistant to definitional controversies and a more stable measure of potential change (ie, abusive head trauma cases in the intensive care unit are probably diagnosed the same over time and the number can be trusted with a high degree of confidence).

Assessment also entails a deeper understanding of the harms of abuse so that it can be known if this is being impacted. Currently the field is not sophisticated enough to compare brain imaging to measure neurological effects[10] or to judge the effect of telomeres,[15] but it is important to know such harms exist and are the final stages in how abuse hurts the child. Health outcomes of adults may also serve as an indirect proxy for reducing abuse in the future; however, this requires substantial longitudinal study and would be difficult to attribute to any single set of interventions, should a reduction in negative health consequences be shown to occur.

Child Abuse Prevention Must be Taken to Scale

Many of the interventions described in the literature, and the many more that are not reported, are based on a community effort. Assume that the intervention was successful. Rarely would it then be seen as a pilot to be developed into a state or national program. Perhaps Healthy Families America, Parents Anonymous, and to a lesser extent, Triple P have tried to have a focus beyond just one community. Yet these efforts have not enjoyed substantial national funding nor have the programs been disseminated as much as desired. Recent substantial increased federal funding for home visitation may be a rare counterexample.

One of the problems in capturing the interest of funders is showing that an intervention not only makes a difference but that it makes a substantial difference. If interventions remain on a small scale they will remain "promising" but will not attract as much attention as an effective effort would warrant. While this might be personally discouraging for the developers, the real loss is the children whose abuse is not prevented.

A small dose of prevention is akin to partially treated meningitis. If a small dose of antibiotics is given, the disease simmers but is not truly cured. While a complex plan of how all the components of a child abuse prevention approach fit together is vital to overall success, interventions that build upon each other over a sustained period of time may fail if the components are not supported financially.

There has been some movement for funders, both government and foundations to recognize that support is needed for evaluation, as well as program delivery, and to move more toward funding outcomes not just programs.

Complex Planning

Child abuse prevention is not as simple as picking a program that seemingly works and replicating it. To truly change human behavior enough to better protect and nurture children requires more sophisticated planning and attention to what it is that is actually hoped to be achieved. CDC's Essentials for Childhood identifies safe, stable, nurturing relationships and environments are essential to prevent child maltreatment and assure children reach their full potential.[16] Essentials for Childhood identifies raising awareness and commitment, using data to inform action, creating the context for healthy children and families through changing norms, programs and policies as important for building a comprehensive foundation of safety, stability, and nurturing relationships for children both in their caregiving and broader social environment. CDC is working with state health departments and their traditional and nontraditional partners to use a collective impact process to identify common strategies in each of the areas to assure safe, stable, nurturing relationships and environments for children in their state and prevent child maltreatment.

Any attempt to modify perceptual or behavioral responses should consider that there is no single point in time that is immutable. Perceptions and behaviors are not constant but change in reaction to the environment and consequences of actions. The person you see now is not the person you will see later. An analogy that has been used in other contexts is to consider a person's life as a stream. Many efforts attempt to understand and to intervene to treat a child and a family as if they were a moment in time rather than changing processes. This can reduce the likelihood of success if strategies do not take this into account.

A key principle of ecological psychology is that change is a fluid process and that in the process of creating change the environment is altered, feedback loops are in play, and the process spirals forward.[17] Thus to say that child abuse is a circular process in this view is wrong. Rather than a cycle that repeats itself over generations, it should be viewed as a spiral capable of modifications. This then presents an opportunity for change, but one that competes with a dynamic organism that is undergoing numerous stimuli (good and bad) far beyond the prevention intervention itself.

In this view, it is simplistic to talk about child abuse prevention as if it was a category, with detection, intervention, and treatment as other categories of human effort. Not only does this detract from the dynamic nature of a child and family's life, but it tends to perpetuate child abuse as an industry. This is contrary to viewing child abuse as a problem to be solved rather than managed.

An alternative way to conceptualize child abuse is not "prevention" per se but in terms of alternate realities. Regardless of whether child abuse prevention programs exist, whether there are nurturing programs, or what the societal environment is, the child will experience a reality. This reality will shape the child's brain by selecting brain cells that are needed for the environment the child actually experiences, neurohormonal axes that are prepared for either benign or hostile surroundings, and corresponding changes that affect diseases and conditions of adulthood. But which reality? In this view, child abuse prevention is any effort that shapes a reality that is judged healthier or more desirable than other alternatives. This approach does not depend on programs or conventional ways to view child abuse prevention. Rather, any creative way to positively impact a child's physical and mental development is the goal. Child abuse is only one of the outcomes if an undesirable alternative reality is allowed to exist. Thus child abuse prevention is perhaps too narrow, and efforts like the CDC's Essentials for Childhood to promote safe, stable, nurturing, and stimulating relationships and environments is the better goal.

If achievement of a more positive alternative reality is the desired outcome, how is it possible to simultaneously intervene both in parallel and sequentially to drive toward multiple goals? And how does this philosophical approach translate into action? Interventions and alterations can take a variety of forms:

1. Intervene at different points in a person's life, knowing that the impact is most long-lasting (by definition) if done earlier. When altering the path of a moving object, for example, a gentle nudge at the beginning has a larger effect than the same force applied later.
2. Shape the individual, family, community, and society, preferably simultaneously. If not, shape as many factors as possible.

3. One highly effective short-term intervention may not have the impact that repeated interventions have over time. Like other organisms, humans often are not 1-trial learners.

4. Because an intervention changes the environment the organism experiences and has an effect on the organism itself, further interventions should build upon this. To prevent child abuse this may mean trying an intervention, determining its effect on a person, and adjusting the next one accordingly. More advanced planning might incorporate multiple synergistic approaches. A community might begin with a media campaign to draw attention to some issue, have live interactive activities to further the awareness (eg, a parade or race), have periodic media reminders (eg, newspapers, TV), have selective interventions for high-risk groups or with people at moments of opportunity (eg, hospital at the birth of a child), have different messages for different ages (eg, middle school program, music messages for young adults), and outcome measures. It is not enough to just have a comprehensive approach, although theoretically desirable, but it is even better to persist with tailored messages and activities that change with the population's attitudes and behaviors.

5. Because the child and family may live in an environment in which negative factors come into play, efforts must be intense and/or prolonged to counter the persistence of the negative factors. For example, substance abuse rehabilitation programs must consider that if the person returns to the same environment that old habits may reinstitute themselves.

6. An alternative is to create an entirely new environment. This disrupts some old habits and better enables new behaviors. The disadvantage is that families cannot easily disrupt their whole lives, cannot always move to a new location with new friends, and often, the goal is for children to live with their families. This may mean changing the environment in the current location.

7. Sometimes alterations in perception or preference have to be incorporated by the caregivers in the dynamic flow of their life. This may not be entirely desired or consensual. A parent may not want to quit smoking, drinking, or using drugs, even if it is harmful to the child, they may want to use harsh punishment to change children's behaviors or to exact retribution, and most difficult to change, they may want to persist in having sex with children. Prevention efforts would be stronger if they not only modified behaviors but exacted real change in the persons themselves.

This last point can be illustrated by examples:

— A caregiver might not perceive that their house is especially dirty and unsafe. Perhaps this is the way they were raised. Visitation programs might help to model a different environment and actually alter the tolerances a person might have for their own house hygiene.

— Some people report that they have no problem with hitting their child and leaving bruises and that they would do it again. Perhaps a subset of those who endorse these ideas would respond to learning about the long-term effect of such actions, particularly in light of work with the Adverse Childhood Experiences study[5] and research showing that physical abuse actually changes the DNA within a person's cells.[15] By creating a different way of viewing the situation, the caregiver might alter future behavior.

— A primary prevention program might be created that would help a person with feelings about having sex with children and create a diversion or model of how to act that would spare children from being sexually abused and the potential perpetrator from severe societal sanctions. To change perceptions or preferences, such an approach would have to diminish sexual arousal to the stimuli (ie, children).

In addition it is important to ask what time frames are involved. A program to help parents cope with crying (eg, Period of Purple Crying) might be effective for those with infants and some toddlers but might not prevent physical abuse in older children. How would that compare to an intervention designed to have parents incorporate the attitudes and behaviors that children are not for hitting (eg, ban on corporal punishment in Sweden)? Measures such as penetrance of the message and effectiveness of the content itself confound comparisons between interventions.

Should a community wish to do something about child abuse prevention (or choosing more desirable alternative realities), the hard part might be to think through the complexities of what is to be accomplished, who is the target, how can sustained change be made for the individuals directly exposed, how might perceptual or behavioral changes ripple to those beyond the direct intervention itself, and how success would be measured.

Child Abuse Prevention System

There is no overarching child abuse prevention in the United States, or in most other countries. The current approach might be likened to a series of small shops rather than a large industry. In general, the industrial revolution benefited from a more systematic approach to manufacturing, with improved quality controls and even cheaper products. The widespread adoption of standardization for prevention is yet to occur. Because there is no single authority, and given the limited successes of child abuse prevention, perhaps this allows for greater experimentation, which is important at this stage in the history of prevention.

"Prevention" among child abuse professionals and agencies is sometimes expressed in ways that are not true primary prevention. Examples might include reducing the number of children in foster care, increasing the percentage of children who remain in the home, decreasing the number of different foster homes a child might live in, or reducing any number of costs. All have been touted as "prevention" when they are in fact program goals that occur after a child has been abused. Whether these are laudable goals or not, they are not primary prevention and do not necessarily achieve the aim to have physically and mentally healthy 18-year-olds. One question might be whether it is more pertinent to "treat" such a statistic or to prevent abuse for a child. And these efforts might siphon money away from primary prevention itself and, thus, pose a potential conflict if resources are limited. The prevention dilemma has been expressed as "treating the invisible"—you don't see what you have prevented. Building a better child abuse system of identification and treatment might be akin to building ever better iron lungs, when the goal should be to develop a vaccine to prevent polio in the first place.

This was the struggle that Dr. Ray Helfer faced when he proposed child abuse trust funds. Knowing that a child abuse victim could not easily be denied, he proposed that money be set aside for child abuse prevention that would not be subject to the perceptions and imperatives of legislative funding. Such a "trust" would ensure that prevention funds not be raided for other needs, and that prevention would be sustained. To a reasonable extent this has occurred in many parts of the United States. Prevention activities in other countries (eg, New Zealand, England), such as home visitation are built into the health or government system and thus have universality, longevity, and viability.

But child abuse prevention often remains with those most committed to child welfare—social work professionals and other professionals with child abuse interests. A criticism could be made that this is self-serving, that child abuse professionals create prevention programs that sometimes pay salaries or increase their domains. However, when considered from the point of view of the child, the main disadvantage of a concentration of child abuse professionals working in prevention is obtaining wider community support. For example, in the 1980s and 1990s the Iowa Child Abuse Prevention Program Advisory Board distributed state monies for child abuse prevention to various counties. Each county was to write a proposal of what they hoped to accomplish and list their community council behind the proposal. The job of the board was to rank which communities got money and how much. If a community had a strong proposal but its community council appeared to be social work professionals from one agency, a question would arise as to whether this proposal is what the community really wanted. In contrast, a council with a banker, media person, union representative, hospital administrator, law enforcement, and a business person had the appearance of more truly representing the community and could therefore speak more convincingly that this is what their community wanted and needed. They were then more likely to receive funding. Community representation in child abuse prevention is important for:

1. ***Public understanding***: Increased appreciation of the wide impact of child abuse and the importance of prevention. Understanding how it impacts me, my business, my community, my children, etc.

2. ***Owning the problem***: However well-qualified and enthusiastic traditional child abuse prevention specialists are, they do not own the problem of child abuse. Rather, it is a community problem affecting everyone. To the extent it is perceived as belonging to a certain subset of professionals, this seemingly absolves others of the responsibility for children and their optimum development.

3. ***Enhancing resources***: Many community prevention programs rely on state prevention dollars through their prevention or trust funds. Some have funding through health entities (eg, hospitals). Some have foundation or some other type of grant money. All of these sources of funding are subject to drying up, especially grant money. Even at their peak, it might be advantageous to have more money for the prevention project. With larger community representation, there is an increased chance that someone will be aware of and connected to additional or novel funding not conventionally considered in traditional child abuse domains.

4. ***Novel thinking***: Much of the social services field is structured with a programmatic approach to solving problems. Ideas are generated for relatively short-term programs (ie, rarely in terms of decades), proposals are processed through agencies, funding is secured for a period of time, and some assessment is made. This approach works well for many traditional service issues, but not necessarily as well for prevention. Prevention need not take the form of programs with the need for constant infusions of money and likely sun-setting of money after a period of time. Community partners may bring alternative experiences and ideas about how to effect changes in behavior and the means to pursue this.

5. ***Dissemination***: Having a media partner would be of considerable help in spreading the message of child abuse prevention in general, and a specific intervention in particular. Such a partner could help identify potential target groups and the means to impact them. For example, it is more likely that teens and young adults listen to music than read trifold brochures. Developing messages in the music world might

have an impact with an audience otherwise inaccessible through conventional educational means. Dissemination also means reporting on success. Human interest stories can help highlight prevention efforts (and periodically do so). Showing a home visitor and how to help a family makes for a watchable and/or readable story. A business leader could share information within the entire company and reach a large audience, institute family friendly work policies, and be an advocate for state and national policies that support families and children.

6. ***Sustainability***: It would be optimal if a child abuse prevention intervention is proven effective, if it can be taken to scale and would be sustained essentially forever. Yet many funding sources, especially those overtly supportive of child abuse prevention, are not set up for long-term funding. Government and health are two domains that are sometimes able to fund themselves for extensive time periods. With a diverse representation in community participation in child abuse prevention, the opportunity to identify funding beyond the initial funding source, or long-term funding itself, are enhanced.

Child abuse prevention would likely profit from a more sophisticated system, even if drawing from existing resources. Schools of public health have considerable talent in research design and assessment, as well as knowledge of what works with other health initiatives. The US Advisory Board on Child Abuse and Neglect recommended in their 1995 report that the National Institutes of Health (NIH) develop a study section on child abuse.[18] While the Office of Child Abuse and Neglect (OCAN), the National Institute of Child Health and Human Development (NICHD), CDC, and others devote some funding for prevention or prevention-related activities, their abilities to intensively study this issue are hampered by fiscal constraints determined by Congress. However, it is not clear whether leadership in prevention should be governmental, health, private, or some hybrid entity.

Proposed Research Agenda

Increased Sophistication of Existing Strategic Approaches

Much of child abuse prevention to date has implicitly adopted the statistical "model" of an intervention and comparison (control) group. The point is to show that the intervention helps to reduce the baseline rate of child abuse. While an important first step in building a more sophisticated approach to prevention, it has the limitation that while an intervention might help a subpopulation, when averaged over the entire group, it might "wash out" the apparent effectiveness. In addition, if a positive effect is shown it is often not clear what aspect was most helpful. This is akin to cancer protocols of the past when a cocktail of perhaps a dozen drugs was shown to be effective. Research after that was often intended to reduce the number of drugs (and side effects) to see what would work equally well.

One example that could benefit from even greater research is home visitation. While an example of modeling (important for human learning), it is not as clear what works. When a nurse is used as the home visitor,[19] health messages and behaviors are often better learned than when a nonmedical professional is used. Is this the desired outcome, or is some other outcome important? Are all aspects of a program important or just some? How big a dose (eg, how often/for how long) of home visitation makes a difference?

Some groups do not respond well to a given approach. For home visitation, a parent who is mentally ill, who has substance abuse problems, or who is in an environment with intimate partner violence is less likely to benefit, presumably because they have larger issues to contend with. Research could help to clarify who is most likely to benefit from a particular approach and who is not.

Research could be done to develop ways to have the recipient be less of a passive learner. Active learning has longer-lasting effects and may increase success. How much intensity in an intervention is important? How would transitions into other interventions work (eg, home visitation into preschool intervention programs)?

Sexual abuse prevention should target the potential or actual perpetrator, as well as building adult and community responsibility for protecting children. Little is known about why some people find children to be their desired sex objects. If such pedophiles exist in all cultures, it is likely that some embryological neurohormone process goes awry, but how can this be recognized and treated, short of incarceration?

Tertiary prevention might also be considered as better helping the child cope with the abuse that has occurred. One aspect would be that treatment might reduce the likelihood that the child becomes a perpetrator now or later in life. If inflammatory chemicals alter the DNA with physical abuse[15] and, therefore, alter the brain,[10] might there be a chemical treatment that would reduce these physical changes? Trauma-focused therapy or cognitive-behavioral therapy seems most beneficial to victims of various abuses. Does it do so by reducing toxic stress–related chemicals in the body or enhancing the repair of damage? Much needs to be learned about the epigenetics of abuse and possible treatment modes to cushion the impact of abuse and increase the safety of others.

Technologies

Historically, teaching has occurred though modeling (ie, direct contact with a parent or mentor who showed how to perform a number of activities, including parenting). This occurs through the mammalian kingdom, if not beyond. With the widespread teaching of visual symbols representing language (ie, writing), books and other enduring written materials provided another source of education. For the last hundreds of years, the major technology to aid in parenting education, and thereby some degree of child abuse prevention, has been the book. Books have an enormous technological advantage in that they require no power, do not easily break, can be shared relatively easily, and can even be annotated. While they supplement modeling, they can also transcend it in some ways.

Electronic means now exist that represent a newer wave of possibilities to educate and assist beyond direct human modeling and books. Electronic technologies also do not have to be passive but can be active or interactive.

Text4baby is an example of a somewhat passive electronic technology with the possibility of high visibility to consumers. Sponsored by US government agencies, the American Academy of Pediatrics, wireless carriers, and many others, this service sends free text messages about parenting issues, including child abuse prevention. When a parent signs up prenatally or around the time of birth, the service sends message appropriate to the child's age until the child is a year old. Other than the initial sign-up, there is nothing else the parent needs to do. Because cell phones are now ubiquitous, an aggressive community program (eg, a birthing hospital that helps all parents sign up) could achieve nearly total penetration. This program is currently undergoing several evaluations, but many more would be possible. In the same vein, similar cell phone applications could be developed and tested that would provide various educational messages in a palatable form with little motivation needed by the end user.

Another approach with technologies is to create more active interactional teaching. Perhaps games could be developed that include aspects of parenting. If online, these might be scored in such a way as to yield data for further analysis. If not, research would still be possible. Such games could be especially useful for physical abuse prevention and some aspects of neglect (eg, players lose points if you forget to feed the baby). It is less clear how to impact primary sexual abuse prevention. Another example is CDC's Essentials for Parenting, a new online interactive initiative for parents of toddlers and preschoolers.

An even more interactive application might be to have the computer, tablet, or cell phone monitor the environment and provide intervention. If an infant cried, it is feasible that a program could monitor the length of crying or even characteristics of crying that might prove more annoying to many people. With various parameters, the device might offer a verbal message to anyone within listening distance with an escalation to a phone call if an even higher parameter is exceeded. User feedback (eg, "How angry/frustrated did you feel with your baby's crying when the device intervened?") could help to reset parameters tailored to more individualized parent reactions. All this data could be gathered, as well information about the content of any device intervention and some sense of effectiveness. At this point, there is no technological barrier to what once would have been considered science fiction, such as a device that could interact with a caregiver in what might be considered stressful and/or crisis situations.

Drownings are a major cause of neglect death in many parts of the country. Possibly technology that requires little action on the part of the caregiver could assist. At this point, reliance on technology seems to be a shirking of parental responsibility, but some serious effort needs to be done to reduce pool and bathtub deaths. Unsafe sleep is another cause of many neglect deaths. Usually this is associated with parental drinking, substance abuse, and/or socioeconomic conditions (eg, low education, limited resources). Perhaps a creative way could be devised to decrease the likelihood that an impaired adult sleeps with a young child. Games could also be created to identify hazards in the home. Professionals sometimes show pictures of a hazardous home and ask the audience to spot as many hazards as possible. For the general public, a similar approach might teach about improved standards—essentially a home safety checklist. This might be coupled with health care visits, perhaps with some sort of incentive.

Primary sexual abuse prevention might be more difficult to imagine with technology. Should a person be self-identified as having such feelings, perhaps part of the therapeutic/prevention process could be a device application that interacts with the user when they are having such feelings. Even if such an approach were not immediately effective, it could provide situational data for a subject that is poorly understood.

Considering the high percentage of people who are abused in their childhood, it would not be unreasonable to have an app for that.

Media

Currently in the United States there are few extensive portrayals in popular television or movies about common problems with children, their normal development, or coping methods for caregivers. Because media likely reaches more people than academic publications (hence advertisers prefer the former), there is a large opportunity to model safe or desirable behaviors in an entertaining way and with considerable repetition.

1. ***Safe sleep***: Children should be placed in a crib or safe sleeping area on their backs without blankets, pillows, toys, or other objects. Nevertheless, this is not how print ads or television shows commonly portray sleeping children, if they address this at all. Media do not reinforce the message that bed-sharing can be unsafe, especially with Western bedding practices. Yet unsafe sleep is one of the leading causes of child neglect deaths.[20]
2. ***Coping with crying/sleep deprivation***: There may be a little attention (usually humorous) to parents of newborns having little sleep and feeling bad as a result.

However, this could be explored to much greater effect. A message that it is OK to put the child down in a safe place and take a 5-minute break would be helpful if it could seep into the culture as a coping mechanism for adults. The advantage of getting support from other adults could also be a key theme. For television, this could take the form of shows in which there are infants who cry and parents who model acceptable behavior. This would not have to be at odds with the entertainment value of the program itself.

3. ***Behavior modification***: In the 1950s, television shows would sometimes talk about spanking a child for misbehavior. This is largely gone now, but it rarely has been replaced by positive behavior management. How would a sophisticated chart for expected and rewarded behaviors look? When parents feel they have to use physical punishment because that is what they are familiar with, extensive doses of television showing alternatives might decrease their negativity to trying what (for them) are unnatural methods.
4. ***Public behavior***: Many people wish they knew what to do if they witnessed a parent verbally or physically abusing a child in public. Fear of confrontation mixes with a general lack of knowing what to do that would be effective and safe for the child. This could be modeled in movies, television, YouTube, print, and other media outlets.

Research about the media could include:

1. What subjects might best be broached educationally within the confines of the perceived nature of the entertainment industry itself? What could be taught while keeping the entertainment interesting?
2. What sells newspapers and how might print media discuss child abuse in a way that has a measurable impact but is prevention-focused, not just reactions to sensational stories of abuse after it has occurred. Presumably, some media outlets would be willing to participate in child abuse prevention if it could be shown that it holds interest and does some good.
3. What are the attitudes of writers on neglect, physical abuse, and sexual abuse? How does this impact on what is seen? What would it take to get them to change if change is necessary?

As with any prevention approach, assessment would be important to be sure that resources are marshaled most effectively.

Research Into Barriers

The advantage of research into barriers is that considerable resources could be devoted to a seemingly important child abuse intervention. However, without knowing the target audience it could be less effective. An analogy would be to medicine, whereby some drugs are known to be effective in some subpopulations but less so in others, requiring individualized therapy.

Considerable frustration is often expressed about making child abuse prevention more effective. Part of this is the impression that public, private sector, and legislative support is not strong. Why is it that legislators don't clamor to give more money for child abuse prevention? Is it because they don't think the science is good enough; there is little public backing (ie, no one votes on this issue, hence their own job is not at risk regardless of what they do); it sounds like just another interest group; it asks for effects measured in the long term, which is of little use for re-election cycles; or some combination of all of these? If any of these contentions are the case, it is researchable. Having effective prevention programs themselves is only part of what is important if children are to be impacted in a wider way.

Studies could be done with state legislators to determine their knowledge and attitudes about child abuse and child abuse prevention. While they likely are against abuse and for prevention, what exactly would they like to see to have it become a higher priority? If given a ranking of the top 20 funding priorities in a state legislature, what would it take to get child abuse prevention on that list? Many who have had even modest experience working with legislators know that if even 3 or 4 constituents from a home district show up at a legislative office, they are likely to be carefully heard. Thus how many in a district would be needed to move the issue forward on average? These answers are not really known, despite advocacy of abuse prevention for years. Would a case history be more compelling than statistics? Are there aspects of prevention that help to address the message more than others? Does the policy maker's own background interact with advocacy success?

Similarly, health administrators could be queried as to priorities in their funding. With increasing emphasis on health outcomes, rather than services per se, this might be an opportunity for increased prevention. The Children's Hospital Association has documented the substantial contribution that their members have made to child abuse identification and treatment.[21] The CDC specifically works on dissemination as one of its aspects of public health, and there is a body of literature from other subject areas that might help inform prevention efforts or suggest research of its own.

For a given message, why are some parents more resistant to intervention than others? Is this a function of family background, cultural norms, or personality traits? What would it take to change messages to be more effective, or would entirely different approaches be needed? Considerable research has been done by corporations in selling products to different markets, and advertising agencies have accumulated extensive data on what works. Some of this, or a parallel approach, might be used to better understand barriers posed by individuals. And is there a "fatigue" factor in the public, whereby one more sad child abuse story creates an increasingly jaded public? If so, positive messages might need to be highlighted more than negative ones. This could be explored by focus groups, but the more compelling research would need to be done with the general public.

More Complex Approaches

Some unconventional system approaches might influence child abuse prevention. Currently, the penalties for abuse are often muted for individuals and there is little incentive for aspects of the system to devote substantial resources. Several examples of unconventional thinking would include:

1. ***Penalties for providing false or misleading misinformation to a medical provider*.** Despite the sometimes medical necessity of knowing exactly what happened to a child, a parent may lie or be deliberately misleading. Examples includes:

   — A 3-month-old with failure to thrive with a parent history of feeding 54 ounces of formula per day

   — A parent denying sexual abuse

   — A parent denying causing loop marks while the 8 year old says they did it

   — A child with abusive head trauma too critical to have another CT scan but with no history by the parent that they were punched hard in the abdomen, which might require life-saving surgery

   It is bad enough that abuse/neglect occurred, but providing false or misleading information to medical professionals compounds the problem. If this could not be easily accomplished by a specific legal penalty, it could be added as a sentencing/

custodial consideration. In practice, this means that it would be to the parent's advantage to tell the truth. This would be tertiary prevention and reduction of harm.

2. *User fees*: If a parent had to pay the actual costs of the abuse/neglect case, there might be a severe financial disincentive to further abuse (tertiary prevention). Currently, most of the costs of a child abuse case (eg, child protective services, medical, law enforcement, legal, therapy) are borne by the taxpayer. If the burden was shifted to the abuser himself or herself, this might have an inhibitory effect. For many cases of abuse, the cost would be hundreds or thousands of dollars. For cases of abusive head trauma, it could be millions.[22] While many abusers could not afford the actual cost of many of the cases, or it would put the child in financial jeopardy as well, some portion could be required. Governmental entities impose substantial parking and traffic fines in the expectation that this modifies future behaviors.

3. ***Insurance responsibility***: If a state required that health insurance pay the state $10 million (or some considerable amount) for every case of abusive head trauma, it would be in the insurance company's interest to invest in primary prevention. This might help the state recover costs of such cases but, more importantly, would prevent some of the cost.

In addition to the need for unconventional approaches and measurement as to whether they work, attention must continually be paid to the end goal: creation of healthy 18-year-olds. This will require neither a single approach to prevention nor an intervention at only 1 point in the life cycle. Continuous pressure will be needed at many points to address different forms of abuse, different ways to enhance physical and mental wellness, and to saturate the populace with key messages and skills.

At the end, this will require changes in the cultural norms for many. It will require a world in which hitting a child is not acceptable. It will require mitigation of substance abuse, alcohol abuse, and intimate partner violence. It will require a world in which reduction of mental health problems occurs and treatment is more available. It will require a world in which children are not used as sexual objects. While addressing each of these problems would substantially help prevent child abuse, the timeline is actually reversed. Preventing child abuse will do more to help these problems that are often the effects of abuse.[5] Education of professionals and the public about the complexities of abuse is one of the key steps to understanding how child abuse prevention can begin.

References

1. Daro D. *Public Opinion and Behaviors Regarding Child Abuse Prevention.* Washington, DC: National Criminal Justice Reference Service; 1999.

2. Labbe J. Ambroise Tardieu: the man and his work on child maltreatment a century before Kempe. *Child Abuse Negl.* 2005;29:311-324.

3. Kempe CH, Silverman FN, Steele BD, et al. The battered child syndrome. *JAMA.* 1962;181:17-24.

4. Adams J. Medical evaluation of suspected child sexual abuse: 2011 update. *J Child Sex Abuse.* 2011;20:588-605.

5. Felitti VJ, Anda RF, Nordenberg D, et al. Relationship of childhood abuse and household dysfunction to many of the leading causes of death in adults. The Adverse Childhood Experiences Study. *Am J Prev Med.* 1998;14(4):245-258.

6. Gilbert L, Breiding M, Merrick M, et al. Childhood adversity and adult chronic disease: an update from ten states and the District of Columbia, 2010. *Am J Prev Med.* 2014;48(3):345-349.

7. Alexander R. *New Hope for Preventing Child Abuse and Neglect: Proven Solutions to Save Lives and Prevent Future Crimes*. Washington, DC: Fight Crime, Invest in Kids; 2003.

8. Fang X, Brown D, Florence C, Mercy J. The economic burden of child maltreatment in the United States and implications for prevention. *Child Abuse Negl.* 2012;36:156-165.

9. Belasco A. *The Cost of Iraq, Afghanistan, and Other Global War on Terror Operations Since 9/11*. Washington, DC: Congressional Research Service; 2014.

10. DeBellis M, Spratt E, Hooper S. Neurodevelopmental biology associated with childhood sexual abuse. *J Child Sex Abuse.* 2011;20:548-587.

11. Frieden T. A framework for public health action: the health impact pyramid. *AM J Public Health.* 2010;100:590-595.

12. Finkelhor D, Jones L. *Have Sexual Abuse and Physical Abuse Declined Since the 1990s?* Durham, NH: Crimes Against Children Research Center; 2012.

13. Sedlak AJ, Mettenburg J, Basena M, et al. *Fourth National Incidence Study of Child Abuse and Neglect (NIS-4)*. Washington, DC: US Department of Health and Human Services, Administration for Children and Families; 2010.

14. Berger R, Fromkin J, Stutz H, et al. Abusive head trauma during a time of increased unemployment: a multicenter analysis. *Pediatrics.* 2011;128:637-643.

15. Shalev I, Moffitt TE, Sugden K, et al. Exposure to violence during childhood is associated with telomere erosion from 5 to 10 years of age. *Molecular Psychiatry.* 2013;18:576-581.

16. Centers for Disease Control and Prevention. *Essential for Childhood Framework: Steps to Create Safe, Stable, Nurturing Relationships and Environments for All Children*. Atlanta, GA: Centers for Disease Control and Prevention; 2014.

17. Gibson JJ. *The Senses Considered as Perceptual Systems*. Boston, MA: Houghton Mifflin; 1966.

18. US Advisory Board on Child Abuse and Neglect. *A Nation's Shame: Fatal Child Abuse and Neglect in the United States*. Washington, DC: US Department of Health and Human Services; 1995.

19. Olds D, Kitzman H, Knudtson M, Anson E, Smith J, Cole R. Effect of home visiting by nurses on maternal and child mortality. results of a 2-decade follow-up of a randomized clinical trial. *JAMA Pediatrics.* 2014;168:800-806.

20. Florida State Child Abuse Death Review Committee. *Child Abuse and Neglect Deaths in Florida: Annual Report 2012*. Tallahassee, FL: Florida State Child Abuse Death Review Committee; 2012.

21. Children's Hospital Association. 2012 survey findings: children's hospitals child abuse services. https://www.childrenshospitals.org/issues-and-advocacy/population-health/child-abuse/reports/2012/2012-survey-findings-childrens-hospitals-child-abuse-services. Accessed November 17, 2016.

22. Miller T, Steinbeigle R, Wicks A, Lawrence B, Barr M, Barr R. Disability-adjusted life-year burden of abusive head trauma at ages 0-4. *Pediatrics.* 2014;134:e1545-e1550.

INDEX

A

Appendix, figures and tables are indicated by a, b, f, and t respectively

B

D

E

F

G

H

I

J

K

L

M

N

O

P

T

U

V

W

Y

Z

www.ingramcontent.com/pod-product-compliance
Lightning Source LLC
LaVergne TN
LVHW060018210926
848481LV00013B/3735